Jaypee's

Dental Dictionary

Disclaimer

The material contained in the book (some of which) has been provided by contributing authors. The publisher and editors disclaim any responsibility about the originality of contents

Jaypee's
Dental Dictionary

Second Edition

Priya Verma Gupta MDS FPFA
Professor
Department of Pedodontics and Preventive Dentistry
Divya Jyoti College of Dental Sciences and Research
Modi Nagar, Niwari Road, Ghaziabad
Uttar Pradesh, India

(Late) LC Gupta MD (Rad) DMRE, MD (PSM), FAMS, DSC (Hon)
Retd Director Medical, Border Security Force
India

Sujata Sarabahi MS, MCh, DNB, MNAMS
Maxillofacial and Plastic Surgeon
Associate Professor
Vardhman Mahavir Medical College and
Safdarjung Hospital, New Delhi, India

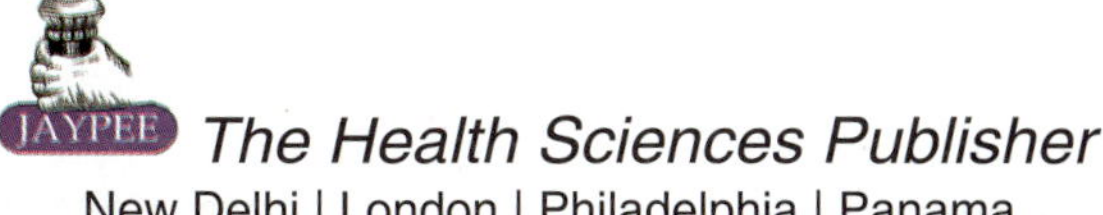

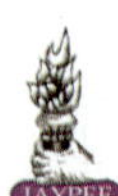

Jaypee Brothers Medical Publishers (P) Ltd

Headquarters

Jaypee Brothers Medical Publishers (P) Ltd
4838/24, Ansari Road, Daryaganj
New Delhi 110 002, India
Phone: +91-11-43574357
Fax: +91-11-43574314
Email: jaypee@jaypeebrothers.com

Overseas Offices

J.P. Medical Ltd
83 Victoria Street, London
SW1H 0HW (UK)
Phone: +44 20 3170 8910
Fax: +44 (0)20 3008 6180
Email: info@jpmedpub.com

Jaypee Medical Inc
325 Chestnut Street
Suite 412, Philadelphia
PA 19106, USA
Phone: +1 267-519-9789
Email: support@jpmedus.com

Jaypee Brothers Medical Publishers (P) Ltd
Bhotahity, Kathmandu, Nepal
Phone: +977-9741283608
Email: kathmandu@jaypeebrothers.com

Jaypee-Highlights Medical Publishers Inc
City of Knowledge, Bld. 235, 2nd Floor, Clayton
Panama City, Panama
Phone: +1 507-301-0496
Fax: +1 507-301-0499
Email: cservice@jphmedical.com

Jaypee Brothers Medical Publishers (P) Ltd
17/1-B Babar Road, Block-B, Shaymali
Mohammadpur, Dhaka-1207
Bangladesh
Mobile: +08801912003485
Email: jaypeedhaka@gmail.com

Website: www.jaypeebrothers.com
Website: www.jaypeedigital.com

Inquiries for bulk sales may be solicited at: jaypee@jaypeebrothers.com

Jaypee's Dental Dictionary

Second Edition: **2016**

ISBN 978-93-85891-49-6

Printed at Sanat Printers

Dedicated to

Padma Shri (Late) Dr LC Gupta
without whom the only existence
of this compilation was not possible

Contributors

Anjula Bhagat, MBBS
USA

Gunjan Gupta, MDS
Assistant Professor
Department of Periodontics
Shree Bankey Bihari Dental College and
Research Centre
Hapur Road, Ghaziabad
Uttar Pradesh, India

Harsh Mohan, MBBS, MD, FIC (Path), FUICC
Prof and Head, Department of Pathology
Government Medical College
Chandigarh, India

Jyoti Gupta, MDS
Prof and HOD, Department of
Oral Medicine and Radiology
Krishna Medical University and
School of Dental Sciences
Karad, Maharashtra, India

Nishant Gupta, MDS
Assistant Professor
Department of Orthodontics and Dentofacial Orthopedics
Shree Bankey Bihari Dental College and
Research Centre
Hapur Road, Ghaziabad
Uttar Pradesh, India

Pooja Ahmad, BDS, MFDSRCS (Eng)
Dental Institute of Guy's, King's and St Thomas's
Kings College
London, United Kingdom

Rishab Malhotra, MDS
Assistant Professor
Department of Pedodontics and Preventive Dentistry
Jaipur Dental College
Jaipur Rajasthan

Ritu Sharma, MDS
Associate Professor
Department of Endodontics and Operative Dentistry
Hindustan Institute of Dental Science
Uttar Pradesh, India

Sakshi Garg, MDS
Reader
Department of Periodontics
Bhojia Dental College and Hospital
Baddi, Himachal Pradesh, India

Shweta Bali, MDS
Professor
Department of Periodontics
Santosh Dental College and Hospital
Santosh Nagar, Ghaziabad
Uttar Pradesh, India

Subhadra H N, MDS
DY Patil Dental College
Mumbai, Maharashtra, India

Sugandha Mohan, BDS
Government Medical College
Rohtak, Haryana, India

Vivek Hegde, MDS
Prof and Head, Department of Endodontics and Operative Dentistry
MA Rangoonwala College of Dental Sciences and Research Center,
Pune, Maharashtra, India

Preface to the Second Edition

It gives us immense pleasure to write the preface for the second edition of Jaypee's Dental Dictionary. We received copious correspondence from the readers commenting about the book and giving suggestions for improvement in past 6 years since the first edition came in to existence. We also kept a record of new researches and techniques that came up in past six years.

Second edition is being divided in three sections, i.e., dictionary, appendices and colour plates. Appendices come with valuable information which will be handy for the students starting their journey in field of dentistry. Addition of latest photographs and figures will help the readers to understand the vocabulary in a better way. As this compilation is a balanced product between dictionary and encyclopaedia, we have tried to incorporate all new updates that will help the students to familiarise themselves with new vocabulary.

We extend our heartfelt gratitude towards all our contributors. We profusely thank Shri Jitender P Vij (CEO) and Mr Ankit Vij (Group President) for their support and encouragement in bringing out the second edition. Lastly but most importantly we thank Dr Ankit Sharma (Senior Editor), Mr Ashutosh Shrivastava (Assistant Editor), Mr Shekhar Bhatt (Typesetter), Mr Manoj Pahuja (Senior Graphic Designer) and Mr Pawan Kumar (Graphic Designer) of Jaypee Brothers Medical Publishers (P) Ltd, New Delhi for their enthusiasm and constant effort in bringing out this compilation.

In spite of our best efforts compilation is bound to have deficiencies. We will be grateful if the readers kindly send their valuable suggestion for further improvement.

Priya Verma Gupta
Sujata Sarabahi

Preface to the First Edition

The world of dental sciences has changed dramatically over the last two decades and simultaneously so has the public awareness about dental health increased many folds. To provide qualified health managers new dental colleges and superspecialities are developing fast.

All learning in science is based on education in vocabulary. Mostly dictionaries are concerned with words while encyclopedias explain the object which describes the word to be understood and used correctly. It is a balanced product of both. We have catered to the needs of postgraduate students by including definitions and diseases which they ought to know.

Editors have made special efforts to include maximum words not only related to dentistry but also all other related medical specialities which have a bearing on dental care. The dictionary has been made pictorial to make the reading more interesting and to give a visual impact to the readers.

Appendices have been added. The main objective was to collect useful and frequently used information from various other sources to make it easily available between the two covers of the book.

We are grateful to Prof Dr Harsh Mohan, a man of pathology and his daughter Dr Sugandha who have provided many of the histological slides to make the dictionary more pictorial and useful. Similarly Dr KD Tripathi who is a milestone in the field of pharmacology has been a source of constant academic encouragement to us.

We are also happy to include some line sketches by master Rohan Gupta for better elaboration of certain terms.

Lastly and most importantly we must express our debt and enduring gratitude to our publisher/family friend and guide Shri Jitendar P Vij, Shrimati Raman Vij and young commander Mr Ankit Vij who have published this book of words in four colors and on art paper at a reasonable price.

We would like to express our thanks in advance to anybody who will spare his valuable time to take the trouble to inform us of any shortcomings in this dictionary and we will surely make the necessary amendments in the next edition.

Priya Verma Gupta
LC Gupta
Sujata Sarabahi

Contents

Section 1: Dental Dictionary

Section 2: Appendices

Section 3: Schematic Representation of Important Anatomic Landmarks

Section 1

Dictionary

A

A (in reference to cephalometrics) is the deepest midline point in curved boney outline from base to alveolar process of the maxilla.

A beta is the type of fibers which carry sensations like touch, pressure and position.

A delta is the type of fibers which carry sharp pain with a speed of 12–20 m/sec.

Abdominal region refers to abdominopelvic cavity that is divided into '9' regions. The central regions are epigastric, umbilical and hypogastric. Epigastric literally means upon stomach. Umbilical is centermost region surrounding umbilicus and hypogastric region, is just below umbilical region. Six regions are on either side, i.e. three to the left and three to the right. These are known as hypochondriac, lumbar and iliac region. Iliac regions are also known as inguinal regions.

Abdominopelvic cavity is a region that is located below diaphragm. Upper portion is called abdominal cavity and contains liver, gall. bladder, pancreas, spleen and kidney. Lower portion is known as pelvic cavity. It extends down from the level of hip and contains rectum, urinary bladder and internal parts of reproductive system.

Abducent nerve is the sixth cranial nerve. It is made up of fibers that arise in the abducent nucleus and supply the lateral rectus muscle of the eyeball.

Abducent nucleus is situated in the lower part of the pons. It lies in the gray matter lining the floor of the fourth ventricle, near the midline. The position of the nucleus in relation to the floor of the fourth ventricle is indicated

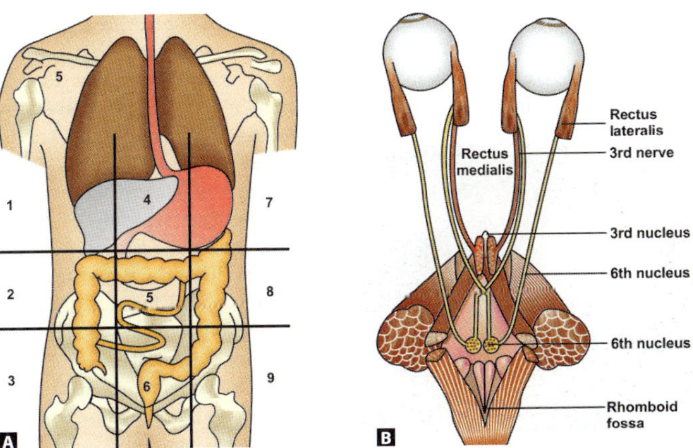

Figs A and B: *(A) Abdominal quadrants; (B) Abducent nerve*

A

by an elevation called the facial colliculus.

Aberrant salivary glands are those salivary gland tissues that develop at a site where they are not usually found. These are frequently seen in cervical region near the parotid gland. Most aberrant glands in neck occur in upper portion of neck.

Abfraction is said to have occurred when minute stresses develop around the cervical margins of teeth as a result of the flexure of the root and the crown of the tooth. The cracks propagate from occlusal forces established along the tooth and from abrasion and erosion.

Abortion means spontaneous or induced termination of pregnancy before the fetus is independently viable or the expulsion of an embryo, or fetus before it has reached to the stage of viability prior to about 20 weeks of gestation. Therapeutic abortion is done to save woman's life. Complication includes shock and sepsis.

Abrasion is wearing away of tooth structure from friction of a foreign object. Most commonly, it is caused by tooth brushing and is seen at the cervical margin of the teeth. It is more common on left side than on the right one. It can be confused with root surface caries. On radiograph, it is seen as well-defined horizontal radiolucency along the cervical margin of a tooth. Habitual cigar holder may cause abrading of an incisal edge. Harder materials tend to be more abrasion resistant than soften ones.

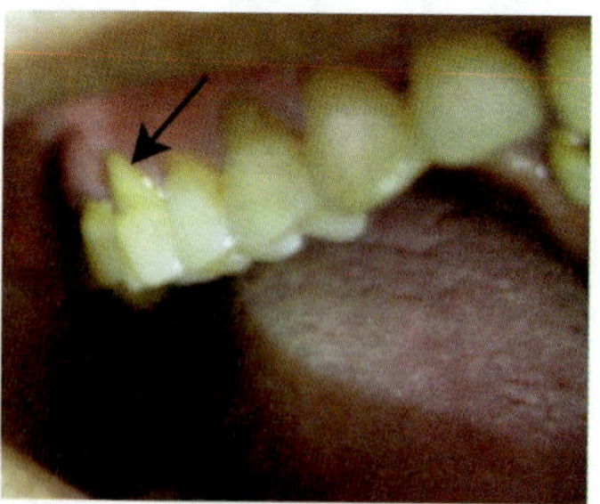

Fig.: *Abrasion cavities with gingival recession*

Abrasive refers to the material which causes wear or abrasion of another material.

Abrasive index is a method of rating the abrasiveness of dentifrices.

Abscess refers to a local infection which can be caused due to severe decay, periodontal disease, or trauma. It is characterized by swelling and pain. If an abscess ruptures, it will be accompanied by sudden relief from pain due to a reduction in pressure. A foul taste may also be noticed.

Absence (Petit mal) seizures: Most common type of generalized seizures occurring in children between 4 and 14 years of age. This type of seizure starts with no warning. They typically last from 10 to 25 seconds. Seizures frequently occur in clusters and may take place up to hundred times a day. There are two types of absence seizures: typical and atypical.

Absent bowel sounds refer to an inability to hear any bowel sounds in every abdominal quadrant. Abdomen distends and risk of perforation or peritonitis develops. It may require immediate attention.

Absent mindedness can be described as habitual inattention marked by preoccupation with thoughts. There is no attention to external stimuli.

Absolute humidity is the weight of water vapor in a unit volume of air. It is expressed as gram per kg or gram per cubic meter of air.

Absolute reliability is quantified by standard error of measurement. It is an extent to which a score varies on repeated measurement.

Absorption (in reference to dental material) can also be described as penetration of one material into another.

Absorption (in reference to radiology) is a process through which X-ray imparts some or all of its energy to the material through which it passes; it depends on the atomic structure of matter and wavelength of the X-ray beam.

Absorption refers to the accumulation of substance at an interface in a concentration different from concentration of substance in bulk.

Absurdity is an idea or expression which is nonsensical, incoherent or meaningless.

Abuse means misuse.

Abutment is a tooth adjacent to an empty space in mouth, which will be used to support the prosthetic device.

Academic refers to pertaining to formal education.

Acanthesthesia refers to the skin sensation in which there is feeling of pinprick.

Acanthosis nigricans may be benign, malignant and pseudoacanthosis nigricans. Benign form seems to be genetic. Malignant form is associated with internal malignancy. It develops after 40 years of age. Pseudoacanthosis is most common form. Tongue and lips appear to be involved more. Lips may be enlarged and covered by papillomatous growths, especially the angle of mouth. Buccal mucosa shows a velvety white appearance with papillary lesions. There develops gingival papillomatosis with periorofacial, mucosal and skin lesions.

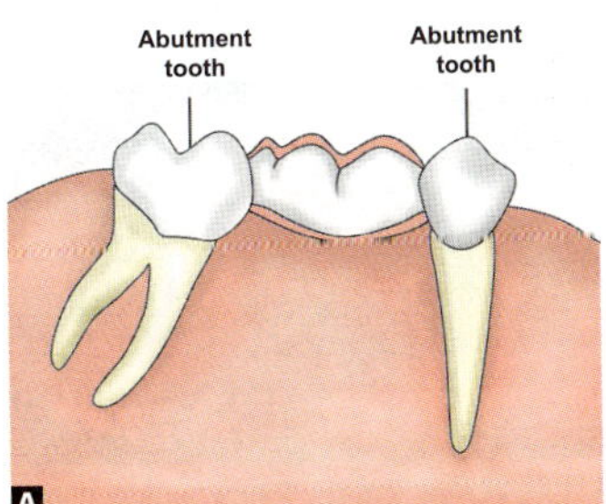

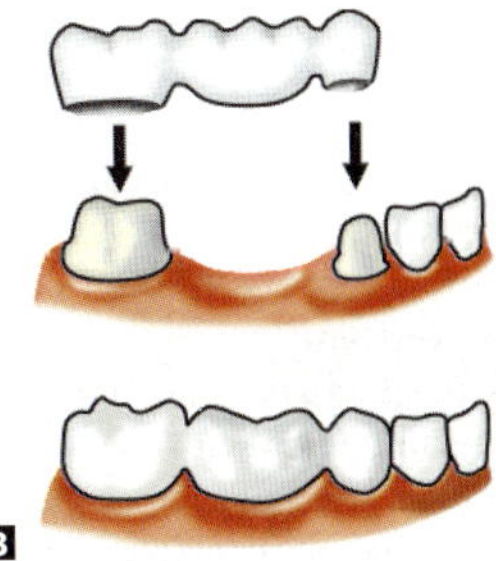

Figs A and B: *Abutment tooth*

Gastric adenocarcinoma may develop. There is no treatment for the disease.

Acatalepsia refers to the inability to comprehend or reason.

Acataphasia refers to the inability to correctly form a sentence.

Access cavity preparation is defined as an endodontic coronal preparation which enables unobstructed access to the canal orifices, a straight line access to apical foramen, complete control over instrumentation and accommodate obturation technique.

Access opening burs are round burs with 16 mm bur shank (3 mm longer than standard burs).

Access refining burs are coarse grit flame-shaped, tapered round and diamond shaped for refining the walls of access cavity preparation.

Accessory canal are lateral branches of the main canal that form a communication between the pulp and periodontium. Accessory canals contain connective tissues and vessels and can be seen anywhere from furcation to apex but tend to be more common in apical third and in posterior teeth. In other words, more apical and farther posterior the tooth, the more likely the accessory canals will be present.

Accessory cusps *see* talon's cusp, dens evaginatus.

Accessory gland is a gland that assists organs in doing their functions.

Accessory muscle refers to the muscle that participates with and assists a major muscle.

Accessory nerve is the eleventh cranial nerve (motor). It consists of two distinct parts, cranial and spinal. Both parts consist predominantly of efferent fibers as follows: The fibers of the cranial part arise from the nucleus ambiguus. These fibers join the vagus nerve and are distributed through its pharyngeal and laryngeal branches to muscles of the pharynx, soft palate and larynx. The fibers of the spinal part arise

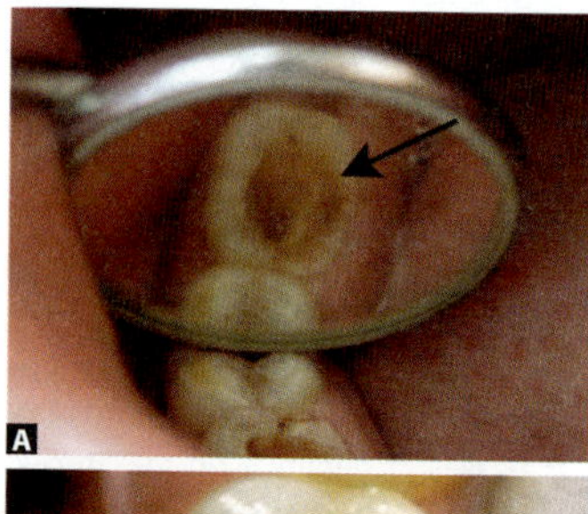

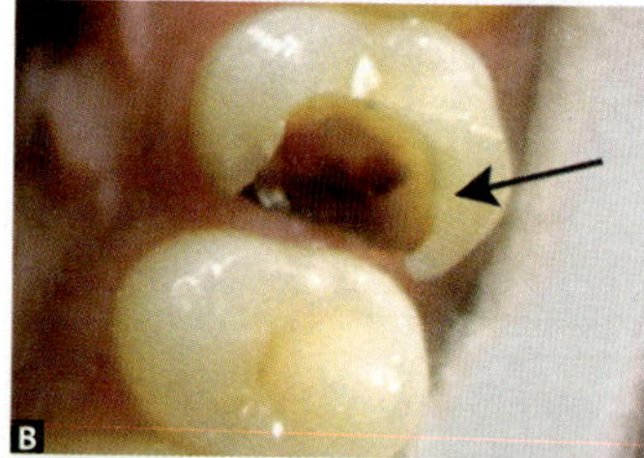

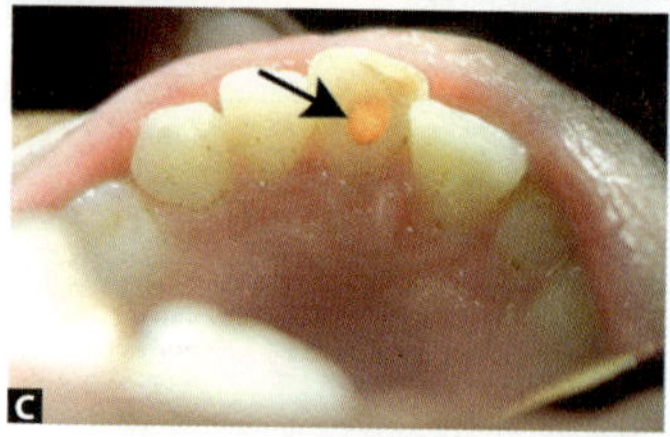

Figs A to C: *(A) Access opening of a molar; (B) Premolar; (C) Incisor*

from the lateral part of the ventral gray column of the upper five or six cervical segments of the spinal cord. They supply the sternocleidomastoid and trapezius muscles.

Acesulfame refers to the non-cariogenic sweetener about 200 times sweeter than sucrose with a pleasant taste and no aftertaste.

Acetabulum is the large cup-shaped cavity on the innominate bone in which femur fits in.

Acetic acid is a chemical found in fixed solution that stops the action of developer.

Acircular refers to the slender needle-like.

Acid is a substance that releases hydrogen ions into a solution. The higher the hydrogen ion concentration of a solution, the greater its acidity.

Acid attack refers to the action of acids that are released from plaque upon enamel.

Acid-base balance refers to the balance of body fluids that is maintained at pH 7.35–7.45 on the alkaline side. Acidic products of the body's metabolism are excreted in urine in combination with bases such as sodium and potassium. These bases are thereby lost to the body and acid-base balance is maintained.

Acid etching is an interim procedure where selective etching of the portions of enamel rods with 37% of phosphoric acid is done in order to increase the surface area and increased surface energy to obtain adhesion.

Acidophilic adenoma refers to the small benign lesion of salivary gland. It is more common in women. The tumor usually measures 3 to 5 cm above the age of 60. It is composed of large cells with eosinophilic cytoplasm. Lymphoid tissue is commonly present. Malignant transformation is rare and it has to be excised.

Acinar cells are those cells that are commonly found in salivary glands.

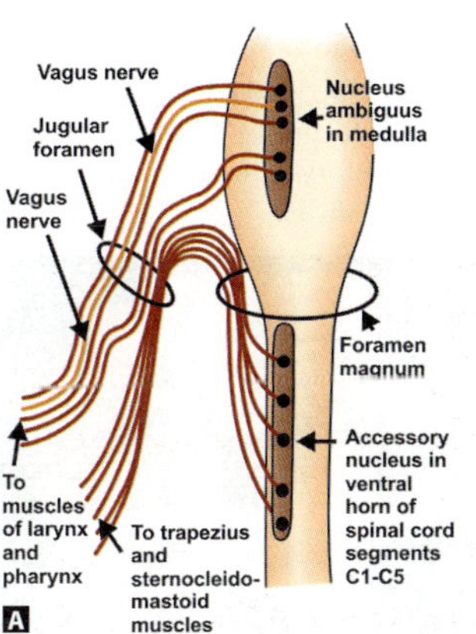

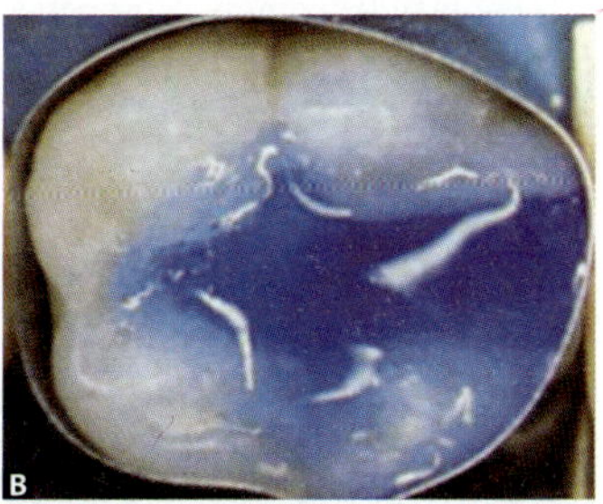

Figs A and B: *(A) Accessory nerve; (B) Acid etching*

The acinar cells are of two types when stained by optical microscopy, i.e. basophilic serous cells and eosinophilic mucous cells. On the basis of their acinar secretory cell composition, the secretions of the parotid and Von-Ebner's gland are classified as serous. The secretions of submandibular and sublingual glands are mixed. The serous and mucous cells also play an important role in protein glycoprotein secretion.

Acini are pancreatic cells that secrete serous fluid with digestive enzyme.

Acinic cell tumor refers to the pleomorphic adenoma; these are not common neoplasm of salivary gland. Parotid is affected and is not frequently seen in intraoral sites. Clinical features: size of lesion is about 3 cm, overlying skin is intact, lesion is well-defined and slow growing, cystic spaces make it fluctuant, rarely lip or cheek may be involved. Surgical excision is the solution.

Acne fulminous is an acute onset of extreme severity. It develops abruptly, numerous large painful papules, nodules and cysts develop. There may be painful arthropathy. Systemic steroids and steroids may be required.

Acne vulgaris refers to the condition where acne develops over face during teenage. Lesions consist of papules and pustules with black and white heads. Face, back and chest are affected. Acne with virilization is due to androgen secreting tumor of adrenal, ovary and testis. Treatment is long and response is slow and uncertain.

Aconite poisoning is mainly used for homicidal purpose. Arrows are poisoned by paste of aconite by hilly tribes to kill their enemies. Powdered aconite is sprinkled in water of tanks and wells so that whosoever drinks, dies. It is extremely unstable, hence is difficult to detect after death.

Acousticophobia refers to the morbid fear of sound or noise.

Acquired congenital reflex is a reflex that develops after the eruption of the posterior primary teeth, i.e. at the age of 18 months or more. The child tends to swallow with the teeth brought together by the masticatory muscle action without tongue thrust.

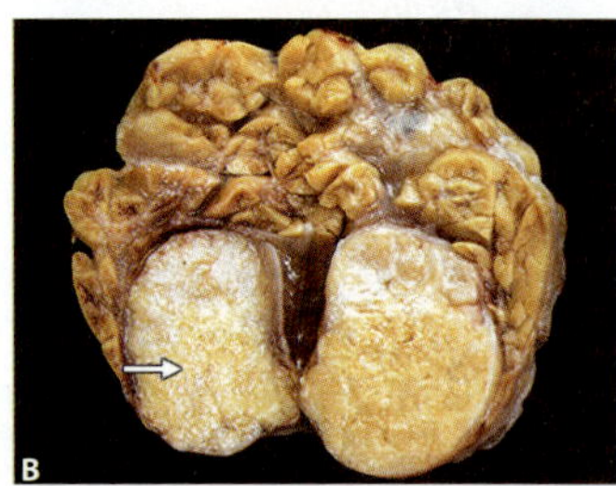

Figs A and B: *(A) Acinar cells; (B) Pleomorphic adenoma*

A

Acquired immunity refers to the immunity that is acquired after birth. It can be described as resistance that is weak or absent in the first exposure but that increases dramatically with subsequent exposures to the same specific pathogen.

Acrocinesia refers to the excessive movement.

Acrodermatitis enteropathica is rare disease affecting childhood and transmitted as an autosomal recessive character. It may be due to zinc deficiency. Zinc supplements are the treatment of choice. Person develops skin lesions, hair loss, nail changes and diarrhea. Retarded body growth and mental changes also occur. Buccal mucosa, palate gingival and tonsils may show red and white spots. Erosions and ulcers are noted and halitosis is severe.

Acrodynia occurs in young infants. There are many cutaneous manifestations. Ear, nose, cheeks become pink and has cold, clammy feeling and the skin over affected area peels off easily. Photophobia, lacrimation, muscular weakness, hypertension and stomatitis are also seen. Drooling of saliva is there, gingiva becomes sensitive to pain, exhibiting ulcer. Mastication becomes difficult. Administration of BAL is helpful.

Acromegaly develops due to excessive growth hormone from anterior pituitary gland. Hands, fingers and feet are enlarged. Face becomes longer. Voice becomes husky. Visual disturbance develops.

Acrosoma is a specialized structure on the sperm containing enzymes.

Acrylic is a material used for prosthesis and various types of appliances. It consists of powder called polymer and a liquid called monomer, when mixed, it sets into a hard acrylic by a process called curing. Heat cured acrylic is used for dentures and orthodontic appliances. While cold cured acrylic is used for denture repairs, impression trays and temporary crowns.

Acrylic faced cast metal crown refers to the crown that can be used as long-term provisional crown during the intermediate stage in a large scale oral reconstruction. However, it has its own disadvantages as it gets deteriorated in the oral cavity by being worn away, discoloring and due to marginal leakage.

Acrylic jacket crowns are used as provisional crowns since they are more permanent than the usual simple temporary procedures and less costly than cast metal crowns. These types of crowns are usually used where other form of treatment, such as periodontal or

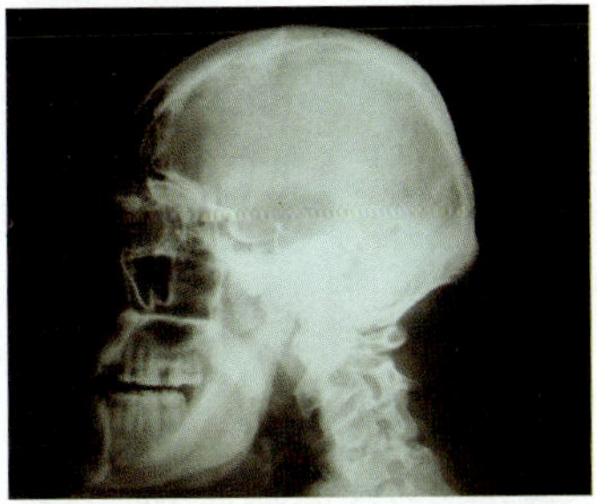

Fig.: *Acromegaly*

orthodontic treatment, is to be done before the final placement of crown.

Actatic speech refers to the uncoordinated verbal communication.

Actin refers to the muscle protein used in contraction.

Actinomyces is a Gram-positive, non-motile, non-spore-forming organism occurring as rods and filaments that vary considering in length. Filaments are usually long and slender and are branching.

Actinomycosis is caused by Gram positive, non-acid fast, branched, filamentous bacteria. It is a chronic granulomatous fibrosing disease. Organism may enter the tissues through the oral mucous membrane and may remain localized or spread to the adjacent soft tissue. Skin over underlying abscess is purplish-red and indurated or often fluctuant. Mandible may be involved.

Action potential is the rapid change in the membrane potential of excitable nerve and muscle cells associated with the conduction of impulses along the cell membrane.

Action tremors *range* in speed between 7 to 11 Hz and more distally than proximally. Such tremors can easily be suppressed by beta blockers. Alcohol may abolish but withdrawal tremors may appear again.

Activation phase Leukocyte chemotactic factors bind to receptors on neutrophils surface and trigger the activation phase of endothelial binding. They include fragments of fibrin/collagen, soluble factors, byproducts of complement cascade, chemokines, PAF, leukotriene

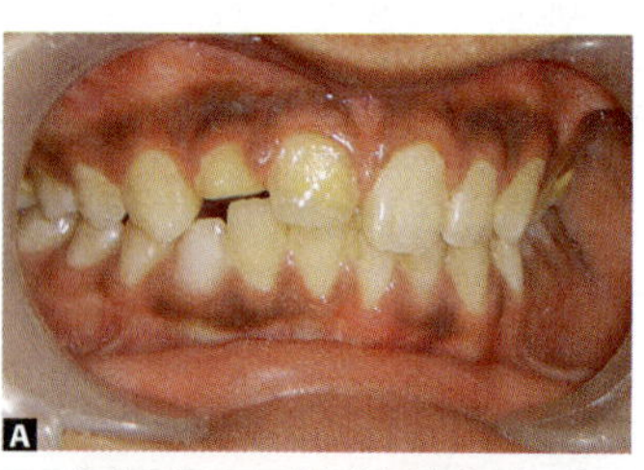

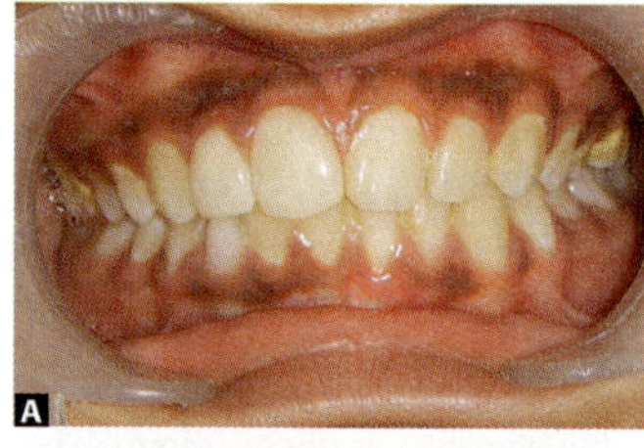

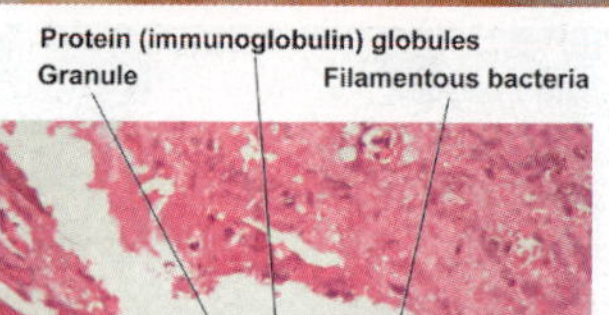

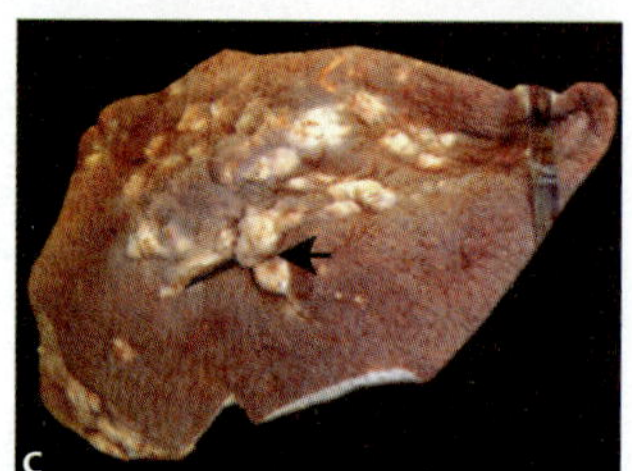

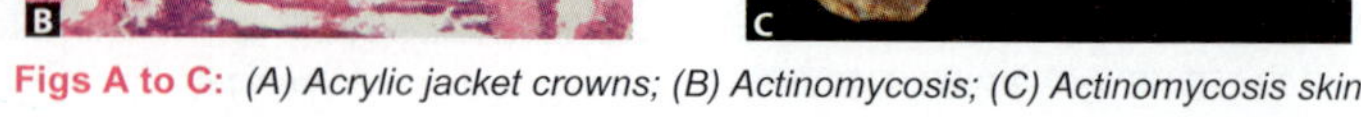
Figs A to C: *(A) Acrylic jacket crowns; (B) Actinomycosis; (C) Actinomycosis skin*

B4, and PGD2. Each leukocyte chemotactic factor is recognized by a specific receptor on the leukocyte surface of the transmembrane receptor family. Contact with even minute amount of such a factor either dissolved in the blood or bound to the endothelial surface triggers diameter changes in the surface adhesion properties of neutrophils. It also induces changes in the conformation of integrins on leukocyte surfaces enabling them to bind specific glycoprotein ligands on endothelium. Chemokines unmask the binding activities of integrins called MAC–1 Leukocyte Functional Ag (LFA), which can each then bind to ICAM-1 on activated endothelial cell.

Active eruption refers to the emergence of the tooth in the oral cavity from its position in the jaw.

Active exercises are movements of body due to voluntary contraction and relaxation of muscle.

Active immunity is of 2 types, active and passive. Active immunity further can be natural or acquired. It occurs naturally when disease is caused by microorganism and protection against further attack by that microorganism is conferred to the individual if the body recovers from the disease.

Active memory refers to the short-term memory.

Acuity is a sharpness of visual perception.

Acupressure is a type of therapy where physician puts light and medium pressure on certain specific points. Their aim is to stimulate the body's electromagnetic energy to help body's own recuperative powers to remove energy blockage. Blockage is due to production of lactic acid and carbon monoxide in muscle tissue resulting in stiff musculature. Removal of blockage relaxes the whole body.

Acupuncture is a system of science where the needles are inserted into patient's skin to treat diseases. Chinese thought that life force flows through the meridians. Flow of force when blocked results in disease. Needles are inserted at specific sites. Acupuncture releases endorphins which act as natural analgesics. Acupuncture has shown successful results in dental surgery and in process of delivery (*see* **Figure on page 12**).

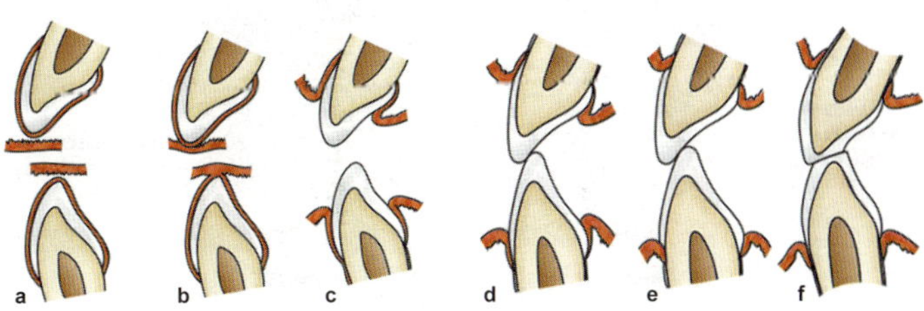

Fig.: *Active eruption*

A

Acute abdomen is a persistent, severe abdominal pain of sudden onset. There may be fever. Abdominal wall may be tense due to appendicitis, salpingitis and peritonitis.

Acute adenitis is a simple inflammation of lymph gland. Glands are bodyguard of specific area and these enlarge when infection develops in their area. In different type of diseases, pattern of gland involvement is different. In infection these enlarge but may remain mobile, in TB. These may be matted, in malignancy these may be enlarged and fixed.

Acute apical abscess is a localized collection of pus in the alveolar bone at the root apex of the tooth, following the death of pulp with extension of the infection through the apical foramen into periradicular tissue.

Acute apical periodontitis is defined as painful inflammation of the periodontium as a result of trauma, irritation or infection through the root canal, regardless of whether the pulp is vital or nonvital. It is an inflammation around the apex of a tooth. The distinctive features of acute apical periodontitis (AAP) are microscopic rather than roentogenographic, symptomatic rather than visible.

Acute atrophic candidiasis is red patch of atrophic raw, painful mucosa which develops with minimal evidence of pseudomembrane. Depapillation of tongue and antibiotic sore-throat may be seen **(*see* Figure on page 13).**

Acute bacterial sialadenitis is caused by *Streptococcus pyogenes* and *Staphylococcus aureus*. Bacteria reach the gland through Stensen's duct. Diabetes, Sjögren's syndrome are the

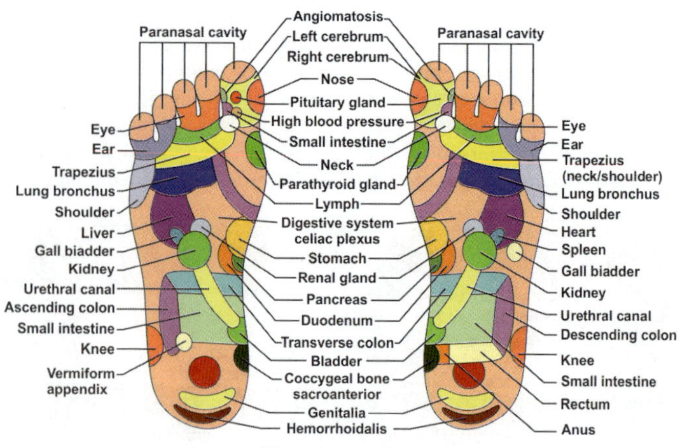

Fig.: *Acupuncture*

causative factors. Clinical features include sudden onset of painful swelling in the preauricular region. One or both sides of parotid gland may be involved. Fever, weakness and redness of skin over parotid are seen. There may be difficulty in swallowing. Antibiotics are helpful.

Acute cholecystitis is an inflammation of gallbladder always associated with gallstones. There is peritoneal pain with overlying skin tenderness and muscle rigidity in right hypochondrium. Referred pain may be radiating to back on right shoulder. Nausea and vomiting may be present. Tenderness and muscle guarding in right upper quadrant. In some cases, palpable mass of globular shape below right costal palpable margin moving with respiration may be felt. Serum bilirubin will be raised. There may be area of hyperesthesia over right subcapsular region.

Acute cold exposure is said to have occurred when body temperature is less than 35°C. Vasodilatation increases the risk of hypothermia. It may result in dizziness, dyspnea, confusion and incoordination. Signs include shivering, dysarthria and altered mental status. Person may suffer from hypotension and respiratory depression.

Acute cystitis is an infection of the bladder most commonly due to coliform bacteria and enterococci. Route of infection is ascending from urethra. Frequency, urgency, dysuria with suprapubic discomfort is common. Ladies may develop hematuria, especially after intercourse. Urine shows pyuria and bacteriuria. Uroflox responds well.

Acute dacrocystitis refers to the condition where patient presents with pain and swelling near the medial canthus of the eye associated with epiphora. Nose appears red, hot, ill-defined and very tender. On pressure on the swelling there is no regurgitation through the puncta. Edema and redness may extend to lower eyelid. Submandibular lymph node may be enlarged and tender.

Acute epididymitis occurs when the route of infection is via urethra to the ejaculatory duct and then down the vas deferens to the epididymis. Symptoms of uretheritis pain at tip

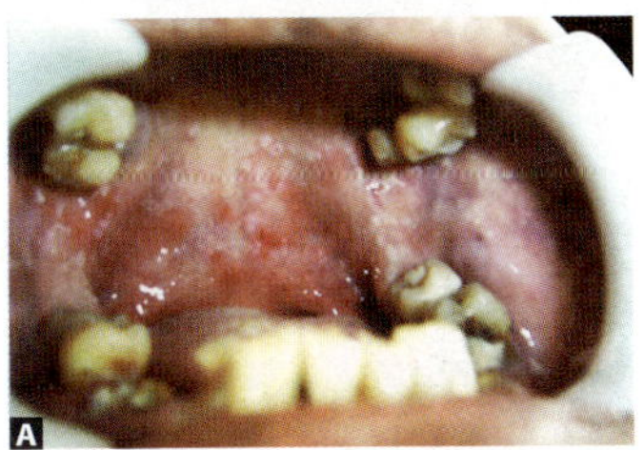

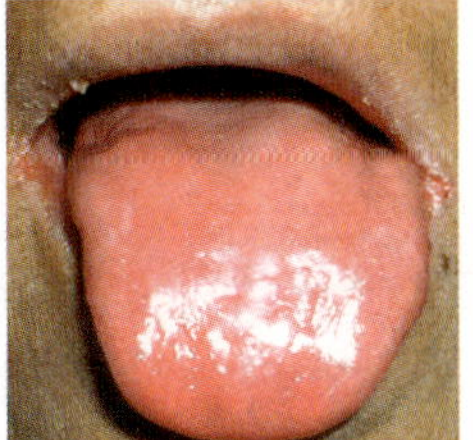

Figs A and B: *(A) Acute candidiasis; (B) Depapillated tongue*

of urethera or cystitis may develop. Pain develops in scrotum radiating to spermatic cord or flank. Prostate may be tender.

Acute gingivitis refers to the inflammation of gingiva, it is the disease of sudden onset and short duration; the condition may be painful in nature.

Acute hepatitis due to bacteria, present within hours or 1–2 days after symptoms. While patients with chronic meningitis present less acutely with a history of months. Mostly, it is tuberculous in origin.

Acute herpes' zoster is the neurotropic virus that travels along the involved nerve. It causes neuritis and vesicular disease of skin and mucous membrane. Eruption is located to a single dermatome. High dose antiviral therapy in acute phase of herpes zoster improves the rate of healing. Intensity of pain also reduces. Post-herpetic neuralgia may continue in old persons.

Acute herpetic stomatitis is an acute viral infectious disease. In 1939, Dodd isolated virus from gingivostomatitis. Person develops fever, irritability, headache, pain and regional lymphadenopathy. Lips, tongue and buccal mucosa are also involved. Painful gingival swelling develops with yellowish fluid filled vesicles, ulcers develop in varying size. These heal automatically within 7–14 days and leave no scar. Isolation can be detected in tissue culture.

Acute illness is the one that comes on suddenly and for a short period.

Acute inflammation: Local signs of acute inflammation are redness, heat, swelling, pain and loss of function. In early stage acute inflammation, edema fluid, fibrin and neutrophils accumulate in the extracellular space of damaged tissue **(*see* Figure on page 15).**

Acute intolerance is a strong negative reaction to a minimal amount of anoxing object.

Acute iritis results from conjuctival injection around cornea. There may be severe pain, blurred vision, photophobia and constricted pupil.

Acute leukemia may be lymphoblastic or myeloblastic. It may be acute or chronic depending upon the nature and progression of disease.

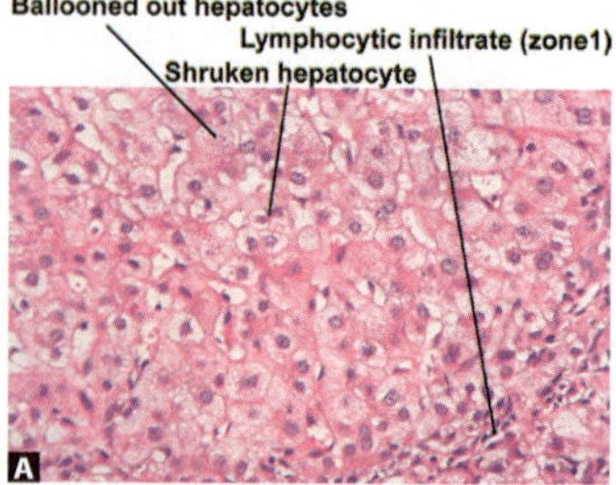

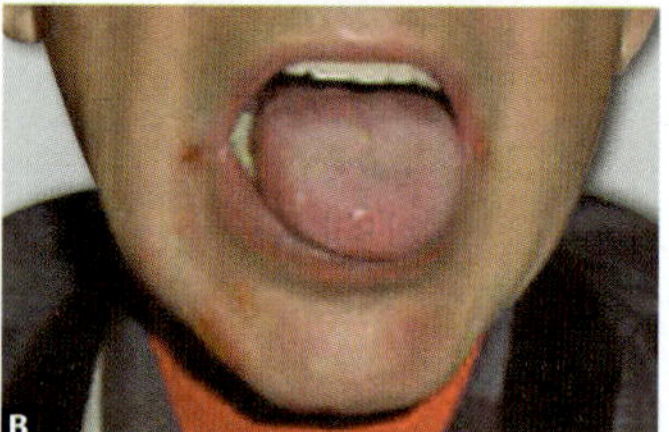

Figs A and B: *(A) Acute hepatitis; (B) Acute herpes zoster, shingles*

Development is sudden with fever, sore-throat, headache, swelling of lymph glands, petechial hemorrhage in skin and mucous membrane. Spleen, kidney and liver become enlarged. Decrease in platelet may lead to hemorrhage. Terminal infection is frequent.

Acute lingual tonsillitis gives rise to unilateral dysphagia and feeling of lump in throat. Lingual tonsil may appear enlarged and congested. It may be studded with follicles. Cervical lymph nodes may be enlarged. Treatment is by antibiotics.

Acute lymphonodular pharyngitis is an acute febrile disease of children. Sore-throat, fever and loss of appetite develop. Symptoms last from 4 to 14 days. Oral manifestation consists of white to yellowish solid papules surrounded

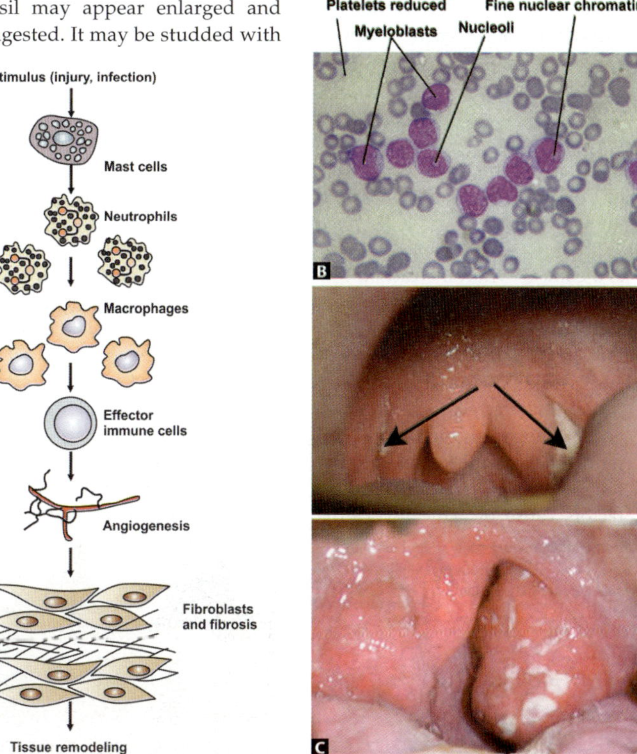

Figs A and B: *(A) Acute inflammation; (B) Acute myeloblastic leukemia; (C) Acute tonsillitis*

by a narrow erythema. It contains packed nodules of lymphocytes.

Acute maxillary sinusitis refers to the periapical infection may involve maxillary sinus. Patient develops pain and swelling over sinus. Pressure over maxillary sinus increases pain. Fever and pain may radiate to the ear. Antibiotics and anti-inflammatory drugs help.

Acute melancholia: Symptoms are constant headache, insomnia, irritability and gastric upsets. Onset is gradual. Hallucinations and delusions are very common. Suicidal and homicidal impulses may be seen. Patient may excite over a minor incident. It may be followed by mania and lucid interval cyclically.

Acute myocardial infarction (AMI) is a clinical syndrome caused by a deficient coronary arterial blood supply to a region of myocardium that results in cellular death and necrosis. This syndrome is usually characterized by severe and prolonged substernal pain but more intense and longer duration than angina pectoris. Predisposing factors cause of acute myocardial infarction in more than 90% of cases is coronary artery disease. Other risk factors include obesity and undue stress, also elevated blood pressure and/or elevated blood cholesterol. Immediate predisposing features for AMI include a significant decrease in blood flow through the coronary arteries, as in coronary thrombosis.

Acute necrotizing ulcerative gingivitis (ANUG) is an endogenous oral infection having necrosis of gingiva. Blood diseases and severe nutritional deficiencies may also result in it. It develops suddenly with pain, tenderness, profuse salivation and spontaneous bleeding. Typical fetid odor develops. Lesion consists of painful, punched out, necrotic ulcers developing on interdental papillae and gingival margin but lips, tongue and palate may also be involved. Gingiva bleeds on touch and is covered by a gray, necrotic pseudomembrane. Patient is not able to eat. Pain is a superficial pressure type. Trench mouth was the term given during World War I in trenches soldiers suffered from

Chronic inflammatory cells
Proliferating capillaries
Fibrous tissue
Viable myocardial fibers
Necrotic myocardial fibers
A

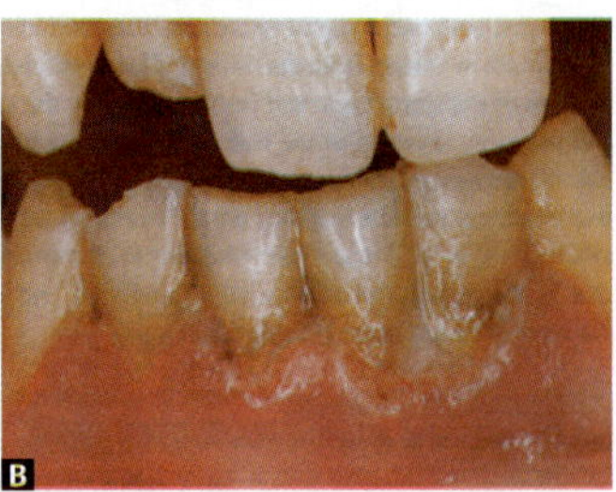

Figs A and B: *(A) Myocardial infarct; (B) ANUG*

acute necrotizing of ulcerative gingivitis. It is an overgrowth of organisms prevalent in normal flora. Disease is not transmissible. Organisms work symbiotically, named *Fusiform*, *Bacillus* and *Spirochetes*.

Acute otitis media is a condition where patient is a young child and complains of pain in ear. There may be hearing loss, fever, vomiting, and diarrhea. Tympanic membrane is bulging. Bloody then serosanguinous and finally purulent otorrhea may follow. Spontaneous perforation of tympanic membrane gives relief.

Acute pain is associated with the pain of sudden onset and short duration.

Acute pancreatitis is an idiopathic condition. Sudden onset of acute excruciating epigastric pain with radiation to back is the main complaint. Pain is more in supine position and there is some relief when patient sits up. Low grade fever, tachycardia and hypotension are common. Bowel sounds are depressed. Green coloration of flanks indicates severe necrotizing pancreatitis. Ultrasound is a good modality to diagnose it.

Acute periapical abscess is an acute inflammation of periapical tissue characterized by localized accumulation of pus at the apex of a tooth. It is a painful condition that results from an advanced necrotic pulp. Patients usually relate previous painful episode from irreversible pulpitis or necrotic pulp. Swelling, tooth mobility and fever are seen in advanced cases.

Acute pericoronitis is an infection associated with a partially erupted tooth or fully erupted tooth that is covered completely or partially by a flap of tissue.

Acute phase response: Most soluble mediators of innate immunity are found in relatively small amount in the serum under normal conditions. Concentration of these proteins can increase 1000-fold during serious injury as part of coordinated protective response called "Hepatic Acute Phase Response". Liver temporarily increases its synthesis of more than a dozen serum proteins that participate in antimicrobial defense. Response occurs when

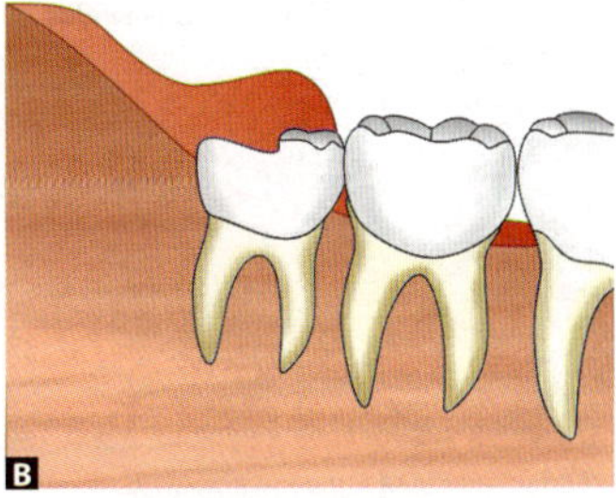

Figs A and B: *(A) Acute otitis media; (B) Acute pericoronitis*

A

hepatocytes are exposed to certain cytokines like IL-6, IL-1, TNF, LPS of bacteria.

Acute proliferative glomerulonephritis is a renal condition where the renal symptoms develop after a period of 10 days. Fifty percent of patients develop hypertension. Urine is of high specific gravity and smoky color. Urinary rudiments contain red cell casts and granular casts. Transient elevation in BUN and serum creatinine may be seen. There may be Frank hematuria with periorbital hematoma. Hematuria may be gross or microscopic with oliguria. Both kidneys are swollen. External surface can be smooth with petechiae.

Acute pulmonary edema is characterized by the accumulation of fluid in the pulmonary interstitium and alveoli due to increase in the pulmonary venous and capillary hydrostatic pressure. The lungs become less compliant, airways resistance increases, and the capillary-alveolar gas exchange is compromised.

Fig.: *Acute proliferative glomerulonephritis*

Acute pulpalgia refers to the development of pulpal inflammation or pulpitis. Increased intrapulpal pressure is the stimulus that is applied to the sensory nerves of the pulp and leads to severe toothache. It occurs with a large carious lesion or with restoration. Severe pain is elicited with thermal changes especially cold. Pain is of lancinating type. Intensity of pain increases when patient lies down, when entrance to the diseased pulp is not wide-pain becomes severe. Pulp contains large number of bacteria. There is no specific treatment and once pulpitis occurs, the damage is irreparable. Tooth involved with acute pulpitis may be treated by pulp therapy.

Acute pyelonephritis condition is uncommon in contrast to acute cystitis. Vesicoureteric infection, pregnancy and instrumentation may predispose to it. Diabetes predisposes to infection. Person develops loin pain, high fever and often rigors. There may be much destruction of cortex sparing of glomeruli and blood vessels.

Acute renal failure is defined as sudden decline in renal ability to maintain fluid and electrolyte homeostasis and to excrete nitrogenous wastes. Clinically, ARF manifests as rising blood urea and serum creatinine levels or decreased urine output over hours or days. Acute renal failure may be oliguric or nonoliguric. In nonoliguric form, the urine output is not reduced, although blood urea and serum creatinine are raised.

Acute retroviral syndrome is a non-specific viral syndrome occurring 1–6 weeks following HIV exposure. Whole features may go unrecognized. Symptoms include fever, sweat, malaise, truncal rash, mouth pain and neck stiffness. Liver and spleen are enlarged. Fever with lymphadenopathy develops.

Acute rheumatic fever (ARF) is a multisystem disorder which follows pharyngeal streptococcal infection. This is the commonest cause of acquired heart disease in childhood and adolescence. Acute rheumatic fever affects children, between 5 to 15 years of age. The manifestations of ARF are fever, lethargy, anorexia and symptoms caused due to involvement of heart, joints, skin and central nervous system. Its diagnosis is based on updated Jone's criteria.

Acute suppurative osteomyelitis is a sequeal of periapical infection. Dental infection is the commonest cause. *Staphylococcus aureus* and *Staphylococcus albus* are the commonest one. Maxilla or mandible may be involved. There will be severe pain and enlargement of lymph glands. WBC count is elevated. Once periostitis develops, there is no swelling or reddening of skin. On X-ray lytic lesion is noted. Individual trabeculae becomes fuzzy and indistinct. Separated fragment of dead bone is called sequestrum. For large sequestrum surgical removal is to be done.

Adaptation refers to the manner in which working end of an instrument is placed against the surface of the tooth to get maximum adaptability or proximity to the tooth surface and avoid soft tissue trauma.

Adaptive immune system is said to have occurred when innate system is breached, a specific response is mounted to each infectious agent and the infectious agent is remembered to prevent it from causing infection later.

Addicted: One who is dependent has a strong psychological reliance.

Addiction is a habit forming and has a compulsive physiological need for it.

Addition polymerization is a polymerization process involving free radicals in which no by-product is formed as the chain grows.

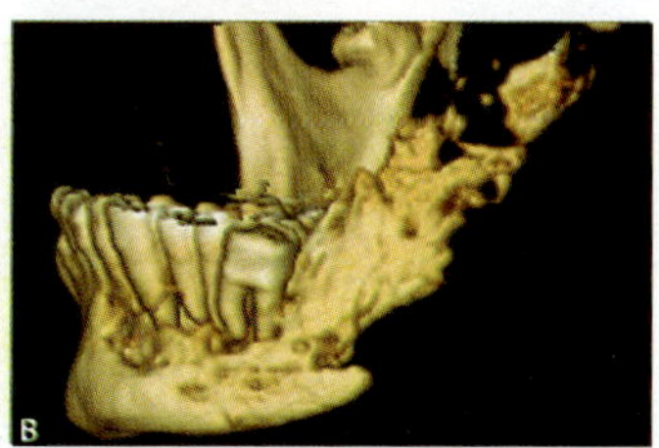

Figs A and B: *Osteomyelitis of jaw (A) Anterior view; (B) Lateral view*

A

Addition silicone is a silicone polymer resulting from free radical polymerization of vinyl group of platinum catalysts.

Adduction is the movement of body part toward the middle of the body.

Adenoameloblastoma arises from residual odontogenic epithelium. In early stage, tumor is completely radiolucent. It may be solid or may contain large cystic areas. It forms duct-like structures. Site of occurrence is more in maxilla. Vast majority measure 1.5 to 3 cm Minute calcifications are also seen under microscope. In advanced stage, sufficient calcification occurs to produce clusters of radio-opaque foci with the radiolucency. Majority occurs in unerupted tooth or in the walls of dentigerous cyst. Mostly involved teeth are maxillary canine, lateralincisors,mandibular premolar. Slow growth expands the cortical plates and produces clinical signs of swelling. Asymmetry is seen. X-ray shows destructive lesions of jaw which may or may not be well circumscribed. Soft tissues are not involved.

Adenocarcinoma occurs more commonly in relation to minor salivary glands. The tumor is slow growing with no surface ulceration. It is a painless mass. Later on tumor grows faster. Swelling becomes painful. Ulceration and loss of sensation develops. Under microscope, one can see numerous proliferating malignant ductal epithelial cells. There will be areas of hemorrhage and necrosis.

Adenocystic carcinoma is a malignant neoplasm arising from glandular epithelium. It is the most common malignant tumor

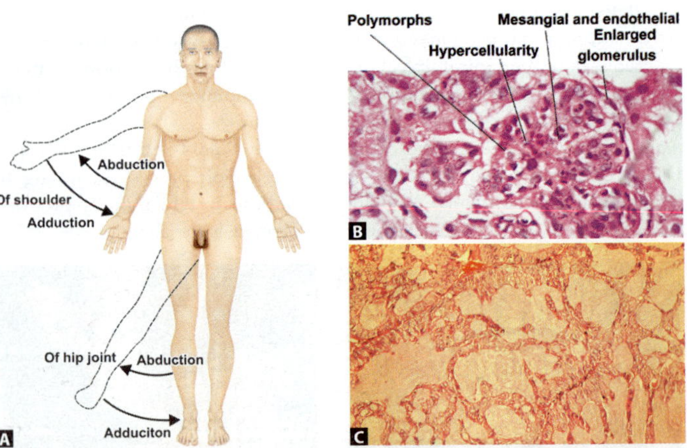

Figs A to C: *(A) Abduction; (B) Adenocarcinoma; (C) Adenocarcinoma high power;*

of submandibular salivary gland. Glands of palate and tongue may also be involved. Parotid tumor produces a subcutaneous mass anterior to or below the external ear. Pain is very common feature in this tumor. There is fixation and induration of tumor. Submandibular gland tumors become quite large. While palatal lesions are often accompanied by delayed healing of socket once tooth has been extracted. If greater palatine nerve is involved, palatal paresthesia will develop. Treatment involves excision followed by radiotherapy because tumor cells are radiosensitive.

Adenofibroma is a frequent neoplasm of youth below the age of 25 years. These are usually small, painless tumors discovered or lobulated. Adenofibroma occasionally undergoes spontaneous infarction and necrosis during pregnancy. Necrosis usually produces no symptoms.

Adenohypophysis is the term collectively used for pars anterior (which is also called the pars distalis) and the pars intermedia, as they both are made up of cells having a direct secretory function.

Adenoid: These are gland-like, adenoid or pharyngeal tonsils. These are paired lymphoid structures in the nasopharynx.

Adenoid cystic carcinoma is a malignant tumor of parotid, submaxillary and accessory glands of palate and tongue. It is composed of deeply staining uniform cell resembling basal cells. Despite of malignant nature, mitotic figures are extremely rare. Surgery is the answer.

Adenoid squamous cell carcinoma develops in younger age. Lesion appears as elevated nodule. It shows scaling, crusting and ulceration. There is a proliferation of surface dysplastic epithelium. Surgical excision helps.

Adenoidectomy is removal of adenoids.

Adenolymphoma is a benign salivary gland neoplasm. It is also known as Warthin's tumor and develops in parotid gland. Tumor lies superficially just beneath the parotid capsule. It is firm but not palpable. It consists of cystic spaces with intraluminar projections.

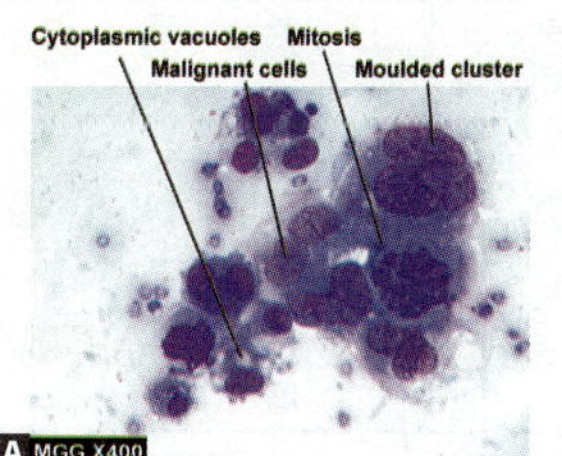

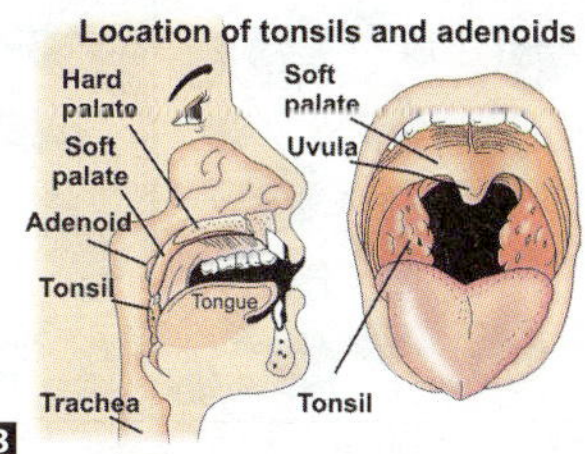

Figs A and B: *(A) Adenocarcinoma and ascitic fluid; (B) Adenoids*

A

It contains a lot of lymphoid tissues. It may develop due to proliferation of ectopic salivary gland tissue. Some think that it is a hemartous growth than a true neoplastic lesion. It comprises 20% of all parotid tumors. *Clinical features:* it is well-encapsulated and movable, is it is slow growing well circumscribed, soft and painless, it can grow up to 2–4 cm in diameter, it gives a compressible and doughy feeling on palpation, on cut surface confluent cystic spaces are seen and chocolate colored fluid comes out. Dense fibrous capsule surrounds it. Malignant transformation is rare. Surgical excision is to be done.

Adenoma thyroid is a solitary discrete nodule. These arise from follicular epithelium known as follicular adenomas. It is well-circumscribed solitary, round, rubbery or firm, and well capsulated. Cut surface is brown and translucent.

Adhesion refers to the sticking together of unlike substances, i.e. force of attraction between the molecules or atoms on two different surfaces as they are brought into contact with one another or it can be described as the surface attachment of two materials.

Adipsia is abnormal absence of thirst. It occurs in hypothalamic injury/ tumor, head injury, cirrhosis and bronchial tumor.

Adjuvant therapy is the treatment given after the primary treatment such as radiation therapy or hormonal therapy.

Admixed alloy is an amalgam alloy containing particles of different

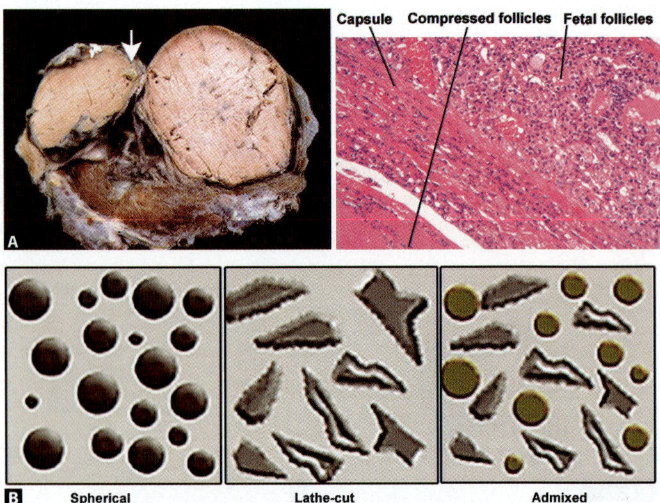

Figs A and B: *(A) Adenoma thyroid; (B) Admixed amalgam alloy*

composition, i.e. silver tin or silver copper particles.

Adolescence is the period of transition from childhood to adulthood, i.e. period of 3 to 4 years after puberty; extending from the earlier signs of sexual maturity until the attainment of physical and emotional maturity.

Adolescent caries: The characteristic features of this type of caries are: Lesions in teeth and surfaces those are relatively immune to caries. There is relatively small opening in enamel with extensive undermining of enamel. Rapid penetration of enamel and extensive involvement of dentin is seen. The rapid progression of the lesion which does not permit an effective pulpal response with little or no secondary dentin.

Adrenal gland is an endocrine gland composed of cortex and medulla. These are two organs situated at upper poles of kidneys and are embedded in perirenal fat. Size of these is 1½ x 3 x ½ an inch. Right is pyramidal in shape while left one is crescent shaped. Adrenal cortex produces and secretes more than 30 steroid hormones, of which cortisol, a glucocorticoid is widely considered the most important. Cortisol helps the body adapt to stress.

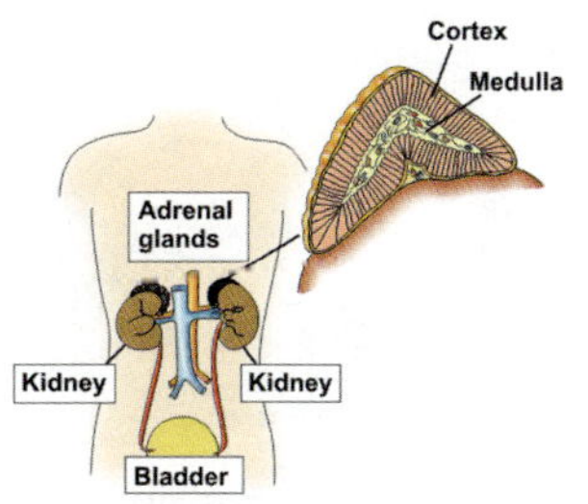

Fig.: *Adrenal glands*

Adrenaline is a hormone secreted by medulla of adrenal glands. It is the first hormone to be discovered. Under emotional stress BP rises due to its liberation. Blood sugar and BMR also rises. It is chemically L4 - (1 - Hydroxy - 2 - (methylaminolethyl) -1, 2- benezenediot.

Adult periodontitis *see* chronic periodontitis.

Adulteration of milk is a process where the milk is adulterated by addition of skimmed milk powder, gelatin or starch with maida or arrow root after extraction of fat to make it thick. Common methods of adulteration of milk are adding water to increase the quantity. Second most common is extraction of cream from milk partially or completely.

Adulthood refers to the stage of growth and development where ossification and growth are virtually completed during early adulthood—18 to 25 years of age. Thereafter developmental changes occur very slowly.

Advanced acute pulpalgia is a stage of pulpal pathology where the pain is very severe—the most excruciating acute pain known to man. Patient may even become hysterical from pain. Relief from this pain is embarrassingly by simple cold water. The history is self-incriminating. Symptoms are violent.

A

The involved tooth usually can be pointed out by patient and is tender to percussion too. Because the inflamed pulp reacts so violently to heat, the most decisive test is the heat test. As soon as the gutta-percha touches the involved tooth, the patient develops subgluteal vacuum and patient rises up in the chair as if stabbed. Cold water is instantly applied and pain subsides. Local anesthesia gives blessed relief.

Advanced interproximal lesion refers to the carious lesion that extends to the DEJ or through the DEJ and into the dentin, but does not extend through the dentin greater than half the distance toward the pulp. An advanced lesion affects both enamel and dentin.

Aerobic training is a process of training when consumption of oxygen develops muscles ability to sustain activity.

Aerobic bacteria are the bacteria which grow in oxygen-rich environment; in the oral cavity the bacteria are found outside the sulcus.

Aerobic is a physiological process in which oxygen is required.

Aerosol refers Mist.

Afebrile is absence of fever.

Afferent fibers (afferent = come towards) are those nerve fibers that carry impulses in the opposite direction, i.e. towards the spinal cord or brain. They are known as the fibers bringing the sensations of touch from the skin, of sight from the eye, or of hearing from the ear. It is through these nerve fibers that we become conscious of such sensations, also called sensory fibers.

Afferent impulse is an impulse traveling toward the central nervous system.

Afferent nerves that carry sensory messages toward the brain.

Aflatoxin is a toxic metabolite in mould of *Aspergillus flavus* discovered in 1960. Infected groundnuts result it in the production of Aflatoxin. Other nuts may also contain it.

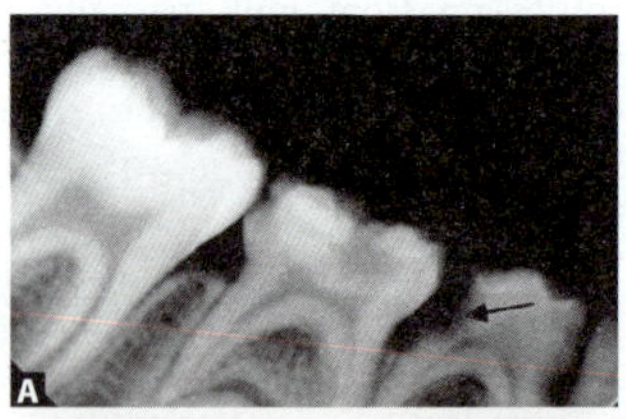

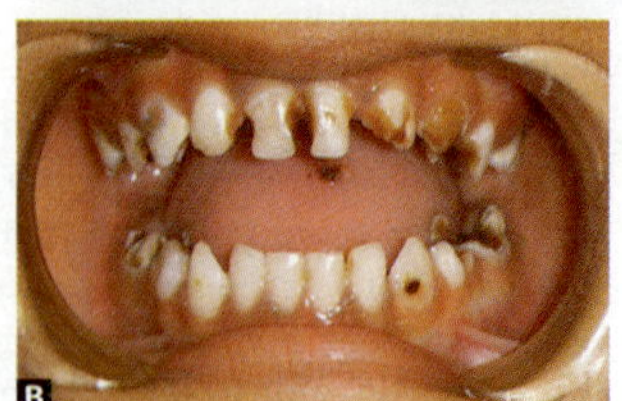

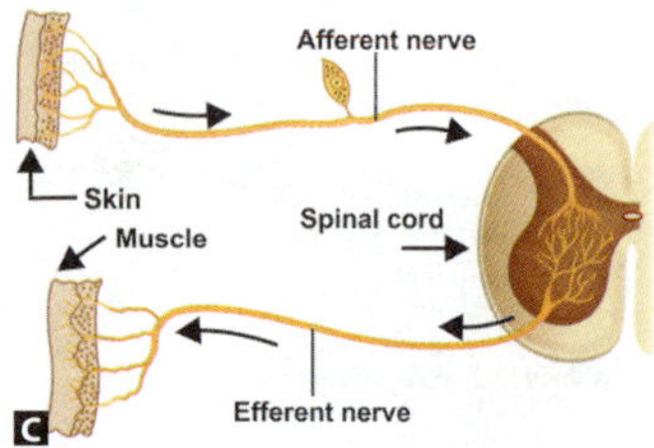

Figs A to C: *(A) Advanced proximal caries; (B) Advanced interproximal caries; (C) Afferent impulse*

Aflatoxin B1 is acutely toxic and carcinogenic. If it is consumed by cows, aflatoxin M1 may be found in milk and cheese.

Agar hydrocolloids are the impression materials that are compounded from reversible agar gels. When heated they liquefy or go into solution state and on cooling they return to gel state. It is usually extracted from seaweed. It is a polysaccharide in nature. Agar impressions are diagonally unstable on standing so model should be made at the earliest.

Age refers to the chronological of date of birth.

Age of abrasion: Fresh abrasion is bright red and oozing. In 24 hours bright red scab forms which becomes reddish, grows and covers the defect under scab. In 7–10 days, scab dries up, shrinks and falls leading to discoloration. For complete healing, it takes 14 days.

Age of bruise: Just after infliction it is red and becomes blue on 3rd day. On 4th day it becomes brown due to hemosiderin. On 5th and 6th day the color becomes green. 7th–11th day color is yellow due to bilirubin and after 2 weeks color becomes normal.

Agglutination is the clumping together of cells distributed in a fluid, generally as a result of antigen-antibody reaction.

Aglycogeusia refers to the condition where the affected individual is not able to distinguish sugar solution from water.

Agnosia refers to the condition where there is the loss of ability to recognize objects by one sense organ while other sense organs may recognize it. Lesions in left angular gyrus produce finger agnosia. Anosognosia is a denial of disease in the affected body part. It is an inability to recognize and interpret sensory stimuli. Auditory agnosia is inability to recognize familiar sounds.

Agranulocytopenia refers to marked reduction in granular leukocytosis. Toxic effect of certain drugs like chloramphenicol, phenyl butazone may result in it. Long-term administration of analgesics, diuretics and anticoagulants may cause it. Ionizing radiation, TB, malaria and typhoid may also induce Agranulocytosis. *Clinical features:* Fever, generally starts with chills and sore throat. Skin becomes pale. Even jaundice may develop, regional lymphadenitis may develop, urinary tract infection may develop, rectal ulcerations are common, severe

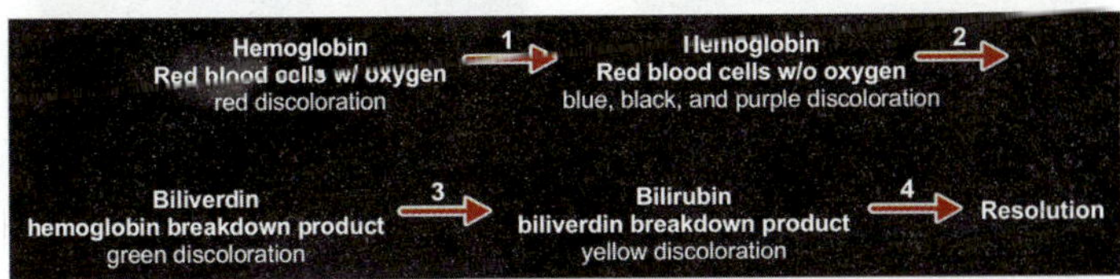

Fig.: *Age of bruise*

leucopenia develops, neutrophils count comes down to 0–2%. Oral manifestations: Agranulocytic angina develops showing necrotizing ulceration over gingival, soft palate and cheeks. Excessive salivation is noted. Ulcers develop which are covered by yellow/gray membrane. Ulcers may start bleeding. Halitosis develops. Opportunistic fungal infections may develop.

Agranulocytosis is a condition where there is marked decrease in the number of circulating neutrophils. In primary agranulocytosis, cause is not known, while in secondary one cause can be traced out. Reaction may be allergic one. It can occur at any age. Disease starts as high fever with chill and sore throat. Patient suffers from weakness and prostration. There develops a necrotizing ulceration of oral mucosa. Salivation increases. Necrosis of gingiva may develop. Rapid destruction of supporting tissues follows.

Agraphia is an inability to express thoughts in writing. It generally occurs due to cerebrovascular accidents.

AIDS is a disabling or life-threatening disease caused by human immunodeficiency virus. Major signs include 10% weight loss. Chronic diarrhea and fever of one month may occur. Minor signs include persistent cough of one month, recurrent herpes zoster, and generalized lymphadenopathy. Most common oral manifestations are hairy leukoplakia, oral candidiasis and Kaposi's sarcoma. Other infections associated with it are orolabial herpes, aggressive pathological periodontal disease and dryness of mouth. It is an epidemic that is now spreading and receiving wide attention throughout the world in the lay of profession. Infection with Immunodeficiency (HIV) has been the most significant disease to affect our society during the last few decades. AIDS stands for the acronym, Acquired Immunodeficiency Syndrome, which is acquired by a retrovirus that causes profound immune suppression rendering the susceptibility of the host and leading to the development of various opportunistic infections and neoplasms. Acute infection occurs 3 to 6 weeks after initial contact

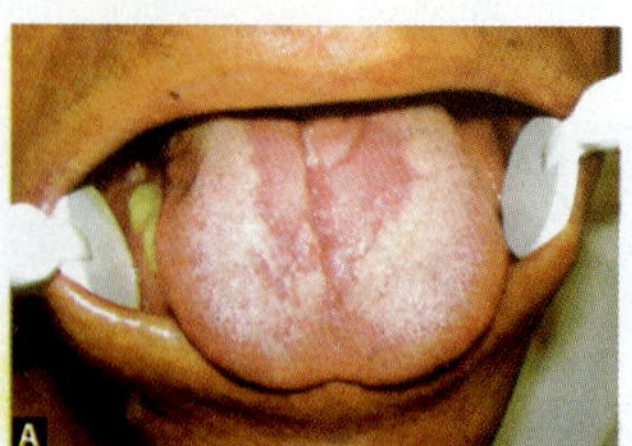

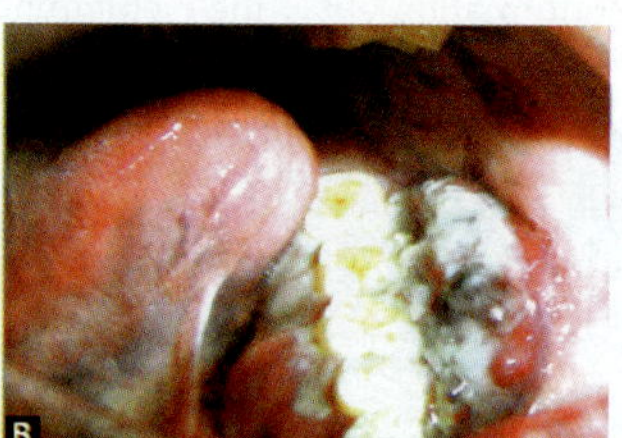

Figs A and B: *HIV patient (A) Oral candidiasis; (B) Kaposi's sarcoma*

with HIV. Non-specific syndrome occurs during which joint pain, gastrointestinal symptoms and a macular rash predominate. These self-limiting symptoms persist for 2–3 weeks. Eight to twelve weeks after infection antibody to HIV can be detected in serum. After acute infection, person enters the symptomatic phase of the disease. The average time from infection to development of disease is 8 to 10 years. During this period, T4 lymphocytes come down from 800 mm^3 to 50 mm^3. Oral manifestations in HIV infected patients or Oral candidiasis occurs in 30% to 90% cases. Persistent ulcers of mouth in AIDS should be biopsied for deep fungal infections. Hairy leukoplakia has been noted in HIV positive homosexuals. Recurrent herpes simple virus progresses to large chronic oral lesions. Ulcers are surrounded by raised white border. Lesions may co-exist with genital and anal lesions. Painful oral ulcers caused by cytomegalovirus may be seen. Kaposi's sarcoma is the most common oral neoplasm in AIDS. Early lesions look like hemangiomas, flat or raised discolorations. Generalized gingivitis and periodontitis.

AIDS of CNS: AIDS has phases of primary infection, asymptomatic infection and established phase. In primary phase, 10% patients have aseptic encephalitis and virus can be isolated from CSF. During asymptomatic phase, there is also aseptic meningitis but virus is not recoverable from CSF. Prednisolone may give relief. In established disease, neurological features are very common when peripheral T4 cell count falls below 500/cmm. Dementia is a well-known feature of HIV disease. These patients have neuronal atrophy and gliosis. There will be slowness of thought, loss of interest and withdrawal from society.

Air velocity is measured by anemometer. At a height of 10 meter velocity is measured. It is measured in meter per second.

Air-water syringe is a device which delivers a stream of water or air and can also deliver a forceful spray of air and water. It is generally used to rinse the patient's mouth.

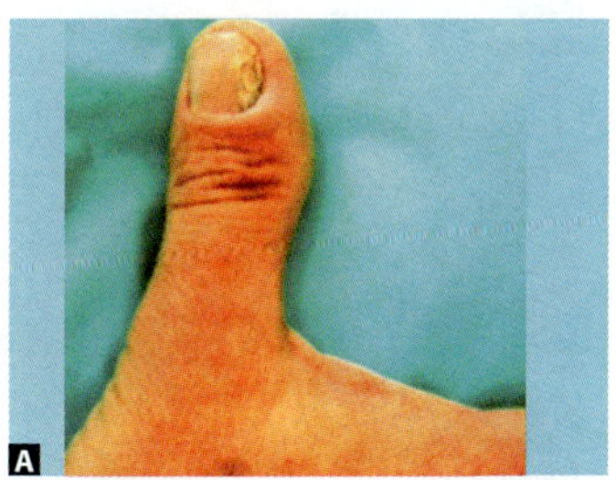

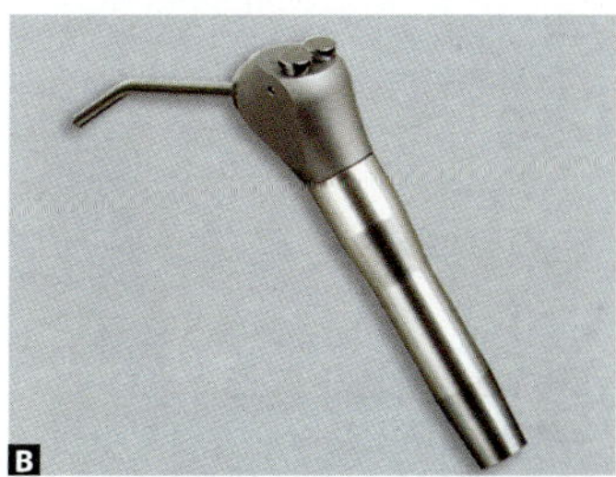

Figs A to B: *(A) Herpes infection in HIV patient; (B) Air-water syringe*

A

Airway obstruction is a condition where partial or complete airway obstruction may occur either due to trauma or any underlying pathology. Dyspnea and cyanosis may occur in seconds and death may occur due to asphyxia or reflex cardiovascular collapse.

ALARA is a concept of radiation protection where radiation is to be kept at minimum. It stands for as low as reasonably achievable.

Albinism is a clinical condition that refers to absence of pigment in skin, hair and eyes of a human being. Absence of chlorophyll in plants.

Albright's syndrome is like fibrous dysplasia of bone. There is replacement of spongy bone by a peculiar fibrous tissue. Radiographs will show radiopacity and radiolucency, some like compact bone other like cystic bone. The cause of endocrine manifestation in Albright's syndrome is not known. Transformation to malignancy occurs. Radiotherapy is not advised.

Albumin is a plasma protein which helps in regulation of the osmotic concentration of the blood.

Albuminuria refers to the presence of albumin in urine usually due to kidney disorder.

Alcohol toxicity refers to the condition where skin becomes cold and clammy. Body temperature is lowered. Respiration is slow, shallow and noisy pulse is weak and accelerated. Pupils become sluggish and various reflexes are generally depressed.

Alcoholic hepatitis is an acute or chronic inflammation and parenchymal necrosis of liver induced by alcohol. It may be a reversible disease or may lead to cirrhosis; liver may be enlarged. Jaundice, abdominal pain, tenderness, splenomegaly, ascites, fever and encephalopathy may be present. AST is usually elevated above 250 units/L. It consists of alcoholic hyaline, hepatic infiltration with polymorphonuclear cell and intralobular connective tissue proliferation. Person may be asymptomatic to mild illness. Hepatomegaly with splenomegaly is common. Fever and jaundice are common.

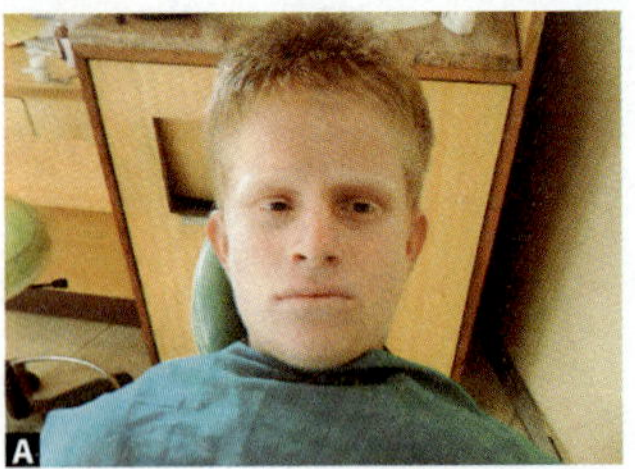

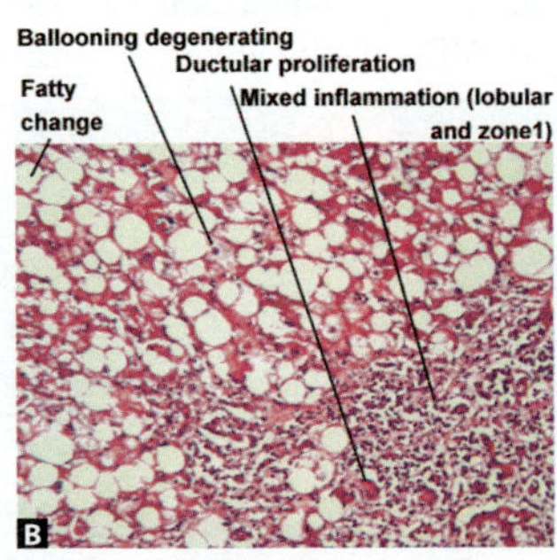

Figs A and B: *(A) Albinism; (B) Alcoholic hepatitis*

Testicular atrophy, parotid enlargement and loss of body hair are often seen. In severe form ascites, edema and encephalopathy are seen. Treatment includes high calorie diet and vitamin supplement. Proteins are restricted and corticosteroids 20–40 mg may be tried.

Alcoholic ketoacidosis occurs after drinking binge by a malnourished, chronic alcoholic, resulting in elevated anion gap acidosis. Symptoms include anorexia, nausea abdominal pain and orthostatic dizziness. There may be odor of ketone on breath, tachycardia and tachypnea.

Aldrich syndrome is a rare hereditary disease transmitted as an X-linked recessive trait. It generally develops in infancy. It develops thrombocytopenic purpura and eczema over face. Eczema is of allergic origin. Spontaneous bleeding of gingiva is frequently seen. There is an abnormality of platelets. There is no specific treatment.

Alginate is an impression material used for dentures. It gives an accurate impression, without distortion. It is mixed by powder and water at room temperature. This sets within a few minutes. Material is an elastic one but the disadvantage is if kept for long it undergoes dimensional changes. So it should be repeatedly rinse in cold running water and dip in sodium hypochloride.

Alimentary canal is a digestive tract consisting of mouth, esophagus, stomach, duodenum and large intestine.

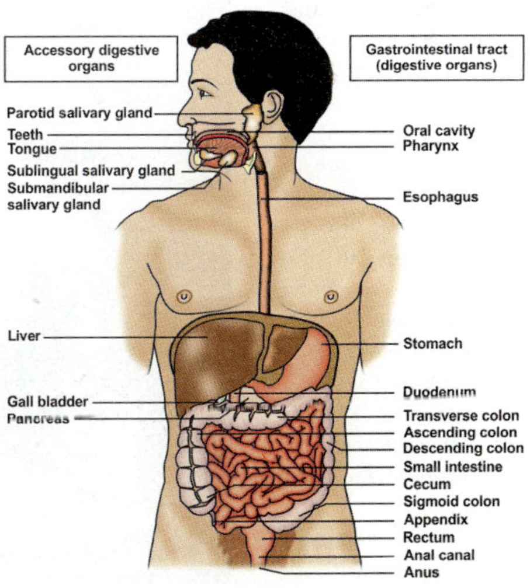

Fig.: *Alimentary canal*

Alitame is an artificial sweetener that is 2000 times sweeter than sucrose, formed from L-aspartic acid and D-alanine. Alitame has a clean taste and is stable. It is derived from proteins.

Alkaptonuria, which is a recessively inherited inborn error of metabolism, is characterized by deposition of dark pigments in bones, joints and nasal cartilages. Occasionally, brownish discoloration of the permanent dentition can also be observed.

All and none phenomenon is said to have occured where nerve or muscle cell will either respond or not respond at all. It responds maximally every time. It is not related with the intensity of stimulus.

Allergic sialadenitis is a non, neoplastic, non, inflammatory enlargement of salivary gland. Enlargement is bilateral and painless. Periauricular portion of enlargement is noted. Salivary potassium content is enlarged and salivary sodium content is reduced. Some may occur due to toxic reaction to drugs. Allergic sialadenitis is a self-limiting disease.

Allergic stomatitis refers to the condition where allergic reactions may cause acute multiple vesicles and ulcers of oral mucosa or a lichenoid reaction. Oral drugs may also cause the condition. The fixed drug eruption is characterized by localized area of erythema, edema and vesiculation at the site of drug contact. Contact allergy is caused by a delayed type hypersensitivity reaction to topical antigen. Contact allergy to dental amalgam is usually caused by mercury. Tooth paste allergy is rare but occurs. It results in fissuring of lips, perioral desquamation edema, angular cheilitis and swelling of gingiva.

Allergy is abnormal tissue reactivity after exposure to a foreign antigen resulting in release of histamine.

Allograft refers to the graft of tissues between individuals of same species but of disparate genotype.

Allopurinol is the xanthine oxidase inhibitor that quickly lowers plasma urate and urinary uric acid concentration. It facilitates topus mobilization.

Alloxan is a pyrimidine derivative that can induce diabetes by destroying islets of Langerhan's.

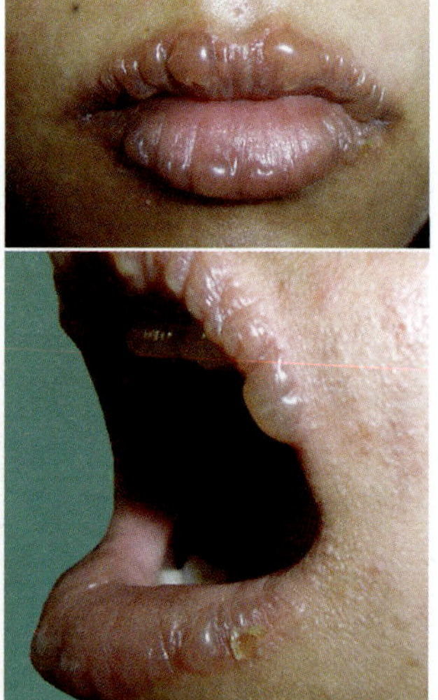

Fig.: *Allergic stomatitis*

Alloy is a mixture of two or more metals. It exhibits metallic properties and is composed of one or more elements, i.e. brass is an alloy of copper and zinc.

Alloy for dental amalgam is a silver-tin alloy containing other metals generally copper and zinc which will be mixed with mercury to form dental amalgam.

Alopecia refers to baldness, loss of hair.

Alopecia areata is the development of well-circumscribed patches of non-scarring scalp alopecia without skin changes. Patches may develop on beared, pubic areas and axilla. This disorder is recurrent.

Alpha-fetoprotein is a normal fetal protein which passes from fetus into the amniotic fluid and maternal serum. At 16 weeks gestation, increased levels suggest fetal spina bifida with Down's syndrome.

Alternate current is a current in which electrons flow in opposite direction.

Alternative medical therapy: Treatment outside the main stream of traditional therapy.

Althesin is a steroid anesthetic agent. It is injected slowly in a dose of 0.05 to 0.075 ml/kg body weight IV, rapid induction of anesthesia occurs. It has a very short duration of anesthesia and recovery is rapid. Extravenous injection does not produce tissue damage.

Alumina slips casting is a process for forming alumina cores that give very high strength values of around 500 MPa. Advantage of it is high strength and good fit. Disadvantages include high initial cost, long processing time and lack of bonding to the tooth structure.

Aluminium is a metal that occurs in rock and clay. It is found in animals and plants. Aluminium cooking vessels are not harmful.

Alveolar bone is the bone surrounding the root of the tooth; loss of this bone is typically associated with severe periodontal disease.

Alveolar bone loss refers to the loss of bone that surrounds and supports the teeth in mandible/maxilla.

Alveolar cavitational osteopathosis refers to the cavity which is not demonstrable on X-ray but is able to locate on surgical procedure.

Alveolar crest fibers refer to the fibers that extend obliquely from the cementum to the alveolar crest. These fibers prevent extrusion and

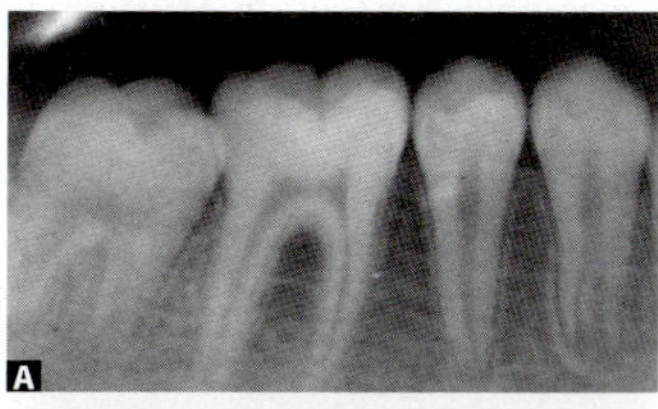

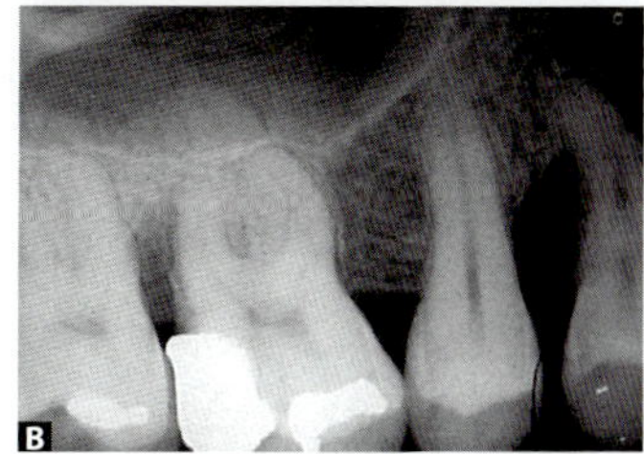

Figs A and B: *(A) Alveolar bone; (B) Alveolar bony defect*

prevent the lateral movements of the tooth.

Alveolar crest is the highest portion of alveolar bone or it is the most coronal portion of alveolar bone found between the teeth, composed of dense cortical bone appearing radio-opaque.

Alveolar eminence is outline of the root on the facet portion of the bone.

Alveolar mucosa is a nonkeratinized epithelium characterized by a smooth and shiny surface. The absence of keratin makes the alveolar mucosa more red than the pink gingival. This tissue has abundance of elastic fibers and is readily movable. Mucosa covers the vestibule and floor of mouth and becomes buccal and labial mucosa. Its width increases with age and eruption of teeth.

Alveolar process is that portion of the mandible or maxilla that surrounds the root of a tooth.

Alveolar soft part sarcoma is a rare tumor. Lesions in tongue and floor of mouth have been reported. Tumor is composed of large cells with fine granular cytoplasm. Lesion is slow growing, well-circumscribed masses with no gross features. Radical surgical excision is an accepted treatment.

Alveolectomy is a surgical procedure that is performed to produce a smooth alveolar ridge, either by removing the sharp bony spicules post-extraction or by augmenting the ridge.

Alveolus is the bony socket in which the root of the tooth sits.

Alveoplasty is a surgical reduction and reshaping of alveolar ridge.

Alzheimer's disease is a degenerative disease of an old age. There is neuronal loss in cerebral cortex with convolution atrophy especially over frontal and temporal lobe. Some amount of ventricular enlargement takes place. There develops thickened neuritic process. Number of plaque in one field is directly correlated with degree of memory loss. Disturbance of speech function takes place. CSF is normal and EEG shows generalized slowing. CT and MRI shows dilatation of lateral ventricles and widening of cortical sulci.

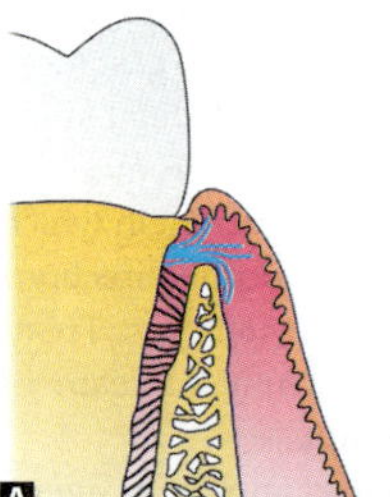

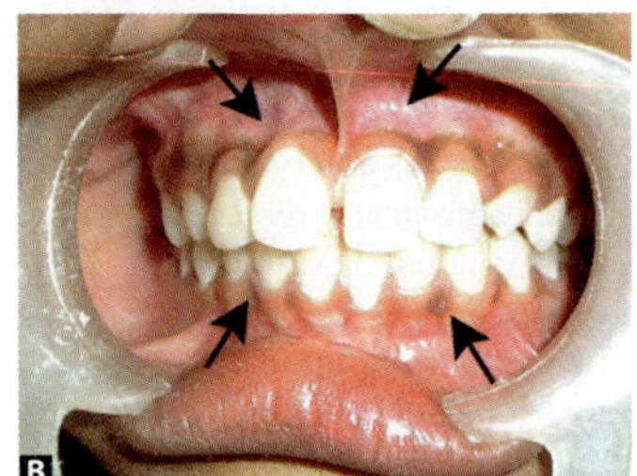

Figs A and B: *(A) Alveolar crest fibers; (B) Alveolar mucosa*

Amalgam is an alloy and the most commonly used restorative material. Its one of the metals is mercury which gives silver color to the filling, thus, it is also known as silver filling. In average depth cavities, the pulp is affected mainly by the cold and hot stimuli that result from the thermal conductive properties of amalgam. In deep cavities, pain is due to unlined cavities and an inflammatory response is seen after 3 days and 5 weeks. Marginal leakage has been shown to cause damage to pulp after the placement of amalgam restorations. Pulpal response to silver amalgam restoration occurs shortly after placement.

Amalgam carrier refers to the dental hand instrument that is used to carry and dispense freshly mixed amalgam into a cavity preparation. The lever forces a plunger to push contained amalgam from the cylinder.

Amalgam carver is a hand instrument used to carve the anatomical features on the occlusal aspect of an amalgam restoration.

Amalgam tattoo is a flat, bluish-gray lesion of oral mucosa resulting from the introduction of amalgam particles into the tissue. The metallic particles disperse in tissue resulting in permanent area of pigmentation. It is mostly seen on gingiva or edentulous ridge.

Amalgam well refers to a small metal disk to hold the mixed amalgam.

Amalgamation is a process of mechanically mixing the dental amalgam alloy with mercury.

Amalgamator is a device used to mix mercury with amalgam alloy.

Ambisexuality refers to the erotic interest toward both males and females.

Amblyopia is a functional loss of vision without any organic defect. There is blurring and inability to focus generally found in alcoholics.

Ameloblastic fibrodontoma is a well-circumscribed lesion. Lesions are small measuring 1 to 2 cm in diameter. Occasionally, these lesions will become huge. It does not evade bone, hence curettage serves the purpose.

Ameloblastic fibroma is an uncommon neoplasm of odontogenic origin. It is a true mixed odontogenic tumor, containing nests and strands of ameloblastic epithelium. Calcified dental structures are not seen. X-ray features are of simple ameloblastoma. There will be well-defined unilocular radiolucency.

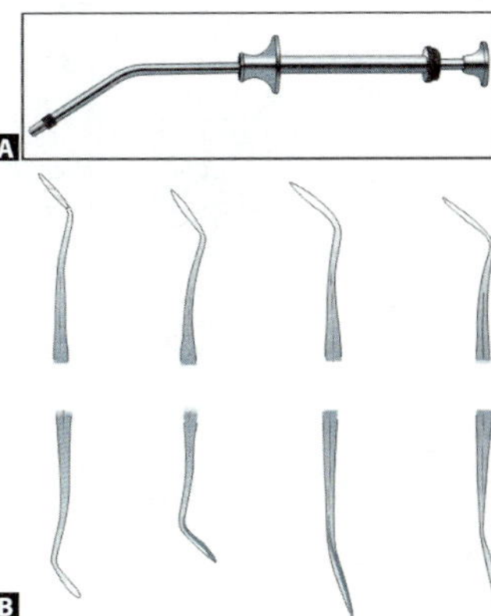

Figs A and B: *(A) Amalgam carrier; (B) Amalgam carvers*

Multilocular lesions may occur. Vast majority occurs in mandible and highest incidence in premolar region. Tumor is often associated with unerupted teeth. Mitotic activity is not common. There may be a paucity of blood.

Ameloblastic odontome is an odontogenic neoplasm characterized by simultaneous presence of ameloblastoma and composite odontoma. Mild pain with delayed eruption of teeth are presenting feature. On X-ray central destruction of cortical plates is seen.

Ameloblastoma is a true neoplasm. It originates in 80% cases from mandible. It develops insidiously as a central lesion of bone which is slowly destructive. It may ulcerate or fungate disfiguring the patients face. Radiographically, it shows multilocular cyst-like lesion of bone. After surgery recurrence is rare.

Ameloblasts are the epithelial cell of the enamel organ. It is responsible for the formation of enamel.

Amelogenesis imperfecta is defined as a spectrum of hereditary defects in the function of ameloblasts and mineralization of enamel matrix that results in teeth with multiple generalized abnormalities affecting the enamel layer only. It is entirely an ectodermal disturbance, since the mesodermal components of the tooth are basically normal. The anomaly occurs in the general population in the range of 1 in 14,000. Three basic type of amelogenesis imperfecta are: Hypoplastic: type in which there is defective formation of matrix,

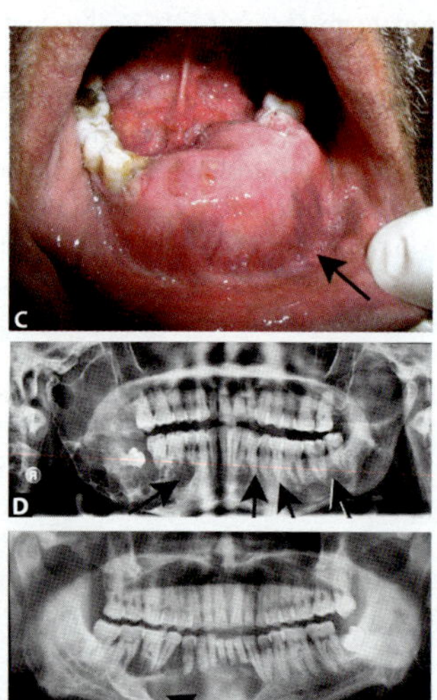

Figs A to E: *(A) Amalgam Hollenback carver; (B) Amalgamator; (C) Ameloblastoma midline; (D) Multilocular-ameloblastoma; (E) Unilocular ameloblastoma*

Hypocalcification type: in which there is defective mineralization of the formed matrix, Hypomaturation type: in which enamel crystallites remain immature.

Amelo-onychohypohidrotic syndrome is characterized by defective nails with subungual hyperkeratosis are seen with sweat gland hypofunction and severe hypoplastic-hypocalcified crowns.

Amino acids are basically proteins in nature. Twenty-two amino acids are known, of which eight cannot be synthesized in our body in sufficient quantity, and hence are to be supplied from outside. Essential amino acid includes isoleucine, leucine, lysine, methionine, phenylalanine, threonine, tryptophan and valine. Growing children need histidine.

Aminoglycosides are bactericidal drugs. They cause misreading of mRNA by the ribosome, leading to abnormal protein production. To enter the bacterium, aminoglycosides need to be actively transported across the cell membrane. This does not occur in anaerobic organisms, which are therefore, resistant.

Amniocentesis is the removal of amniotic fluid for analysis. It is a procedure to detect birth defects.

Amoebiasis, *Entamoeba histolytica* exists in two forms, the trophozoite form and the cystic form. Later is involved in transmission by food, fingers and flies. In intestine, it results in amoebiasis. Hepatic amoebiasis is the commonest manifestation of extra intestinal amoebiasis. Large liver abscesses contain-reddish brown fluid and cellular necrotic tissue.

Amoebiasis is an infection caused by the intestinal protozoan *Entamoeba histolytica*. The infection is spread by cysts which are present in water and uncooked food contaminated by human feces. About 90 percent of infections are asymptomatic.

Amoebic liver abscess is a condition where E. histolytica invades colonic mucosa and carried to liver by portal circulation to form microabscess. Microabscesses confluent to make larger one. Posterior lobe is the commonest site to form abscess.

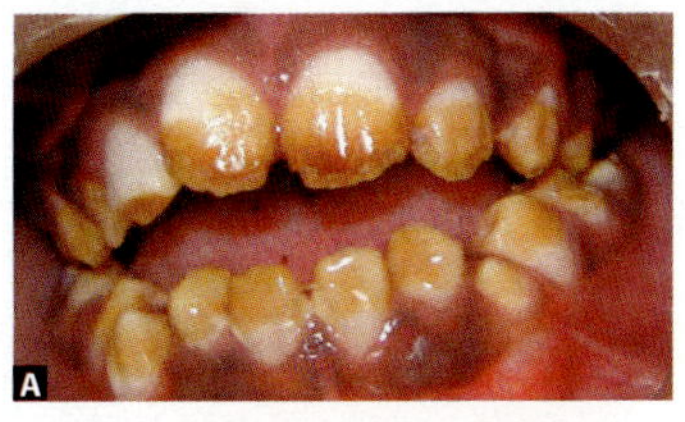

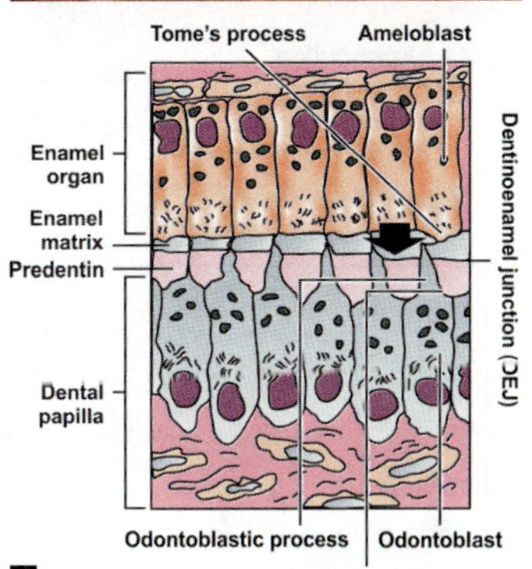

Figs A and B.: *(A) Amelogenesis imperfecta; (B) Ameloblast*

A

There will be abdominal pain, fever, rigor and sweating. In pleural irritation, one will develop intercostals tenderness and cough. As complication, it may rupture into pleural, pericardial sac or into peritoneal cavity. Radiograph will show elevated right dome with restricted mobility. Metronidazole and ampicillin in high doses is effective.

Amoebic lung abscess develops by spread across the diaphragm from liver. It is more common in liver. Prior to rupture of amoebic abscess there is generally a non-suppurative effusion. It is known as sympathetic effusion. Amoebic abscess may show troptozoites of *E. histolytica* along the margins of healthy and necrotic tissue.

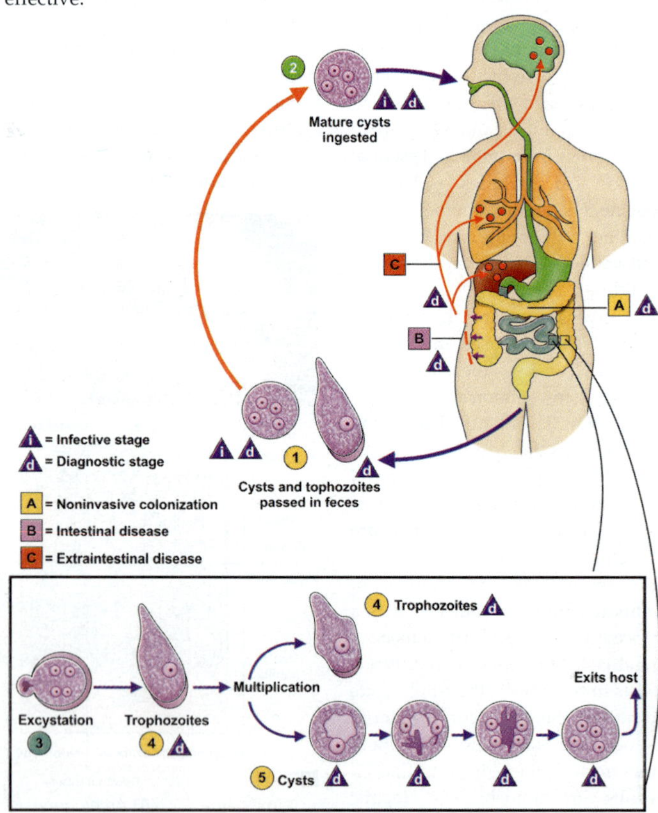

Fig.: *Life-cycle of amoebiasis*

Amorphous is without any long range order of atoms or groups of atoms.

Amperage is the number of electrons that pass through a conductor, the strength of electric current.

Amplitude is defined as the total height of the wave oscillation from the top of the peak to the bottom. A measurement of the amount of energy in the wave: larger the amplitude, greater the amount of energy that can do useful work.

Amylase is an enzyme that converts starch into sugar.

Amyloid spleen follicles appear as small granules gross inspection known as sago spleen. In another variety, follicles are spared and amyloid is deposited in the wall of sinusoid.

Amyloidosis kidney can result in enlargement of kidney. Pathologically, glomeruli are filled with amorphous deposits staining with congo red. Primary amyloidosis results in end-stage renal disease within 2–3 years. Renal transplantation is an option.

Anabolic therapy is use of testosterone or analogs to build lean body mass.

Anacrotic pulse refers slow rising pulse.

Anaerobic bacteria are those bacteria that do not need oxygen to grow; they are generally associated with periodontal disease.

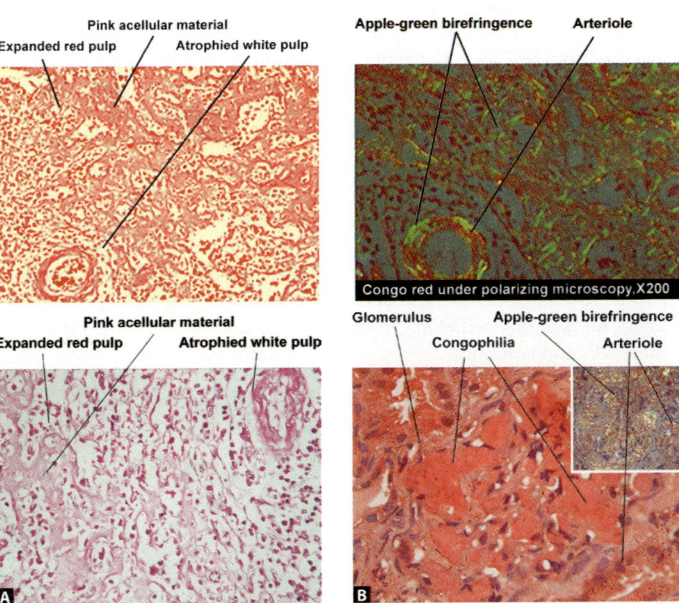

Figs A and B: *(A) Amyloidosis spleen; (B) Amyloidosis kidney*

A

Anaerobic culture is the culture which is carried out in the absence of air.

Analgesia is the absence of sensitivity to pain. It indicates a specific type of spinal cord lesion. It always occurs with loss of temperature. These fibers travel together in spinal cord. It can occur with paresthesia. It can be classified partial or total below the level of lesion. When develops abruptly, it is due to trauma.

Analgesics are drugs used to eliminate or reduce sensation of pain. These drugs are used to alter the central perception of pain. Site of action is cortex. These can be narcotic or narcotics.

Analog image is a radiographic image produced by conventional film.

Analysis of variance Group of statistical tests used to analyze differences between two or more groups based on positioning the sum of squares into that attributable to between group differences and that attributable to within group differences.

Anaphylactoids are non-immunologic release of mediators from mast cells and basophils.

Anaphylaxis is Type I hypersensitivity reaction or an acute, severe, allergic reaction characterized by sudden collapse, shock or respiratory/circulatory failure following an injection of an allergen where there is exaggerated immunologic reaction resulting from the release of vasoactive substances, such as histamine. There is an increased susceptibility to an allergen resulting from previous exposure to it.

Anaplasia is a growth of abnormal cells.

Anatomic apex is "tip or end of root determined morphologically".

Anatomic crown: Entire crown, extending from cusp tip to the cementoenamel (CE) junction.

Anatomic mouth breather is one whose lip morphology does not permit complete closure of mouth, such as patient having short lower lip. Removal of any nasopharyngeal obstruction, rapid maxillary expansion, Vestibular screen may be the treatment of choice.

Anatomic tongue thrust occurs in persons having enlarged tongue, these can have an anterior tongue posture.

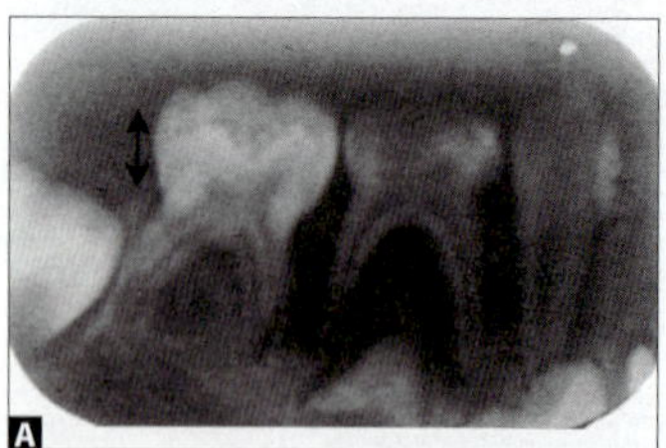

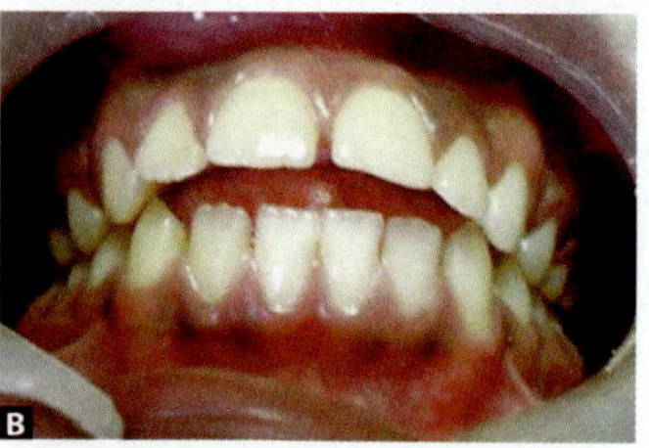

Figs A and B: *(A) Anatomic crown; (B) Mouth breathing and tongue thrust*

Anchor sutures are the type of suture that are used to close the facial and the lingual flaps and adapt them tightly against the tooth. The needle is placed at the line angle area of the facial or lingual flap adjacent to the tooth, anchored around the tooth, passed beneath the opposite flap and tied.

Anergy: Non-responsiveness to antigen T cells may become anergic when exposed to antigen in the absence of activation signal.

Anesthesia is a medication which relieves the sensation of pain.

Anesthesia testing is a procedure to localize pain when patient is not able to specify the site of pain and when other pulp testing techniques are inconclusive, the selective anesthesia may be used. The main objective of this test is to anesthetize a single tooth at a time until the pain is eliminated. It should be accomplished by using intraligamentary injection. Injection is administered to the most posterior tooth in the suspected quadrant. If the pain persists, even after tooth has been fully anesthetized, then repeat the procedure to the next tooth mesial to it. It is continued until. Site of pain is specified.

Aneurysmal bone cyst is a solitary lesion of young adults below 20 years of age. X-ray shows that bone is extended. Lesion is cystic and may show soap bubble appearance. Bone is eccentrically ballooned. It consists of fibrous connective tissue stroma with blood filled spaces. Numerous young fibroblasts are seen. Surgical curettage and excision is treatment of choice.

Aneurysm is a localized dilatation of blood vessel due to weakening, thinning and stretching of wall. In aorta, it is more common. It may be saccular, fusiform, mycotic and dissecting aneurysm.

Angina pectoris: Angina is a Latin word describing a spasmodic, cramp like, choking feeling or suffocating pain, pectoris is Latin for chest. Angina is defined as a characteristic thoracic pain usually substernal, precipitated chiefly by exercise, emotion or a heavy meal; relieved by vasodilator drugs and a few minutes rest and result of a moderate inadequacy of coronary circulation. Angina pectoris is classified into stable angina/classic angina—is usually the result of coronary artery disease. Stable angina is triggered by strenuous activity, emotional stress or cold weather. The 'pain' of stable angina lasts for 1–15 minutes and builds gradually. The pain of stable angina is relieved by rest or administration of nitroglycerin. Variant angina/ Prinzmetal's angina—more likely to occur when patient is at rest than during physical exertion or emotional stress. Coronary artery spasm is the cause of variant angina. Variant angina is more common in women under the age of 50 years. Signs apart from chest pain, syncope, dyspnea and palpitation. Nitroglycerin usually provides prompt relief of pain.

Unstable angina—lies intermediate between stable angina and acute myocardial infarction. Unstable angina is the result of progression of atherosclerosis. Episodes of pain associated with unstable angina may persist for up to 30 minutes. Three characteristics used to define unstable angina, i.e. angina of recent onset, caused by minimal exertion, increasingly severe, prolonged or frequent angina, angina both at rest and with minimal exertion.

Angiedema is an occasional manifestation of hypersensitivity in man. It presents as an intense edema of face, pharynx and larynx. It may cause respiratory obstruction needing tracheostomy. It is due to release of histamine from sensitized mast cells in face and buccal cavity.

Angiedema collections refer to the collection of fluid in the skin, mucous membrane or viscera due to over-production of anaphylatoxin.

Angio-neurotic edema is a non-hereditary form and is due to food allergy. It manifests itself as a smooth diffuse edematous swelling involving face, lips, chin and eyes. There is a feeling of itching or pricky sensation. Skin is of normal color. Hereditary form has visceral involvement and is serious. Edema develops due to vascular swelling.

Angioplasty is a medical procedure in which vessels occluded by arteriosclerosis are opened. This technique was developed in 1977. This is done in patients who don't respond to medical treatment as well as don't require by-pass surgery also.

Angiosarcoma is the malignant vascular neoplasm. These are rapidly proliferative and present as nodular tumors. These can arise from lymph or blood vessel. Oral cavity is the rare site. Even after radical excision they have a poor prognosis.

Angle A is a figure formed by two lines diverging from common.

Angle of facial convexity is formed by the intersection of glabella—subnasale line and subnasale—soft tissue pogonion line. Mean value is 12° and SD is ± 4°. A smaller positive or negative value suggests a class III relationship. A high positive value reflects a class II relationship. The value of this angle, however, does not reveal the localization of the deformity.

Angle of mandible is an area of mandible where body meets the ramus.

Anglo-saxon system, for diagnosing pit and fissure caries, which consist of certain "liberal" criteria was described by Horowitz, HS, in 1972. Description of the system: The pits and fissures on the occlusal, vestibular and lingual surfaces are

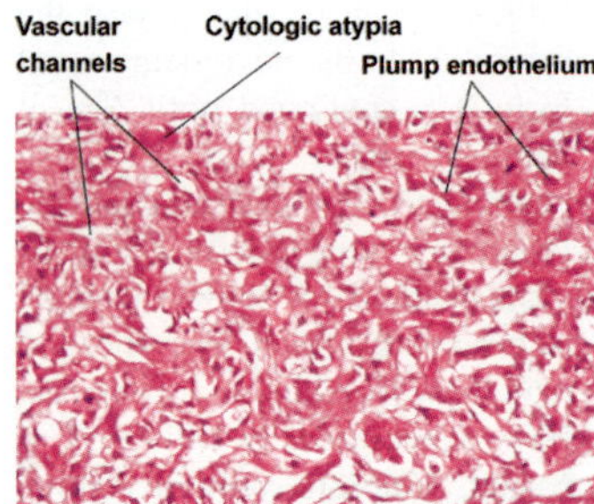

Fig.: *Angiosarcoma*

carious when the explorer "catches" after insertion with moderate to firm pressure and when the "catch" is accompanied by one or more of the following signs of decay: Softness at the base of the area. Opacity adjacent to the area provides evidence of undermining or demineralization. Softened enamel adjacent to the area that may be scraped away by the explorer. *Note:* These areas should be diagnosed as sound when there is apparent evidence of demineralization, but no evidence of softness.

Angular bone loss *see* ***vertical bone loss.***

Angular cheilitis is also known as angular cheliosis. It may be caused by *Candida Albicans*, streptococci or staphylococci. Riboflavin folate and iron deficiency may cause it. General protein deficiency can also result it. Recurrent trauma from dental flossing may also be implicated.

Angular defects *see* vertical defects.

Angulation refers to the angle formed between the blade of the instrument and the tooth surface.

Anhidrosis is an abnormal deficiency of sweat. It can be localized or generalized. Localized anhidrosis being limited to a part rarely affects thermo- regulation. Anhidrosis may develop due to neurological or skin disorders.

Ankyloglossia is the fusion between tongue and floor of mouth. Partial ankyloglossia is known as tongue tie. Restricted movement of tongue results in difficulty in speech. Clipping of the lingual frenum is part of treatment.

Ankylosing spondylitis is a chronic inflammatory disease affecting joints of axial system. Disease starts insidiously in sacroiliac joints with

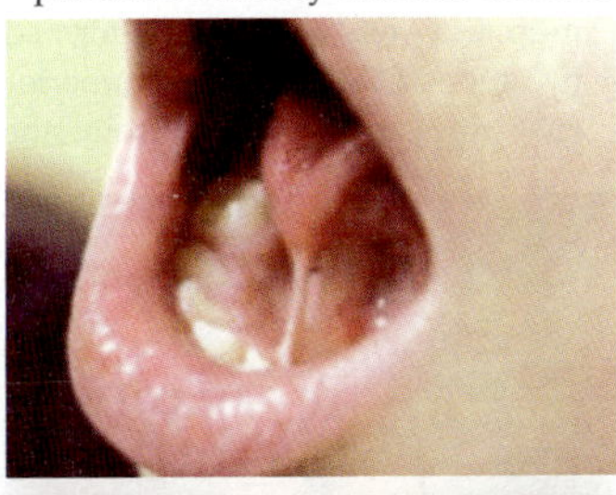

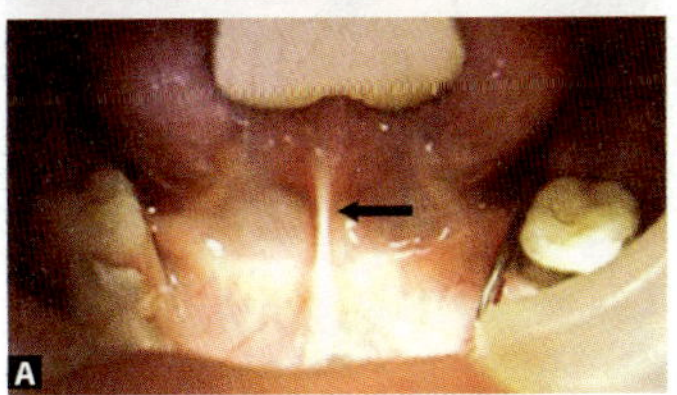

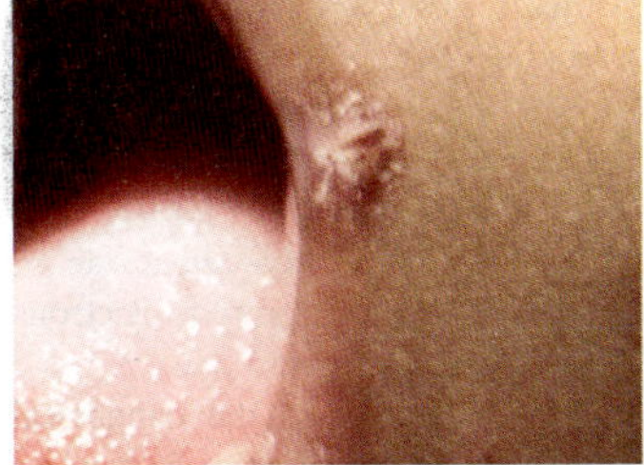

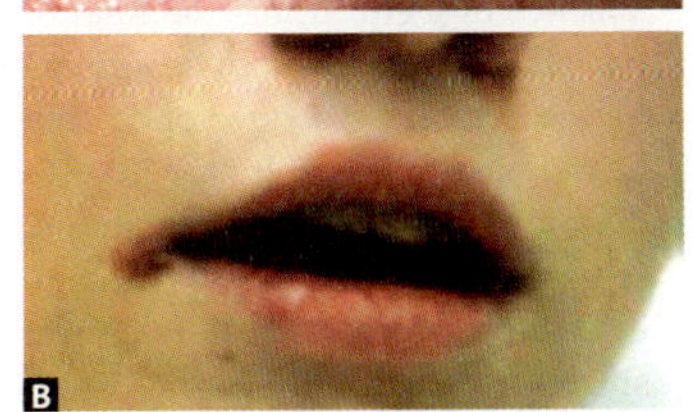

Figs A and B: *(A) Ankyloglossia; (B) Angular cheilitis*

pain and stiffness. There is progressive limitation of back motion. Eventually the entire spine becomes fused. Chest expansion becomes limited. ESR is high. Erosion and sclerosis of sacroiliac joints are first to be noticed. Peripheral joints when involved don't show any demineralization or erosion. Non-steroid anti-inflammatory drugs are used.

Ankylosis is the term given to the fusion between cementum of teeth and the underlying bone. Generally, the deciduous teeth are affected in which bone has fused to cementum and dentin preventing exfoliation of tooth and eruption of underlying permanent tooth. Tooth erupts into oral cavity but does not reach the occlusal plane. In addition, adjacent permanent teeth are taller occlusocervically. Ankylosed tooth sounds solid on percussion.

Annealing ***is a low temperature heat treatment*** for removing residual stress, e.g. heating of a direct gold filling to remove gaseous impurities from the surface.

Anode is the positive electrode in the X-ray tube. It converts electrons into X-ray photons.

Anodontia refers to the congenital absence of teeth. It may be total or partial. This term cannot be applied to teeth that have developed, but have failed to erupt. It may involve dental or permanent dentition. False anodontia develops due to extraction of all teeth. Etiology of single missing tooth is unknown. It may have family history too.

Anomaly is a deviation from the normal or expected outcome.

Anorexia nervosa is an eating disorder or an abnormal psychic condition in which person loses all desire for food and even develops nausea due to self-starvation. Girls think that they are overweight and will do excessive exercise and cut their consumption of food. Patient has low esteem.

Anosmia is a loss of smell and is called anosmia and perverted smell as persomia. Anosmia is due to common cold and nasal energy, unilateral anosmia occurs due to brain tumors. Olfactory hallucination occurs in lesions of uncus, hippocampus and psychosis.

Ansa cervicalis is also called the ansa hypoglossi. It is a nerve loop lying in front of the common carotid artery. Branches arising from the ansa cervicalis innervate sternohyoid, sternothyroid and the omohyoid muscles. Ansa cervicalis is formed by union of two roots. The superior root appears to arise from the

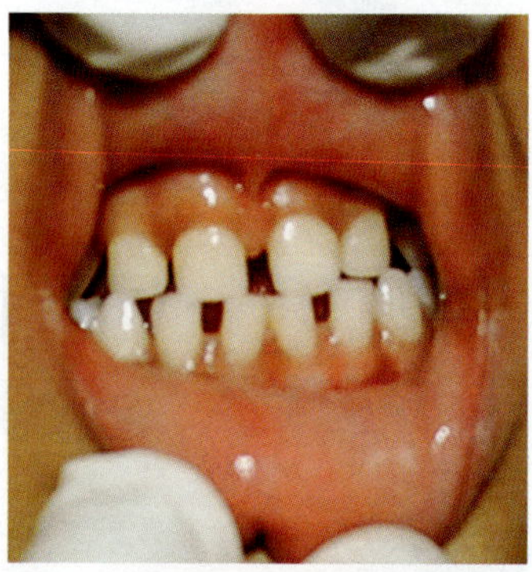

Fig.: *Partial anodontia*

hypoglossal nerve. However, the root is generally made up of fibers derived from the first cervical nerve.

Ansa subclavia is a nerve cord that descends from the middle cervical sympathetic ganglion to the front of the first part of the artery, and looping round it ascends behind it to reach the inferior cervical (cervicothoracic) sympathetic ganglion.

Antagonists are reflected to teeth in opposing arches that usually contact each other in occlusion.

Anterior cerebral artery occlusion: Anterior cerebral artery is a branch of internal carotid and supplies medial surface of frontal and parietal lobes and corpus callosum. Occlusion of it affects motor and sensory cortices representing contralateral leg causing motor weakness and sensory loss.

Anterior situated in front of.

Anterior cord syndrome: In this syndrome, analgesia and thermoanesthesia occur bilaterally below the level of lesion. There is flaccid paralysis.

Anterior cranial base length (Se-N) is the measurement of the anterior cranial base. It can be performed using the center of the superior entrance to the sella tursica as a set point. The correlation of this criterion with the length of the jaw bases enables the assessment of the proportional averages of these bases.

Anterior cranial fossa, is the part of the base of the skull that is the floor, is formed by the (right and left) orbital plates of the frontal bone. The right and left halves of the frontal bone are divided by projection called the frontal crest. Posteriorly, floor of the anterior cranial fossa is formed by the sphenoid bone called the jugum sphenoidale.

Anterior cross bite is a condition characterized by reverse overjet where one or more maxillary anterior teeth are in lingual relation to the mandibular teeth. Anterior cross-bites should be intercepted and treated at an early stage so as to prevent a minor orthodontic problem from progressing into a

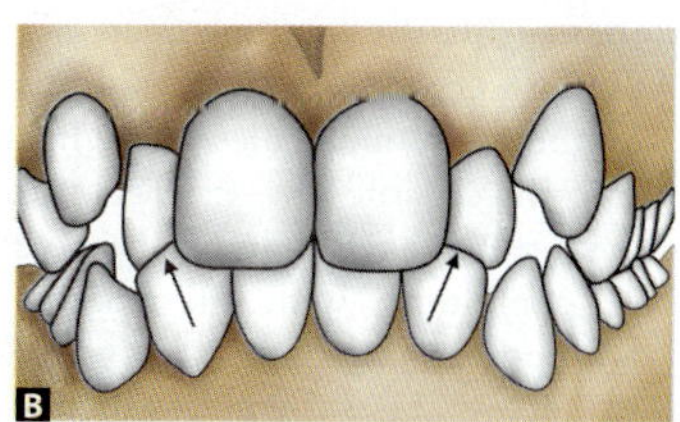

Figs A and B: *(A) Ansa cervicalis; (B) Anterior crossbite*

A

major dentofacial anomaly. An old orthodontic maximum states. "The best time to treat a cross bite is the first time it is seen".

Anterior partial crown: In the earlier days before the use of metal ceramic crowns, when there was no satisfactory facing material, partial crowns were the only alternative to restore individual teeth.

Anterior teeth refer to the front teeth, i.e. incisors and canines.

Anterograde amnesia refers to the loss of memory following the accident.

Anthropometry: Various landmarks established on dry skull are measured viewing individuals by using soft tissue points overlying the bony landmarks.

Anti-embolic stockings: Elastic stockings.

Antisialalogue is a drug or substance that prevents salivation.

Antibiotics are the drugs or substances that are produced by or derived from bacteria that may either kill the microorganism (bactericidal) or may retard their growth (bacteriostatic) so that the body's own immune system can overcome the infection.

Antigen is any foreign substance that elicits an immune response (e.g. the production of specific antibody molecules) when introduced into the tissues of a susceptible animal and is capable of combining with the specific antibodies formed.

Antimicrobial is a chemotherapeutic agent that works by destroying or reducing the number of bacteria present.

Antiseptic is a chemical disinfectant that can be diluted sufficiently to be safe for application to living tissues like intact skin, mucous membranes and wounds. These inhibit the growth and multiplication of bacteria. Generally, it does not kill bacteria but does not stops their growth.

Antitoxin is a specific type of antibody produced by body in response to a toxin.

Antivitamins are substances known as vitamin antagonists, which block the synthesis or metabolism of vitamins. Drug methotrexate is antagonist of folic acid; antibiotics interfere with vitamin K synthesis. These are known to be present in natural foods, e.g. thiaminase in raw fish. Some synthetic antagonists of vitamins are used as drugs in the therapy of neoplasm, e.g. methotrexate infections e.g. pyrimethamine. Neoplastic cells and micro-organisms are much more sensitive than normal cells, but high doses of antivitamins may led to a conditioned vitamin deficiency.

Anxiety disorder is a clinical condition. Patient shows excessive anxiety and worry about a number of events and activities for at least 6 months. Symptoms include restlessness, fatigability, difficulty with concentration, irritability and sleep disturbances. Person may develop hypertension.

Anxiety tremors: Tremor is fine and rapid. It is seen in thyrotoxicosis.

Anxiolytics: Substances or drugs reducing anxiety.

Aortic dissection: There is an entrance of blood into aortic media. Underlying conditions associated include, hypertension and atherosclerosis. Person will develop severe abrupt pain. Pain is sharp and tearing. Systolic BP is higher than 150 mm Hg. One may hear aortic insufficiency murmur and pulse deficit is increased.

Aortic regurgitation is a cerdiac manifestation that is ruled out during ECHO. It is usually asymptomatic until middle age persists with left side failure or chest pain. There will be wide pulse pressure with left side failure or chest pain. There will be wide pulse pressure with associated peripheral signs. There will be hyperactive enlarged pulse pressure, hyperactive enlarged left ventricle. Diastolic murmur along left sternal border will be heard. ECG shows left ventricular hypertrophy.

Aortic stenosis: There will be delayed and diminished carotid pulses with soft, absent or paradoxically split S2. Harash systolic murmur with thrill along left sterna border often radiating to neck is heard. ECG shows left ventricular hypertrophy. Angina pectoris frequently occurs.

Apathy is an absence or suppression of interest in the external environment and personal affair. It may be caused by alcohol, drug abuse, neurological or psychological disorder.

Apex the pointed extremity of a structure.

Apexification is a root induction procedure of a non-vital tooth where a medicament is applied within a root canal which allows a calcified barrier to form across the open apex.

Apexogenesis is a root induction procedure in a vital tooth where the normal development of the apex of a root is expected by placing a medicament within the pulp chamber of tooth. Treatment of a vital pulp by pulp capping or pulpotomy.

Apexum is a procedure used for enucleation of periapical tissue by minimally invasive technique through root canal access, thereby enhancing the healing kinetics of periapical lesions. For apexum procedure, after completing biomechanical preparation, apical foramen is enlarged with No. 35 rotary file about 1 to 2 mm periapically. This is done for insertion of apexum device which is a nickel-titanium wire into periapical area. This device rotates and minces the tissue. After this a biodegradable fiber is rotated at

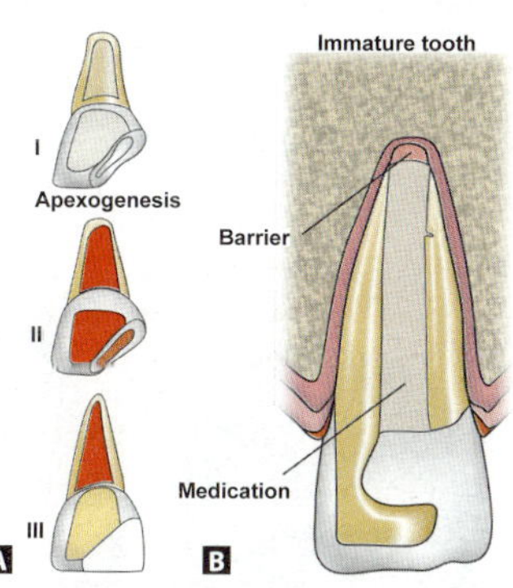

Figs A and B: *(A) Apexogenesis; (B) Apexification*

A

high speed so as to make this tissue into thin suspension. This can be later removed with normal saline irrigation.

Aphasia is a defect of language function secondary to brain damage.

Aphrodisiac is a substance that stimulates the sexual desire and activity but claims have not been proved scientifically.

Aphthous stomatitis is an idiopathic, non-infectious inflammatory disease. Ulcers develop recurrently on non-keratinized oral mucosa. There are three types of ulcers: Minor aphthous stomatitis produces small ulcers which heal within 10 days. Major aphthous ulcers produce larger ulcers and takes longer time to heal. It heals by scarring and at least one ulcer is always present. Herpetiform aphthae present multiple painful ulcers of 1 to 20 cm affecting non-keratinized area. Ulcers are superficial with an erythematous halo. These are non-indurated and painful. Reiter's syndrome is an immune mediated disease. It produces lesions like oral aphthous ulcers, polyarthritis, urethritis, and conjunctivitis.

Apical constriction is apical portion of root canal having narrowest diameter. It is usually 0.5 to 1 mm short of apical foramen. The minor diameter widens apically to foramen, i.e. major diameter.

Apical curettage is the surgical removal of infectious material surrounding the apex of a tooth root.

Apical fibers are the periodontal fibers that radiate in the apical portion from the cementum to the bone and keep the tooth intact within the socket.

Apical foramen is an aperture at or near the apex of a root through which nerves and blood vessels of the pulp enter or leave the pulp cavity. Normally, it is present near the apex but, sometimes, opening may be present on the accessory and lateral canals of root surface forming the accessory foramina.

Apical heart rate refers to the number of ventricular contractions per minute.

Apical periodontal cyst is a true cyst because cavity is lined by epithelium. It is asymptomatic. Tooth is rarely painful or even sensitive to percussion. Apical periodontal cyst

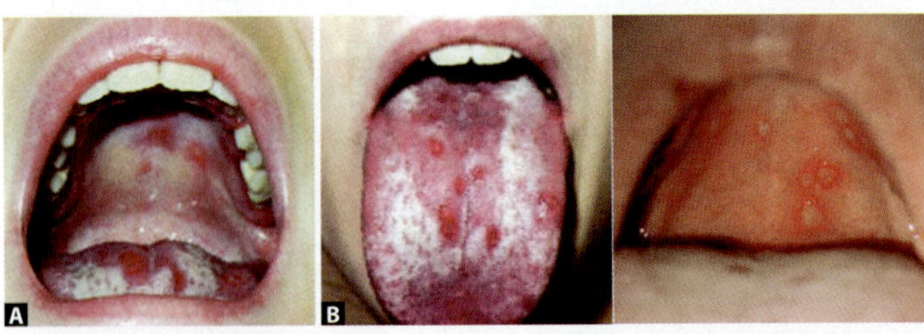

Figs A and B: *(A) Stomatitis affecting palate; (B) Stomatitis affecting tongue*

is a lesion due to chronic inflammatory process. On X-ray, cyst may be of greater size, occasionally apical periodontal cyst exhibits a thin radiopaque line around radiolucent area.

Apicectomy (Apicoectomy) is a surgical procedure done to remove the apical portion of tooth. Main purpose is to save the tooth where root filling is not feasible. It is the final alternative to extraction.

Aplasia of mandibular condyle is the abnormality associated with other abnormalities also. If it is one sided, facial abnormality is seen. Shift of mandible towards affected side occurs during opening. In bilateral cases shift is not there. Osteoplasty is the treatment.

Aplasia of salivary glands refers to any one of the glands that may be missing. Cause is not known. It may result in dry mouth. Oral mucosa looks dry and pebbly. Cracking of lips and fissuring of corners of mouth is seen. Food debris may accumulate around tooth. There is no particular treatment.

Aplastic anemia is a dramatic decrease in all circulating blood cells because of depression of bone marrow activity. Primary is congenital, while secondary may be due to ionizing radiation, benzene, cyclophosphamide and viral hepatitis. Higher doses of chemotheraphy destroy stem cells which are not recovered. Lymphadenopathy is not seen. Platelet count falls gradually. Skin rashes, nose bleed and gum bleeding are common.

Apocrine sweat glands are associated with hair follicles and are found in axillary and genital areas. These respond to emotions and become active when person is frightened, upset in pain or is sexually excited. It does not have a strong odor.

Apparent density is a mass of sample divided by volume it occupies.

Appendicitis *lies* one inch below the ileocecal valve. All the taeniae of colon converge at the base of appendix. As appendicitis progresses the organs swell up due to accumulated pus within the lumen. It leads to compromise in blood supply, gangrene and perforation.

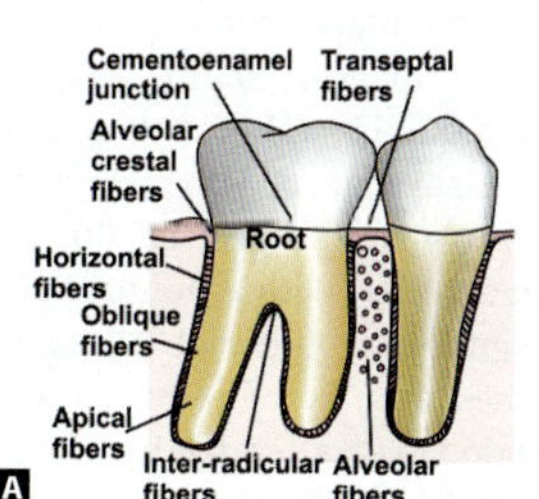

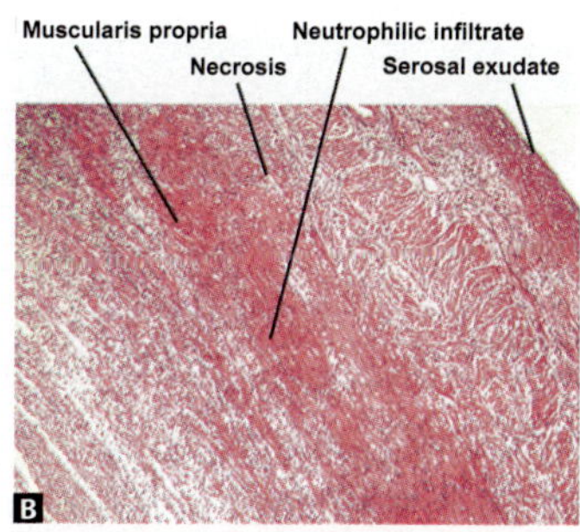

Figs A and B: *(A) Apical fibers; (B) Acute appendicitis;*

A

Appendicular skeleton is a part of skeleton that includes the bones of upper extremities, the lower extremities, the pelvic girdle and the pectoral girdle.

Appetite center is a cluster of neurons in the lateral hypothalamus whose impulses cause an increase in appetite.

Apposition is the laying down of.

Apraxia is an inability to carry out an organized voluntary movement despite the fact that motor and sensory pathways are normally intact. There is no paralysis. It is due to loss of acquired motor skills.

Aqueous humor is a watery fluid that fills the anterior chamber of the eye in front of lens.

Arch a curvature: both the maxillary and mandibular ridge form a horseshoe-shaped arch.

Arch bars are the prefabricated form of metal bars which are used for mandibular fixation particularly when the patient has an insufficient numbers of suitably shaped teeth to enable other effective wiring to be carried out. After reduction, the teeth on the main fragments are tied together to a metal bar which has been bent to conform to dental arch.

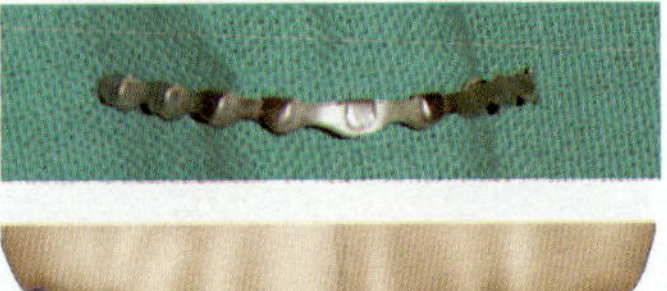

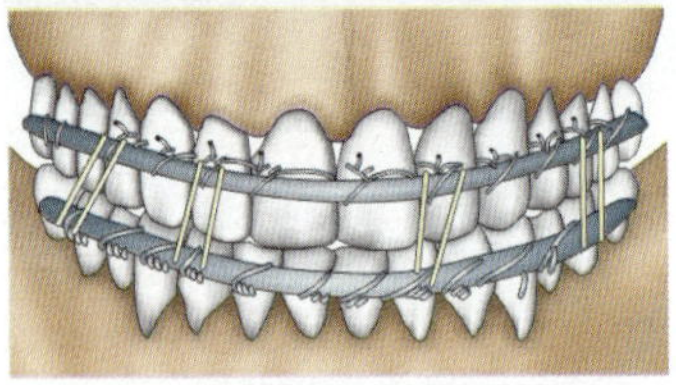

Fig.: *Arch bars*

Argon lasers have an active medium of argon gas that is fiber optically delivered in continuous—wave and gated—pulse modes. Two emission wavelengths, and both are visible to the human eye 488 nm (blue in color) and 514 nm (blue—green). Both wavelengths are not well-absorbed in dental hard tissues and are poorly absorbed in water. It can be used as an aid in caries detection. The diseased, carious area appears as dark orange-red color and is easily discernible from the healthy structures.

Ariboflavinosis is a deficiency of vitamin B_2 showing swollen, cracked, bright red lips, enlarged tender magenta red tongue, cracking at the corners of mouth and congested conjunctiva.

Armamentarium includes equipment, books, materials and instruments essential to professional practice.

Arsenic is colorless, tasteless and odorless. Small quantity is required to kill a man, i.e. 0.2 g. A pinch of white arsenic about 20 g. Fatal period is 12–48 hours. It is tasteless so easily mixed with sweats. It has cumulative properties. But it can be detected with absolute certainty from each of burial place, burnt ashes and hair/teeth for a long period even after death.

Arterial hemorrhage: Woundly bleed profusely and lost blood is bright red in color and blood comes out in jet. The rise and fall of which synchronize with the pulse of the patient.

Arterio-venous malformations deve-lop due to a mesh of abnormally thin vessels. Larger ones are seen in posterior half of hemispheres forming a wedge-like lesion. Bleeding of AVM is principally intraparenchymal. Patient may develop seizure, focal neurological deficits, impaired higher functions and headache. X-ray skull will show calcification in AVM while MRI will show pattern of blood flow in lesion and will spot the thrombus too.

Arthralgia refers to pain in a joint without swelling or other sign of arthritis.

Articular angle (S-Ar-Go) is a constructed angle between the upper and lower parts of the posterior contours of the facial skeleton. Its size depends on the position of the mandible, it is larger if the mandible is retrognathic but small if the mandible is prognathic. It decreases with anterior positioning of the mandible, closing of the bite, and mesial migration of the posterior segment teeth and increases with posterior relocation of the mandible, opening of the bite and distal driving of the posterior teeth.

Articular cartilage is a layer of hyaline covering the joint surface of epiphysis.

Articular prominence is a rounded projection of temporal bone located anterior to glenoid process.

Articulate to come together.

Articulating head rest can be moved in multiple directions.

Articulating paper refers to carbon paper; placed between the upper and lower teeth to mark contact.

Articulation refers to the point where two or more adjacent bones create a joint.

Articulator is a mechanical device used to replicate functional movements of the jaw to casts.

Artifacts are physical evidence within a qualitative research design which contributes to the understanding of research question.

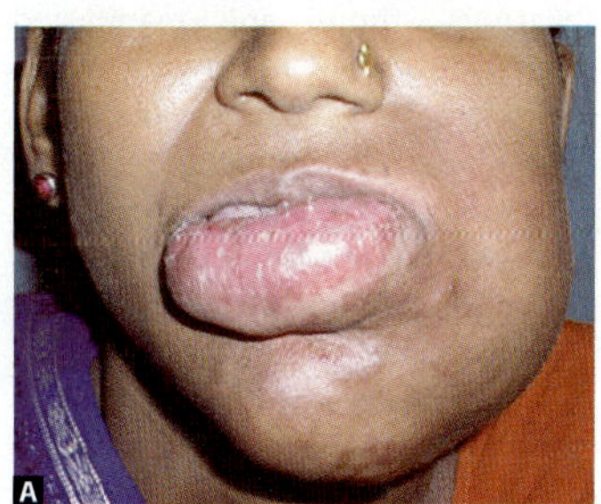

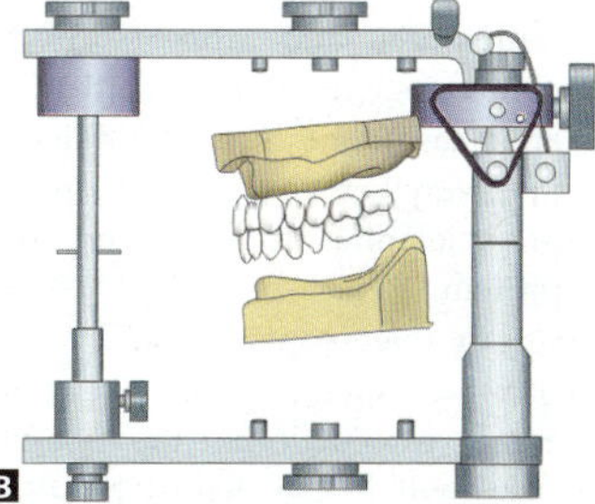

Figs A and B: *(A) Arterio-venous malformation; (B) Articulator*

A

Artificial insemination is an artificial introduction of semen into vagina, cervix or uterus. Artificial insemination homologous is the process in which husband's semen is used. In artificial insemination donor—semen of donor other than husband is used while in pooled donor, semen of husband is added.

Aryl acetic acid is a drug whose pharmacological effects are similar to other NSAIDS, i.e. inhibition of synthesis of prostaglandins. Its potency is greater than indomethacin. It is rapidly absorbed. It is better for joint fluid, is 8 times to that of plasma concentration.

Aseptic meningitis refers to non-infective inflammation of the meanings of brain that is common and is not generally fatal in children. It is caused by one of the enteroviruses like poliovirus. Other common cause is virus infection. CSF shows lymphocytosis.

Aseptic technique refers to measures taken to reduce or eliminate micro-organisms.

Aspartame is better known as nutrasweet and appears to be non-cariogenic. It is devoid of an after taste but is contraindicated in phenylketonuria as it contains phenylalanine. It is derived from protein.

Aspirate refers to withdraw.

Aspirator refers to an apparatus employing suction or the tube-like straw which the dentist places in your mouth for suction.

Assistant's stool is the chair used by assistant to provide dental treatment to the patient.

Assistant's zone is the part of work circle where the dental assistant is positioned during the delivery of dental treatment. Best position is 2 to 4 o'clock position.

Asthma is a disease of the airways in which there is a chronic inflammation and increased responsiveness to a wide variety of stimuli, leading to reversible airway obstruction. Patients generally have paroxysms of cough, wheeze and dyspnea, interspersed with symptom free periods. Severe life-threatening attack of asthma was previously known as status asthmaticus. The patient may additionally have tachycardia, pulsus paradoxus, cyanosis and active accessory respiratory muscles. The air entry is drastically reduced (silent chest on auscultation). The patient may become confused or drowsy. It is characterized by an increased responsiveness of the trachea and bronchi to various stimuli and manifested by wide spread narrowing of the airways that changes in either spontaneously or as a result of therapy. Acute asthmatic episodes are usually self-limiting, however, clinical entity termed "status asthmaticus" characterized by a persistent exacerbation of asthma. Individuals who suffer from status asthmaticus experience wheezing, dyspnea, hypoxia and other symptoms that are refractory to two or three doses of adrenergic agents. Asthma can be manifested if there is a coughing spell, with or without sputum production and wheezing. Breathing during an asthmatic attack is labored. Blood pressure may rise in acute episode attacks, also heart rate increases—rate of more than 120 beats/minute. If left untreated, acute asthmatic episode may last minutes or hours. Termination of attack is usually heralded by a period of intense coughing with expectoration of a thick, tenacious mucus plug. This is followed immediately by a sensation of relief and a clearing of the air passages.

Asymmetric tonic neck reflex: When the body is at rest and not crying, the patient keeps his head on one side, the arms and the legs on the same side extend, while the opposite limbs go into flexion. The reflex is prominent between 2nd and 4th month. Persistence of the reflex beyond the age of 6 to 9 months or a constant neck posture is abnormal and usually indicates spastic cerebral palsy or poor control over the motor functions.

Asymmetry refers to the discrepancy in the two sides of the body.

Asynergy is an impaired coordination of muscles or organs that normally function harmoniously. It may develop due to disorder of basal ganglion and cerebellum.

Ataxic is a forming cerebral palsy where the movement, balance and posture are involved, often fine motor skills such as hand writing and eye movements are affected.

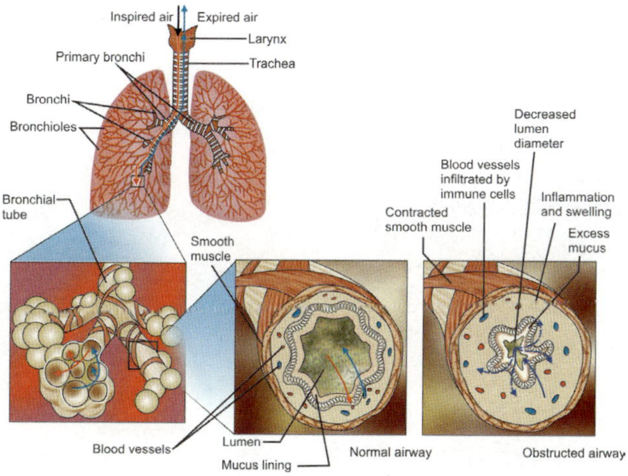

Fig.: *Pathophysiology of Asthma*

A

Atherogenesis is the formation of atherosclerotic lesion on the walls of arteries.

Atherosclerosis is a generalized and slowly progressive disorder of aorta and large and medium sized muscular arteries. It is the main cause of arteriosclerosis. Lesion develops slowly over years. Atherosclerosis is known to undergo ulceration, hemorrhage, calcification and thrombosis. Hypertension acceleration atherosclerosis in turn increases the risk of ischemic heart disease.

Athetoid includes involuntary movement such as arm, legs and hand.

Athetosis is a slow, purposeless writhing movement of limbs, face or tongue. These movements increase when patient carries out voluntary movements. Posthemiplegic athetosis is unilateral. Some amount of rigidity brings slowness. Discrete individual movements of lips, tongue and hand are abnormal.

Athletes' foot is a fungal infection characterized by vesicles, fissures, ulcers and itching. It commonly affects toes.

Atlanto-axial joints refer to joint that forms from the articulation between the atlas and axis vertebrae. They articulate with each other at three joints, one median, and two that are lateral. There are two types of atlanto-axial joint, i.e. median atlanto-axial joint is a synovial joint of the pivot variety and lateral atlanto-axial joints are synovial joints of the plane variety.

Atlas vertebra is the first cervical vertebra and is called the atlas. It has a different look from cervical vertebra. It has no body, and no spine. Anteriorly, it is joined by a short anterior arch; and, posteriorly, by a longer posterior arch. The vertebral bodies are small in the cervical vertebrae. In shape, the body is oval.

Atomic weight is the total number of protons and neutrons in nucleus of an atom.

Atonic seizures or drop attacks manifest as a sudden loss of muscle strength. As a result, the

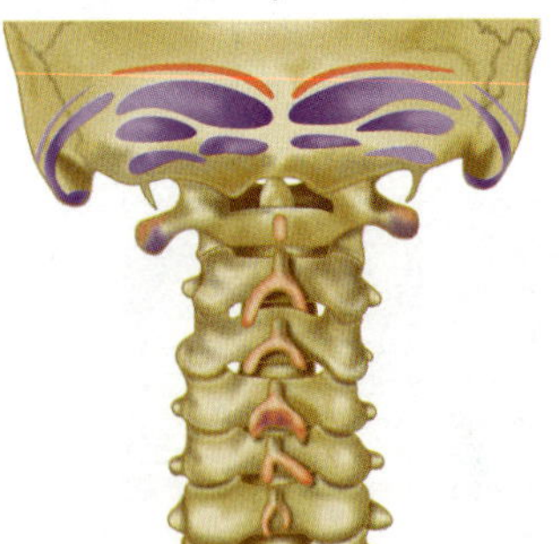

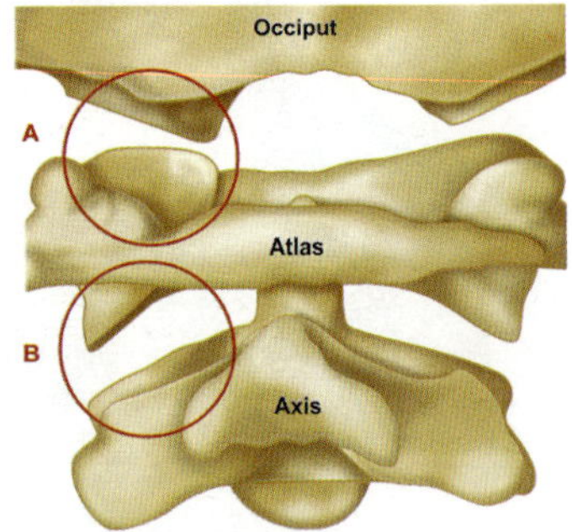

Fig.: *Atlanto-axial joint and Atlas vertebra*

person collapses to the ground. Such seizures are associated with an increased risk of head or jaw injury. Generally, these seizures begin in childhood and typically last less than five seconds. They are associated with change of consciousness. Usually, there are no postictal symptoms. Atonic seizures are a defining feature of symptomatic generalized epilepsies.

Atopic dermatitis is a chronic, itching superficial inflammation of skin. There may be family history too. Exact cause is unknown. Patients have high serum levels of IgE antibodies; child may develop red, weeping, crusted lesions on the face, scalp and extremities. Itching is a constant feature. Later dermatitis may become generalized. Secondary bacterial infections and regional lymphadenitis are common. Diagnosis is entirely clinical.

Atresia refers to closure or absence of a usual opening.

Atrial fibrillation can be manifested as an irregularity in ventricular beats created by inconsistent impulses through AV node transmitted to the ventricles at irregular intervals.

Atrial septal defects are small and moderate defects that may be asymptomatic. With large shunts exertional dyspnea or cardiac failure may develop. Right ventricular and pulmonary artery pulsations are palpable and visible. S2 is widely split.

Atropine is named after one of leading fates called 'atropos'. It is well-absorbed from body surface. It reduces all secretions except milk. Smooth muscles are relaxed. Its side effects include dry mouth, tachycardia, urinary retention and constipation.

Attached gingiva is the part of gingiva which is in continuation with the marginal gingiva. It is firm and resilient and tightly bound to the underlying periosteum of the alveolar bone. In children, it appears less dense and redder than in adults due to less keratinized epithelium with its greater vascularity. The attached

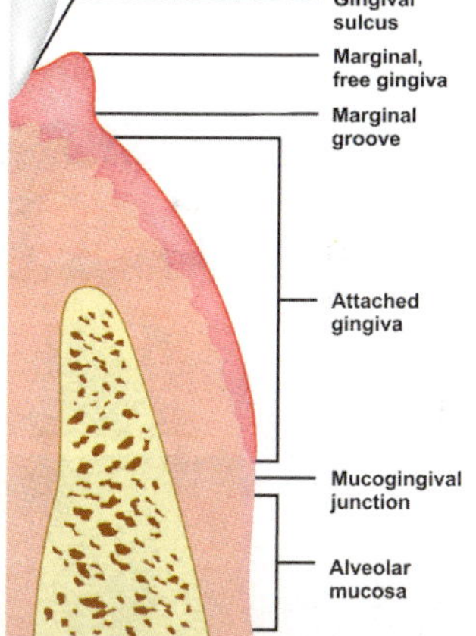

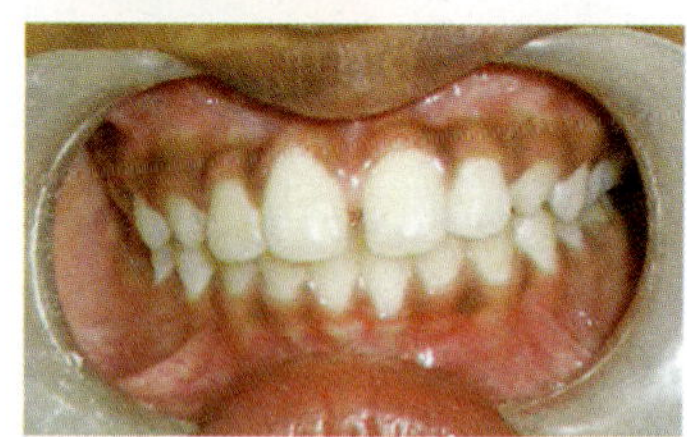

Fig.: *Attached gingiva*

A

gingiva is more blacked because of lesser connective tissue density and its texture is less stippled. The two unique characteristics of the attached gingiva in children are the interdental clefts and the retrocuspid papilla. The interdental clefts are normal anatomic feature found in the interradicular zones underlying the saddle areas. The retrocuspid papilla is found approximately 1 mm below the free gingival groove on the attached gingival lingual to the mandibular canine. It occurs in 85% of children and apparently decreases with age.

Attached subgingival plaque is a bacterial plaque located below the gingival margin that is attached to tooth.

Attenuated live vaccine refers to live vaccine containing organism of reduced virulence due to culturing under unfavorable conditions.

Attrition is a physiological or mechanical wearing down of a tooth due to contact of another tooth as during mastication in old age. There develops flattening of an incisal edge. There is slight mobility of teeth in their sockets. Man shows severe attrition than woman.

Atypical facial neuralgia is a dull, aching and throbbing pain due to vascular component. It is accompanied by muscle pain. Pain is diffusely located even though

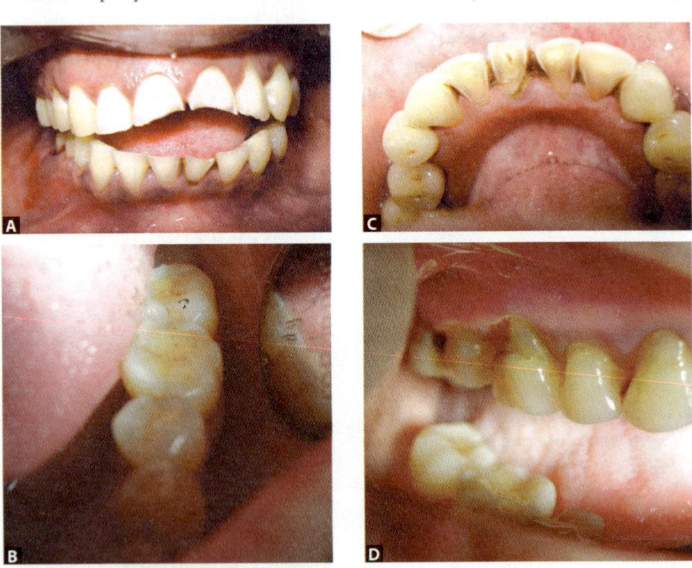

Figs A to D: *(A) Attrition; (B) Attrition and abrasion; (C) Severe attrition; (D) Attrition on posterior teeth*

persistent and variable. Quality of being acute, sudden, intense exacerbations gives it a neuralgic quality.

Atypical facial pain occurs usually in middle aged depressed females. It is a constant pain often burning type which is centered on the maxilla, but may spread to the rest of the face on the affected side. Sometimes it may involve other side of the face, neck or back of the head. Tricyclic antidepressant, analgesics, carbamazepine or phenytoin may be tried. The response to therapy is poor.

Atypical odontalgia is a persistent pain in tooth with no abnormality found in tooth on any type of examination. Odontalgia word comes from Greek word odont means tooth and algo means pain. Cavity and exposure of nerve causes pain. But tooth pain which occurs when there is no dental disease is called atypical odontalgia. It generally occurs after root canal treatment or tooth extraction.

Atypical orofacial pain is a condition where patient is not able to locate and identify the quality of pain. Emotional breakdown, tears and hysteria are not uncommon. On account of pain, person does not leave work place. Referred pain also may be poorly localized and pain of vascular origin in head becomes difficult to separate from atypical facial pain. Atypical facial pain is not associated with trigger zones.

Augmentation material: The three primary augmentation materials in dentistry are intramucosal, endodontic and bone substitute materials. Material should be easy to fabricate, biocompatible, sterilize and shape intraoperatively.

Auricle refers to the portion of external ear which looks like ear.

Auricular lymph nodes refer to the lymph nodes associated with ear. These can be palpated bilaterally in front and behind of ears.

Auriculotemporal nerve arises by two roots that form a ring through which the middle meningeal artery passes upwards. The nerve runs backwards deep in the infratemporal fossa; and crosses deep to the neck of the mandible. It then turns laterally behind the temporomandibular joint. In this part of its course it is closely related to the upper part, of the parotid gland.

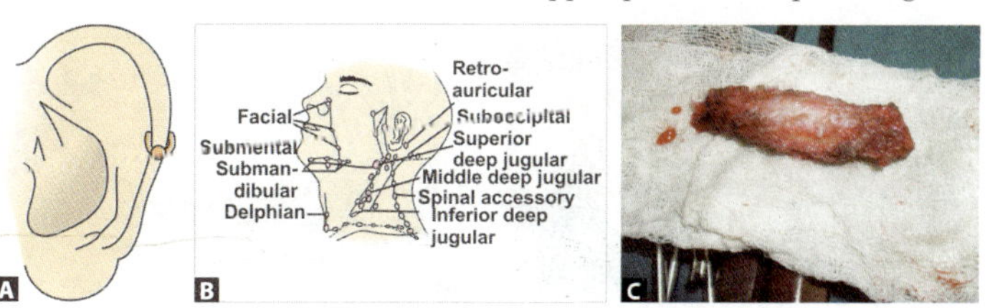

Figs A to C: *(A) Auricle; (B) Auricular lymph nodes; (C) Autograft*

The nerve finally turns upwards into the scalp and ends by dividing into branches that supply the skin over the temple.

Autograft is the graft taken from patient's own skin which is best used to cover the wounds. The best donor site is the patient's thighs or upper arm. But in case of extensive burns, these areas can be reused to obtain grafts again after 2 weeks because usually thin grafts are taken. In case the area is extensive, scalp is a good donor site because it can be reused many times as a donor area.

Autoimmune disease is a disease that is characterized by tissue injury caused by a cell mediated immune response against constituents of body's own tissues.

Autoimmunity is a protection against mechnism by pathogenic immune reactions against self antigens.

Autotransformer is a voltage compensator that corrects for minor fluctuations in current flowing throughout the X-ray machine.

Autoclave is a sterilization machine that provides the most efficient and reliable method of sterilization for all dental instruments. It involves heating water to generate steam in a closed chamber resulting in moist heat that rapidly kills micro-organisms.

Autogenous refers to self-generated, self propagated. It originates within an organism.

Automatic processing is the method used to process films in which all film processing steps are automated.

Autonomic nervous system is a part of nervous system that controls involuntary body functions, such as salivation, sweat and heart beat.

Autonomic seizures are the types of epileptic seizures that cause changes in the autonomic nervous system. This may manifest as a change in the heart and breathing rates, cause sweating, or an unpleasant sensation in the abdomen, chest, or head.

Autopsy postmortem examination.

Autotransplant refers to the procedure where the transfer of a tissue or organ to some other part in same person is performed.

Avascular refers to the absence of blood supply.

Avidin is a protein present in white of an egg which combines with vitamin H and makes it available to the body. It is inactivated in cooked eggs.

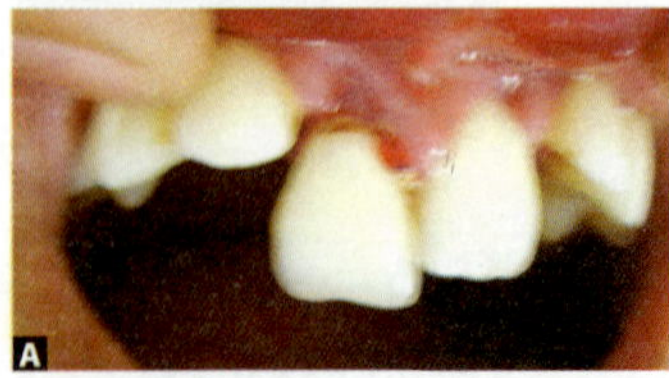

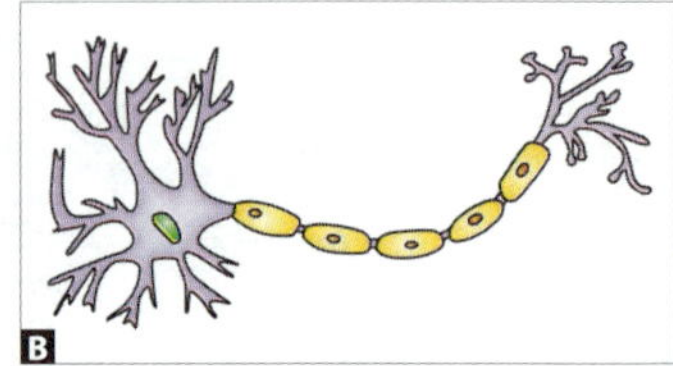

Figs A and B: *(A) Avulsion; (B) Axon*

Avitaminosis means without vitamins.

Avulsion is the tearing away of a tendon or ligament attachment from bone.

Axial wall is the vertical axis of a tooth.

Axis vertebra is the second cervical vertebra having thick finger-like projection arising from the upper part of the body.

Axial is opposite of appendicular. It is pertaining to the central portion of the body.

Axon the process that carries impulses away from the cell body of a nerve.

B

Babinski's reflex refers to the stroking of the lateral surfaces of the planter surface of the foot from the head to the toe that results in flexion of the toe.

Backache refers to the pain occurring in the back due to any reason. Malignant tumors will have night rest pain. Mechanical pain is worse with activity. There will be weight loss, malaise and loss of appetite.

Backward decay or caries refers to that kind of carious progress where caries process in dentin progresses much further than it does in enamel, i.e. when the spread of caries along the DEJ exceeds the caries in the contagious enamel, from the junction and is termed as backward caries.

Bacteremia refers to presence of bacteria in blood stream.

Bacterial infections are classified as plants but without chlorophyll. These can cause dental decay, periodontal disease, TB, typhoid, tetanus, diphtheria, etc. In presence of unfavorable conditions these develop a protective mucoid coating which helps them to survive. And in favorable condition these become virulent again. Killing of spores is difficult.

Bacterial plaque is a dense, organized matrix of microorganism that forms on the teeth, gingiva and restorations. It is a cause of poor oral hygiene, dental caries and periodontal diseases. In a recently cleaned mouth, it contains leukocytes, epithelial cells and a few Gram-positive cocci, 2–14 days old plaque will contain leukocytes, rods, Gram negative bacteria white cells and Gram-positive cocci.

Bacterial sialadenitis refers to infective inflammation salivary glands. There will be unilateral/bilateral swelling of parotid gland. Swelling

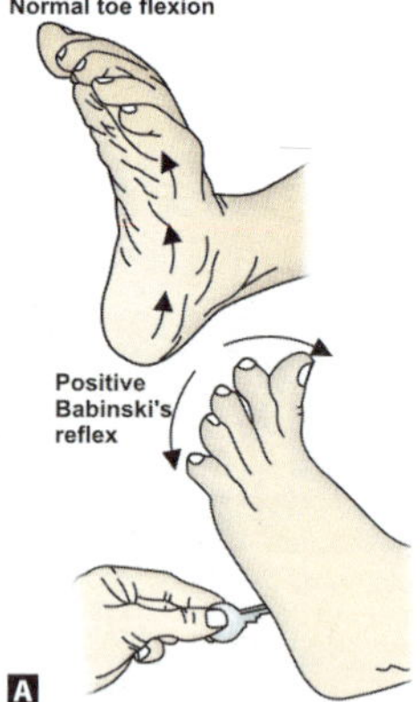

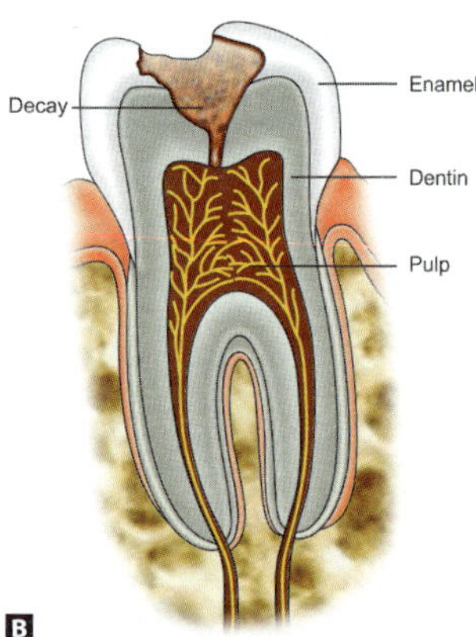

Figs A and B: *(A) Babinski's reflex; (B) Backward decay*

may involve pre-and post-auricular areas. Trismus results from pain and swelling. Occasionally, fever, chill and leucocytosis may be seen. In chronic infection, recurrent bouts of acute exacerbation may be seen. Antibiotic helps.

Bacterial spore is a resistant form of bacteria encapsulated by a thick wall which enables the cell to survive in unfavorable environment of growth.

Bactericide is an agent that is capable of destroying bacteria.

Bacteriocins are proteins produced by certain bacteria that can kill other bacteria.

Bacteriophage is a virus that infects a bacterium also known simply as a growth of bacteria.

Bacterium is a microorganism capable of causing disease, a primitive single-celled organism without membranous organelles.

Baking powder is a mixture which liberates CO_2 when moistened/heated. Sodium bicarbonate is the source of CO_2 and an acidic substance is required such as tartaric acid. Quick acting powders contain tartrate and liberate CO_2.

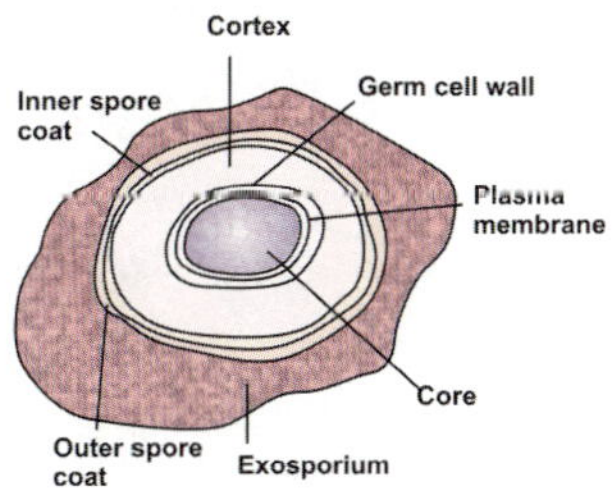

Fig.: *Bacterial spore*

Balanced diet is defined as a diet which provides adequate amount of energy, amino acids, carbohydrates, fats, vitamins and minerals to maintain health and general well-being. The diet should also provide extra amount of nutrients to meet the demands during shortage.

Balanced force technique involves oscillation of instrument right and left with different arcs in either direction. Instrument is first inserted into the canal by moving it clockwise with one quarter turn. Then to cut dentin, file is rotated counter-clockwise, simultaneously pushing apically to prevent it from backing out of the canal. Finally, the file is removed by rotating file clockwise, simultaneously pulling the instrument out of the canal. It involves the use of instrument with noncutting tip. Since the K-type files have pyramidal tips with cutting angles which can be quite aggressive with clockwise rotation. For this technique, use of triangular cross-sectioned instruments should be done. The decreased mass of the instrument and deeper cutting flutes improve the flexibility of instrument and decrease the restoring force of the instrument when placed in curved canals.

Ball scaler number b2–b3 is a popular heavy sickle with wider and heavier blades used for removing granulation tissue, fibrous interdental tissue and tenacious subgingival deposits.

Bar over denture is a male portion of appliance that provides stability and is attached to another tooth in the same dental arch.

Barbed broaches are disposable hand instruments for removing the pulp. It is made of fine wire with multiple barbs. When broach is inserted in a root canal and rotated, it engages the pulp which can be taken out with broach. After use, these are thrown out.

Barbiturates are drugs that depress all areas of CNS but reticular activating system is most sensitive, its depression is primarily responsible for inability to maintain wakefulness. Barbiturates do not have selective antianxiety action. They can impair learning, short-term memory and judgment. These drugs are widely used in treatment of mild anxiety. These produce sedation and drowsiness and less of concentration.

Barbiturates-antidotes best antidotes are bemegride or megemide and daptzol. They are given with IV 5% glucose drip in a dose of 15 mg of daptozol and 50 mg of bemegride every 5 minutes until pharyngeal and laryngeal reflexes return.

Barlow's sign: An indicator of congenital dislocation of hip detected during first 6 weeks of life.

Baroreceptor reflex is a nervous reflex which senses sudden change in blood pressure and then stimulates heart and blood vessels to bring hypertension in normal range.

Barre's pyramidal sign is an inability to hold the lower legs still with the knees flexed. Place the patient prone and his knees at 90°. Then ask him to hold his lower legs still. If he cannot maintain this position, you have observed the cause of pyramidal tract disease.

Barre's sign is a delayed contraction of iris seen in mental deterioration.

Basal cell adenoma is a tumor that develops in major salivary glands especially parotid gland. These are painless and grow slowly. It has a well-defined connective tissue capsule. Cells are isomorphic. Cytoplasm is scanty and ill-defined. Tumor has to be removed.

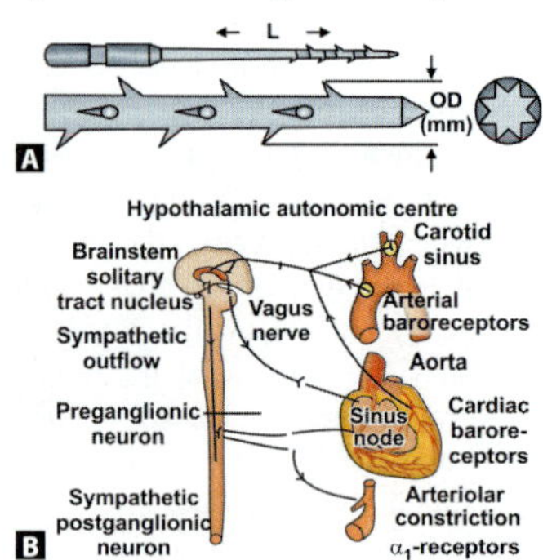

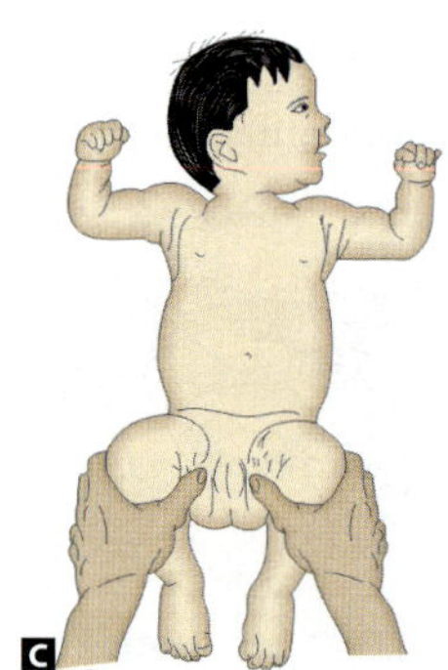

Figs A to C: *(A) Barbed broach; (B) Baroreceptor reflex; (C) Barlow's sign*

Basal cell carcinoma is a locally aggressive malignant neoplasm that develops on the sun exposed surface over skin. It does not metastasize. It generally involves middle one-third of face in 4th decade of life. It arises from basal layer of epidermis or from hair follicle. Direct strong sun light is the causative factor. It starts as a small, elevated papule which ulcerates, heals over and then breaks down. Untreated lesion grows on. Common site involved includes upper lip, nasolabial folds, cheek, forehead, etc. It does not arise from oral mucous membrane. *Clinical features:* It starts as a slow growing small nodule. It develops into central crusted ulcer with an elevated but smooth rolled border. It develops as a sole lesion. If not treated, it invades adjacent structures. There is basaloid cell's proliferation but cells don't show any mitosis. In some cases, squamous cell may occur in tumor. Surgical treatment followed by radiotherapy gives good results.

Basal metabolic rate refers to the process when body is at complete rest, 12 hours after meal energy is needed to maintain the heart beat, respiration, etc. But largely to maintain body temperature and tension of muscle, is known as BMR. It is related to muscle mass and surface area of body. For infants BMR is 50–70 k cal per square meter per hour. Average BMR is about 1500 k cal per day. It is under control of thyroid gland and is increased in fever and hyperthyroidism.

Base metal refers to the metal that oxidized readily. It is an alloy composed of metals that are neither precious nor noble. It was developed in 1970 based on nickel and chromium. A thin invisible chromium oxide layer provides a complete and impervious film. It does not dull the surface finish. They are low in cost but their hardness makes occlusal adjustment, polishing and crown removal very difficult.

Base plane angle (pal-mp) is the angle between the maxillary and mandibular jaw bases, also is used to determine the inclination of the mandibular plane. In horizontal

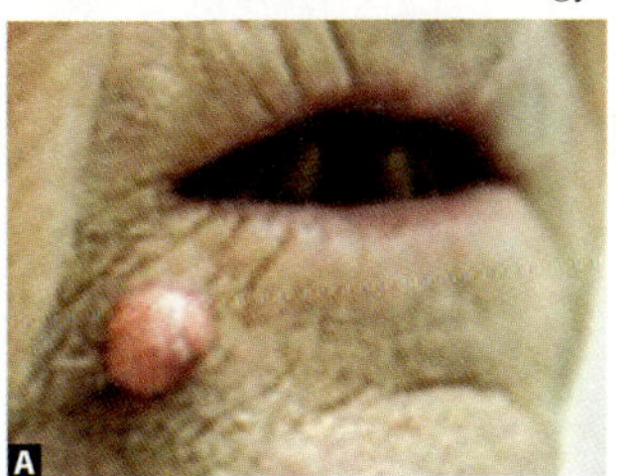

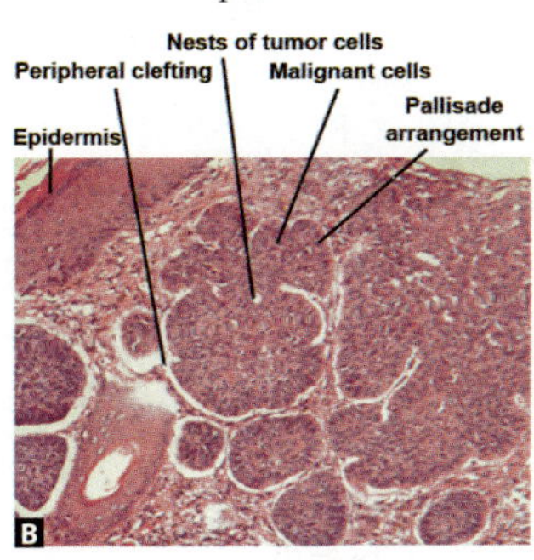

Figs A and B: *Basal cell carcinoma (A) Gross presentation; (B) Microscopic presentation*

growth pattern, this angle is small (23.4° at 9 years and 20.5° at 15 years), whereas in vertical growth pattern it is larger (329° at 9 years and 30.9° at 15 years).

Basic research is the systemic application of scientific method leading to the establishment of new knowledge or theory.

Basilar migraine is the headache of occipital region and is very severe. Aura includes disturbance of vision. Numbness, tingling of lips, hands and feet occur. Some may have vertigo, diplopia, dysarthria and aggressive outbursts. Basilary artery spasm is responsible for it.

Basophils are white blood cell that stain the basic dyes. It consists of coarse granules in the cytoplasm.

Bass method is a method of tooth brushing where the tooth brushes are oriented in a 45° angle to the long axis of the tooth and a vibratory motion is used to remove debris/plaque.

B-cell is a b-lymphocyte that produces and secrets antibodies.

B-cell lineage is an ability to synthesize protein called immunoglobulin. Mature B cells can express Ig in two different forms.

BCG vaccination: Importance of BCG vaccine in prevention of tuberculosis was understood in 1948 after its universal acceptance. It is given intradermally. It gives protection for 20 years. After about 239 subcultures over a period of 13 years Albert calmette and Camille guérin were able to evolve a strain known as Calmette-Guerin or BCG.

Beau's lines are transverse white linear depression on the finger nails. These lines may develop after severe illness or due to toxicity. It may also be seen in malnutrition,

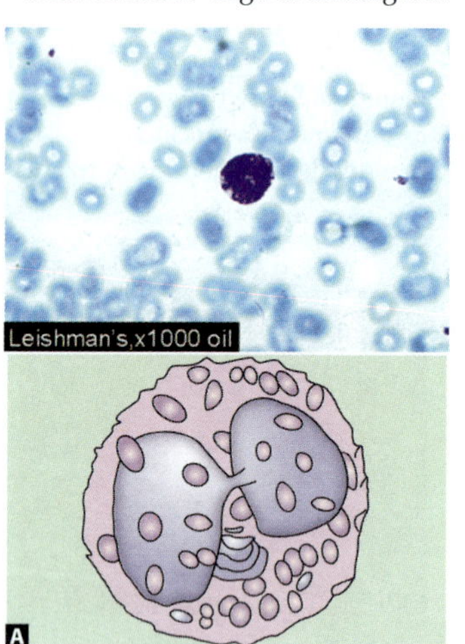

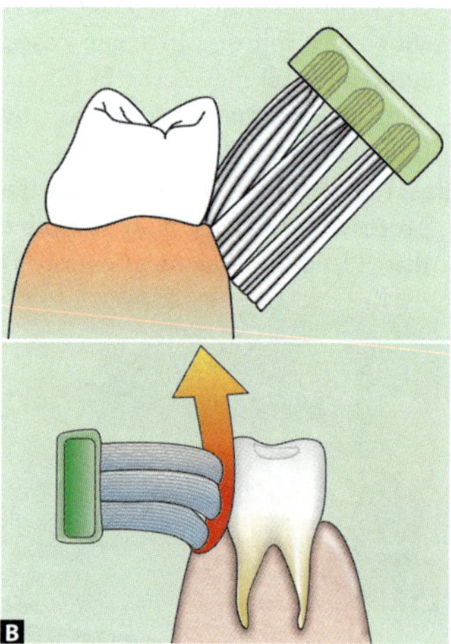

Figs A and B: *(A) Basophil; (B) Bass technique*

nail bed trauma and coronary artery disease.

Bed bath: Washing with a basin of water at the bedside only.

Bedsore is a type of ulcer that is situated over a pressure point. Size and shapes of ulcers are variable. It may extend up to the bone. It is covered by pale dirty slough. Edge is clean-cut and sloping. There may be sero purulent fluid.

Beer is an alcoholic beverage produced by fermentation of cereals. First step is malting of barley. On sprouting, enzyme amylase develops which hydrolyzes starch into dextrin and maltose. Sprouted barley is dried and extracted with hot water to produce wort. Then hops are added to ferment. A slow fermentation is continuously increasing the alcoholic content and forming CO_2. Beer contains 3–7% alcohol and 30–60 k cal per 100 mL.

Behavior learning theory (Palermo1956) habit is a learned behavior and confirm to the laws of learning theory with no underlying causes and no more emotional or psychologic problems. The learning theory advocates that non-nutritive sucking stems from adaptive response. According to this theory, since habit behavior is learned, it can presumably be unlearned. For instance, an infant associates sucking with pleasurable feelings such as hunger, satiety and being held. These events will be replaced in latter life by transferring the sucking action to the most suitable objects available namely, the thumb or fingers. Learning theorists say that conditioning results in the development of habit (Pavlov 1928). A conditioned reflex is a reflex response, acquired by repeated pairing of one stimulus with another stimulus that normally does produce the response. This is an example of one stimulus to another. Conditioning and stimulus generalization can intimate a habit, which if continuously repeated or reinforced will become a learned pattern.

Behavior therapy is an application of interventions based on an understanding of learning principles.

Belief is a concept that a person holds to be true.

Bell's palsy is the most common cause of facial palsy. It is a type

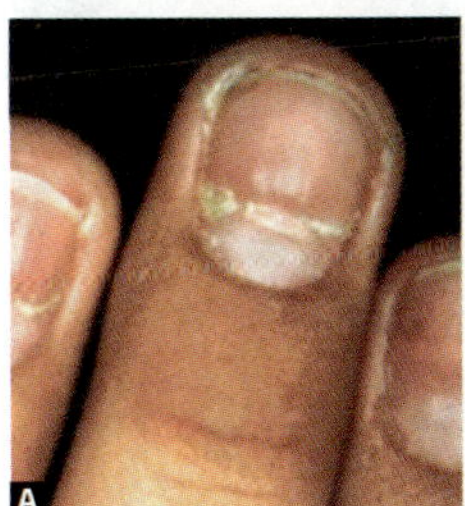

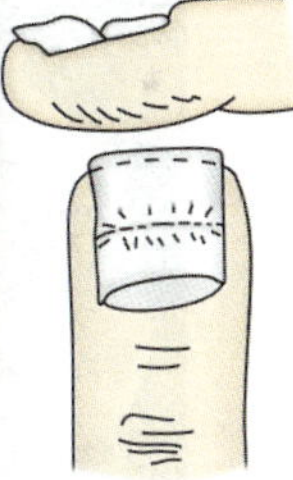

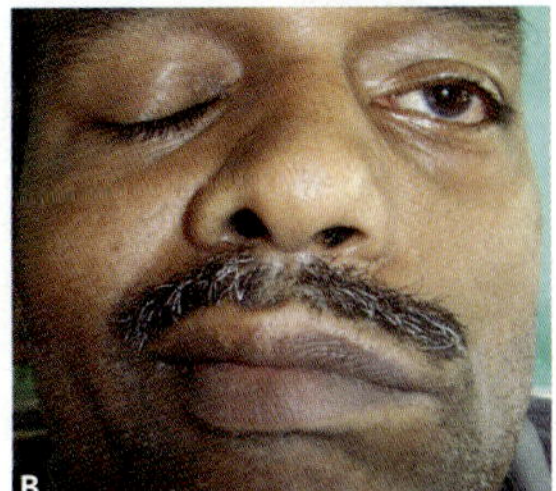

Figs A and B: *(A) Beau's lines; (B) Bell's palsy*

of idiopathic infranuclear (lower motor neuron type) facial palsy, the cause of which is not known. Bell's palsy has been associated with reactivation of herpes simplex type I infection, but its causal role is not established.

Benign cementoblastoma is a true neoplasm of functional cement blasts. These develop in younger age group. Mandible is affected more. Radiographically, tumor mass is attached to the tooth root and appears as a well-circumscribed dense mass. It is outlined by thin radiolucent line.

Benign chondroblastoma develops between the age group of 5–25 years of age. It is composed of closely packed, polyhedral cells with occasional foci of chondroid matrix. Surgical excision is advised, recurrence is common.

Benign cystic teratoma of ovary contains several types of tissue representing two or three embryonic layers. Tumors are unilateral with cystic spaces.

Benign fibrous histiocytoma lesion develops in skin over breast. They may develop on a previous scar on the skin. Lesion is a firm nodule covered by shiny pink epithelium. Wide local excision is required.

Benign neonatal convulsions refers to the familial benign neonatal convulsions that are dominantly inherited. Most cases are mapping to chromosome 20q and some to 8q. The onset is on 3rd day of life. Short duration attacks with tonic syndromes and ocular symptoms. Ocular remissions occur. Between seizures infants are well.

Benign osteoblastoma was first described in 1954 by Dublin and Johnson. Vertebral column is mostly involved. Lesion is well circumscribed. Actively proliferating osteoblasts pave the irregular trabaculae of new bone. Conservative surgical excision is the treatment.

Benjamin theory (1960): Says, "Thumb sucking arises from the rooting (or) placing reflex seen in all mammalian infants. Rooting reflex is the movement of the infant's head and tongue towards an object

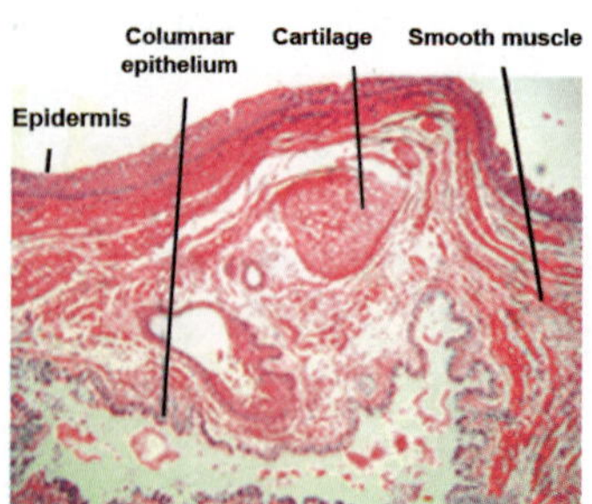

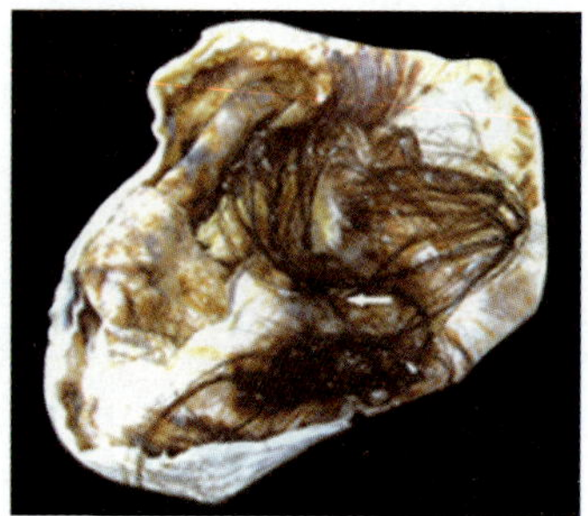

Fig.: *Benign cystic teratoma ovary*

touching his cheek. The object is usually the mother's breast but may also be a finger (or) a pacifier. This rooting reflex disappears in normal infants around 7–8 months.

Beri beri is a condition that occurs due to severe persistent deficiency of thiamine (B_1). Heart is enlarged due to dilatation and some hypertrophy of all chambers, especially right ventricle. Muscle fibers show varying degrees of degeneration.

Beta-titanium orthodontic wires the composition of titanium-molybdenum is 77.8% titanium, 11.3% molybdenum, 6.6% zirconium and 4.3% tin. Molybdenum results in excellent formability or capability for permanent deformation. These wires have true ability to weld.

Bezold's sign is a swelling and tenderness of the mastoid area. It indicates mastoiditis.

Bicuspidization refers to hemisection.

Bicuspid refers to a type of tooth that has two cusps, i.e. premolars. The first and second bicuspids; they are the fourth and fifth teeth from the center of the mouth, respectively. These are the posterior teeth that are used for chewing.

Bifid cleft into two parts and branches.

Bifid tongue *see* cleft tongue.

Bifurcation having two branches, or dividing into two parts.

Bilateral both sides.

Bilateral condylar neck fractures refer to the bilateral bony injury to the condylar neck of the mandible. In such fractures, usually there is considerable displacement of one side or the other.

Bilateral extracapsular fractures refer to the condylar neck fractures occurring on both the sides and are of two types: low condylar neck fractures and high condylar neck fractures. Operative reduction of at least one side of fracture to restore ramus height is desirable. In case of high condylar neck fracture intermaxillary fixation (IMF) is done for up to 6 weeks and maintained until bony union has occurred.

Bilateral fracture occurs on both sides of the body due to combination of direct and indirect violence. Condylar neck and canine regions are the most common sites.

Bilateral intracapsular fractures are the fractures occurring in the condyle. The occlusion is slightly deranged in these cases and

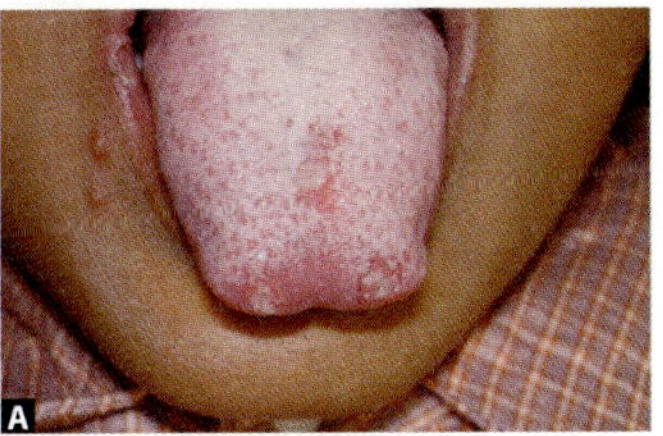

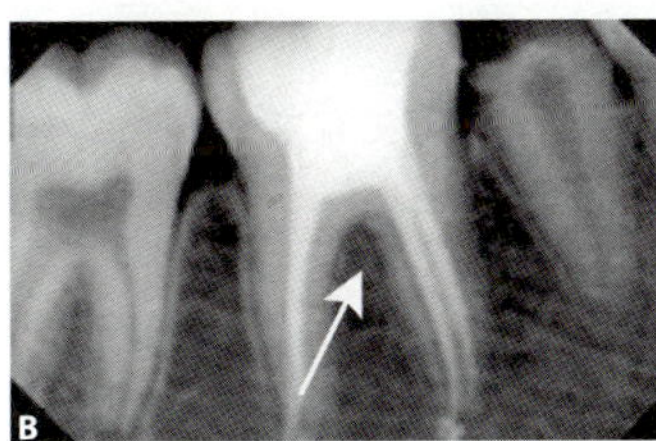

Figs A and B: *(A) Bifid tongue; (B) Bifurcation*

immobilization of 3–4 weeks may be required to achieve stable union.

Bilateral renal artery occlusion produces anuria or severe oliguria. Person may develop low back pain, fever, flank tenderness and hematuria.

Bile is produced by liver and is stored in gall-bladder. It consists of bile salts sodium glycocholate and sodium taurocholate. Bile pigments are bilirubin and biliverdin. Bile salts are used in digestion of fats and bile pigments being waste are excreted in feces.

Bimanually examination using both hands.

Binangle an instrument having two offsetting angles in its shank.

Binary alloy is an alloy that is composed of two elements.

Bioavailability is the amount of drug reaching the systemic circulation in the unmetabolized form by absorption through bodily surfaces.

Bioburden refers to any visible organic debris in dentistry.

Biofilm can be defined as a sessile multi-cellular microbial community characterized by cells that are firmly attached to a surface and enmeshed in a self-produced matrix of extracellular polymeric substances. Bacterial biofilms are very prevalent in the apical root canals of teeth with primary and post-treatment apical periodontitis. First stage adsorption of macro-molecules in the planktonic phase to the surface, leading to the formation of a conditioning film. Second stage adhesion and co-adhesion of microorganisms and attachment may be strengthened through polymer production. Third stage multiplication metabolism of attached microorganisms that ultimately will result in a structurally organized mixed microbial community. Fourth stage involves detachment of biofilm microorganisms. According to (Costerton, et al—1995). Biofilm is a community of bacteria embedded in exopolysaccharide that adhere out an inert or living surface.

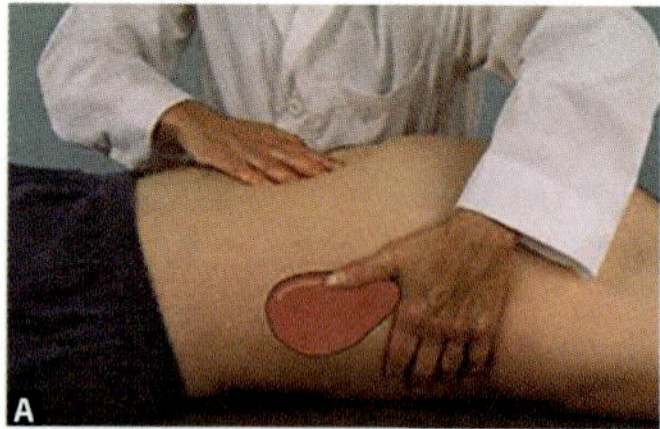

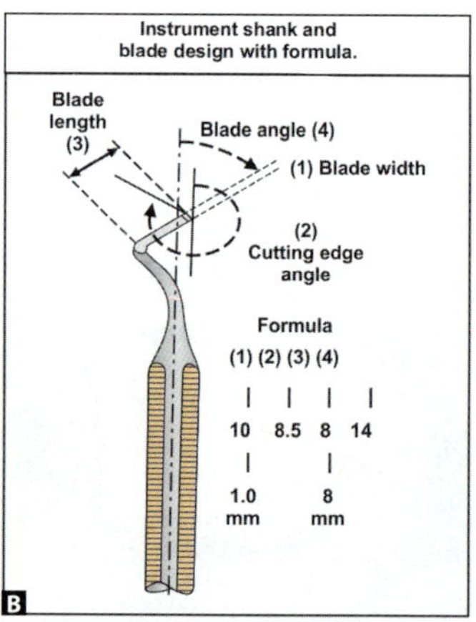

Figs A and B: *(A) Bimanual examination; (B) Biangle instrument*

The slime layer that forms on rocks in streams is a classic example of a biofilm. So is the plaque that forms in the oral cavity. Biofilms are everywhere in nature. They form under fluid conditions. It is estimated over 95 percent of bacteria existing in nature are in biofilms. Sometimes biofilms are seen as positive, such as their use for detoxification of waste water and sewage. More often biofilms provide a challenge for humans. Human biofilm infections include dental cavities, gum diseases, ear infections and some infections of the prostate gland and heart. When bacteria in a biofilm aggregate on surfaces, they produce copious amounts of a sugary, mucus coating. In the case of our mouth, teeming bacteria can, in just a few hours, erect the microscopic equivalent of a coral reef on our teeth. However, the term biofilm describes the relatively undefinable microbial community associated with a tooth surface or any other hard, non-shedding material. Biofilms are obliquities; they form on virtually all surfaces immersed in natural aqueous environments. Form particularly fast in flow systems where a regular nutrient supply is provided to the bacteria. Rapid formation of visible layers of microorganisms due to extensive bacterial growth accompanied by excretion of copious amount of extracellular polymers is typical for biofilm.

Biologic pocket depth is the distance measured between the gingival margin and the base of the pocket.

Biological indicator is also known as spore test to know whether sterilization has been done or not.

Biological therapy is a treatment to stimulate or restore the ability of the immune system to fight infection.

Biomaterial centered infection (BCI) occurs when bacteria adheres to an artificial biomaterial surface, such as root canal obturating materials and forms biofilms. Presence of biomaterial in close proximity to the host immune system can increase the susceptibility to BCI. BCI usually reveals opportunistic invasion by

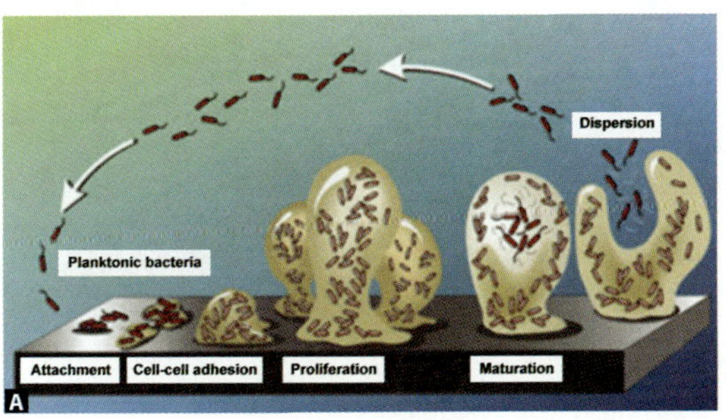

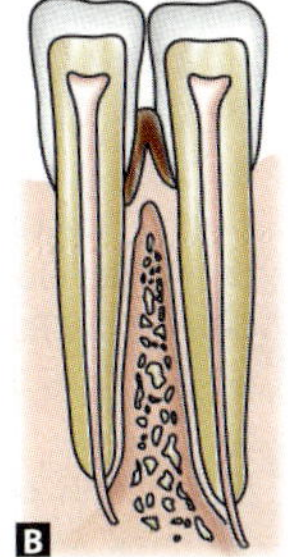

Figs A and B: *(A) Formation of biofilm; (B) Biologic pocket depth*

nosocomial organisms. Coagulase-negative *Staphylococcus, S. aureus,* enterococci, streptococci, *P. aeruginosa*, and fungi are commonly isolated from infected biomaterial surfaces. Three phases of bacterial adhesion to biomaterial surface. **Phase 1:** Transport of bacteria to biomaterial surface; **Phase 2:** Initial, nonspecific adhesion phase; **Phase 3:** Specific adhesion phase.

Biometrics is defined as the science of statistical biology, the collection and statistical analysis of data regarding a living organism.

Biopsy is the removal of tissue from the living organism for the purpose of examination at microscopic level. It not only helps in diagnosis but determines the nature of any unusual lesion. Total excision of a small lesion for study is known as excisional biopsy when only a small part is removed for diagnostic biopsy.

Biostimulation is a photochemical interaction which describes the stimulatory effects of laser light on biochemical and molecular processes that normally occur in tissues, such as healing and repair.

Biotin was obtained from egg yolk in 1936. It is known as vitamin 'H' also. Its daily requirement is one microgram. Its deficiency rarely develops. Use of antibiotics destroys it. Raw white egg prevents its absorption. It is required in the synthesis of hemoglobin and production of glycogen. Raw egg contains avidin which binds with biotin preventing its absorption.

Bipolar: Having two poles.

Birth history is the history of newborn during birth that includes the type of delivery, occurrence of any complication during birth, such as Rh incompatibility or neonatal jaundice.

Bisferiens pulse is a combination of collapsing pulse and low-rising pulse.

Bisque the first firing of porcelain.

Bitewing vertical is an intraoral film used to examine the level of alveolar bone in mouth. It is placed with long portion of a film in a vertical direction.

Bite block is a device used to hold the mouth open during mouth surgery.

Bite marks are the marks given by convict with teeth. A classical bite mark is circular or oval with the canines leaving the deepest and most prominent marks. The normal distance between the maxillary canine teeth in adults is 2.5 to 4.0 cm. It is an unintentional condition and occurs due to lack of awareness. Child neglect is prevalent globally, affecting all ethnicity, religion,

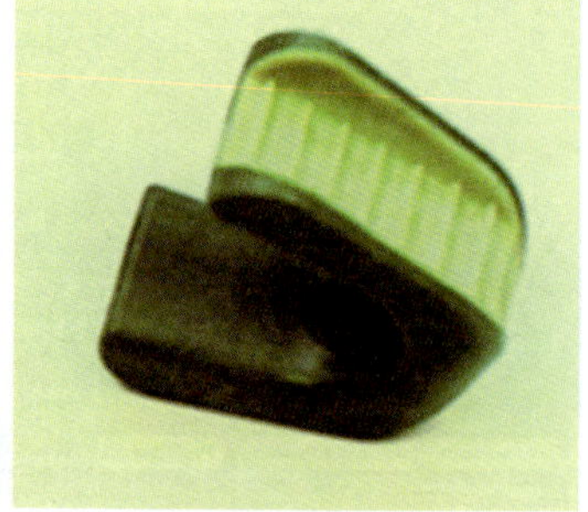

Fig.: *Bite block*

socio-economic status and different religions. WHO defines neglect as inattention or omission on the part of caregiver to provide for the development of child in all sphere; health, education, nutrition, emotional, development, shelter and safe conditions. NCANDS defines neglects as maltreatment that refers to failure of care given by the caretaker to provide needed, age appropriate care although financially be able to do so. People in close contact are frequently the ones to know and report it. Polansky defines neglect as a condition in which caretaker is responsible for the child, either deliberately or extraordinary inattentiveness permits the child to experience avoidable suffering and fails to provide things that is essential for developing person's physical, intellectual and emotional capacities.

Bite plane a fixed appliance made of acrylic used to correct crossbite.

Bite registration is a procedure used to orient upper and lower models of the teeth in proper bite relationship during fabrication of crown.

Bite test helps in identifying a cracked or fractured tooth. This is done if patient complains of pain on mastication. Tooth is sensitive to biting if pulpal necrosis has extended to the periodontal ligament space or if a crack is present in a tooth. In this, the patient is asked to bite on a hard object such as cotton swab, tooth pick or orange wood stick with suspected tooth and the contralateral tooth.

Bitewing film is an intraoral radiograph used to examine crowns of both maxillary and mandibular teeth biting surface on the same film.

Biting habits refer to the self-inflicting habits such as nail biting, pencil biting and lip biting.

Bitot's spots are triangular, foamy, rough and raised patches seen on bulbar conjunctiva in vitamin A deficiency. These don't interfere with vision. These are generally bilateral. If more than 2% children between 0–5 years show Bitot's spot in community, it is known as community xerosis.

Black lesions are the lesions thatoccur due to foreign body deposition.

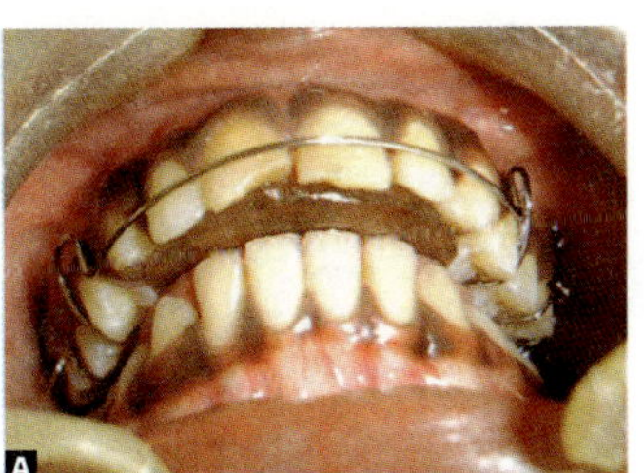

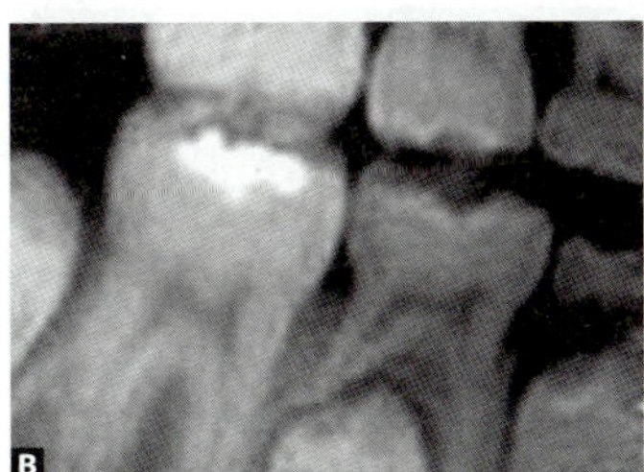

Figs A to B: *(A) Anterior bite plane; (B) Bitewing*

It may be developed due to altered blood pigment and necrosis. If an alteration in blood pigment occurs with oxidation and drying, black color may appear in crust. Gangrene gives a black color. As dead tissue sloughs a depressed lesion with a black periphery develops.

Black stain refers to black deposit, takes the form of thin line or band just above the free gingiva. Black stain is dominated by actinomyces. These are highly retentive calculus-like stain, black or dark brown in color, occurring on the gingival third along the gingival margin also known as brown stain. The stain appears as a continuous or interrupted line following the gingival margin. This line may be 1 mm wide with no appreciable thickness or it may also appear as heavy deposits which will be slightly elevated from the tooth surface and is easily detectable. The teeth frequently appear clean and shiny with a lower tendency to bleed. Black stain has a calculus-like appearance and is generally composed of microorganisms embedded deep in a matrix. These stains can occur at any age but are more common in childhood, females and frequently found in clean mouth. These stains tend to recur despite maintenance of personal hygiene but the severity may reduce with meticulous plaque control methods.

Black's cavity classification is the classification system given by Dr GV Black used to code cavities according to location on the tooth.

Blastocyst is a stage in embryology following morula.

Blastomycosis is a fungal infection caused by blastomyces dermatitidis. It is a normal habitant of soil. In chronic form, low-grade fever and mild cough may develop. Oral lesions are rarely the primary lesions, but if occurs, it is non-specific painless verrucous ulcer with indurated borders. Patients will show pulmonary lesions on X–ray. It may cause shortness of breathing, weight loss and blood tinged sputum. There will be development of painless ulcer with indurated borders. In some cases, hard nodules and radiolucent jaw

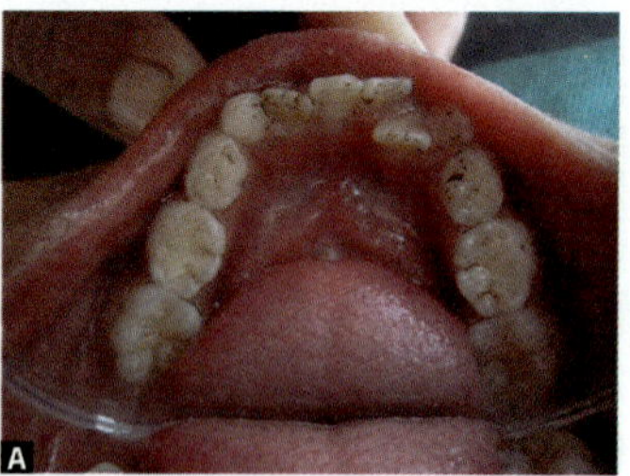

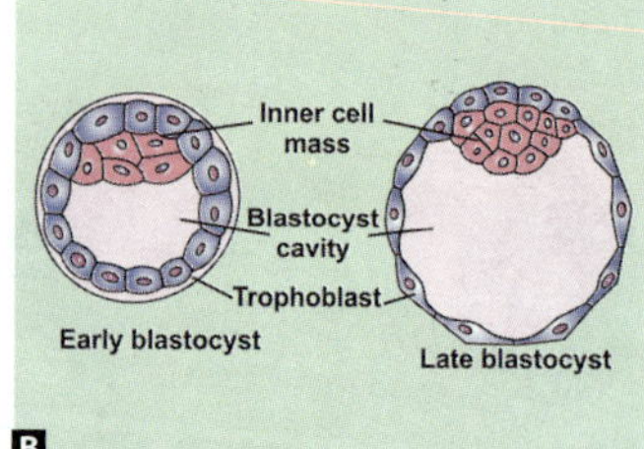

Figs A and B: *(A) Black stain; (B) Blastocyst*

lesions can be seen. Diagnosis is made on biopsy.

Bleaching is the lightening of the color of a tooth through the application of a chemical agent to oxidize the organic pigmentation in the tooth.

Bleeding index is an index that is used to score the status of gingiva where presence or absence of bleeding is recorded by inserting a periodontal probe into the sulcus.

Bleeding time is a diagnostic test that provides an assessment of adequacy of platelet function not the number. It means the time taken by a standardized skin incision to stop bleeding by formation of clot. It is 1–6 minutes.

Blephroclonus is an excessive blinking of eyes. This extrapyramidal sign occurs with disorders of basal ganglia and cerebellum.

Blind spot is the area on retina that has no rods or cones. So any image that focuses on blind spot cannot be seen.

Blink reflex is a neonatal reflex, when we gently tap the glabella (junction between the nose and forehead), both eyelids of the neonate blink.

Blocking is a cognitive disturbance resulting in interruption of a stream of speech or thoughts. Blocking may occur in normal individuals but most commonly occurs in schizophrenia.

Blood borne pathogens are the microorganisms present in blood that cause disease.

Blood brain barrier: It is a structural and functional barrier formed by astrocytes and blood vessel walls in the brain. It prevents some products diffusing from the blood into brain tissue.

Blood pressure is a measurement of two blood vessels. The first is the pressure of the blood against the arterial blood vessels and second is the pressure against the blood vessels as the heart relaxes between contractions. It is known as diastole.

Blood sugar is a test used to assess the level of sugar in blood. Fasting blood sugar is 80–100 mg/100 mL. The level rises after meals to 140 mg/100 mL, but rapidly returns to normal unless person is suffering from diabetes. Glucose provides energy and is stored in liver as glycogen.

Blue color weakness develops from diminished or absent blue receptors.

Blue grass appliance (1991) was introduced by Haskell, this is

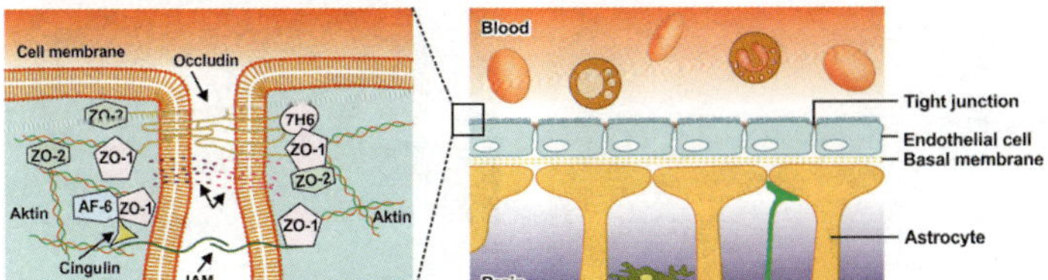

Fig.: *Blood brain barrier*

a habit breaking appliance for children with a continued thumb sucking habit, which is affecting the mixed or permanent dentition. It consists of a modified six-sided roller, machined from teflon to permit purchase of the tongue. This is slipped over a 0.045 stainless steel wire soldered to molar orthodontic bands. This appliance is placed for 3–6 months. Instructions are given to turn the roller instead of sucking the digit. Digit sucking is often seen to stop immediately.

Blue lesions there is no biological blue pigment. Some cystic lesions containing clear fluid appear blue and some vascular lesions may also look blue when blood within the lesion contains a large amount of reduced hemoglobin. Shade of blue color may be altered by the thickness of overlying mucosa. Darker blue is seen in most superficial lesion.

Blue nevi these are due to benign proliferation of melanocytes. Nevocellular nevi arise from basal layer melanocytes early in life. Proliferation is minimal and is macular, classified as junctional nevi. These are feat, round or oval in outline. Such nevi assume dome shape. Blue nevi blue are in color on the skin. The melanocytes of blue nevus differ morphologically from nevocellular nevus being spindle-shaped. These may be seen at any age. Biopsy is needed, simple excision is the treatment of choice.

Blue nevus is a common pigmented lesion of oral cavity. *Clinical features:* These are commonly seen on the mucosal surfaces of hard palate. It is a dome-shaped dark blue papule. Cells of blue nevus are elongated, bipolar and spindle-shaped. Few pigmented macrophages may be present. These do not change into malignancy and hence surgical resection serves the purpose. Compound nevus presents the combined features of intradermal nevus and junctional nevus.

Blunderbuss canals refer to immature canals with open apex. Blunderbuss canals are characterized by flared out apical foramen. So a special procedure, like apexification, is required to ensure apical closure. For complete obturation of such canals, tailor made gutta-percha

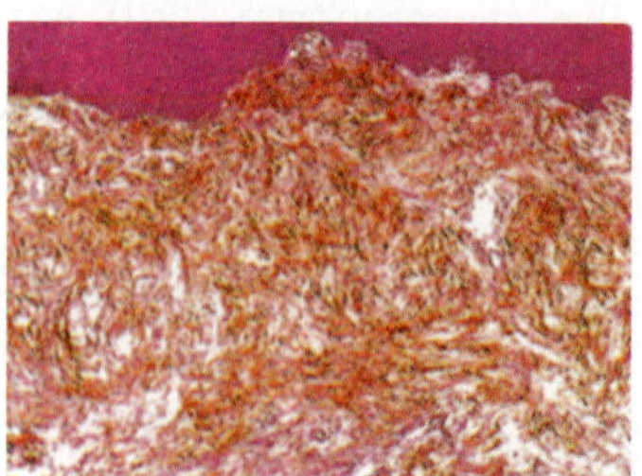

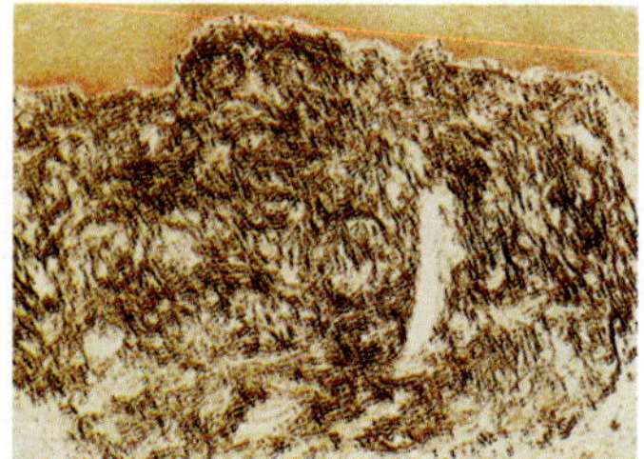

Fig.: *Blue nevus*

or warm gutta-percha technique is preferred.

B-lymphocytes are the components of WBCs that matures without passing through the thymus and matures into plasma cells that produce antibodies.

Body language is the communication of feelings and attitudes/desires through gesture, postures and facial expression. It is an important relationship between two sexes.

Boil is a single or multiple painful swelling. It is present in hairy areas and does not occur on palm of hand. Swelling is small and conical having a point. A black dot may be present in the center of swelling.

Boiling is a process of sterilization. When other proper facilities for sterilization are not available boiling for 20 minutes may be done. Boiling does not render spores nonviable, hence is not very reliable and effective. Needles and syringes are generally sterilized this way.

Bolus refers to chewed up mass of food and saliva.

Bonded modified orthodontic brackets are used for fracture with minimal displacement where the fracture can be immobilized with the help of placement of bonded modified orthodontic brackets onto the teeth and applying intermaxillary elastic bands.

Bonding the covering of a tooth surface to correct stained or damaged teeth.

Bonding-dentin establishment of micromechanical bond between cut dentin and the bonding agent.

Bone clamps are another form of external fixation of mandibular fractures. Here instead of pins, the bone clamps are used to secure the fragments of the bone. The clamps are secured on the lower border of the mandible. Pins that project from the clamp, are connected by a system of external rods and universal joints as it is done in external pin fixation.

Bone marrow aspiration is a procedure done to conduct biopsy. Posterior iliac crest is the preferred site for both marrow aspiration and biopsy. Sternum should be used

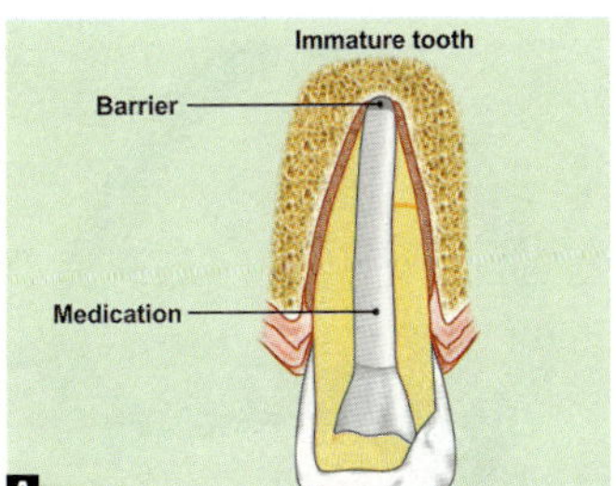

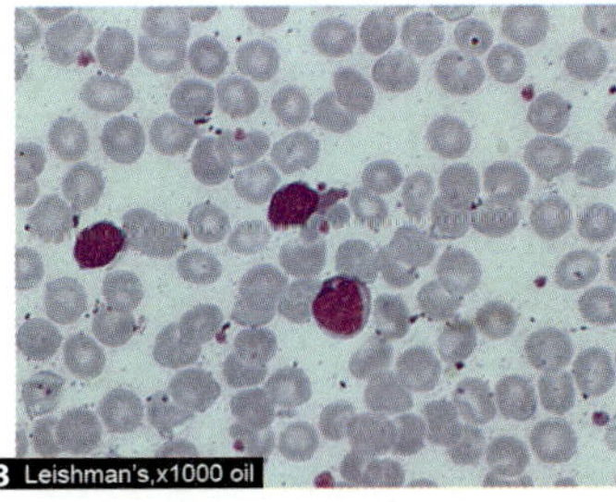

Figs A and B: *(A) Blunderbuss canal; (B) B-lymphocytes*

for aspiration only. Anteromedial surface of tibia is an ideal for infants. Marrow should be examined when blood picture is not clear about hematological disorder. Marrow biopsy is useful in monitoring the progress of disease.

Bone scan is a tracer element study of technetium 99 and then patient is scanned. The tracer localizes to areas of increased metabolic activity such as fracture, infection and cancer.

Bonnet's sign is the pain noted on adduction of thigh, seen in sciatica.

Border molding is a technique used in removable denture to adopt the border of the partial or complete denture to the patient's soft tissue.

Botulinum toxin inhibits acetylcholine release at the neuromuscular junction causing reversible chemodenervation. The general indication for botulinum toxin injection in cerebral palsy is the presence of a dynamic contracture, interfering with function, in the absence of a fixed muscular contracture. If botulinum toxin injections are started at an early age and repeated as necessary, they can help to prevent the development of muscle contractures and bony deformities.

Bowel obstruction: Mostly it develops due to hernias and 5 to 15% by strangulated hernias and 10% by neoplasms. Symptoms include abdominal pain, nausea, vomiting, and no passing of flatus and distension of abdomen. Abdomen will be tender. In case of hernia, tender palpable mass will be palpated.

Bowen's disease is localized, intra-epidermal squamous cell carcinoma. It may develop into invasive carcinoma over years. Clinically, it is a slow enlarging erythematous patch. Histologically, epithelial cells are seen in complete disarray. Many will be of hyperchromatic nuclei. This disease may develop in genital mucosa. Erythroplakia and Bowen's disease both are hairy red patches.

Brachial plexus is a network of nerve fibers formed from the ventral branch of nerves C5-C8 and T1.

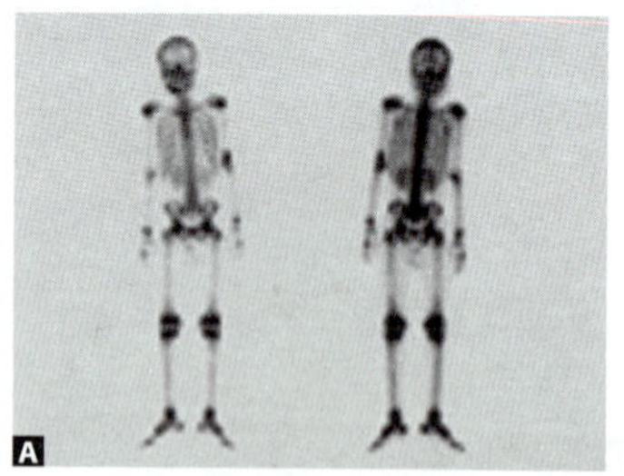

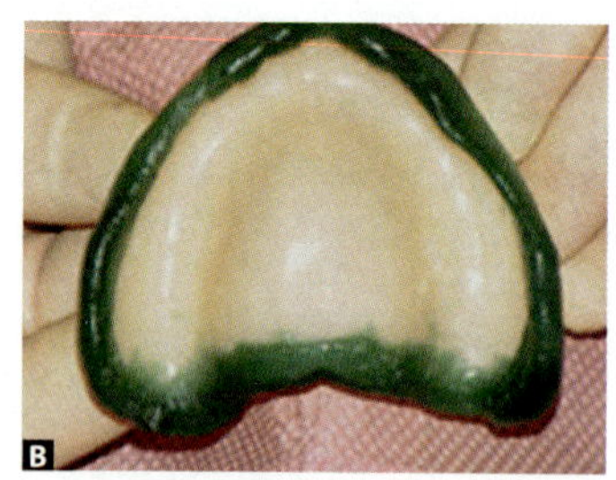

Figs A and B: *(A) Bone scan; B) Border moulding technique*

Brachial pulse is a throbbing sensation that is felt over the brachial artery located on the inner side of the elbow.

Bracket is a small device attached to the teeth that hold the arch wire to the teeth.

Bradykinesia is the slowness of all voluntary movement and speech. It is due to reduced level of dopamine. It is noted in Parkinsonism. Certain drugs may also cause it. There may be tremor and muscle rigidity.

Bradykinin is an endogenous polypeptide released from the inflammatory reaction site. It serves as a powerful vasodilator and excites all types of receptors, sensitizing some high threshold receptors to respond to otherwise innocuous stimuli. It acts only in the presence of prostaglandin.

Bradypnea is a life-threatening apnea or respiratory arrest. Respiration is regular but rate is 12 per minute. It may result due to drug overdose.

Brain abscess encapsulated pus in brain is known as brain abscess. It may directly extend from mastoid, skull bones or paransal sinus. Metastatic brain abscess is secondary to bronchiectasis, empyema or lung abscess. Brain abscess is caused by *Staphylococcus aureus, Staphylococcus viridians* and hemslytic streptococci. Abscess manifests with headache, vomiting and convulsions. Hemiplegia may develop. In raised intracranial pressure, puncture is not done. It may extend from face or middle ear. There will be localizing signs of irritation of brain. Cerebral malaria can also give similar symptoms, but in brain abscess total white cell count and pus cells in CSF will help in diagnosis. Lung abscess is generally a complication of lobar pneumonia. There will be high fever with rigor, chest pain and bronchial breathing. X-ray will help in reaching a diagnosis.

Brain hemorrhage accounts a majority of case of stroke. Hypertension is the main culprit. Blood may be more than 5 cm in diameter.

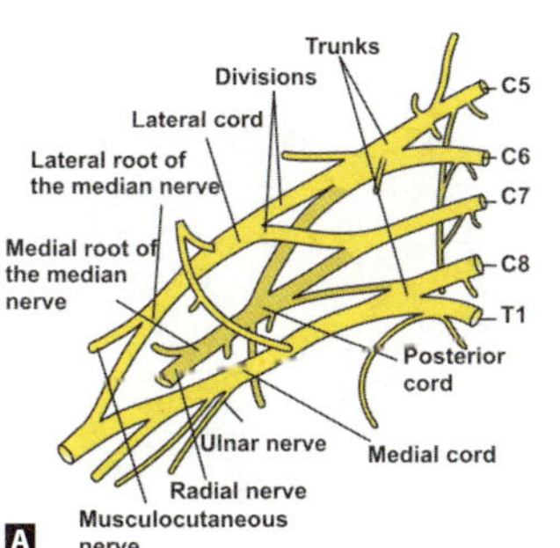

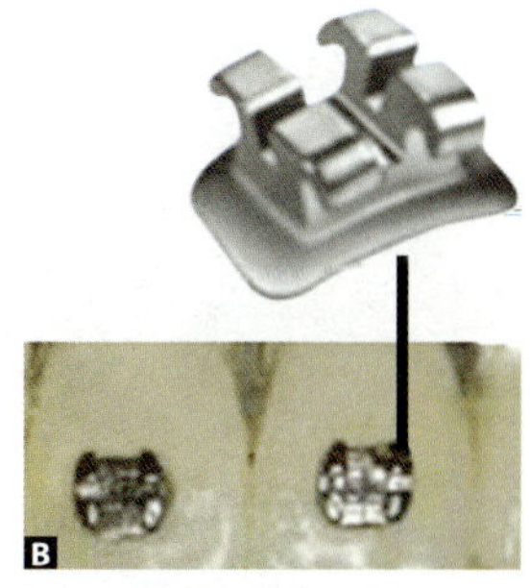

Figs A and B: *(A) Brachial plexus; (B) Bracket*

B

Brain stem is a lower part of brain which connects the brain with spinal cord. It consists of mid-brain, pons and medulla.

Brain tumor headache rapidly growing brain tumor produces headache. Once CSF circulation stops, it produces headache. It is worst on awakening and is aggravated by sitting, standing and coughing. Supratentorial masses produce frontal or temporal headache, while occipital lesions produce occipital headache. Pituitary tumors produce fronto-temporal headache. Meningiomas and meningeal sarcomas cause headache at the site. AVMs produce sentinel headache.

Brain wave is a fluctuating electrical activity occurring in brain.

Branchial (pharyngeal) arches: During the late somite period (4 weeks iu) the mesoderm lateral plate of the foregut region becomes segmented to form a series of five distinct bilateral mesenchymal swellings known as the branchial (pharyngeal) arches.

Branchial cleft cyst develops in lateral aspect of neck in young adults. These are slow growing and symptom free. Cyst is usually lined by stratified squamous epithelium. Surgical removal is a part of treatment.

Branchial efferent fibers are the special visceral efferent fibers that supply skeletal muscle developing in branchial arch mesoderm. The muscles supplied include those of mastication, face, pharynx and larynx.

Brazilian pemphigus is found on tropical regions. It is similar to pemphigus foliaceus.

Breaking cough indicates edema of larynx and surrounding tissue. It may become an emergency.

Breast lipoma is a beingn neoplasm. It devops generally as a single lesion. These are soft movable and fairly well delineated. Treatment is an excision.

Breast pain and nodularity women with benign breast disease present with complaints of physiological swelling, nodularity and mastalgia. Breast pain is related to menstrual cycle.

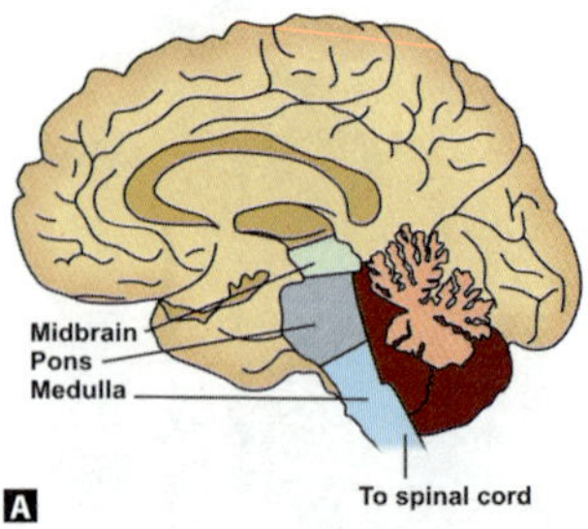

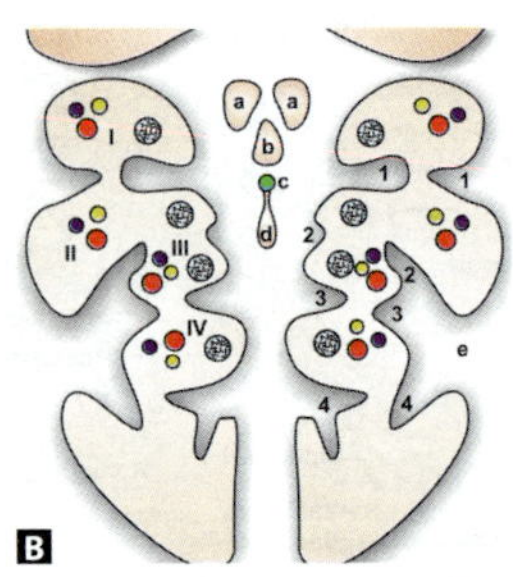

Figs A and B: *(A) Brain stem; (B) Branchial arch*

Breast traumatic fat necrosis occurs when bulky breasts are exposed to trauma. It may stimulate carcinoma. Occult fat necrosis is asymptomatic and goes undetected. Such women have large, dependent breastes. Skin over lesion is red. If tumor develops, it is firm and often relatively fixed to the surrounding breast tissues. Symptoms resemble that of breast abscesses.

Bridge is a fixed appliance (prosthesis) that replaces missing teeth. A bridge is a series of attached crowns (abutments and pontics). Artificial tooth is called pontic and supporting teeth are called abutments. The crown and inlays on abutment teeth are called retainers.

Bridge threader is a flexible plastic device used to floss under a fixed bridge to remove plaque from the interproximal surfaces.

Bridging the creation of voids and pits in a restoration by improper stepping and condensation.

Bristle brush an attachment to the handpiece to remove stain from occlusion surfaces of teeth.

Broach is a sharp instrument used to extripate pulp from the root canal. Broaches are available in variety of sizes, from triple extrafine to extra coarse. Broach does not cut the dentin but can effectively be used to remove cotton or paper points which might have lodged in the canal. It is triangular, square or rhomboidal in cross-section, manufactured from stainless steel wire, which is grounded into desired shape. Smooth broach: It is free of barbs. Previously it was used as pathfinder, but at present flexible files are used for this. Barbed broach: It is one of the oldest intracanal instruments with specifications by ANSI no. 63 and ISO no. 3630-1. It has ADA specification no. 6. Broach is short-handled instrument meant for single use only. It is made from round steel wire. The smooth surface of wire is notched to form barbs bent at an angle from the long axis.

Bristle brushes are cleansing and polishing instrument available in wheel and cup shapes.

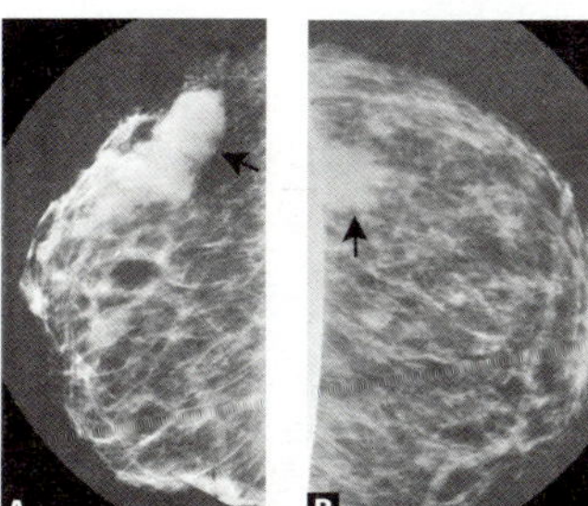

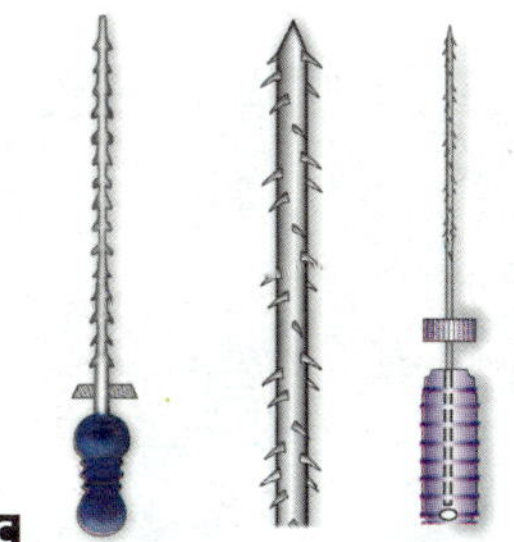

Figs A to C: *(A) Breast nodularity; (B) Breast traumatic fat necrosis; (C) Broach*

These brushes are used with handpieces along with a polishing paste.

Broadbent's inverted sign: These are the pulsations in the left posterolateral chest wall during ventricular systole. Put your palm over areas of visible pulsation while hearing for ventricular systole. Rate, rhythm and pulsation will be high. It is due to gross dilatation of left atrium.

Broca's aphasia there is striking difficulty with speech though they fully understand what is being said. They can make nonverbal responses. Milder form results in hesitancy of speech.

Brodies abscess patient is between 10–20 years of age upper end of tibia and lower end of femur are the common sites. A deep boring pain is the main symptom which may be worst at night. X-ray shows oval lucent area. Treatment is by operation.

Bronchial breathing is a type of breathing that originates from large airways when lung between these airways and chest wall is airless due to consolidation, collapse or fibrosis. Sound resembles as listening over trachea. Quality of sound is harsh and of higher frequency. It becomes inaudible just before the end of inspiration.

Bronchiectasis is a congenital or acquired disorder of dilation and destruction of bronchial wall. Caused due to cystic fibrosis and recurrent infection. Symptoms include chronic cough, production of copius amount of purulent sputum, hemoptysis and recurrent pneumonia. Clubbing is frequent and copious foul smelling purulent sputum is characteristic. It occurs due to abnormal and permanent dilatation of bronchi.

Bronchodilator is the dilatation of the bronchi in order to facilitate breathing.

Bronchogenic carcinoma is mostly amongst smokers. Patient presents with anorexia and weight loss. There develops new cough or changes in cough. 25% will show hemoptysis. Some may develop pneumonia or pleural effusion. Sputum cytology is highly specific but not sensitive. CT helps in diagnosis. 5 years survival is only in 5% cases.

Bronchopneumonia is a multifocal process which starts in terminal and respiratory bronchioles and

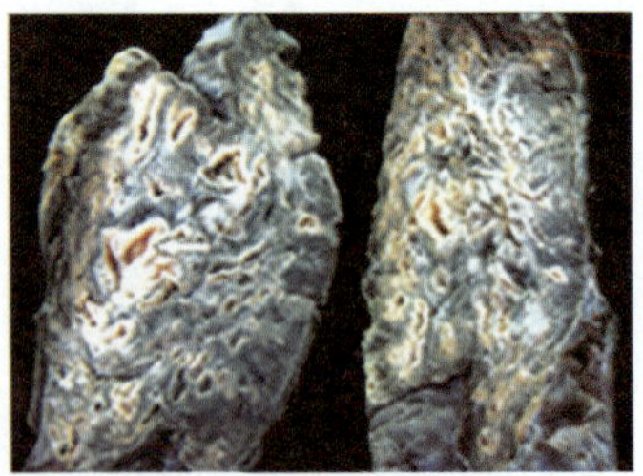

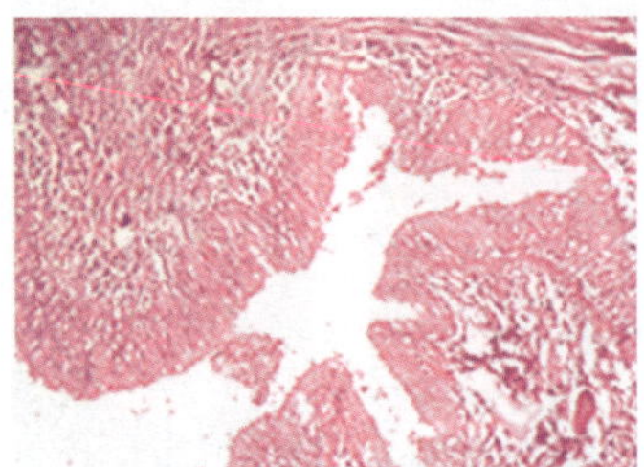

Fig.: *Bronchiectasis*

produces patchy consolidation caused by *S. aureus* and Gram-negative organisms. The lesion occurs in scattered nodular fashion around the bronchi. Lesion may be of a few mm to 1 cm. Bronchioles show exudates and lining may show ulceration. Bronchiole is surrounded by a zone of consolidation.

Bronchoscopy is a procedure where trachea or bronchi are directly visualized by flexible or rigid bronchoscope. Samples from airways can also be obtained by bronchial washings, aspiration, or biopsy. Foreign body can be removed (therapeutic bronchoscopy).

Bronchospasm is a generalized contraction of smooth muscles of bronchi and bronchioles resulting in constriction of bronchi and mucosal edema. Expiratory phase is more involved and may become life-threatening.

Brown lesions may be caused by melanin or hemosiderin. Melanin is a substance produced within melanocyte by melanosomes. An increase in brown pigmentation may be brought by increased number of melanocytes. Increased number of melanocytes forms different benign and malignant neoplasms. Heat, ultraviolet rays and X-rays may increase melanin synethesis. Brown color resulting from hemosiderin is associated with crusting and drying of ulcerated lesions.

Brown sataining of tooth, it is a thin, brown, delicate pellicle-like structure. It may be composed of salivary mucin.

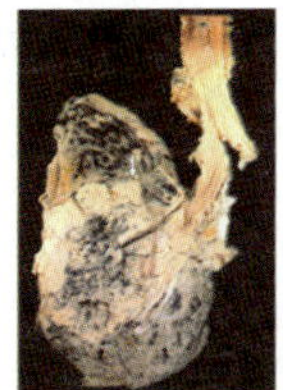

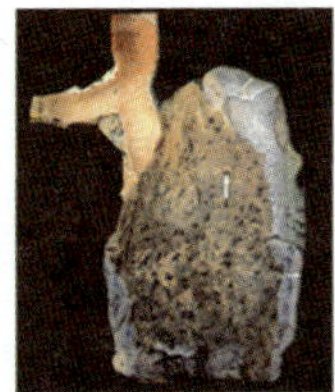

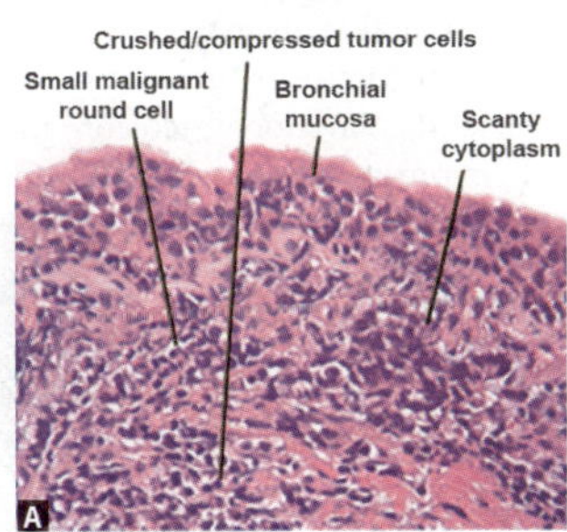

Figs A and B: *(A) Bronchogenic carcinoma; (B) Bronchopneumonia*

Brown stains due to betel leaf: Use of betel leaf will give rise to stains which can vary in color from dark brown to deep mahogany brown to black. These stains generally contain microorganisms and mineralized content which has the characteristic resemblance to the sub-gingival calculus.

Bruises are reddish-blue marks that occur due to any form of blunt injury, a very common form of physical abuse, however, it is also very common in accidental form especially in active children. One must learn to differentiate between international and accidental abuse.

Brown stains due to brown pellicle is smooth and structureless and recurs readily after removal. The pellicle can take on stains of various colors.

Brown stains due to chlorhexidine mouth rinses: Chlorhexidine mouth rinses are the excellent agents for the plaque control, but repeated use of these agents may give rise to brownish stains on the tooth surfaces, generally affecting the proximal surface of the tooth.

Brown stains due to food pigments: Stains resulting from pigments leaching out of the food such as turmeric stains, stains from tea, coffee, and use of artificial colors give rise to various stains.

Brown stains due to stannous fluoride: Stains appear sometimes as light brown or light yellow, which form onto the tooth surface after the prolonged or the repeated use of stannous fluoride product which results in the formation of brown tin oxide due to the reaction of the tin ion and fluoride compound.

Bruxism is an involuntary grinding, clinching of teeth, especially done during sleep mostly as a result of stress and tension. It causes abnormal wear of teeth. It can be explained as deleterious habit of grinding the teeth. It is defined as the grinding of teeth for non-functional purposes. Some authors refer to nocturnal grinding as bruxism and grinding during the day as burxomania, which could be due to psychological and emotional stresses. Occlusal interference or discrepancy between centric relation and centric occlusion can predispose to grinding, pericoronitis and periodontal pain may also trigger bruxism. Occlusal disturbance may cause it. Emotional tension may be expressed through a number

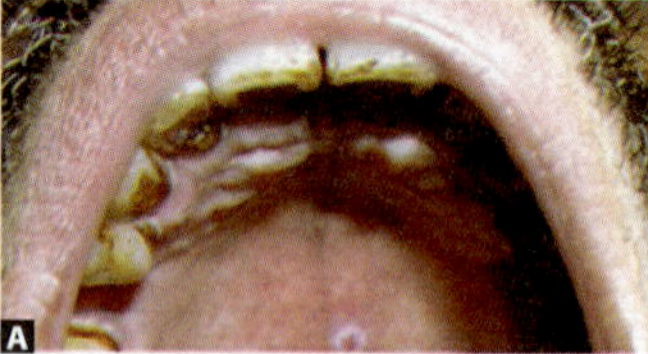

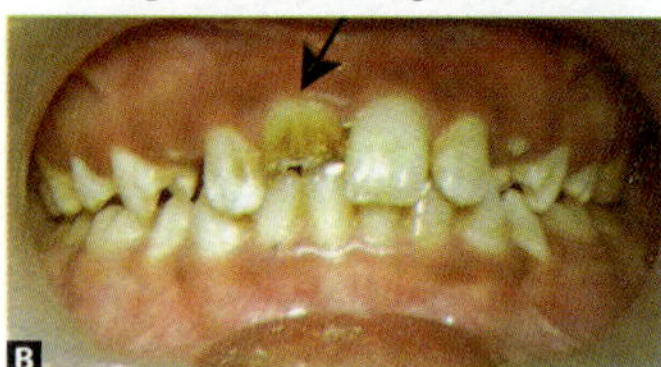

Figs A and B: *(A) Betel leaf stains; (B) Stains due to trauma*

of nervous habits, bruxism is one of them. It may be associated with grinding or grating noise.

Buccal pertaining to cheek.

Buccal nerve block an injection to provide pain control to the soft tissues, facial to the mandibular molars.

Buccal object rule a rule for the orientation of structures seen in two radiographs exposed at different angles used to determine buccal lingual relationship of an object.

Buccal pouch keratosis habit of tobacco chewing may be maintained for decades giving rise to keratosis where there is white thickening and wrinkling of buccal mucosa. Malignant change can follow after decades.

Buccal space refers to the space existing between buccinator and masseter muscle. Infection of this space may lead to swelling of the cheek and may extend to temporal or submandibular space, with which the buccal space communicates.

Buccal wall cavity wall nearest to cheek.

Buccinator that forms the muscular basis of the cheeks. It is a thin quadrilateral muscle occupying interval between maxilla and mandible. It is supplied by lower buccal branches of facial nerve. It compresses the cheeks against the teeth.

Buccinator muscle the cheek muscle.

Bud stage is initial stage where epithelial cells of dental lamina proliferate and produce a bud-like projection into adjacent ectomesenchyme.

Bullous pemphigoid is a skin lesion and has limited life of 5 years. Initial defect is in lamina lucida of basement membrane. There is no acanthylosis. Bullae do not extend to periphery. Lesions remain localized and heal spontaneously. Oral lesions are smaller, mild painful and grow slowly. Histologically, one can only notice bulla formation in subepithelial region. Systemic corticosteriods are useful. It is a disease of an old age. Generalized non-specific rash develops. Vesicles and bullae are thick-walled and remain intact for some days.

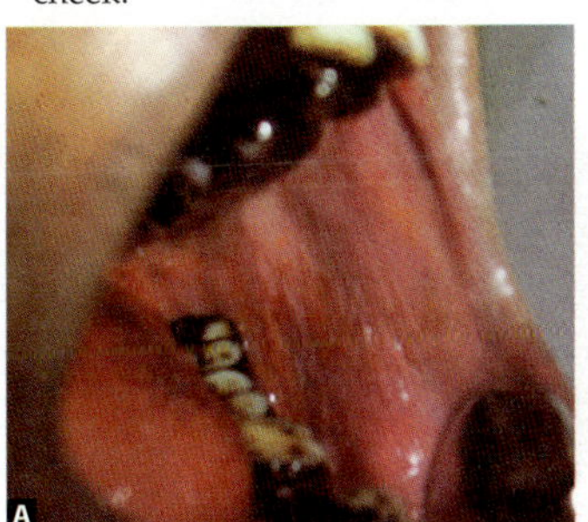

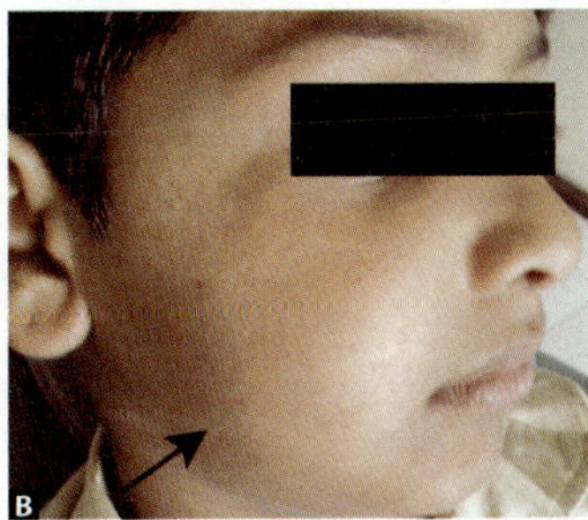

Figs A and B: *(A) Buccal pouch keratosis; (B) Space infection involving buccal and infraorbital spaces*

Gingival involvement generally occurs much and is painful.

Bundle bone is the bone present adjacent to the periodontal ligament that contains large number of Sharpey's fibers.

Bur is a small instrument that has coated tip for the pursose of cavity preparation, crown cutting, finishing the tooth.

Burn of oral mucosa, it is a frequent cause of transient nonkeratotic white lesion. Saliva protects mucosa from chemical and thermal burn. Ingestion of caustic liquids results in oropharyngeal burns. Mild thermal burn of anterior tongue is the result of accidental ingestion of hot food. Application of 70% ethyl alcohol to dry mucosa will result in sloughing.

Burning mouth syndrome: Painful, burning sensations localized in the tongue or affecting other areas of oral mucosa. The pain of burning tongue is rated similar to that of toothache. Tongue temperature is decreased. Some evidence suggests the existence of oral somatosensory and special sensory deficits.

Burning tongue paresthesia of oral mucous membrane is a common clinical finding. Pernicious anemia, diabetes, gastric disturbances and psychogenic factors may result in it. Tongue is commonly involved, pain, burning, etching and stinging of mucous membrane are felt. No satisfactory treatment is available.

Burnishing soothing the surface of a dental amalgam after initial carving by rubbing with a metal instrument having a broad surface.

Burns is any injury to skin by an energy source. This source of energy could be heat, which could be by fire or by hot liquids, chemicals, electricity, lasers, friction, and radiation. Burns may involve the different layers of skin and has varied effects on the skin and may be the deeper structures. The amount of damage will be directly proportional to the amount of energy released by the energy source which will depend upon the temperature of the source and the duration of contact. The higher the temperature, greater is the degree and depth of damage.

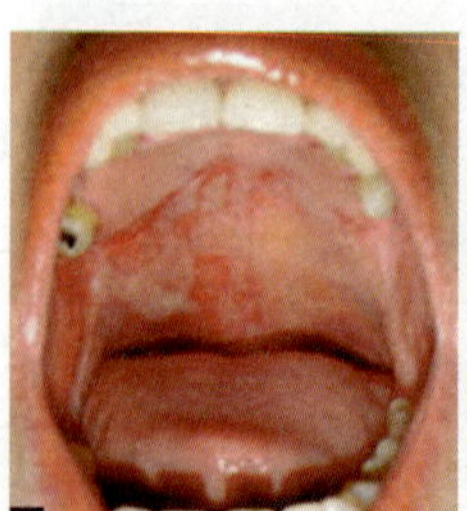

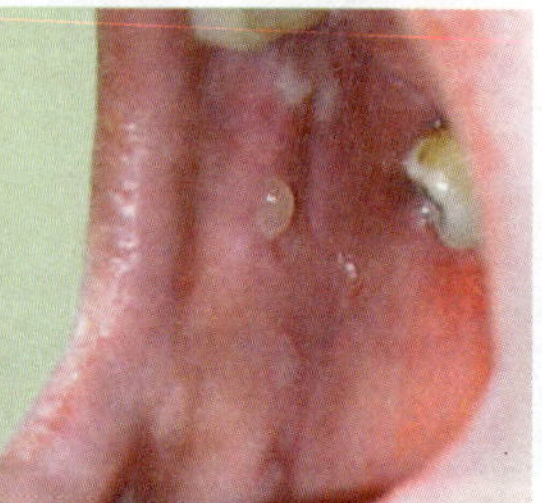

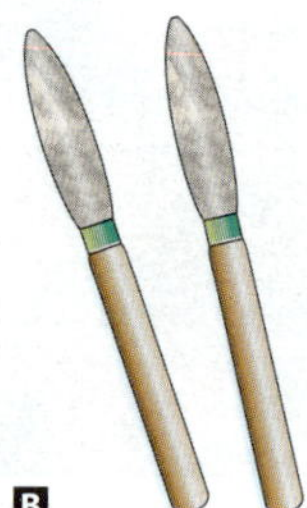

Figs A and B: *(A) Bullous pemphigoid; (B) Diamond bur*

Burnishing is a process of (burnisher) smoothening the surface of a dental amalgam after initial carving by rubbing with a metal instrument having a broad surface.

Burs for low speed pieces burs are made up of steel. These are used to remove caries, trimming dentures and cutting dentin. Burs for air turbine have diamond or tungsten carbide.

Bursa fluid sac which reduces friction between two structures.

Burst fracture of vertebra; it results due to compression force. Fracture is unstable. It may be associated with neurological deficit.

Butterfly cannula is a special needle having flange to facilitate insertion of it and allow it to be taped to the skin. It has a flexible tube into which syringe nozzle fits. It arrows additional injections to be given immediately.

Bypass surgery operation in coronary vessels which have been blocked through atheromatous plaques are literally by-passed. Part of vessel is used to connect aorta to a point beyond occlusion in coronary vessel. Vessel can be a vein of leg or an internal mammary artery. It is generally done when at least 3 vessels are blocked.

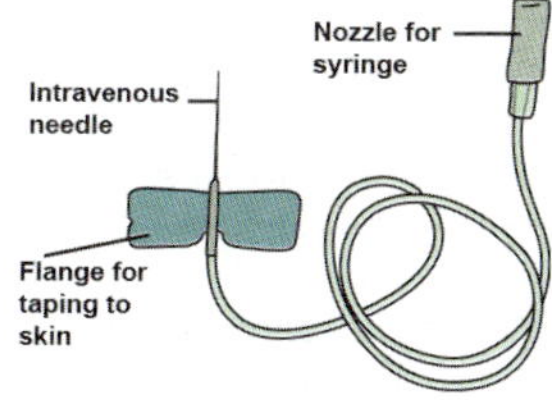

Fig.: *Butterfly intravenous needle (butterfly cannula)*

C

C fibers are the fibers which carry pain with a speed of 2–3 m/sec.

Cachexia refers to the loss of anorexia due to psychological factors. Anxiety and depression may cause the condition. It may also result in lack of nutrition, wasting, may develop in course of chronic disease. General weakness is usually associated with cancer.

Caffey's disease generally affects children. High fever, raised ESR and pleural exudate is seen. Child is hyper-irritable with soft tissue swelling and pain. There is patchy distribution of lesion characterized by remissions and relapses. Marked cortical thickening of mandible is seen.

Calcific metamorphosis is defined as a pulpal response to trauma that is characterized by deposition of hard tissue within the root canal space. Calcific metamorphosis occurs commonly in young adults because of trauma. It is evident usually in the anterior region of the mouth and can partially or totally obliterate the canal space radiographically. Tooth darker in hue than the adjacent teeth and exhibits a dark yellow color because of decrease in translucency from greater thickness of dentin under the enamel. The radiographic appearance of calcific metamorphosis is partial or total obliteration of the pulp canal space with a normal periodontal membrane space and intact lamina dura.

Calcification prolonged heating of a substance just below its melting temperature.

Calcifying odontogenic cyst is a non-aggressive cystic lesion lined by odontogenic epithelium with ghost cell keratinization. Occasionally, it may show aggressive behavior. On X-ray, it appears as a well-defined intrabony lesion that can present as unilocular or multilocular radiolucency. It is well-circumscribed. Calcification can occur as radiopaque areas. It is treated by conservative surgical enucleation.

Calcination prolonged heating of a substance at some temperature below its melting point.

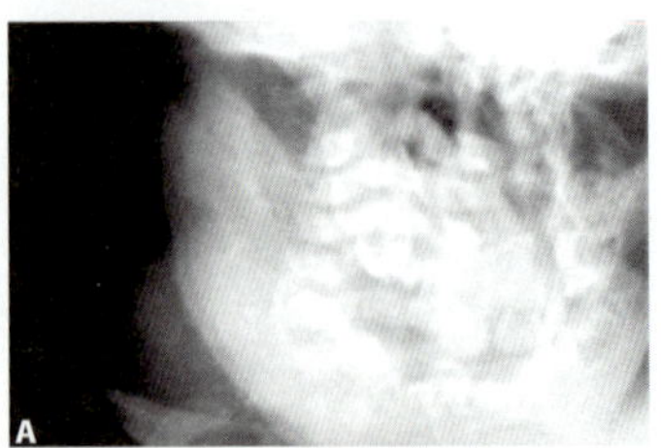

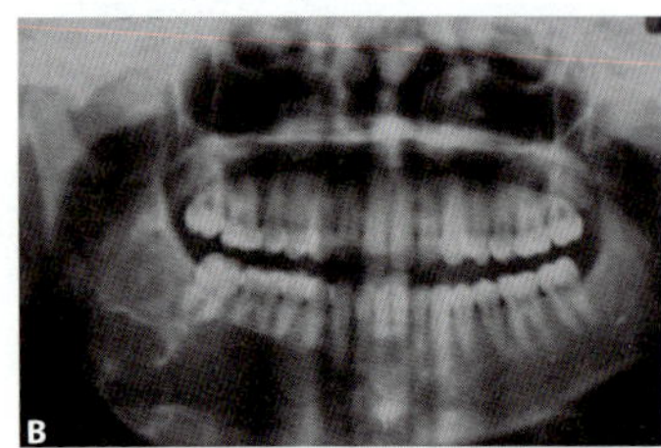

Figs A and B: *(A) Caffey's disease (infantile cortical hyperostosis) showing gross periosteal thickening of mandible; (B) Calcifying odontogenic cyst*

Calcined refers to the powdery, friable, dry substance formed by application of heat.

Calcinosis is the calcification in or under skin. It is of 2 types, calcinosis universalis and circumscripta.

Calcitonin is a peptide hormone secreted by the thyroid gland. It regulates calcium homeostasis.

Calcium 1.5 to 2 percent of total body weight is made up of calcium. More than 90% is in bones and teeth. About 1 g of calcium is found in extracellular fluids and 4-5 g in soft tissues. For adults calcium/phosphorus ratio should be 2:1. Daily requirement is 0.5 g. Milk and dairy products are good sources. Soyabean is a significant source of calcium. In children, lack of calcium affects their growth adversely.

Calcium also plays large role in formation of bones and teeth. In blood, it ranges from 9 to 11 mg/dl. Low concentrations below 8 mg/dl may produce convulsions. Daily requirement in adults is 500 mg, growing child may require a little more. Absorption is hardly 30% of its consumption. Oxalate interferes with calcium absorption forming calcium oxalate. Lactose or milk sugar increases calcium.

Calcium homeostasis refers to the process where calcium participates in neuromuscular function, blood coagulation membrane function and multiple enzyme reactions. Human body contains 25 g/kg of lean body mass. 90% of it is present as calcium phosphate. Daily calcium loss in stool is 100–200 mg as a part of intestinal secretion. D3 helps in absorption of calcium.

Calcium hydroxide is a dental material where it can be used both as a cement for both direct and indirect pulp capping and as a protection barrier beneath composite restoration or it can also be used as antibacterial, root canal medicament, root induction material or an obturating material for primary teeth. The material has an alkaline pH of 11–12 and it functions by stimulating the formation of reparative dentin.

Calculus is an adherent calcified or calcifying mass that forms on the surface of natural teeth and dental prosthesis. Ordinarily calculus consists of mineralized bacterial plaque. It is classified according to its relation to the gingival margin as supragingival and subgingival. It consists of inorganic matter, some water, an organic component made up of desquamated epithelial

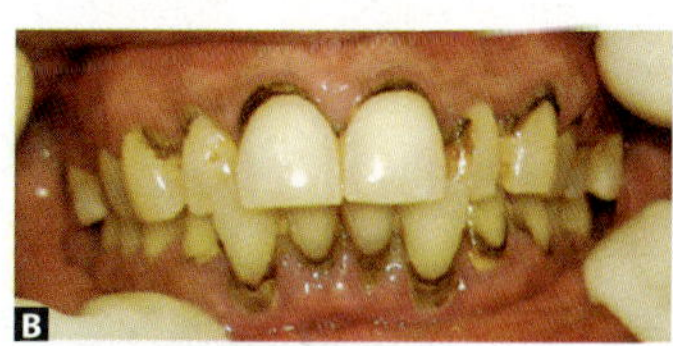

Figs A and B: *(A) Supragingival calculus; (B) Subgingival calculus*

cells, Gram-positive filamentous microorganism such as leptotrichia, some Gram-negative filamentous forms and cocci, leukocytes and an amorphous ground substance. The inorganic component consists mainly of calcium phosphate as hydroxyapatite and other crystalline forms of calcium phosphate such brushite, whitlockite and octacalcium phosphate. There is also a small amount of calcium carbonate and magnesium phosphate as well as fluoride.

Callus is the structure that unites the two broken ends of the bone. It is composed of fibrous tissue, cartilage and bone. Internal callus is new bone arising from marrow cavity, while external callus is new bone formed around two fragments. As callus formation progresses the cartilage cells begin to mature and cartilage begins to mature. Cartilage begins to calcify.

Calorie equivalent is the number of kilo calories produced per liter of oxygen consumed.

Calorie: In Physics, energy is defined as capacity to do work. The body needs energy to maintain body temperature for metabolite purposes, to support growth and for physical activity. One kilocalorie is the amount of heat required to raise the temperature of one kilogram of water from 15° to 16°C.

Canal blockage is obstruction in a previously patent canal system that prevents access to the apical constriction or apical stop.

Canal orifices are openings in the floor of pulp chamber leading into the root canals.

Canal transportation apical canal transportation is moving the position of canal's normal anatomic foramen to a new location on external root surface.

Cancellous bone see trabecular bone.

Canalicular adenoma develops in intra-oral accessory salivary glands and in upper lip in elderly age group. It is a slowly growing, well-circumscribed, firm nodule, especially in lip. It is not fixed and

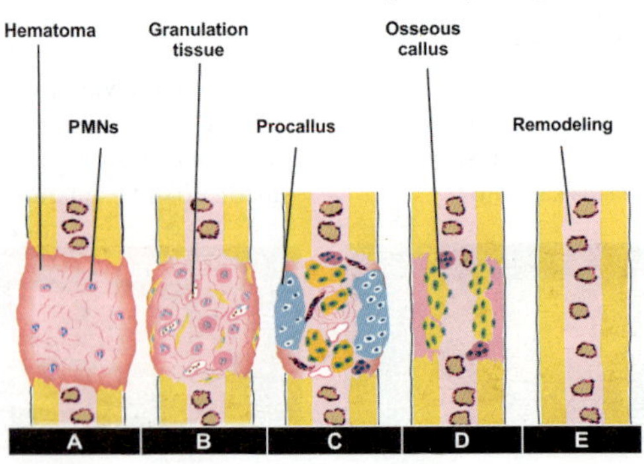

Fig.: *Callus formation*

is composed of long strands or cords of epithelial cells arranged in double row. Enucleation of lesion is the treatment of choice.

Cancer refers to an abnormal growth of cells that can invade and destroy surrounding normal tissues and sometimes spread to other parts of the body.

Candida associated denture stomatitis is a common ailment in wearers of full denture. It is also common in patients wearing orthodontic appliances or obturators for cleft palate. Patient may be symptom free.

Candida hypersensitivity syndrome is a triad of symptoms that includes fatigue, headache/rashes oral or vaginal infection with Candida. Nystatin therapy generally does not help.

Canine refers to the third incisor tooth from the midline of the oral cavity. It has the longest crown root with the sharp cusp which performs the tearing action.

Canophile is an organism that grows best in the presence of increased concentration of CO_2.

Cap splints are the silver–copper alloy type of splints which fit on-to the tooth in a cap or crown form along with locking plates and connecting bars for the immobilization of all types of jaw fractures. The technique is time consuming both clinically as well as in the laboratory.

Cap stage is the second stage of tooth development where cells of dental lamina proliferate to form a concavity which produces cap-like appearance. It shows outer and inner enamel epithelia and stellate reticulum. The rim of the enamel organ, i.e. where inner and outer enamel epithelia are joined is called cervical loop. As the cells of loop proliferate, enamel organ assumes bell stage.

Capillary hemangiomas are well defined hemangiomas that appear from bright-red to purple patches. Common sites are skin, subcutaneous tissue and mucous membrane of oral cavity and lips. Hemosiderin represents the ruptured vessels. These may also be found in liver, bones, stomach and small intestine.

Capillary hemorrhage refers to the bleeding occurring from the capillaries. The wound bleeds slowly. The blood is bright-red in color and oozes from many points.

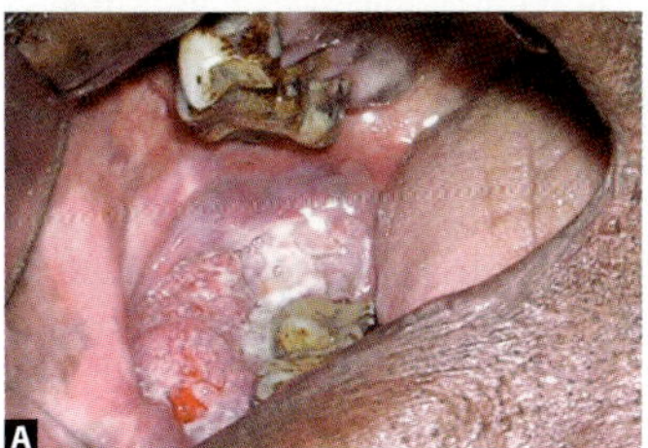

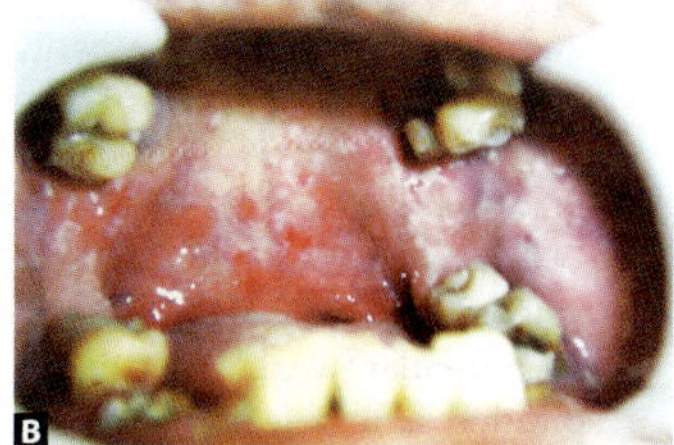

Figs A and B: *(A) Carcinoma of lower alveolus; (B) Candida associated stomatitis*

C

Capillary penetration is the movement of a liquid into crevice or tube because of capillary pressure.

Capsule is a fibrous or membranous connective tissue envelop.

Carbohydrate intolerance is the inability of the body to completely process the nutrient carbohydrate (a classification that includes sugars and starches) into a source of energy for the body, usually because of the deficiency of an enzyme needed for digestion. Lactose intolerance, the inability to digest the sugar found in milk, is widespread and affects up to 70% of the world's adult population.

Carbohydrates are the richest source of energy. About 70-80% of total energy is supplied by carbohydrate. It contains carbon, hydrogen and oxygen. Each gram of it provides 4.1 calories minimum of 100 g of carbohydrate is needed in diet.

Carbon monoxide is a colorless, odorless and non-irritant gas which cannot be perceived by senses. Whenever carbon is burnt some carbon monoxide is formed. It is highly poisoning gas which is absorbed through lungs.

Carbon monoxide poisoning develops by breathing air which is contaminated by coal gas in badly ventilated room. Below 10–20% concentration causes lassitude, headache and shortness of breath; 20–30% concentrations menifests as will have severe throbbing headache, muscular weakness, hurried respiration and defective memory and might faint. 30–40% concentration produces uncoordinated movement, mental confusion, defective sight and hearing. 40–50% concentration results in behavior like that of a drunken person and loss of power. Increasing confusion and hallucination will also develop. 50–60% concentration results in comma followed by convulsions. Skin will become pink. 60–70% results in deep coma. Incontinence of urine and feces will develop. 70–80% concentration results in quick death.

Carbon steel refers to an alloy of carbon and iron with less than 2% carbon present.

Carbuncle is a lesion where there is swelling of short duration. It is present commonly on the neck. It may be bluish-red in color. There are multiple openings with pus giving a sieve like appearance. It is diffuse and tender and can be commonly seen in diabetic patient.

Carcinoma in situ is a premalignant condition where it is very difficult to differentiate it from dysplasia. There is no individual cell keratinization, no epithelial pearl formation and no hyperkeratosis. Lesions may be flat, red, velvety and granular. Severe dysplastic changes in white lesion are an indication of precancerous state. More severe grade of dysplasia is carcinoma in situ. Lesions of carcinoma in situ are to be treated vigorously with local excision. Wider surrounding area should also be removed, regional nodes are generally not removed. Majority of these lesions occur in floor of mouth.

Carcinoma of buccal mucosa refers to the malignant ulcer affecting buccal mucosa. Chewing of tobacco is commonly involved. Verrucous carcinoma develops in case of chewing tobacco. Leukoplakia is a common predecessor of it. Cheek biting and dental irritation from jagged teeth may rarely cause it. Lesion is painful ulceration. Superficial lesions may grow outwards. Incidence of metastases is high. Maxillary lymph glands are commonly involved.

Carcinoma of floor of mouth refers to the lesion affecting floor of the mouth. Smoking pipe or cigar is the main etiology. Generally, there is indurated ulcer of varying size situated on one side of midline. It may be painful. Carcinoma may invade deeper structure and may involve submaxillary or sublingual gland. Involvement of tongue results in slurring of speech. Metastases spread to submaxillary group of lymph nodes. Even small tumors recur after surgical excision, otherwise prognosis is fair.

Carcinoma of gingiva generally develops after extraction of tooth. Carcinoma initiates as ulceration, purely erosive lesion. Fixed gingiva is more commonly involved.

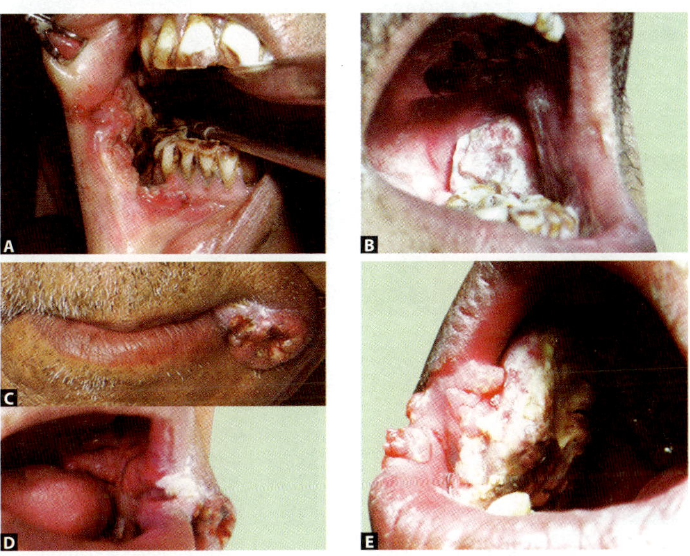

Figs A to E: *(A) Carcinoma of buccal mucosa; (B) Carcinoma of buccal mucosa near retromolar pad; (C) Advanced carcinoma of buccal mucosa involving angle of mouth; (D) Advanced carcinoma of buccal mucosa (intraoral view); (E) Carcinoma of buccal mucosa involving angle of mouth*

It generally involves maxilla. Mandibular gingiva metastasis occurs more than maxillary gingiva. Metastasis is a common sequel of gingival carcinoma. Prognosis is not very good.

Carcinoma of lip refers to the malignant lesion occurring on the lip. Pipe smokers are commonly involved. It involves vermillion border of lip of one side. It starts as area of thickening, indurations and irregular ulceration. Later, it may produce an exophytic proliferative growth. Carcinoma is slow to metastasize. Sub-mental and sub-maxillary nodes of same side are involved. Surgical excision followed by radiotherapy may help.

Carcinoma of maxillary sinus is often hopelessly advanced before patient comes to know about it. There is development of swelling and bulging of alveolar ridge, mucobuccal fold and elongation of maxillary molars. Patient complains of unilateral nasal stiffness along with discharge. Various walls of antrum may be involved. Ulceration into oral cavity may develop. Metastasis generally does not occur.

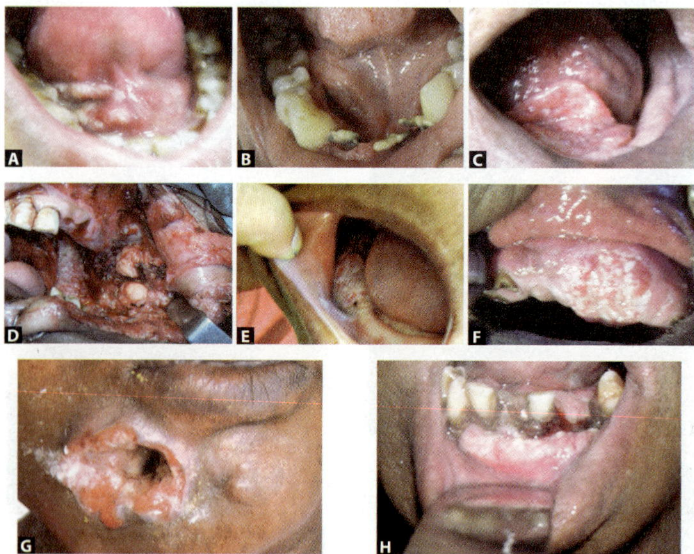

Figs A to H: *Carcinoma (A) Floor of mouth; (B) Floor of mouth and lower gingivobuccal sulcus; (C) Tongue involving floor of mouth; (D) Upper gingival sulcus; (E) Lower gingival mucosa in an edentulous patient; (F) Upper gingival mucosa; (G) Advanced carcinoma of lower GB sulcus with oro-cutaneous fistula; (H) Carcinoma of lower gingivolabial sulcus*

Carcinoma of palate is poorly defined ulcerated painful lesion on one side of midline. It may invade bone and nasal cavity. Metastasis to regional lymph nodes is common. As treatment, both surgery and radiotherapy has been used.

Carcinoma of pancreas occurs most commonly in 50–60 years of age. Tumors of head of pancreas present with weight loss, obstructive jaundice and gastric pain. When mass is palpable surgery loses its use. Liver is enlarged. Gallbladder is palpable. Elevated alkaline phosphatase and bilirubin reflect common duct obstruction or hepatic metastasis. Carcinoma of distal common bile duct present with weight loss, obstructive jaundice and palpable gallbladder.

Carcinoma of tongue is common carcinoma of oral cavity. Leukoplakia may predispose it. There is formation of painless mass or ulcer. Pain develops on infection. Developed mass can be exophytic or may infiltrate to deep layers of the tongue. It results in indurations and fixation. It develops on lateral border or ventral surface of tongue. Treatment is complicated and prognosis is not good.

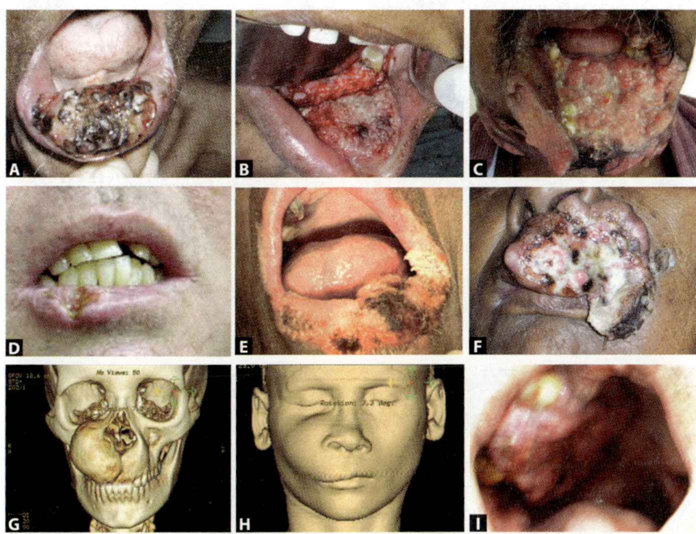

Figs A to F: *(A and B) Carcinoma of lower lip; (C) Carcinoma lower lip; (D) Carcinoma of lip; (E) Carcinoma of lower lip also involving angle of the mouth; (F) Advanced carcinoma of upper lip; (G) Carcinoma of maxillary antrum; (H) Carcinoma of palate and uvula; (I) Carcinoma of maxilla with involvement of hard palate*

Carcinoma stomach may be associated with H. pylori. Adenocarcinoma comprises 95% of cases with variable degree of differentiation. Polyoid type is well differentiated.

Cardiac arrest refers to the most serious complication of collapse followed after angina or myocardial infarction. Signs of cardiac arrest include sudden unconsciousness, absence of breathing and pulse and dilated pupils.

Cardiac impulse is an action potential that occurs in the cardiac conduction tissue.

Cardiac edema refers to the right ventricle failure edema, systemic in distribution and all tissues and organs. In left ventricle failure, the lungs are primarily affected. Edema is in lungs. Cardiac edema is a generalized edema.

Cardiac muscle, involuntary muscles, found in heart. Like skeletal muscle, cardiac muscle is striated. Cardiac muscle cells are long branching cells and fit tight. These tight fitting junctions promote rapid conduction of electrical signals throughout

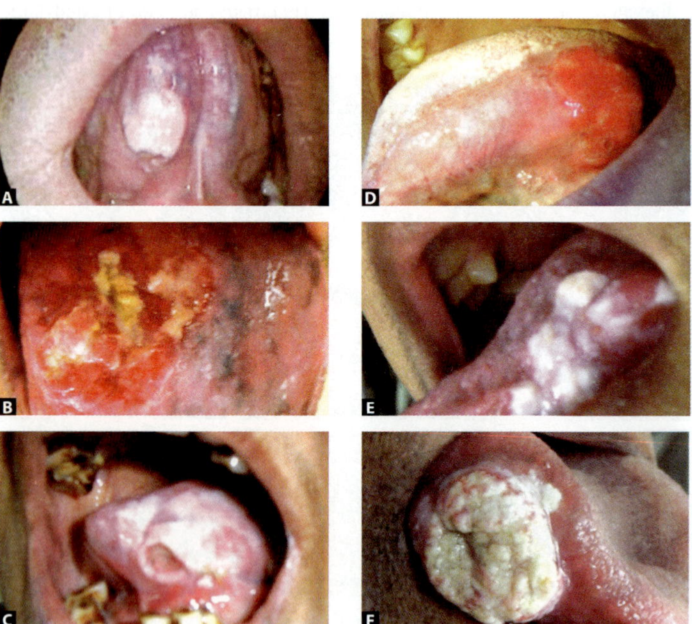

Figs A to I: *(A and B) Carcinoma of tongue; (C) Carcinoma of tongue—ulcerative growth; (D) Carcinoma of tongue—ulceroinfiltrative growth; (E and F) Carcinoma of tongue—exophytic growth*

heart. Cardiac muscle is not under voluntary control.

Cardiac toothache severe referred pain felt in mandible and maxilla from area outside the head and neck region is most commonly from the heart. Cardiac pain is clinically characterized by heaviness, tightness or throbbing pain in the substernal region which commonly radiates to left shoulder, arm, neck and mandible. Cardiac pain is most commonly experienced on the left side rather than right. In advanced stages, the patient may complain of severe pain and rubs the jaw and chest. In present time, dentist should be aware of incidence of jaw pain, which is occurring in a number of patients secondary to cardiac pain. Sometimes, patient presents dental complaints as the chief complaint rather than having pain in substernal region, it creates confusion in diagnosis for dental pain. A lack of dental cause for dental pain should always be an alerting sign. Anesthetizing the lower jaw or providing dental treatment does not decrease the tooth pain, it indicates that primary source of pain is not the tooth. Usually, the cardiac toothache is decreased by taking rest or a dose of sublingual nitroglycerin.

Cardinal leprosy presentation includes hypopigmented skin lesions with loss of sensation or absence of sweating. Nerve involvement is manifested by nerve thickening and/or tenderness. Skin smear may be positive for M. leprae. When the skin smear is negative presence of other 2 cardinal sign is sufficient to make a diagnosis of leprosy.

Cardiogenic shock in systolic BP falls to less than 80 mm Hg or 30 mm Hg less than baseline. It will result in narrowed pulse pressure. There may be rapid, weak and occasionally irregular pulse. Peripheral vasoconstriction causes cyanosis of extremities giving pale, cool and clammy skin. Person may become restless and anxious. Oliguria and confusion develops.

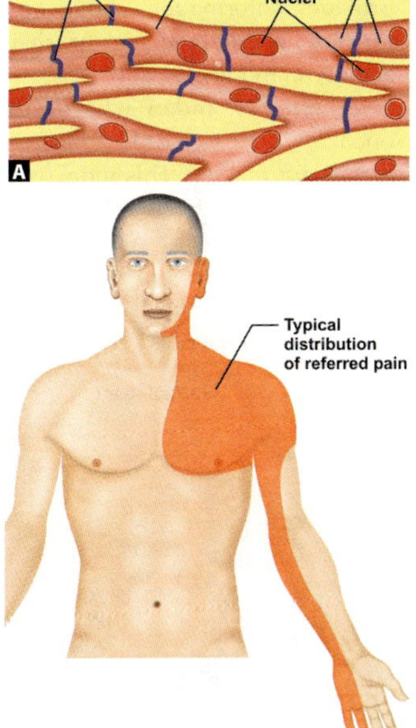

Figs A and B: *(A) Cardiac muscle; (B) Cardiac toothache*

Cardiomyopathy is a group of diseases involving primarily the heart muscle.

Cardiospasm refers to the weak or peristalsis through lower esophagus and failure of relaxation of cardiac in response to peristaltic wave of swallowing. There develops gradual or sudden onset of dysphagia. To start with, food regurgitates and later on when dilation of esophagus takes place food accumulates. Pain is relieved by drinking cold water. Endoscopy shows chronically inflamed mucosa.

Caries activity test is a quick test that provides information about acid forming microorganisms or their activity in mouth.

Caries severity index was developed by Tank Certrude and Storvick Clara in 1960. This index was developed to study the depth and extent of the caries surfaces and the extent of pulpal involvements. The progress of the dental caries in stages as described by Massler and Schour in 1952, were modified and this caries severity index was devised to measure the extent and depth of decayed surfaces and pulpal involvements based on clinical and radiographic examinations.

Caries susceptibility index was developed by Richardson in 1961, for assessing caries susceptibility. This index is based on Bodecker and Mellanby caries indices. There are two factors involved in measuring caries susceptibility using the dynamic survey, namely:
a. Amount of tooth surfaces at risk,
b. Amount of caries developing during the period of observation.
'b' divided by 'a' will give a measure of susceptibility.

Caring skills are the nursing skills to maintain patient's health.

Cariogram is a new method of illustrating an interaction of factors contributing to the development of caries. It has been introduced by Bratthall, et al. (1999). A pie circle diagram is divided into 5 sectors in the following colors:

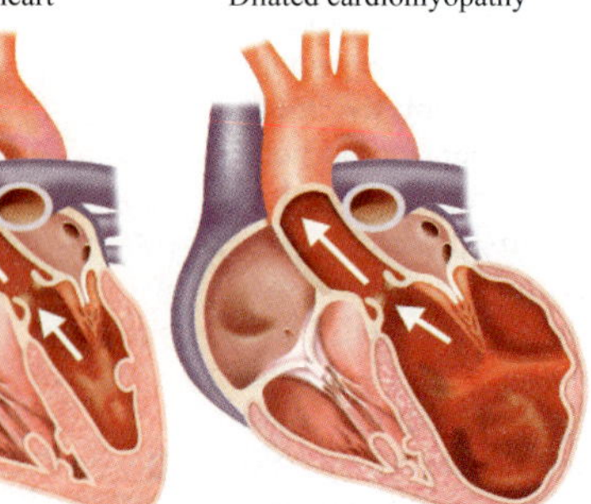

Fig.: *Cardiomyopathy*

Green—shows an estimation of the chance to avoid caries. Dark blue—'diet' is based on a combination of diet contents and diet frequency. Red—bacteria are based on a combination of amount of plaque and mutans streptococci. Light blue sector—'susceptibility' is based on a combination of fluoride program, saliva secretion and salivary buffering capacity. Yellow sector—'circumstances' is based on a combination of past caries experience and related disease.

Carotid artery syndrome refers to the transient cerebral ischemia with contralateral weakness of arm and leg. Mental confusion and phemisensory disturbance will take place.

Carotid sinus is the term applied to a dilated segment of the common carotid body located at its bifurcation. The dilatation usually extends onto the initial part of the internal carotid artery, and may be confined to it.

Carpus is the proximal portion of hand that contains the eight bones.

Carrier is one who is carrying a disease without being aware of it or is not having clinical symptoms.

Carrying angle is the angle forming at elbow between center line of humerus and forearm. Angle in normal person is 5° in men and 10 to 15° in women. Carrying angle bilaterally should be symmetrical.

Cartilage is a firm, elastic, flexible connective tissue that is attached to articulate bone surfaces forming certain part of skeleton.

Carver is an instrument used to shape restorative material.

Case fatality rate represents the killing power of a disease. It is simply the ratio of death to cases. It can be calculated.

Case study is a method of structuring a qualitative research project by detailed analysis of a well-defined unit or case.

Castable ceramic is used to case crowns by the lost wax process. It is used in single anterior and posterior crowns.

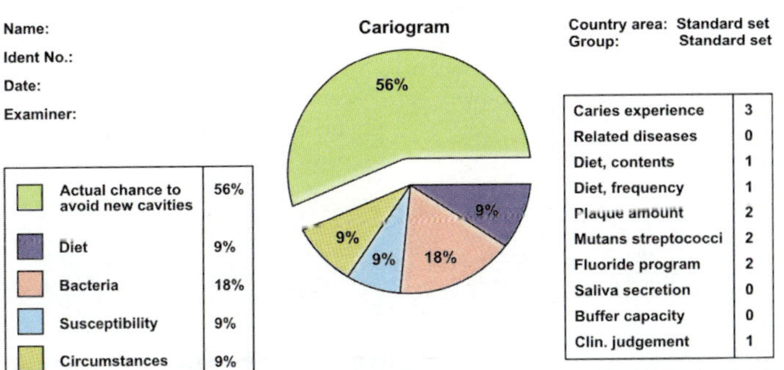

Fig.: *Cariogram*

C

Casts in urine are portion of gelled protein like material which are moulds of interior of tubules. Hyaline casts appear as clear cylinders in febrile illness. Red cell casts are RBCs seen in subacute glomerulonephritis. White cell casts are hyaline casts with WBCs seen in chronic pyelonephritis. Epithelial cell cast is seen in tubular necrosis while granular cast is seen in chronic glomerulonephritis. Fatty cast is composed of epithelial cells. Waxy cast is more opaque.

Casual comparative research is a non-experimental research in which assignment to groups is based on pre existing characteristic or attributes of subjects.

CAT stands for computerized axial tomography.

Catabolism is a metabolic breakdown of complex molecules into simpler molecules, i.e. there is the breakdown of food compounds or cytoplasm into simpler compound. Process releases energy.

Catalyst is a chemical that speeds up reactions without being changed. When proteins play a role of catalysts, these are known as enzymes.

Catamenia menstruation.

Catarrh is an inflammation of mucous membrane of nose and throat. It is a non-productive cough.

Catatonia is marked inhibition or excitation in motor behavior developing in psychotic disorder.

Catatonia stupor and muscle rigidity seen in schizophrenia .

Catheterization is a process where the passage of flexible tube into bladder through the urethra is performed for the withdrawal of urine.

Cathode is a negative electrode in X-ray tube. It supplies the electrons necessary to generate X-rays.

Cation refers to the positively charged particle.

Caudal means towards the tail.

Cauder equine syndrome is a syndrome caused by compression of cauda equine. There will be bladder complaints as well as motor anesthesia with incontinence or urinary retention. Symptoms include low back pain, incontinence of urine and bilateral sciatica. Person may develop fecal retention and saddle anesthesia.

Causalgia is an unpleasant burning type of continuous pain following peripheral nerve injuries. It is more common in hand and arm. Skin of the affected area has spontaneous pain and perspires excessively.

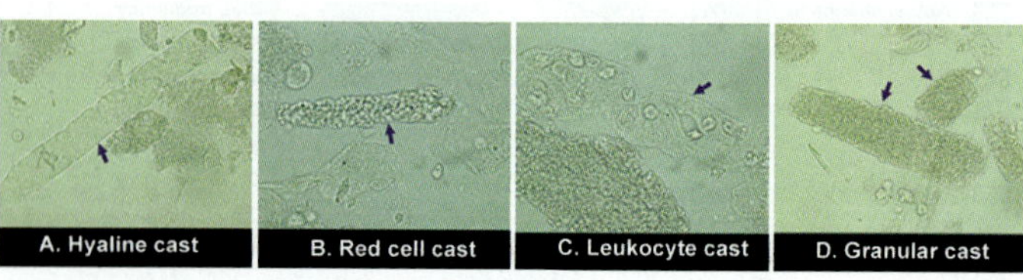

Figs A to D: *Cast in urine*

Patient will not allow skin to be touched.

Cauterize is to burn, corrode or destroy living tissue by means of caustic soda, heated metal or electric current.

Cavitation is a cavity in a tooth resulting from caries process. It appears as radiolucent lesion on radiograph.

Cavity liners are liquid suspensions of zinc oxide or calcium hydroxide. It can be applied in a thin film to the surface of cavity. Cavity liners neutralize the free acid of zinc phosphate and silicate cements.

Cavity preparation is a mechanical alteration of defective, injured or diseased tooth in order to best receive a restorative material which will reestablish a healthy state for the tooth including esthetic correction where indicated, along with normal form and function.

Cavity primers are solutions that are used to increase the adaptation of methylmethacrylate filling materials to cavity walls. It seals the margins.

Cavity varnishes are solutions of one or more resins from natural gums, synthetic resins. It reduces postoperative sensitivity by sealing the open ends of dentin tubules with a glaze-like covering, but being thin it is insufficient to provide thermal insulation. Varnishes check the microleakage of fluids around the margins of restorations.

Cavosurface margin is the contact between the cavity surface. The tooth surface location where the walls and line angles meet the unaltered tooth surface.

CCD technology is usually made of a chip of pure covalently bonded silicon atoms. When the chip is exposed to visible light or X-ray radiation, bonds are broken, and charged electron hole pairs are formed. The electrical charge created is captured, amplified, converted, and displayed as an image.

CD_4: Promote proliferation, maturation and immunologic function of other cell types.

CD_{44} are the hematopoietic progenitor cells express the most truncated form of cd_{44}, which bind hyaluronic acid, a gag found in extracellular matrix (ecm). Therefore a wide variety of adhesive interactions between cell-cell and cell-ecm are critical for hematopoiesis.

CD_8/cytotoxic t-cells/tc are those cells that have an ability to kill cells and have foreign molecules on their surface.

Cell culture is an in vitro growth of cells, although the cells proliferate they do not organize into tissue.

Cell mediated immunity is a resistance to disease organisms resulting from the actions of cells especially sensitized T cells.

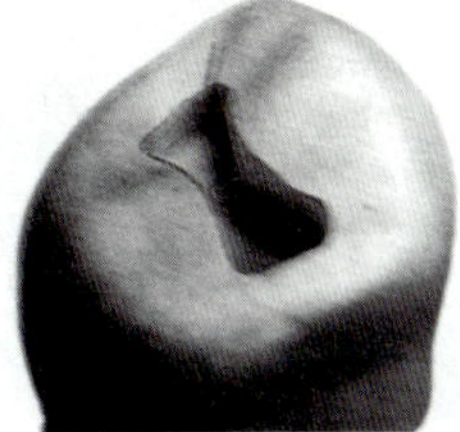

Fig.: *Cavosurface margin*

C

Cell-free zone of weil is located immediately subjacent to the odontoblast layer, which is 40 mm in width and is relatively free of cells. It is traversed by capillaries and unmyelinated nerve fibers. This zone may or may not be apparent in young pulps, where dentin forms rapidly or in older pulps, where reparative dentin is being produced.

Cell-poor zone see cell-free zone of weil.

Cell-rich zone of pulp, this layer is located immediately subjacent to the cell-poor zone. It is much prominent in the coronal pulp than in the radicular pulp. This zone is richly populated with fibroblasts, along with macrophages, dendritic cells and lymphocytes. It forms as a result of peripheral migration of cells populating the central regions of the pulp, commencing at the time of tooth eruption. Although cell division within the cell-rich zone is a rare occurrence in normal pulps, death of odontoblasts causes a greater increase in the rate of mitosis. It acts as a reservoir for the replacement of irreversibly damaged odontoblasts.

Cellulitis refers to an inflammation of soft tissues. It is a local pain ana swelling of acute onset with pyrexia and general debility. Streptococci are particularly potent producing hyalurodinase and causing cellulitis. Cellulitis of face and neck develops mostly due to dental infection. Person is ill with fever and increased WBC count. There is painful swelling of soft tissue. Its boundaries are not very well defined. Skin is of pinkish color and lymph glands are enlarged. Cellulitis is treated by antibiotics. Infection of sublingual space produces swelling of the floor of mouth.

Cement base is a layer of cement commonly used beneath a permanent dental restoration with purpose to encourage recovery of injured pulp or otherwise protect pulp against injury. Better cement base is zinc oxide eugenol and calcium hydroxide. Glass ionomer cement is polyacrylate based and has anticarinogenic properties.

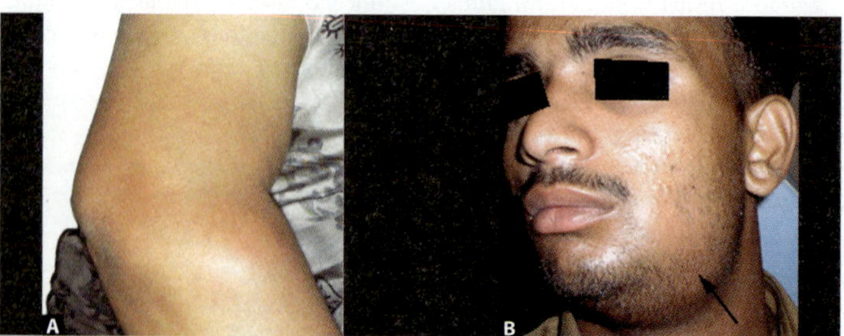

Figs A and B: *(A) Cellulitis of hand; (B) Cellulitis involving floor of the mouth*

Cement sealer is a compound used in filling of a root canal. It is put in plastic form which solidifies after placement. It fills the irregularities of canal.

Cementation is the process where the appliance is glued on to the associated area.

Cementicles are small foci of calcified tissue not necessarily true cementum. It lies free on periodontal ligament. These are developed by calcification of nests of epithelial cells. The pattern of calcification gives appearance of a circular lamellated structure. Cementicles may arise from focal calcification of connective tissue sometimes calcification occurs as small, round or ovoid globules of calcium salt. Cementicles are of no clinical significance.

Cementodentinal junction(CDJ) is the region where cementum and dentin are united, the point at which cemental surface terminates at or near the apex of tooth. Actually it, is also known as neck or cervix of tooth. It is not always necessary that CDJ always coincide with apical constriction. Location of CDJ ranges from 0.5 to 3 mm short of anatomic apex. Working width is defined as, "initial and postinstrumentation horizontal dimensions of the root canal system at working length and other levels". The minimum initial working width corresponds to initial apical file size which binds at working length. The maximum final working width corresponds to the master apical file size.

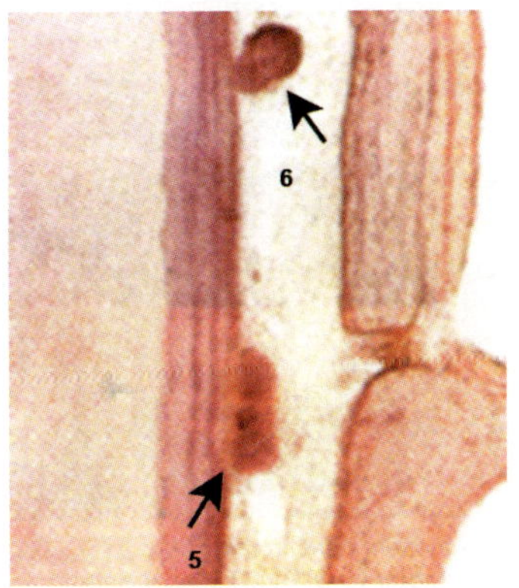

Fig.: *Cementicles*

Cementum can be defined as hard, avascular connective tissue that covers the roots of the teeth. It is light yellow in color and can be differentiated from enamel by its darker hue and lack of luster. It is very permeable to dyes and chemical agents, from the pulp canal and the external root surface. The main function of cementum is to provide attachment of the tooth to alveolar bone. Union of cementum and dentin is known as dentino-cemental junction. Like dentin, cementum also shows continuous growth. Junction between the enamel and cementum is called cemento-enamel junction. Cementum has the same hardness as that of bone. Composition—50% of inorganic substance, 50% of organic and water.

Cemento-ossifying fibroma is uncommon and a well-circumscribed lesion. It undergoes slow expansile growth usually in mandibular or molar region. It causes painless swelling between 20–40 years. It is radiolucent with varying degree of calcification in center. Roots of related tooth can be displaced. It may have a definable capsule so can easily be enucleated.

Center of gravity is the center of one's weight, half above and half below. Similarly, it is half on left and half on right.

Central buttressing bone formation is the process of compensatory bone formation occurring within the jaw in an attempt to buttress bony trabaculae which is weakened by bone resorption.

Central cementifying fibroma is a neoplasm of bone and may develop at any age. Mandible is more affected. Radiographically one can notice radiolucent area with no radio-opacities. It is composed of delicate interlacing collagen fibers arranged in discrete bundles. Mitotic figures

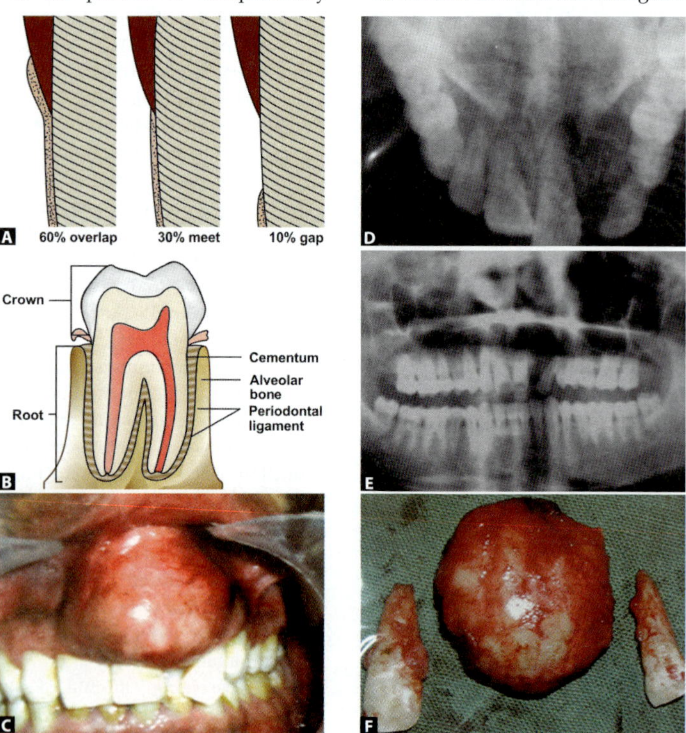

Figs A to F: *(A) Cementoenamel junction; (B) Cementum; [(C to F—C) Cemento-ossifying fibroma) Intraoral view; (D) Occlusal view; (E) Panoramic view; (F) Surgically excised]*

may be present in small number. It has to be excised carefully.

Central giant cell granuloma generally develops in younger age group. Pain is not a common feature. Slight bulging of jaw is noted. On X-ray, it is a destructive lesion showing radiolucent area. Borders may be smooth or ragged. Larger lesions show loculations. Cortex is thin and extended. Teeth may be displaced. It is made up of connective tissue stroma and many interspersed proliferating fibroblasts and small capillaries. It is a benign intraosseous destructive giant cell lesion. Generally, anterior part of jaw bone is affected. It is a reactive lesion. Clinical features: It affects mandible more than maxilla. Some lesions may cross the midline. It is a small, slow enlarging, and bony hard swelling of jaw. Lesion may cause perforation of cortical plate. Teeth in affected region are always vital. Radiographically, lesion shows multilocular radiolucent area in jaw and it gives a soap bubble appearance. When unilocular, it will show a drop-shaped appearance. Histologically, central giant cell granuloma shows multinucleated giant cells. Several areas of hemorrhage and hemosiderin pigmentation are also seen. Around these blood capillaries are also found. Treatment includes excision and curettage.

Central hearing impairment is an abnormality of the auditory system in the brain associated with sensorineural hearing loss.

Central incisors are used for cutting or biting food, these are the first of the four anterior teeth.

Central nervous system includes brain and spinal cord.

Central ossifying fibroma represents a well-demarcated expansile jaw lesion. It is well-encapsulated. Children and young adults are affected. Clinical features: There is usually a single lesion. There is localized painless non-tendered bony hard swelling in jaw. Tumor is slow growing but may disfigure the face. In some cases, displacement of teeth may be seen due to expansion and distortion of cortical plates. Histopathologically, highly cellular fibroblastic stroma with 'whorled pattern' collagen fibers may be noted. It may occur at any age.

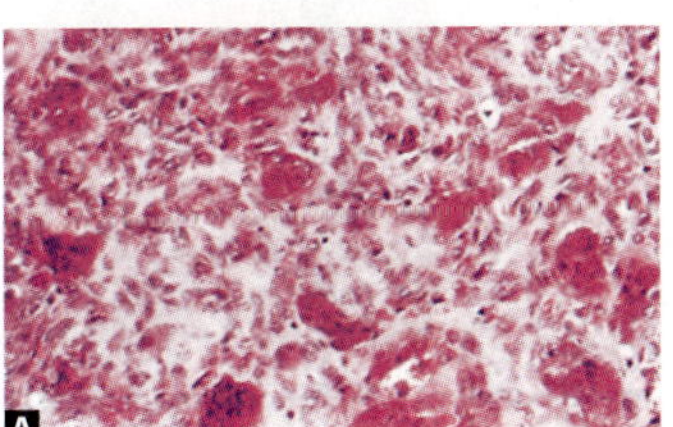

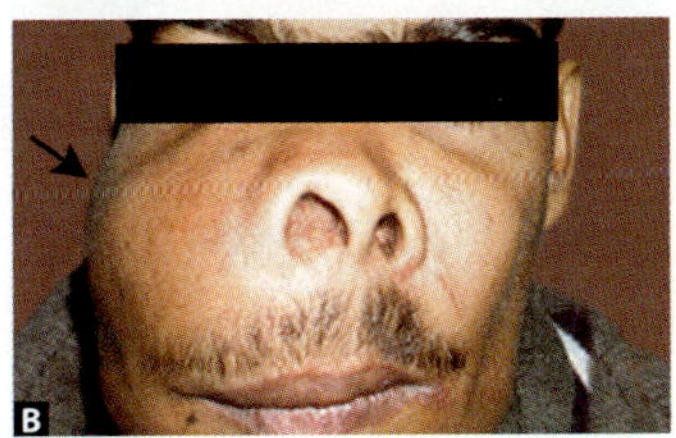

Figs A and B: *Central giant cell granuloma (A) Histologic view; (B) Extraoral view exhibiting a disfigured face*

There is predilection for mandible. Until swelling develops symptoms does not develop. Displacement of teeth may be one of the early features. It is slow growing. Lesion contains delicate interlacing collagen fibers. Mitotic figures may be present.

Central ray is the central portion of the primary beam of radiation.

Centric occlusion is the relationship of the occlusal surfaces of one arch to those in the opposing arch at physical rest position.

Centric occlusion refers to the closing of jaws in a position that produces maximum stable contact between the occluding surfaces of the maxillary and mandibular teeth.

Centric relation is the relationship of the maxillary arch to the mandibular arch when the condyle is in its most retracted position or the most cranial position of the mandible along the retruded path of closure.

Cephalic vein one of the four superficial veins of upper limb.

Cephalocaudal gradient of growth is an axis of increased growth extending from head towards the feet. In the fetal life, at about the third month, the head takes up almost 50% of total body length. At this stage, cranium is large relative to the face and represents more than half of total head. In contrast, limbs are still rudimentary and the trunk is underdeveloped. By the time of birth, the trunk and limbs are grown faster than head and face so that the proportion of entire body devoted to head has decreased about 30%. The overall pattern of growth, thereafter follows this

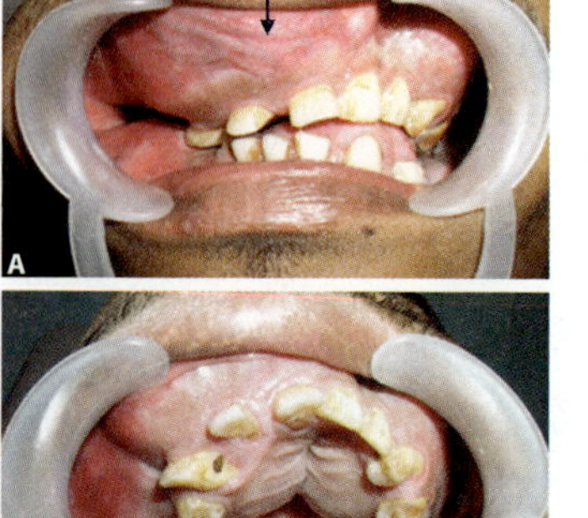

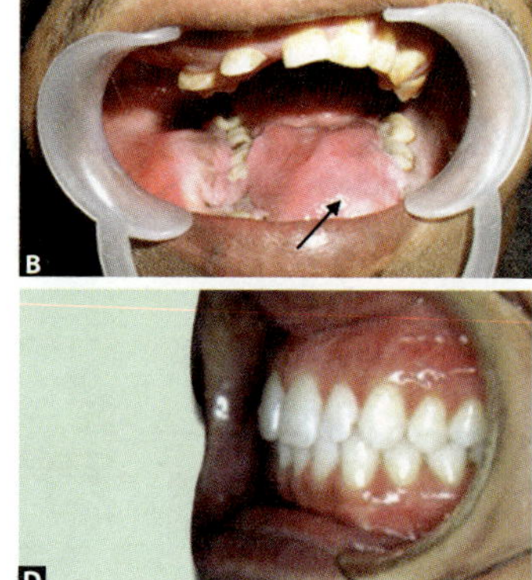

Figs A to D: *(A) Giant cell granuloma intraoral view showing movement of maxilla along with the displacement of tooth; (B) Giant cell granuloma intraoral involving palate; (C) Giant cell granuloma intraoral view involving mandible; (D) Centric occlusion*

course with progressive reduction of relative size of the head to about 12% of adult.

Cephalometric, this technique has contributed significantly to the knowledge of human cranio-facial skeletal growth. Cephalometry makes it possible to take serial radiographs of a patient's skull in order to study the growth changes taking place.

Cephalometric film an extra oral X-ray film used to view bony and soft tissue areas of facial profile.

Cephalosporin is a bactericidal drug that contains a beta-lactam ring. These are broad-spectrum antibiotics. There are many different cephalosporins with varying side chains; these side chains alter the pharmacokinetics, spectrum of activity and beta-lactamase resistance. Cephalosporins are relatively expensive and, although a good alternative to penicillin when a broad-spectrum drug is required, should not be used as first choice unless the organism is known to be sensitive.

Ceramic is a compound of metallic and non-metallic elements. Its fully oxidized materials are, therefore chemically stable. So these don't elicit adverse biological response. However, metal do oxidize. Two types of 'inert' ceramics of interest are carbon and alumina; dental gypsum, zinc phosphate and porcelains are example of ceramic material.

Cerebellar ataxia appears in druken patient. Patient walks on a broad base. Feet are planted wide apart and placed irregularly. Ataxia is severe in open as well as in closed eyes.

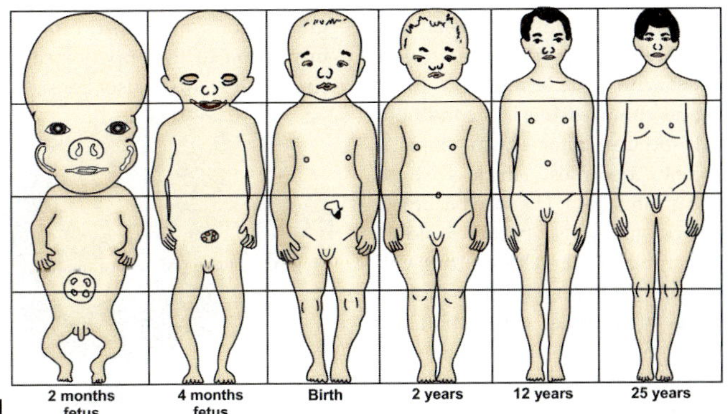

Figs A and B: *(A) Central Ray; (B) Cephalocaudal gradient of growth*

C

Cerebellar gait the main feature of this gait is wide base, unsteadiness and irregularity of steps. On getting up from chair, irregular swaying of trunk takes place. Standing heel to toe in a straight line is difficult. With lesions of thalamus and midbrain ataxic signs on opposite side develop. It is common in alcoholics, long-term dilantin intake and multiple sclerosis.

Cerebellum is a part of the brain that is located in posterior fossa and is separated by tentorium cerebella. It comprises median vermis and two lateral cerebellar hemispheres. It is comprised by a layer of cortex and an internal mass of white matter in which cerebellar nuclei are located. The lesion of flocculonodular lobe causes trunk ataxia, swaying and staggering. Paleocerebellum controls antigravity muscles. Neocerebellum controls fine coordinated movements of hands. Extensive lesion of anterior lobe causes hypotonia, postural abnormalities, ataxia and mild weakness of ipsilateral arm and leg. Hypotonia is more apparent with acute lesions.

Cerebral compression is a condition that occurs after head injury. Patient becomes restless and passes into coma. His face becomes flushed and pulse becomes slow. On paralyzed side-temperature will be more. Pupil on the side of lesion dilates after initial contraction. In last stage, both the pupils dilate and become fixed.

Cerebral dura mater is a thick fibrous membrane. It can be divided into a cerebral part lying in the cranial cavity. A spinal part lying in the vertebral canal. The arachnoid mater is a thin membrane. There are no blood vessels in it. The arachnoid mater is separated from the dura mater by the subdural space. On both sides (dural and arachnoid), the surface lining this capillary interval is smooth. This facilitates slight movement between the dura and arachnoid. Pia mater is thicker than the arachnoid mater. In contrast to the arachnoid mater, it is highly vascular, and the blood vessels in it are important for supply of the underlying brain. The pia and arachnoid are separated by the subarachnoid space. At places, such projections are microscopic and are referred to as arachnoid villi. At other places, these villi form aggregations that are visible to the naked eye and are then called arachnoid granulations. Arachnoid villi can be identified in all intracranial sinuses. Arachnoid granulations are most numerous in relation to the superior sagittal sinus. They may also be seen in

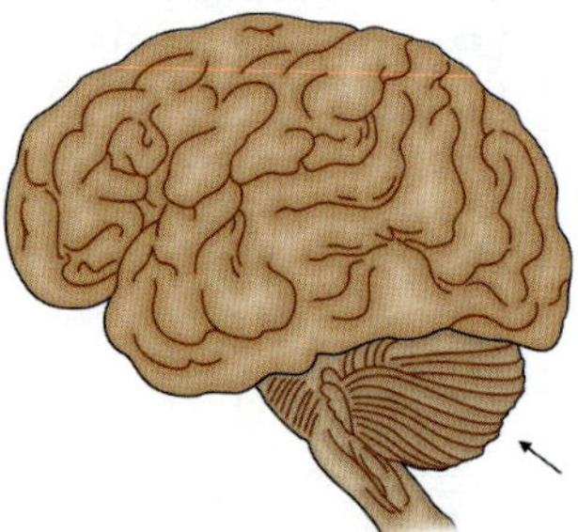

Fig.: *Cerebellum*

lateral extensions (lateral lacunae) present in relation to this sinus. The masses of vascular pia mater covered by ependyma are referred to as choroid plexuses. They are the sites where the cerebrospinal fluid is secreted into the ventricles of the brain. The part of the vertebral canal below the level of the spinal cord contains several roots of spinal nerves that collectively form the cauda equina. In anterior cranial fossa, there is a median bony projection called the crista galli. The lowest part of the spinal cord is conical and is called the conus medullaris. The conus is continuous with the filum terminale. The gray matter of the right and left halves of the spinal cord is connected across the middle line by the gray commissure.

Cerebral edema the normal water of gray matter is 80% and of white matter 60% of weight. Brain may also swell due to increase in cerebral volume known as congestive brain swelling.

Cerebral infarction: In this disease, contralateral athetosis is accompanied by altered level of consciousness. There may be paralysis of face/limbs of opposite side.

Cerebral ischemia brain derives the energy from oxidative metabolism of glucose. In brain there is no glucose store. Once the CBF falls below 20 mL/100 g of brain tissue/minute, EEG becomes flat and evoked response disappears signifying the starving neurons. CBF below 10 mL/100 g of brain tissue per minute leads to infarction, and restoration of circulation is of no value as pet shows complete cessation of glucose metabolism. Around the infarcted zone, there is potentially viable zone of brain tissue where blood flow is low, function is depressed but recovery is possible. Vasogenic edema starts due to dilation of vessels in infarcted zone. Edema stays maximum for 2–4 days and then subsides.

Cerebral malaria is caused with falciparum infection. Multiple petechial hemorrhages are responsible for CNS symptoms. High fever may be followed by convulsions or unconsciousness. Sensory motor deficits and mental symptoms may occur. Parasite may be recovered from peripheral blood. Mortality is 20–40%. It is a medical emergency. Quinine hydrochloride 600 mg in 5% dextrose is given IV. Oral quinine 350 mg 2 tablets three times a day along with tetracycline is given. Plenty of IV glucose is necessary.

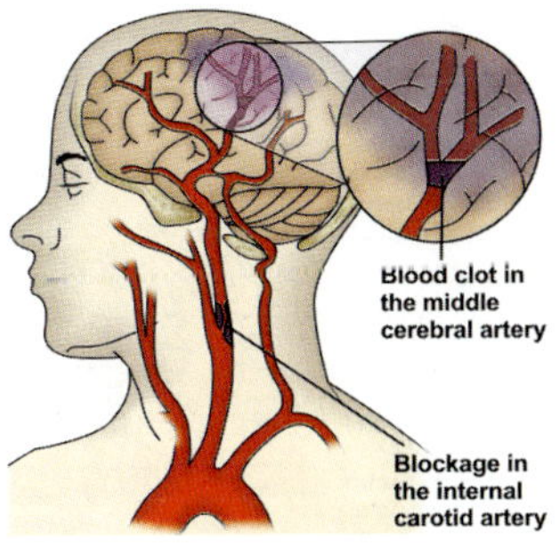

Fig.: *Cerebral infarction*

C

Cerebral nuclei are islands of gray matter located in cerebral cortex which are responsible for automatic movements and postures. These are known as basal ganglion.

Cerebral venous thrombosis may develop after pyogenic meningitis, collagen disease, and trauma. When superior sagittal is involved, it may cause papilledoma and hemorrhagic infarction. Patient may develop papilledema, extensive bilateral hemorrhagic infarction not confirming to any specific vascular territory. Headache and seizure may develop.

Cerebrospinal fluid is a clear fluid of the brain and spine. About 500 ml of it is produced daily from choroid plexuses of 3rd, 4th and lateral ventricles. It is clear and colorless with slightly opaque hue due to globulin. Specific gravity ranges from 1003–1009.

Cerebrospinal rhinorrhea refers to the escape of cerebrospinal fluid into the nasal cavity due to communication of ethmoidal bone which occurs due to Le fort II and Le fort III fractures and the fracture involving nasal complex, which may lead to a dural tear in the cribriform plate region of ethmoidal bone.

Cerebrovascular accident (CVA) is a focal neurologic disorder caused by destruction of brain substance as a result of intracerebral hemorrhage, thrombosis, embolism or vascular insufficiency. CVA is also known as stroke, cerebral apoplexy and brain attack. There are 2 major classes of stroke, hemorrhagic and occlusive. The most prevalent form is the occlusive stroke that commonly results from atherosclerotic disease and cardiac abnormalities. Thrombosis of intracranial and extracranial arteries and cerebral embolization from various origins throughout the body are the primary causes of cerebral infarction. Thrombus formation is more likely to occur in other atherosclerotic vessels. Cerebral embolization is also a causative factor. A major source of emboli is in the heart of individuals with

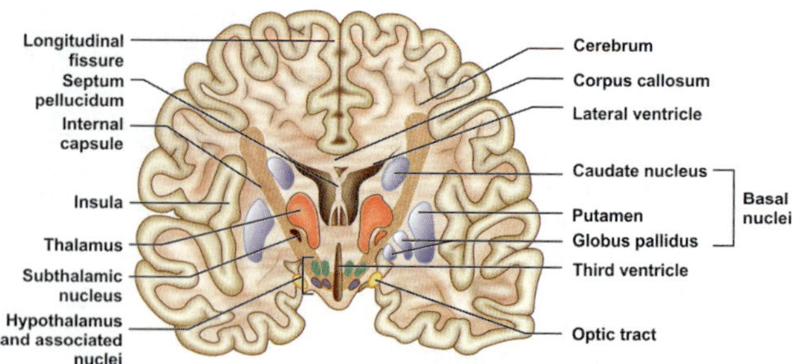

Fig.: *Cerebral nuclei*

impaired flow or damaged valves—rheumatic heart disease with mitral stenosis and atrial fibrillation are most common cases.

Cervical refer to neck.

Cervical burnout is a radiolucent artifact seen on dental X-ray. It may be confused with dental caries and appears as collar or wedge-shaped radiolucency.

Cervical collar is the splint made of foam or rigid material around the neck.

Cervical erosion is the wearing away of cementum that has been exposed as a result of gingival recession.

Cervical nerve root compression is the compression of cervical nerves supplying upper arm; produces chronic arm and neck pain. Prolonged sitting worsens the pain. There will be muscle weakness, paresthesia and decreased reflex response.

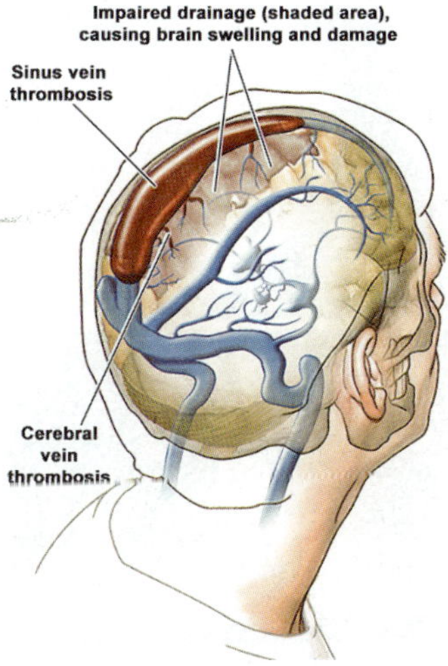

Fig.: *Cerebral venous thrombosis*

Cervical plexus is formed by the ventral rami of the first, second, third and fourth cervical nerves. With the exception of the ramus of the first cervical nerve, each of them divides into ascending and descending branches. The ascending branch of the second nerve joins the first nerve; and its descending branch joins the ascending branch of the third nerve. Similarly, the descending branch of the third nerve joins the ascending branch of the fourth nerve.

Cervical radiculopathy in Latin, radiculitis refers to 'by the roots' and when root of nerve is pinched, it is called radiculopathy. It causes numbness, and/or weakness in arm. Common causes of pinched nerves are calcium deposits from arthritis or herniated disc.

Cervical rib is a congenital disorder. Lowest cervical vertebra is over-developed to form a rib. It may be partially or completely developed. It may be symptom free or may cause numbness and tingling.

Cervical spin disc herniation: Symptoms include neck pain which may radiate to scalp, shoulder or to extremity certain position may increase the symptoms. One may develop numbness in distal upper extremity. It may result in fasculations, loss of deep tendon reflex and atrophy of muscles.

Cervicogenic headache describes head pain and occurs as an abnormality in neck. The work genesis means 'to come pain'. So cervicogenic literally means pain coming from neck area. Generally, headache is experienced as pain in neck on one side. Certain neck movements may relieve pain.

Cervix is the area that refers to the neck of the tooth; the area where the crown joins the root or the enamel joins the cementum.

Characteristics of lymph, node enlargement gives diagnostic clue. In tuberculosis, nodes are matted due to periadenitis. Infected nodes are tender and firm. Lymphomas produce symmetrical large, firm and rubbery nodes. These are movable, discrete and non-tender. In metastasis, one finds fixed, stony hard, localized glands. In children, due to throat infection cervical glands are enlarged. Bilateral cervical glands are enlarged in tuberculosis, lymphoma, and leukemias. Nodes in Hodgkin's disease are rubbery, discrete and mobile.

Charcot's joint is more frequently seen in diabetic neuropathy, syringomyelia, spinal cord injury, leprosy and peripheral nerve injury. Prolonged administration of hydrocortisone in bone may cause it. Normal muscle tone and protective reflexes are lost. It is a painless joint with extensive cartilage erosion.

Charter's tooth brushing is a method designed to increase cleaning effectiveness and gingival stimulation in the interproximal areas. Bristles are pointed toward the crown of the tooth rather than apically. Tooth brush is positioned horizontally and parallel with the arch in all areas except the lingual area of anterior teeth and the occlusal surfaces. Bristles are placed at gingival margin. These are directed toward the occlusal surface at a 45° angle to the long axis of tooth. Back and forth motion is used for activation. It is good for patients with orthodontic brackets.

Cheatle forceps is a heavy stainless steel forceps without locking system. It is used to hold sterilized items like bandage, gauze and gloves. It is kept in bottle dipped in savlon solution.

Chediak higashi syndrome is an uncommon genetic disease and is

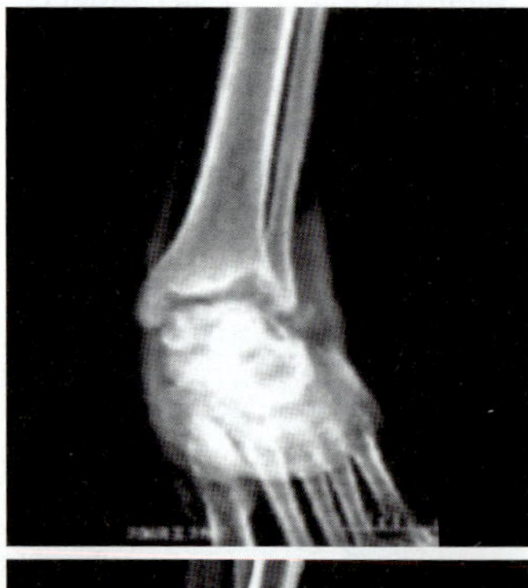

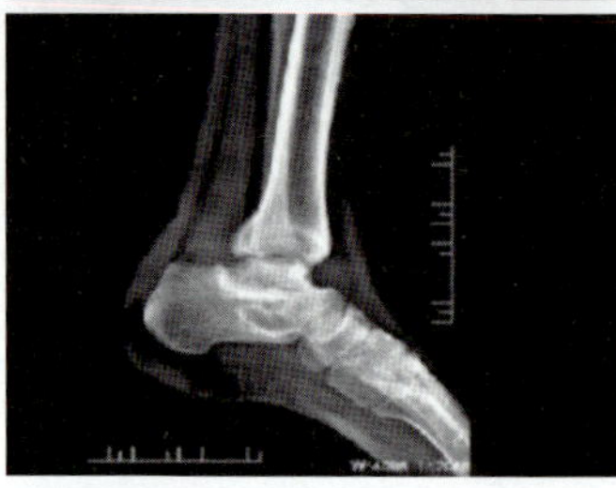

Fig.: *Charcot's joint*

fatal in early life. It is transmitted as an autosomal recessive trait. Defect is of granule containing cells as granulocytes and melanocytes. Hypopigmentation is seen on skin and hair. Some may develop neuropathy. Child dies before the age of 10 due to recurrent infection. Lymph nodes, spleen, liver and bone marrow are infiltrated with lymphohistiocyte cell. There may also be photophobia; nystagmus and albinism. Oral lesions include glossitis, gingivitis and ulceration of oral mucosa. Blood shows giant abnormal granules in peripheral circulating leukocytes. There is no specific treatment.

Cheek pouch is the area of the mouth inside the cheek.

Cheilitis granulomatosa develops as a persistent swelling of a lip, facial nerve palsy and fissured tongue. Cause is unknown.

Chelation refers to removal of ions from the surfaces so that they are not available for biological reaction.

Cheilitis glandularis is a condition where lower lip becomes enlarged, firm and finally everted. Cause is unknown. Labial salivary glands are enlarged. They may become nodular. Orifices of secretory ducts are inflamed and red. These are of three types, simple type, superficial suppurative type, deep suppurative type. Simple type is multiple, pin-head size lesion. Central part is depressed. Superficial suppurative type is having painless, induration and crusting ulcerations.

Chemical burn the gingival becomes white and necrotic following injudicious use of caustic agent.

Chemical cure is a method where the restorative material bonds to the tooth by the means of chemical. It gives good esthetics, more complete cure and curing light is not needed. Disadvantage of it is more porosity, poor color stability and less working time available. Light cure gives better color quality.

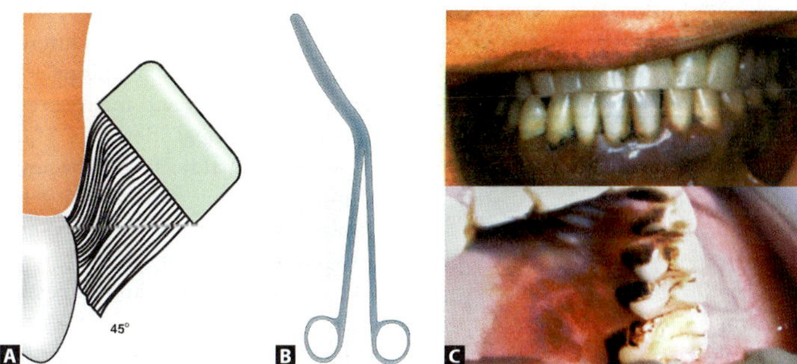

Figs A to C: *(A) Charter's tooth brushing method; (B) Cheatle forceps; (C) Chemical burn*

Chemical diabetes refers to the asymptomatic diabetes mellitus without any symptoms.

Chemical name refers to the name by which a chemist knows the drug.

Chemical reaction is a process where atoms of molecules or compounds interact to form new chemical combination, e.g. Glucose interacts with oxygen to form CO_2, water and energy.

Chemical sterilization is a process where combination of formaldehyde, alcohol, acetone, ketone and steam serves as an effective sterilizing agent microbial destruction results from dual action of toxic chemicals and heat.

Chemical theory given by Parmly (1819) rebelled against the vital theory and proposed that an unidentified "chemical" agent was responsible for caries. Support for the chemical theory came from Robertson (1835) and Regnart (1938), who actually carried out experiments with different dilutions of organic acids (such as sulphuric and nitric) and found that they corroded enamel and dentin. He stated that caries began on the enamel surface in locations where the food putrefied and acquired sufficient dissolving power to produce the disease chemically.

Chemical vapor sterilization refers to sterilization by chemical vapor under pressure. In this, special chemical solution is heated in a closed chamber, producing hot chemical vapors that kill microorganisms. Temperature, pressure and time required for completion of one cycle is 270°F (132°C) at 20 lb for 30 minutes. Chemical vapor sterilizer is also known as chemiclave.

Chemoattractant refers to activation phase.

Chemo–parasitic theory is a blend of the two theories, i.e. chemical theory and parasitic theory because it states that caries is caused by acids produced by microorganisms of the mouth. In a series of experiments, Miller demonstrated the following facts, acid was present within the deeper carious lesions, as shown by reaction on litmus paper. Different kinds of foods (bread, sugar, but not meat) mixed with saliva and incubated at 37° centigrade could decalcify the entire crown of a tooth. Several types of mouth bacteria (at least 30 species were isolated) could produce enough acid to cause dental caries. Lactic acid was an identifiable product in carbohydrate–saliva incubation mixtures. Different microorganisms (filamentous, long and short bacilli and micrococcus) invade carious dentin. Miller concluded that no single species of microorganism caused caries but rather the process was mediated by an oral microorganism capable of producing acid and digesting protein.

Chemoreceptors are the receptors that respond to chemicals and are responsible for taste and smell.

Chemotaxis is a process in which substance attracts cells or organism in its vicinity.

Chemotherapeutic is an agent of a chemical nature which exerts an antimicrobial effect.

Chemotherapeutic agent is a term used for a chemical substance that provides a therapeutic benefit.

Chemotherapeutic index is the ratio of minimal effective dose to the minimal tolerated dose.

Cherubism is an uncommon disease involving teeth. It appears at the age of three. It generally develops bilaterally. Mostly mandible is involved. Deciduous teeth shed suddenly at the age of three. Permanent dentition is defective with the absence of numerous teeth. Oral mucosa remains normal. Some teeth look like floating in cyst like space.

Chest pain is a most common cause in winter was fibrositis. Chest pain may be caused by pleurisy and pneumonia. Most prominent is the pain of angina and myocardial infarction. Myocardial pain may be referred to arm. Pain of pericarditis is felt in center. In some cases, anxiety and stress may also cause chest pain.

Chickenpox is a highly contagious disease. The spread of infection is through inhalation of infected droplets (aerosol) or through contact with the skin lesions. Incubation period is 10–21 days. It is mild but is highly infectious. Rash shows centripetal distribution. Fever is mild and develops along with rash. Disease may start with exanthem on buccal mucosa and soft palate. Rashes appear as crops on face, scalp and trunk. Extremities are less involved. Rash is macular or maculo-papular which, within a few hours changes into vesicular, one can see all the stages at one point of time. Rash goes on appearing for 3 to 5 days and then goes to crust formation. Most of the scrubs fall in 2 weeks. Generally, it does not leave permanent scars. Mortality is lower but eyes require special care.

Chief complaint is complaint recorded by a medical professional in patients, own words. It gives information which promoted patient to visit a clinician. Phenomenon symptoms or signs of deviation

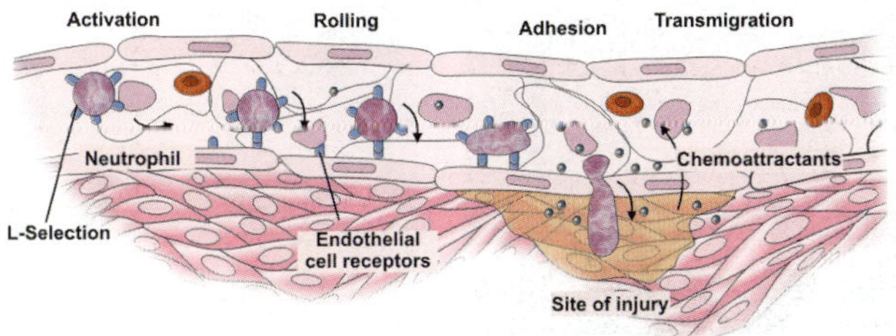

Fig.: *Chemotaxis*

from normal are indicative of illness. The form of notation should be in patient's own words.

Child abuse may be defined as an act by parents or caregivers who endanger a child's or young person's physical, emotional, educational or medical health and development. For the purpose of child protection, one can recognize a child or young person as an individual less than 17 years of age.

Child psychology is the science that deals with the mental power (or) an interaction between the conscious and subconscious element in a child.

Child sexual abuse involves an inappropriate sexual behavior that includes reaching out to child genitals/getting them to touch genitals of adults, indecent/vulgar language, use of inappropriate words, rape, exhibitionism or sexual explanation and touching them done by a stranger/caretaker/baby sitter/teacher/parent. Penetrative Sexual Assault (PSA)—Penetration of an organ or any other object into vagina, urethra, anus or mouth or making the child do vice-versa. Aggravated Penetrative Sexual Assault (APSA) is considered when the same is done by police officer, public/government servant, member of armed forces, staff of private hospitals or staff of an education institution if a child is part of it. Sexual Assault (SA) is if a person touches the private parts of child with sexual intent without penetration or makes the child do vice versa. Aggravated Sexual Assaults (ASA) is considered when the same is done by police officer, public/government servant, member of armed forces staff of private hospitals or staff of an education institution if a child is part of it. Sexual Harassment (SH) when a person with sexual intent uses inappropriate words, pornographic video/pictures and questions. Emotional Abuse defined as the continuous emotional maltreatment of a child's that hampers child emotional development. Emotional abuse has long-term deteriorating effects on the child's personality. It may range from making fun of the child normally to frightening and isolating the child. Emotional abuse

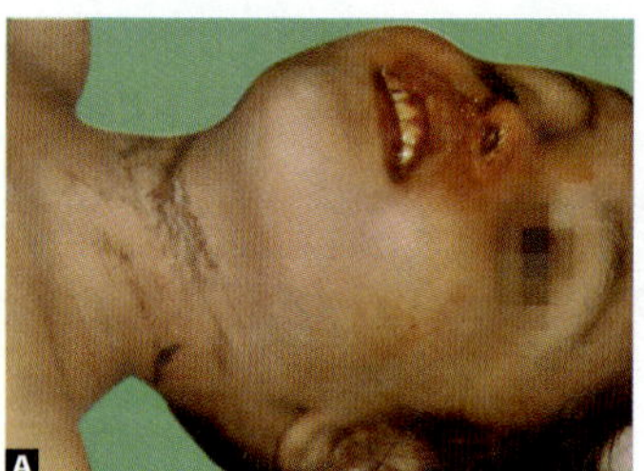

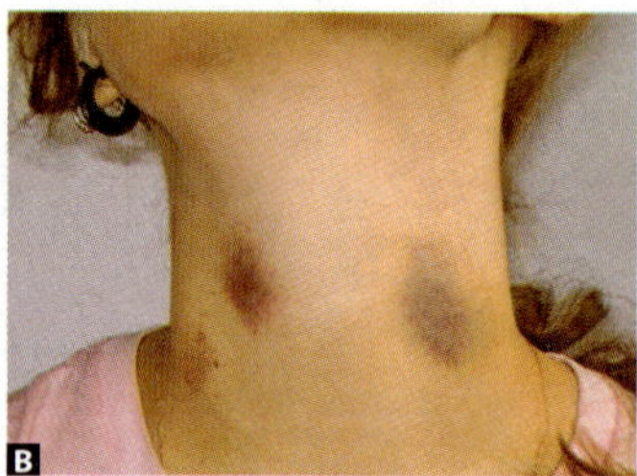

Figs A and B: *(A) Child abuse; (B) Child sexual abuse*

has always been a part of some or the other abuse and neglect.

Child trafficking is refers to when the child is abducted illegacy and used for unlawful purposes one of the most important dimensions of child abuse and neglect of missing children in the country; it is more prevalent in children than adults. Studies have indicated that child-trafficking is more common in developing nation rather than the developed ones.

Childhood is the period from 15 months until 12–13 years. During early childhood there is active ossification, but the child grows older, the rate of growth slows down.

Chills are extreme, involuntary muscle contractions. There may be violent shivering and teeth shattering and fever. Pneumonia produces a single chill and malaria produces a recurring chill with high fever. Chill can be produced by transfusion reactions and exposure to cold. Certain drugs may also cause it.

Chime is partially digested food mixture leaving the stomach.

Chin-neck contour is the mentocervical angle formed by the intersection of the e-line and a tangent to the submental area (110–120°). The submental neck angle is formed between the submental tangent and a neck tangent at points above and below the thyroid prominence.

Chiropractice was known to Hippocrates 2500 years ago too. It is concerned with treatment of mechanical disorder of joints, especially spinal joints.

Chisel scalers are the set of double ended instruments with the curved shank at one end and straight shank at the other end, although the blades are slightly curved and have a straight cutting edge bevelled at 45 degrees.

Chitin is a polysaccharide found in fungal cell wall but not in any other microorganism.

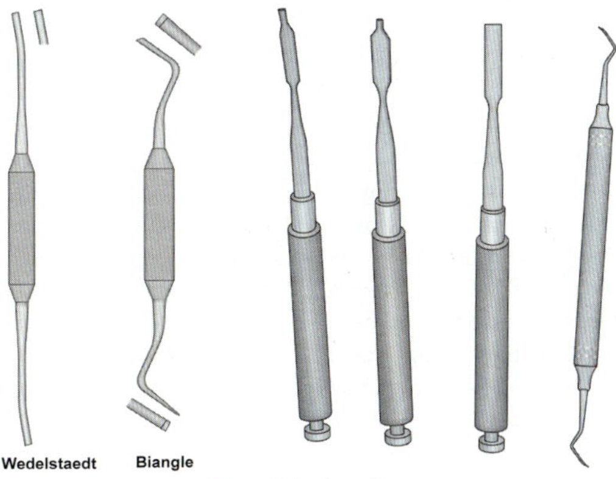

Fig.: *Chisel scalers*

C

Chloasma is the hypopigmentation of skin, especially cheeks. Ladies taking estrogen tablets as family planning measures may also develop it. Lesions are distributed symmetrically over bridge of nose, upper lip, cheeks and forehead. Disease is asymptomatic. Local use of hydrogen peroxide may be useful. Lesions may disappear after delivery.

Chloramphenicol is a broad spectrum antibiotic with a range similar to tetracycline. Side effects include agranulocytosis. It is used in the treatment of typhoid fever.

Chlorhexidine digluconate is effective against both Gram-positive and Gram-negative bacteria due to its ability to denaturate the bacterial cell wall while forming pores in the membrane. It kills E. faecalis cells in 30 seconds in less concentrations of 0.2 to 2 percent. Although in vitro studies have demonstrated the antibacterial effect of CHX against E. faecalis to be superior to that of NaOCl, there are no in vivo studies yet available that would confirm the better activity of CHX against this resistant species in the infected root canal also.

Chlorhexidine was developed in the late 1940s in the research laboratories. Chlorhexidine is the most potent of the tested bisbiguanides. It has strong base and is most stable in the form of its salts, i.e. chlorhexidine gluconate. It acts by binding to the hydroxyl apatite of enamel, the pellicle, the bacteria, extracellular polysaccharides and the mucous membrane owing to its cationic nature. After binding, the agent is slowly released in an active form over a 12–24 hour period. This property of chlorhexidine is an attribute to its substantiality. It can be delivered as a rinse, a syringe for subgingival application and incorporated in chewing-gum. Disadvantages: brownish-black discoloration of the teeth, restorations and tongue, temporary aberration of taste sensation (dysgeusia), burning lips, mucous membrane discoloration. It is a potent antiseptic which is widely used for chemical plaque control in the oral cavity in concentrations of 0.2%. It shows optimal antimicrobial action between pH 5.5 and 7.0. For using it as an irrigant, it should be used as 2% in concentration.

Chlorhexidine stain is extrinsic stain caused by prolonged use of a mouth-wash containing chlorhexidine.

Chloride compounds are oxidizing agents and end-products are inactive chlorides. Strong hypochlorite solutions have a penetrating and irritating odor due to release of chlorine gas. It may corrode metals.

Chloride shift is a diffusion of chloride ions into red blood cells as bicarbonate ions diffuse out. It maintains electrical neutrality of red blood cells.

Chlorine is closely related to potassium and sodium maintaining water balance. Average daily consumption is 6–9 g. It is excreted through kidney. Normal blood plasma concentration is 550–650 mg/dl. It activates salivary amylase. Large quantities may lead to convulsions. In reference to dentistry, chlorine is a potent germicide widely used as disinfectant of water. Sodium hypochlorite in 0.5% solution is an effective antiseptic and will dissolve necrotic tissue. It is useful for irrigation of root canals. One percent solution of sodium hypochlorite diluted with 3 times hot water is useful for irrigating dry sockets.

Chlorine dioxide is a stronger oxidizing agent than other chlorine disinfectants. Sporicidal action is independent of pH over 6–10.

Chloroquine is a drug used for the prevention of malaria. It may be used as antirheumatic drug. It is the main drug in case of acute malaria. Side effects include nausea, headache, diarrheal and abdominal cramps.

Chloroxylenol is a 0.2% chloroxylenol with menthol and diluted 1 in 50 is a pleasant mouthwash as reported by Dilling and Hallam. It is active against streptococci and less active against staphylococci.

Chlorpromazine is a drug that induces emotional sedation. Patient becomes completely isolated form outside environment. These develop apathy lethargy and reduced motor activity. Largactil produces fall in body temperature. It has a moderate anticholinergic and antihistaminic effect. It is rapidly absorbed from of GIT.

Choking agents include ammonia, chlorine, hydrogen chloride and chemicals which irritate throat, airway and lungs. Onset may be immediate or delayed. There will be irritation to eyes, coughing chest tightness, shortness of breath and dizziness. Cyanosis and ventilation failure may develop.

Cholecystectomy is a surgical removal of gallbladder.

Cholecystitis is the inflammation of gallbladder.

Cholecystokinin is a peptide hormone secreted by intestinal mucosa. It regulates several gastrointestinal activities including motility.

Cholera is caused by coma-shaped actively motile flagellated Gram negative bacillus Vibrio cholerae. The bacilli proliferate in small intestine without invasion producing a potent protein. Incubation period varies from a few hours to 6 days. Disease has 2 phases. Evacuation phase is of acute, painless, profuse diarrhea with vomiting. Stool is watery nd odorless. In collapse phase, there develops cold clammy skin, hypotension and tachycardia. Patient becomes dull and apathetic, prompt rehydration is the only remedy. Chemoprophylaxis with 500 mg helps.

Cholesterol is present as free sterol in most tissues except for adrenal cortex, plasma and athermatous plaques. Most of the tissues are capable of synthesizing cholesterol; most of plasma cholesterol originates from liver and distal small intestine. Increase in LDL and decrease in HDL cholesterol are related to atherosclerosis independently.

Cholesterolemia refers to the increased amount of cholesterol in blood, more than 225 mg%.

Choline is a precursor of acetylcholine, phospholipids, and betaine. It is also necessary for the integrity of cell membrane. Deficiency can lead to fatty liver and elevated transaminases levels. Vitamin C is a potent antioxidant which is involved in many oxidation-reduction reactions. It is also required for the synthesis of collagen and conversion of dopamine to norepinephrine. Vitamin C promotes iron absorption because it reduces ferric iron in diet to ferrous form, which is better absorbed. Choline was first used in 1939 when it was shown to relieve a condition known as fatty liver. Prevention of fats and cholesterol in the body is the function of choline. It maintains integrity of myelin sheath. Daily requirement is 10 mg.

Cholinergic nervous systems are nerve fibers which release acetylcholine as a neurotransmitter.

Cholinesterase is an enzyme which splits acetylcholine into acetate and choline.

Chondral fracture is a fracture of an articular surface in a synovial joint.

Chondrocyte: Cartilage cell.

Chondrolysis is a degeneration of cartilage cell.

Chondroma is a painless slowly progressive swelling of jaw and is composed of mature cartilage. It seldom develops in membranes. It may develop at any age. Radiographically, it shows an irregular radiolucent or mottled area. Root resorption may be seen, surgical excision is advanced because it is resistant to X-rays.

Chondromyxoid fibroma was first described by Jaffe in 1946. Majority of cases develop in long bones. It exhibits swelling and pain is severe. Foci of calcium are sometimes found. Conservative surgical exci-sion is done.

Chondrosarcoma is a malignant neoplasm of bone. In this abnormal cartilage tissue is formed but no osteoid bone is produced. Peak age is 30–40 years. Males are more affected.

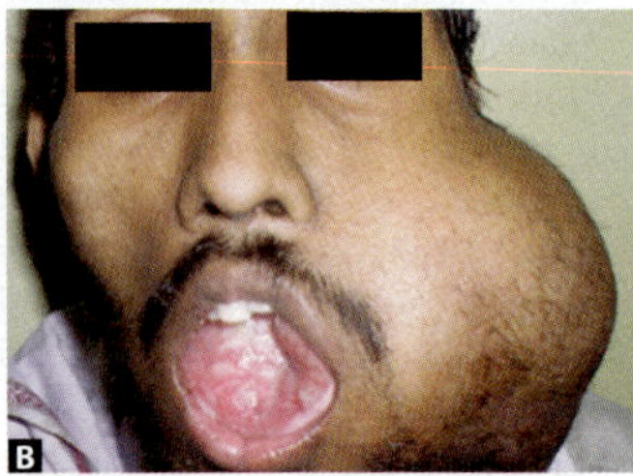

Figs A and B: (A) *Histologic view of chondrosarcoma;* (B) *Chondrosarcoma of jaw involving mandible*

In mandible, it develops in posterior region. Clinical features: It produces a painless swelling of jaw. Later on it becomes painful and tender. It is very fast enlarging causing severe expansion. Radiologically, it shows moth-eaten radiolucent area in bone with ill-defined borders. Blotchy areas of radiopacities are also found. Even wide surgical excision gives poor prognosis.

Chorea is a rapid, involuntary, non-repetitive, irregular and arrhythmic contraction that can affect any part of body but are more pronounced in digits. It may be hereditary with Wilson's disease. Anticonvulsants, cocaine and amphetamine may also result in this condition.

Choroid plexus is a specialized group of capillaries in ventricles of the brain that secrete cerebrospinal fluid.

Chrome refers color intensity.

Chromosome analysis is a test that is undertaken at 16–18 weeks of pregnancy. The amount of desquamated fetal cells is obtained and cell culture is necessary before a chromosomal diagnosis is made.

Chronic alveolar abscess is a local mild inflammation of infection. It occurs around the roots of tooth. It may result due to pulpitis. Sinus may be present and pass through alveolar bone to open into mucosa.

Chronic atrophic rhinitis is of two varieties, simple atrophic rhinitis and ozena associated with fetor. In ozena, fetor comes from presence of dry cysts formed from viscid secretions. Surface epithelium is thinner than normal. The overlying crusts are made up of dense inspissated neutrophilic exudates, necrotic debris and bacteria.

Chronic bacterial sialadenitis is a non-specific inflammatory disease of salivary gland, generally occurs in children after the obstruction of duct. Usually, parotid gland of one side is affected. There is sudden onset of unilateral swelling at the angle of mandible. Fever or leukocytosis is not marked. There is mild pain and disease responds to antibiotics. There may develop recurrent, tender swelling. Salivary flow is decreased. Treatment includes massage and antibiotics.

Chronic cholecystitis is a condition associated with gallstones. There will be ill-defined epigastric discomfort and a dull ache in right hypochondrium. Fat intolerance may occur. Plain X-ray may show

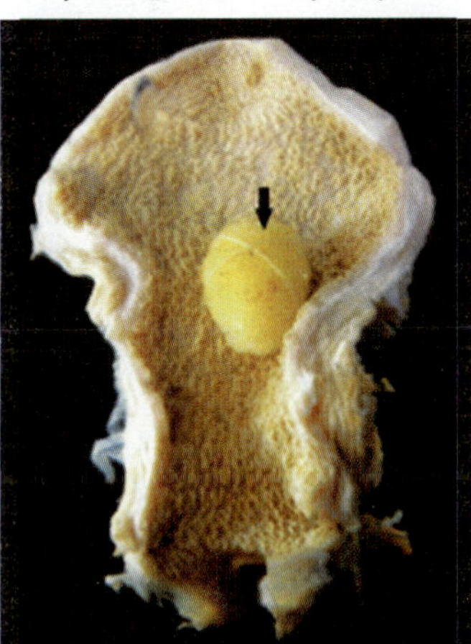

Fig.: *Chronic cholecystitis with cholelithiasis*

gall-stones. Sometimes cholecystectomy may be done.

Chronic desquamative gingivitis was first recognized in 1894, but the term was coined by Prinz in 1932, who described this term as a desquamative and ulcerative lesion of free and attached gingiva, the lesion is generally limited to gingiva though the involvement of other areas are also reported. Gingiva is red, swollen and glossy with multiple vesicles. Distribution is patchy buccal mucosa may also be involved. Patient is not able to eat hot, cold or spicy food. It is more commonly found in women between the age group of fourth to fifth decade of life.

Chronic diffuse sclerosing osteomyelitis may develop at any age. There may be chronic infection. Person may develop vague pain and bad taste. Radiographs show diffuse sclerosis of bone. Lesion may be bilateral. Look is of 'cotton wool' appearance. Lesion shows dense, irregular trabaculae. Focal areas of osteoclastic activity are seen polymorphs are in plenty. Lesion is too big to be removed surgically.

Chronic discoid lupus erythematosis can be described as irregularly thickened red plaques with well-defined margins develop is an important localizing stimulus. After sometime atrophy or scarring may develop in these areas, these can also be seen as hyperkeratosis and warts.

Chronic focal sclerosing osteomyelitis generally develops in adults. First molar of mandible is involved. Radiograph will show well-circumscribed radiopaque mass of sclerotic bone. It consists of dense mass of bony trabaculae with interstitial marrow tissue.

Chronic gingivitis is long-standing gingivit is that has slow onset, it is a painless condition unless complicated by acute exacerbations.

Chronic glomerulonephritis these patients develop loss of appetitie, weakness, hypertension and vomiting. In terminal stage, proteinuria may diminish but specific gravity of urine is fixed at 1010 which is otherwise of plasma. Kidneys

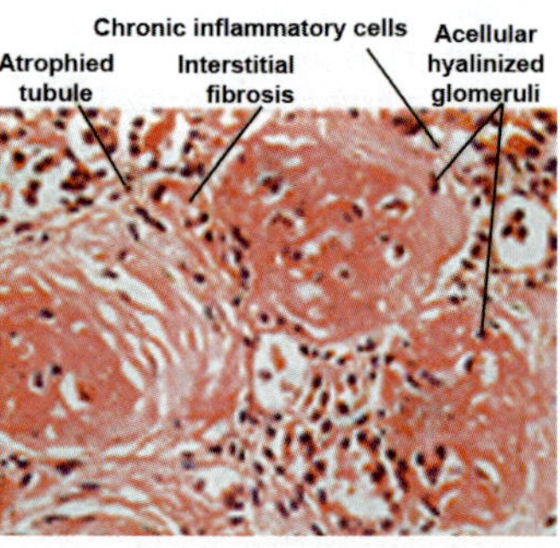

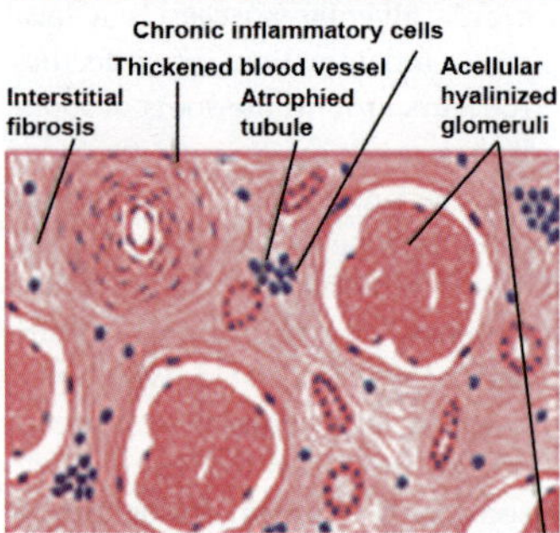

Fig.: *Chronic glomerulonephritis*

are symmetrically contracted and diffusely granular cortical surfaces.

Chronic hyperplastic pulpitis generally occurs in young children. Affected pulp appears pinkish. Deciduous molars are affected more. Hyperplasic tissue is a granulation tissue made up of delicate connective tissue fibers with small capillaries. Condition is irreversible and extraction of tooth to be done.

Chronic laryngitis refers to the repeated acute attacks that may develop due to singing, teaching, speaking, nasal obstruction and mouth breathing.

Chronic leukemia refers to the increased number of WBC count in children. Disease may be present for months. It may be diagnosed incidentally. Patient may look healthy. Lymph node enlargement is common in lymphatic leukemia but is uncommon in myeloid leukemia. Enlargement of salivary glands and tonsil may take place. Skin may show petechiae or ecchymosis. Finally, nodular lesions composed of leukemic cells may occur.

Chronic lymphocytic leukemia is a malignant condition due to lymphocytic infiltration of the leukemic cells never seen in children. There is a permanent lymphocytosis. Half of CLL patients show decreased immunoglobulin production. High-risk patients require chemotherapy.

Chronic lymphedema swelling starts from most dependent part. Swelling pits on pressure to start and later on edema pits less and less due to fibredema. Overlying skin becomes thick and rough.

Chronic maxillary sinusitis is an infection of maxillary sinus that may be manifested as pain and stuffiness on the affected side. Breath may be fetid. Sinus mucosa is thickened and polyps may develop may not be symptomatic and may

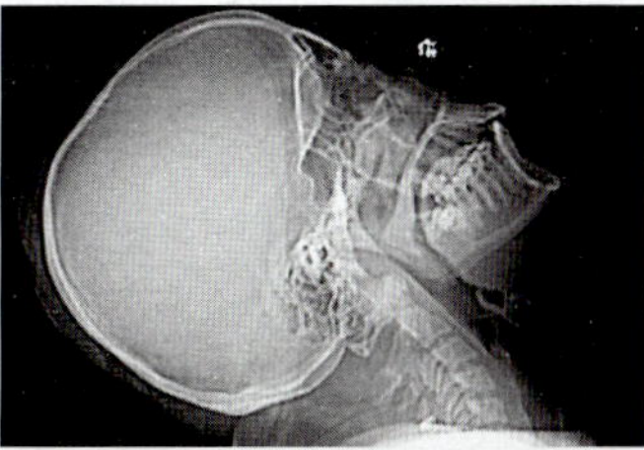

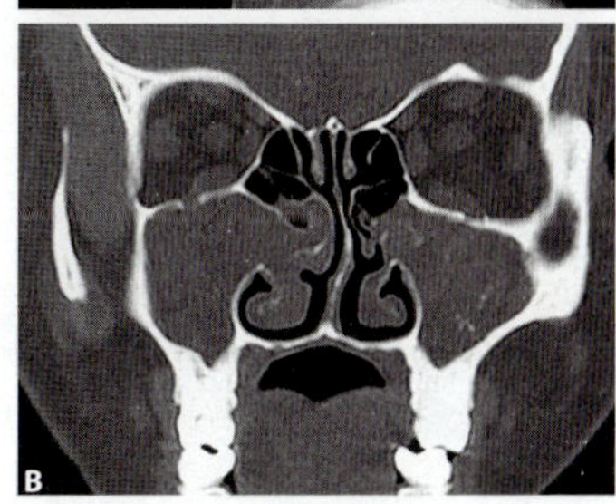

Figs A and B: (A) *Chronic lymphocytic leukemia; (B) Maxillary sinusitis*

be discovered radiographically. Antibiotics help.

Chronic mercurial poisoning is a condition that occurs due to presence of excessive amount of mercury in the body. Symptoms include loss of appetite and colicky pain in the abdomen and occasional vomit are common complaints. Gums become tender, swollen and ulcerated. Tongue and cheeks are ulcerated. There may be necrosis of jaw. Teeth become loose, anemia develops and skin eruptions are common. Speech becomes stammering, muscles of arm and leg may have tremor.

Chronic myelocytic leukemia is a malignant condition where cells retain the capacity for differentiation and are able to perform essential function. There is marked shift towards granulocytic differentiation at the expense of erythroid differentiation. Anemia is present. Mass of myeloid tissue is greatly increased. Myeloid cells have a striking propensity for malignant blastic transformation. It has three phases: (i) Chronic phase lasting for 3 years; (ii) Accelerated phase which lasts for 1½ years; (iii) Final phase of 3–6 months which usually ends in death.

Chronic obstructive pulmonary disease is the chronic lung disease that results in narrowing of airways, emphysema and bronchitis.

Chronic osteomyelitis also known as Garre's osteomyelitis in 1893. Garre described the lesion as thickening of periosteum. Maxilla and mandible are often affected in children. Patient complains of pain in tooth and jaw. Radiograph will show caries tooth against bony mass. X-ray shows focal growth of bone. Mass is smooth and well calcified. Periosteal reaction of carious tooth is the remedy.

Chronic pain is associated with longstanding disease and may persist for a longer period of time.

Chronic pancreatitis is a condition that results due to excessive alcohol consumption. There is deposition of protein plugs within pancreatic ducts. Chronic pancreatitis is not reversible. Only it can be arrested. There will be a chronic pain radiating to back. It is deep seated and antacids don't give any relief. Protein plugs calcify to give pancreatic calcification. Pain is to be controlled and surgical resection may be needed.

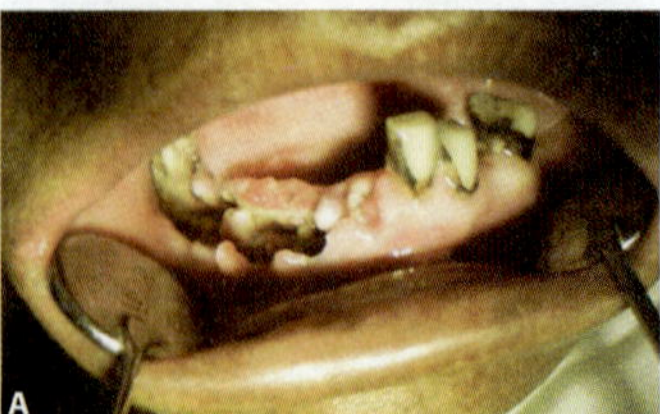

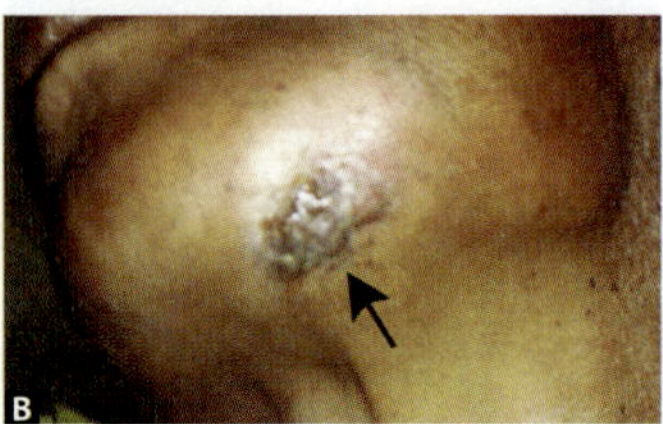

Figs A and B: Chronic osteomyelitis (A) Intraoal view; (B) Extraoral view

Chronic periodontitis is a slowly progressing disease and is defined as an infectious disease resulting in inflammation within the supporting tissues of the teeth, progressive attachment loss and bone loss. Clinically supragingival and subgingival plaque accumulation can be seen which is frequently associated with calculus formation, gingivitis, pocket formation, loss of periodontal attachment and alveolar bone. Loss of stippling along with spontaneous bleeding and suppuration can be appreciated.

Chronic adult periodontitis see Chronic periodontitis.

Chronic pulpalgia refers to the pain of pulpal origin. The pain is diffuse and patient may not be able to locate the site of pain. The pulp involved is not affected by cold. Pain persists till irritant is there. These are the lesions which cause pain until irritant is dislodged. Radiograph often reveals interproximal or root caries or recurrent caries under a restoration. The apices of involved roots also show external resorption. Thermal tests are of little value in a positive sense. Pulp extirpation and endodontic therapy if the tooth is to be saved, otherwise extraction is the line of treatment.

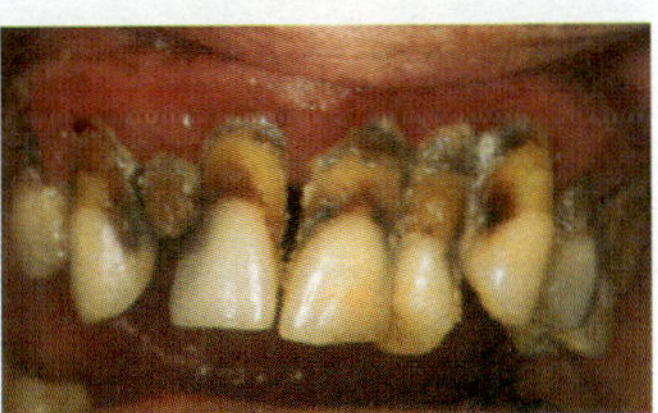

Fig.: *Chronic periodontitis*

Chronic pulpitis is an infection of pulpal origin where pain is not an important feature of chronic pulpitis. Reaction to thermal change is dramatically reduced. Pulp may become totally necrotic without pain. There is infiltration of pulp tissue by varying number of mononuclear cells specially lymphocytes and plasma cells.

Chronic pyelonephritis is a chronic tubulointestinal disease resulting from repeated attacks of inflammation and scarring with pelvicalyceal damage. Most of patients develop hypertension. Kidneys are small and irregularly scarred. Involvement is symmetrical in both kidneys. Hallmark of disease is coarse, discrete large scars with flat surface. Pelvic and calyceal walls are thickened and distorted mucosa becomes granular or atrophic.

Chronic sclerosing sialadenitis is a chronic inflammation of salivary gland tissue. It results in degeneration and subsequent replacement of acini by fibrous tissue. Trauma, infection and autoimmune all may cause it. Major or minor gland all may be affected. Affected gland is enlarged and remains freely movable. More the fibrosis develops, more the firm it becomes. Once the acini are lost, the gland parenchyma undergoes progressive sclerosis. Then sialoadenectomy has to be done.

C

Chronic suppurative osteomyelitis is a chronic form of acute stage. Symptoms will be mild with slight leukocytosis. Tooth may not be loose and patient may be able to chew food. Symptoms may develop periodically. Fistula may be formed.

Chronological age refers to the age in years.

Chuck is a small screwdriver type of instrument to replace burs in hand piece.

Chvostek's sign is an abnormal spasm of facial muscles which can be elicited by lightly tapping the patient's facial nerve. It can develop in lower calcium level.

Chyle is a fatty material taken up by the central lacteals in the villi of duodenum after a fatty meal.

Chyle is a milking fat containing lymph in the lymphatic of intestine.

Cicatricial pemphigoid is an autoimmune disease and is also known as benign mucus membrane pemphigoid. Mucus membranes including oral and conjuctival surfaces develop lesions. There develops transient vesicles and bullae formation which on rupture gives ulcers. Ulcers of cicatricial pemphigoid tend to heal more with scarring. Oral lesions can be widespread. Long-term management requires local and systemic corticosteroid.

Cicatrix refers to a scar, fibrous tissue left after healing of a wound.

Cicatrization refers to the formation of scar tissue.

Cingulum refers to a raised area on the lingual surface of anterior teeth.

Circular fibers are those which through the marginal and interdental gingiva and encircle the tooth in a ring-like fashion.

Circumcision is a surgical removal of foreskin or prepuce.

Circumferential wiring is technique for intermaxillary fixation where oblique fractures of the mandible can be managed by passing a soft stainless steel wire circumferentially.

Cirrhosis of liver is an irreversible pathological state of liver with widespread hepatic cell necrosis.

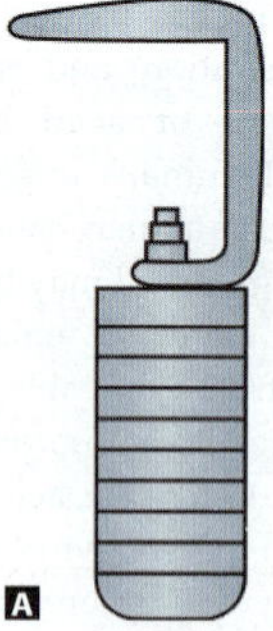

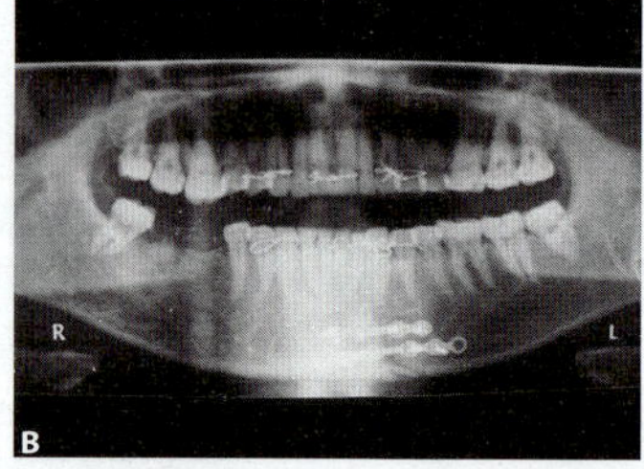

Fig.: *(A) Bur chuck; (B) Circumferential wiring*

Diffuse scarring, shrinkage and nodular regeneration is seen. Alcohol, hepatitis B, C, biliary cirrhosis all may lead to it. Regenerating nodules are smaller than 3 mm is called micronodular

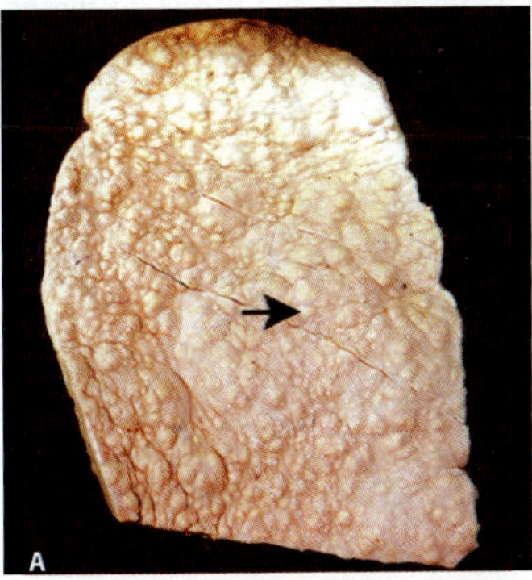

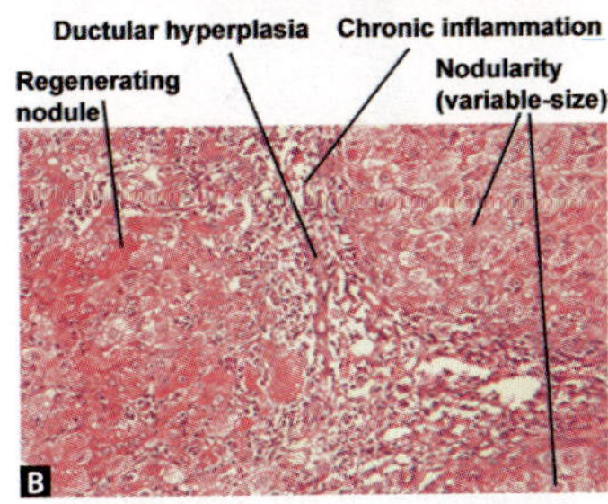

Figs A and B: *Cirrhosis of liver*

cirrhosis and when larger than 3 mm it is known as macronodular. Liver may be large or shrunken, firm to hard in consistency. Hepatocellular dysfunction includes jaundice, palmar erythema. Raised aminotransferases, low serum albumin, raised serum bilirubin helps in diagnosis. Prothrombin time may be prolonged.

Class I caries refers to the lesions that occur in pits and fissures of all teeth, but this class is essentially intended for bicuspid and molars.

Class I molar relationship is the mesiobuccal cusp of the maxillary first permanent molar occludes with the buccal groove of the mandibular first molars. This is considered as the normal relationship of these teeth.

Class II caries refers to the lesion that can involve either mesial and distal surfaces or only proximal surface of a tooth and is referred to as a mesio-occlusal (MO), disto-occlusal (DO) or mesio-occlusodistal (MOD).

Class II molar relationship is the mesiobuccal cusp of the maxillary fist permanent molar occludes mesial to the buccal groove of the mandibular first molar.

Class III caries refers to the cavity may occur on mesial and distal surface of any incisor/cuspid.

Class III molar relationship is the mesiobuccal cusp of the maxillary first permanent molar occludes distal to the buccal groove of the mandibular first molar.

Class IV caries refers to the lesions that are found on the proximal surfaces of anterior teeth that involve the incisal edge—is a lesion on the proximal surface of an anterior tooth, in which the incisal edge is also involved.

Class V caries found at the gingival third of the facial and lingual surfaces of anterior and posterior teeth—can occur on either the facial or the lingual surfaces; however, the predominant occurrence of these lesions is adjacent to the lip and cheeks rather than tongue.

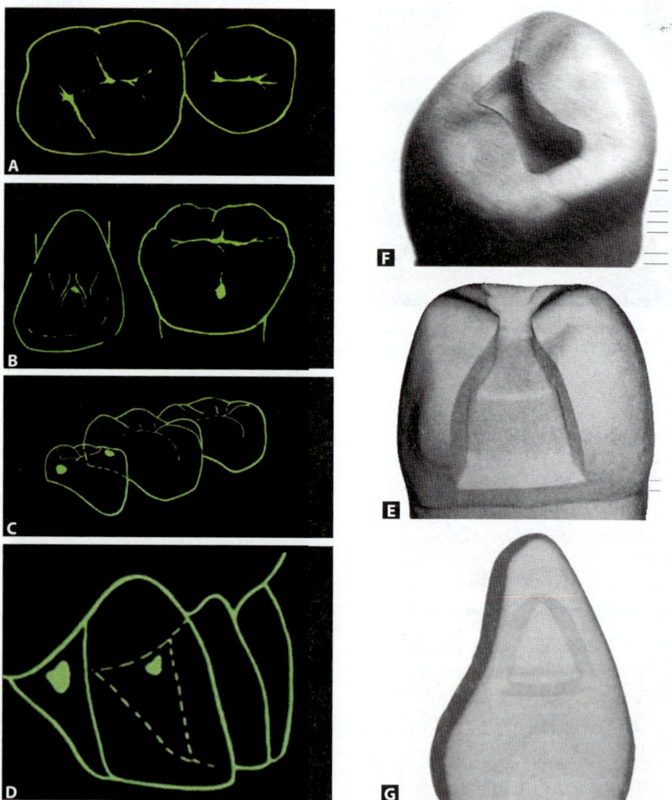

Figs A to G: (A) *Class I (carious lesion) involving occlusal surfaces;* (B) *Involving buccal and lingual pit; (C) Class II carious lesion; (D) Class III carious lesion; (E) Class I cavity preparation; (F) Class II cavity preparation; (G) Class III cavity preparation*

Class VI caries refers to the lesion that involves occlusal cusps of posterior teeth and incisal edge of anterior teeth. Defects found on incisal edges and cuspal tips. Also found on premolars and molar cuspal tips.

Classical conditioning is a behavioral theory put forward by a Russian physiologist. Ivan Pavlov in 19th century. During his studies of reflexes that apparently unassociated stimulus could produce reflexive behavior. Pavlov's classic experiment involves a presentation of food to a hungry animal, along with some other stimulus like ringing of a bell. The sight with sound of food elicits the salivation by reflex mechanism. If a bell is rung everytime the auditory stimulus is associated with food presentation stimulus. In short time, the ringing of a bell by itself will elicit salivation classical conditioning then operates by the simple process of association of one stimulus with another. It is unusual for the child to see the people with white coat if the unconditioned stimulus of painful treatment comes to be associated with conditioned stimulus of white coat, a child may cry withdraw immediately of first sight of white coat. Later on child learned to associate these stimuli on seeing white coat is enough to produce a pain.

Classical migraine is described as periodic headache, usually unilateral in onset but which later on becomes generalized. It is associated with nausea, photophobia or diarrhea. Prodromic phase includes visual disturbance. Usually it attacks half the visual field. At times, it induces typical toothache. It may last from a few hours to several weeks and may occur at any age.

Classification variable is a variable created not by manipulation but through division of subjects

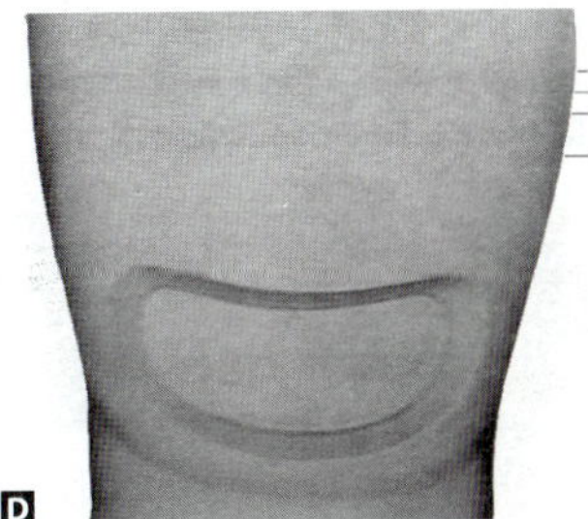

Figs A to D: (A) *Class IV carious lesion; (B) Class V carious lesion; (C) Class VI carious lesion; (D) Class V cavity preparation*

into groups based on an existing attribute such as sex or age.

Claude's hyperkinesias signs refers to increased reflex activity of paretic muscles elicited by painful stimuli.

Clavicle sign is a swelling, puffiness or edema at the medial third of right clavicle seen in congenital syphilis.

Cleaning see prophylaxis.

Clear cell carcinoma is found in major salivary glands especially parotid. Clear cell carcinoma is composed of cluster of cells surrounded by thin septa of fibrous connective tissue. These are treated by surgical excision.

Cleft tongue is rarest. Partial cleft is the result of incomplete merging and failure of groove obliteration by mesenchymal proliferation.

Cleidocranial dysostosis is a autosomal dominant disorder caused by mutation of chromosomes. Person presents with large head, small face and drooping shoulders. Chest is narrowed. There is delayed or absent ossification of calvaria. Pelvis is small or underdeveloped. There may be agenesis of middle or lateral portion of clavicle.

Clenching is the term used when the person holds the teeth together firmly with significant force.

Cleoid refers to a dental hand carving instrument with a blade-shaped like a pointed spade.

Clinical crown refers to that portion of the tooth visible in the mouth, extending from the occlusal or incisal edge to the crest of the free gingiva. Any unerupted area is not a part of clinical crown.

Clinical pocket depth is a distance to which probe penetrates into the pocket. The measurement of this depth is dependent on variable factors such as size, force, direction of probe penetration and resistance given by the tissues.

Clinician refers to practicing physician.

Clip true copy refers to the clones of cells are descended from one original cell. Clones of organisms can be produced by removing the nucleus from a cell of one individual and transplanting it into egg cell of another individual.

Closed anchor suture is used to close a flap in edentulous area present mesial or distal to the tooth and consists of tying a direct suture that closes the proximal flap, carrying

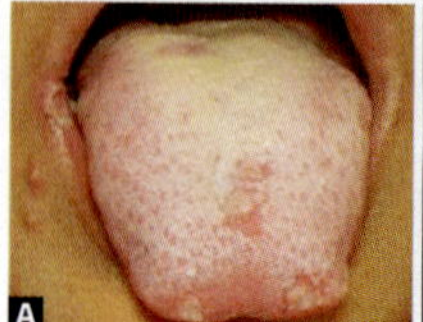

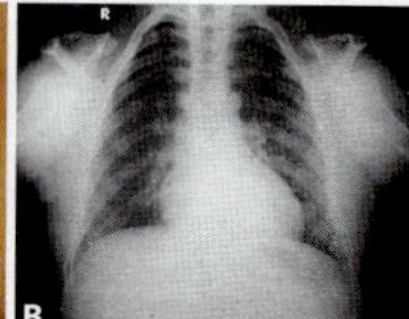

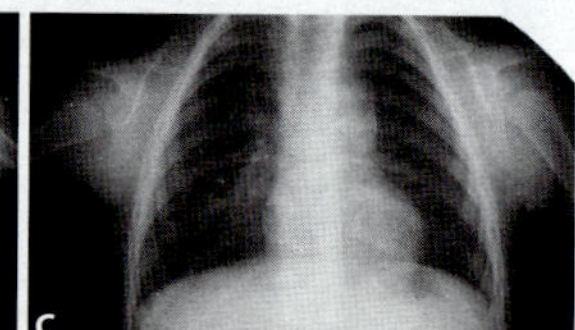

Figs A to C: (A) *Cleft tongue; (B) Cleido-cranial dysostosis showing hypoplastic absent clavicles; (C) Cleido-cranial dysostosis with nearly absent clavicles*

one of the threads, around the tooth to anchor the tissue against the tooth.

Closed chain exercise refers to exercise in which distal segment of extremity is fixed to the ground.

Closed coil spring refers to orthodontic springs that are stretched between teeth and exert a pulling force on selected teeth.

Closed format item questionnaire refers to items which require a speci-fic type of response such as yes or no.

Closed wound is the one in which there is no outside opening to skin/mucous membrane.

Cluster headache is a recurrent unilateral headache. Pain starts 2–3 hours after falling asleep during the phase of REM sleep. Headache is intense, nonthrobbing, unilateral and around the orbit. Stress, strain and alcohol may precipitate it. Prednisolone 60-80 mg daily helps.

Cluttering produces abnormal speech characterized by excessive speed, repetition, and interjections. Cause is unknown.

CO_2 laser is a gas active medium laser that must be delivered through a hollow-tube like wave-guide in continuous or gated pulse mode. It has a wavelength – 10,600 nm. It is well-absorbed by water, second only to er series of lasers, there is rapid soft tissue remover and has a shallow depth of tissue penetration, which is important when treating mucosal lesions especially useful for cutting dense fibrous tissue—focused onto the surgical site in a non-contact fashion. Loss of tactile sensation is disadvantageous, but the tissue ablation can be precise with careful technique.

Coadaptation refers to proper adaption of ends of fractured bone or the edges of a wound without overlap.

Coaggregation is the ability of 2 genetically distinct bacteria to recognize and adhere to one another is called co-aggregation and the term was first coined in 1970. Coaggregation is based on specific interaction of a proteinaceous adhesion produced by one bacteria and a respective carbohydrate or protein receptor found on the surface of another bacterium.

Coagulation refers to it is changing of a soluble into an insoluble protein process of changing into a clot.

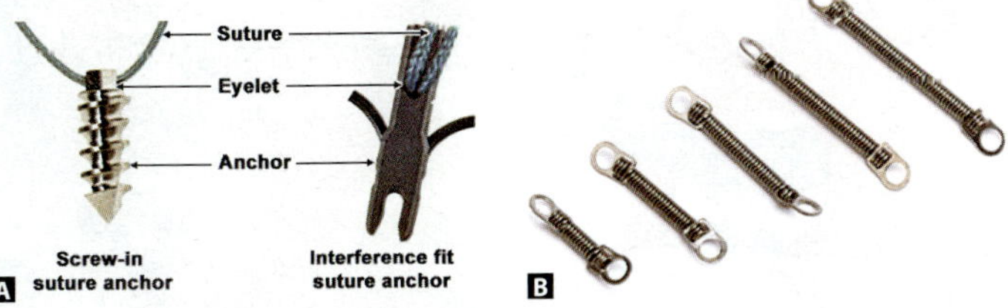

Figs A and B: *(A) Closed anchor suture; (B) Closed coil spring*

C

Coarctation of aorta (COA) is a congenital heart disease where infants may have severe heart failure. Adults may have only hypertension. There will be absent or weak temoral pulses. Systolic pressure is higher in upper extremity then lower and diastolic pressure remains the same. Harsh systolic murmur may be heard in back ECG shows left ventricular hypertrophy.

Coated hairy tongue is a yellow, whitish or pigmented covering on all or a portion of the tongue's dorsal surface. Normally keratinized surface layers of filliform papillae are continuously desquamated due to friction of food and anterior upper teeth. These are replaced by new epithelial cells from below. When tongue movements becomes restricted during illness the papilla enlarges and becomes heavily coated. Longer papilla entangles food particles of different colors. Tobacco smoke colors it black. Mid-dorsum is first to be affected. Dehydration and terminally-ill patients also develop thick coatings. Nicotinamide deficiency may produce black hairy tongue in experimental animals. Systemic antibiotics may also produce hairy tongue. Through scrapping and cleaning of tongue is advised.

Cobal-chromium-nickel wire constitutes 40% cobalt, 20% chromium, 15% nickel, 15.8% iron, 7% molybdenum, 2% manganese, 0.15% carbon and 0.04% beryelium. These are available in four temples, soft, ductile, semi-resilient and resilient. Soft temper wires are popular with clinicians because they are easily deformed and shape into appliance. Heat treated wires have increased values of yield strength and resilience.

Cobalt is part of vitamin B_{12} molecule and is incorporated in many enzymes. Human body contains 100 to 150 mg of it. Generally there is no deficiency of cobalt in human being. Daily requirement is of 2 microgram. Its deficiency leads to anemia, abnormalities of hair and skin pigmentation. Its deficiency may cause hepatolenticular degeneration. Acute cobalt poisoning leads to diarrhea, tinnitus and loss of hearing.

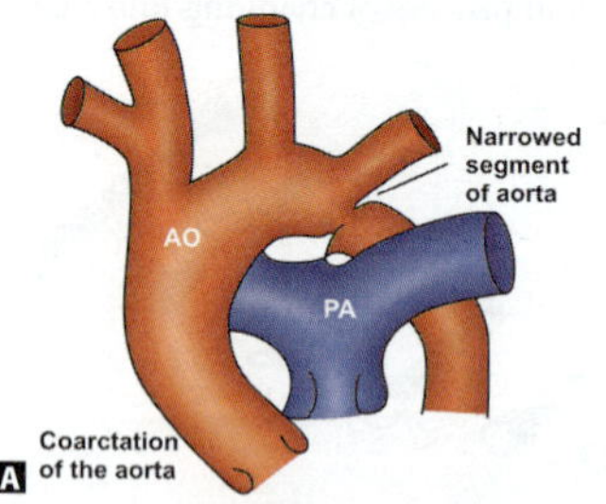

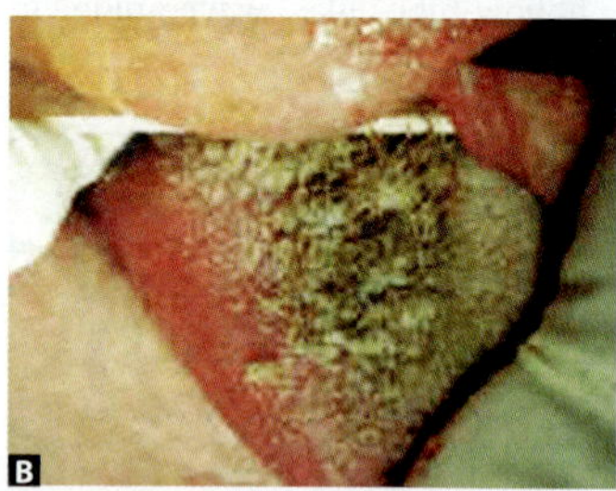

Figs A and B: *(A) Coarctation of aorta; (B) Hairy tongue*

Chronic administration may cause polycythemia.

Cocaine is an alkaloid derived from leaves of erythroxylon coca and its varieties. It is a colorless, odorless, crystalline substance and has bitter taste causing numbness of tongue and mucous membrane of mouth. It is slightly soluble in water but dissolves readily in alcohol. It reduces hunger. Small doses develop euphoria. There is exhilaration, excitement and restlessness.

Cocaine poisoning: It first stimulates then depresses the central nervous system, paralyses the nerve centers of the brain and spinal cord. Small doses develop euphoria. There is exhilaration excitement, restlessness, talkativeness and reflexes are increased temperature may suddenly rise with rigor. Later on dryness of mouth and throat, feeling of numbness and tingling in hand and feet, quick irregular pulse develops. Lastly person may start gasping, convulsion and coma may follow. 10 to 15 grains orally is sufficient to kill a person. A grain injected hypodermically may kill an adult. Death may occur within a few minutes to a few hours.

Coccidioidomycosis causative organism is Coccidioides Immitis. It is of 2 types, primary nondisseminated and progressive disseminated. Patient develops cough, pleural pain, headache, and loss of appetite. Disease may be self limiting in nature.

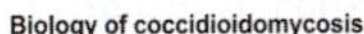

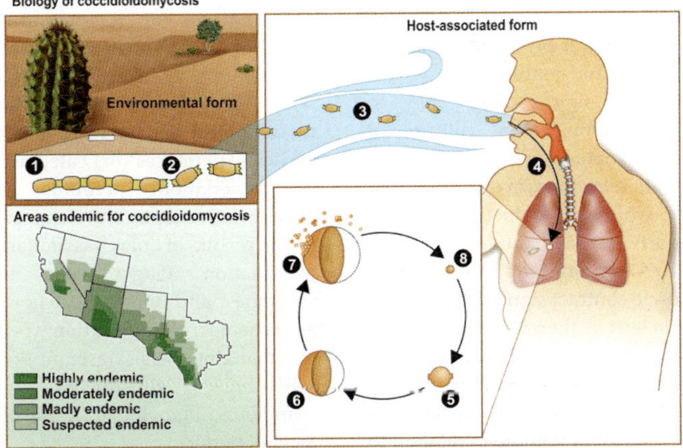

In the environment, Coccioides ssp. exists as a mold (1) with septate hyphae. The hyphae fragment into arthroconidia (2). Which measure only 2–4 μm in diameter and are easily aerosolized when disturbed (3). Arthroconidia are inhaled by a susceptible host (4) and settle into the lungs. The new environment signals a morphologic change, and the arthroconidia become spherules (5). Spherules divide internally until they are filled with endospores (6). When a spherule ruptures (7) the endospores are released and disseminate within surrounding tissue. Endospores are then able to develop into new spherules (6) and repeat the cycle.

Fig.: *Coccidioidomycosis*

C

Coccus means spherical bacterium

Cochlear nuclei are somatic afferent nuclei that are two in number: dorsal and ventral. These nuclei receive fibers from end organs in the cochlea that are concerned with hearing.

Cocoa is obtained from the seeds of plant theobroma cacao. Fat content of seeds is removed and then dried. Theobromine is stimulating principle. It is nutritive as well as stimulating. It has a palatable taste. Chocolate is a preparation of it which is made from ripe seeds of cocoa beans. It lessens the feelings of hunger but does not prolong life in starvation.

Codeine is poor analgesic. It is an effective antitussive and is useful in controlling diarrhea due to its spasmogenic effect on gut. Overdose of it produces, vomiting, dizziness and confusion.

Codman's sign occurs due to pain resulting from rupture of supraspinatus tendon. Have the patient relax the arm on the affected side while you abduct it. If patient reports no pain until you remove your support and the deltoid muscle contract sign is positive.

Coefficient of thermal expansion all metals when cooled they shrink or contract when heated they expand. Coefficient of thermal expansion is the change in volume in relation to change in temperature.

Cofactor is a nonprotein factor attached to an enzyme molecule that enables the enzyme to function well.

Coffey's disease affects children with high fever, raised ESR and pleural exudate. Child is hyper-irritable with soft tissue swelling with pain. There is patchy distribution of lesion characterized by remissions and relapses. Marked cortical thickening of mandible is seen.

Cognition refers to giving attention.

Cognitive theory: In the year 1952, Jean Piaget; A Swiss psychologist formulated a theory on how children with adolescent think and acquire knowledge. He derived his theories from direct observation of children by questioning about their thinking. Like other theories, it also passes through relatively distinct stages and its development is based on one dominant individual. This process of adaptation is made up of 3 functional variants. Assimilation: concerns with observing, recognizing taking up an object and relating it with earlier experiences (or) categories. Accommodation: accounts for changing concepts and strategies as a result of new assimilated information Piaget calls the strategies and mental categories as schemes. Equilibration: refer to changing basic assumptions following adjustments in assimilated knowledge so that the facts fit better.

Coherency is a property unique to lasers. The light waves produced by a laser are a specific form of electromagnetic energy. A laser produces light waves that are physically identical. They are all in phase with one another; that is, they have identical amplitude and identical frequency.

Coherent scatter is one of the interactions of X-radiation with matter in which the path of X-ray photon is altered by matter without a change in energy.

Cold abscess is a slow forming abscess. It can develop anywhere in the body. Patient is usually a young person with swelling of insidious onset. It is hemispherical, smooth, soft and non-tender. Edges are soft and may not be well-defined. Fluctuation may be present. Patient may have an evidence of tuberculosis.

Cold injury develops due to localized tissue damage due to cold. Frost bitten area becomes hard and white. At high altitude in snow it may develop so. Blood restriction to the area may cause gangrene. Amputation has to be done.

Cold intolerance happens due to damage of body's temperature regulating mechanism. Hormonal deficiency may result it. It may happen in old age too.

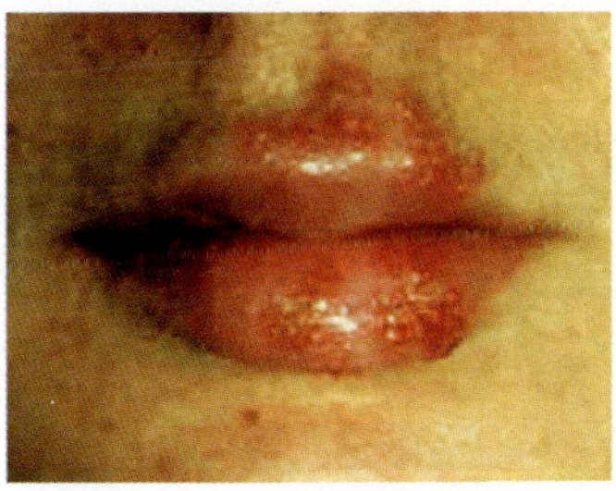

Fig.: *Cold sores*

Cold sterilization is a process of disinfecting instruments by using a liquid chemical germicide. It requires exposure up to 10 hours. Aseptic rinsing with sterile water and drying should follow.

Cold sweat refers to the sweat not associated to high temperature sweating is regulated by sympathetic nervous system. When person is emotionally upset sympathetic nervous system is stimulated and it results in sweating. This sweating is not associated with exercise. It is called a cold sweat.

Cold therapy is the application of cold in the tissues after injury is an old technique. Now ice therapy is done to reduce pain, spasm and spasticity. It reduces pain, spasm and spasticity. It reduces swelling, promotes repair and provides excitatory stimulus.

Colitis is any inflammatory condition of colon or rectum.

Collagen is a protein which is basically composed of different type of aminoacids such as glycine, proline, hydroxylysine and hydroxyproline. The cells mainly responsible for the synthesis of collagen are fibroblasts, chondroblasts, osteoblasts and odontoblasts.

Collagenase is a bacterial enzyme that causes the breakdown of collagen.

Collapsing pulse refers to water hammer pulse.

Collimation refers to the beam having specific spatial boundaries. These boundaries ensure that there is a constant beam size and shape that is emitted from the laser unit.

Colloid is a material in which a constituent in a finely divided state is invisible to the eye but is capable of scattering light is suspended.

Colon is a part of large intestine that is 2.5 inches wide and 4.5 feet long M-shaped loop in abdomen. It is irregular in outline. It consists ascending, transverse, descending and sigmoid colon. Ascending colon starts at caccum and extends upto liver. Point is known as hepatic flexure. Then it passes to spleen and bend is known as splenic flexure. From here it comes to pelvis and becomes 's' shaped sigmoid colon.

Colorado stains was the name given by Dr Frederick S Mckay for the condition dental fluorosis and described it in the literature as mottled enamel. Ingestion of excessive fluoride leads to enamel hypomineralization due to toxic damage to the ameloblastic cells. This may lead to development of pitting or crack in the tooth. The stains may range from isolated white flakes to smudged dark brown stains.

Colostomy is the opening of the colon.

Color content relative intensity at each wave-length.

Color Doppler of heart is a diagnostic test that shows patterns and direction of flow. It is better for evaluation of heart disease. It can frequently detect clinically insignificant valvular regurgitation.

Color fatigue refers to decrease in response to one color due to constant stimulus.

Color rendering index is a measure of the degree to which illuminant can impart the color of an object as compared to the reference source.

Colubrine snake bite symptoms develop within 15 minutes. Patient complains of burning pain which passes off with local redness, erythema and local paresis. There will be nausea, progressive weakness, staggering gait and feeling of intoxication

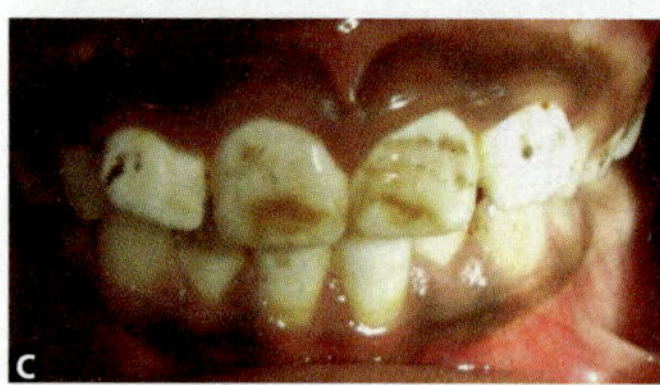

Figs A to C: (A) *Collimator*, (B) *Colon; (C) Colarado stains*

with loss of power. There may be general paralysis of all voluntary muscles and person will not be able to swallow. Death occurs due to paralysis of respiratory center in medulla.

Coma is the stage of unconsciousness resembling deep sleep and involves stoppage of action of brain. Consumption of excess of barbiturates, alcohol, and opium or brain injury may result in it. In the actual stage of coma reflexes are absent. Sphincters are relaxed and there is intoxication of urine and feces. Body temperature becomes subnormal and breathing becomes slow and irregular.

Comfort control syringe (CCS) is an electronic, pre-programmed delivery system for local anesthesia that dispenses the anesthetic in a slower, more controlled and more consistent manner than traditional manual syringe. The comfort control syringe has two-stage delivery system in which injection begins at a very slow rate to decrease the discomfort associated with rapid injection. After ten seconds, CCS automatically increases injection rate for the technique which has been selected. There are five different injection rates to choose from that are preprogrammed into CCS system. As a result, CCS can be adapted for any intraoral injection and still deliver an injection that can be less painful than with a manual syringe.

Communited fracture involves compound fracture with extensive communition.

Commissural lip pits are epithelium lined blind tracts located at corners of mouth. Tracts may be shallow or of several millimeters deep. These are common developmental anomalies. No treatment is advised.

Commissures refer to the corner of mouth.

Common bile duct is a duct from liver going to duodenum. It is made up of right and left hepatic duct.

Common carotid artery is a branch of the brachiocephalic trunk, while on

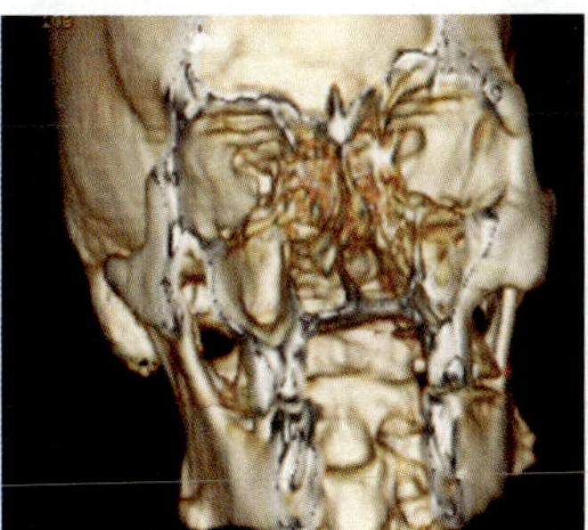

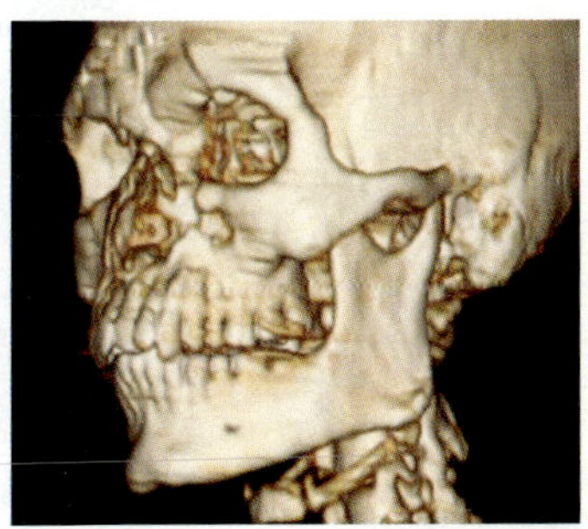

Fig.: *Communited fracture*

the left side, it is a direct branch of the arch of the aorta.

Common cold is a viral disease and lasts for 5–7 days. Large virus of 5 um causes upper respiratory tract infection. Smaller than this causes pneumonitis and bronchiolitis. Person develops sore-throat and nasal obstruction. Diagnosis is on the basis of symptoms so is the treatment.

Communicable is a term which signifies a capacity for the maintenance of infection by various means of spread such as by direct contact or by air-borne route.

Communicable diseases are capable of being transmitted from one person to another.

Communication is a two-way process of exchanging and shaping feelings, ideas and information. It is more than mere exchange of information. It is an interdisciplinary science. Communication gaps produce problem.

Community dentistry is a speciality that encompasses the dental health of the public and use of dental services by public. It involves identifying and addressing the oral health needs of a particular population.

Community oral health is the oral health education and promotion aimed at meeting the specific oral health needs of a people, group, community, state or nation.

Community organization is a process aimed at developing the skills and abilities for the betterment of group.

Community water fluoridation is defined as the controlled adjustment of the concentration of fluoride in a communal water supply so as to achieve maximum caries prevention and a clinically insignificant level of fluorosis (Gordon Nikiforuk).

Compact bone is a dense bone, contains structural units called Haversian systems.

Complement (c) pathway is an interacting network of about 30 membrane associated cell receptors and soluble serum of about 30

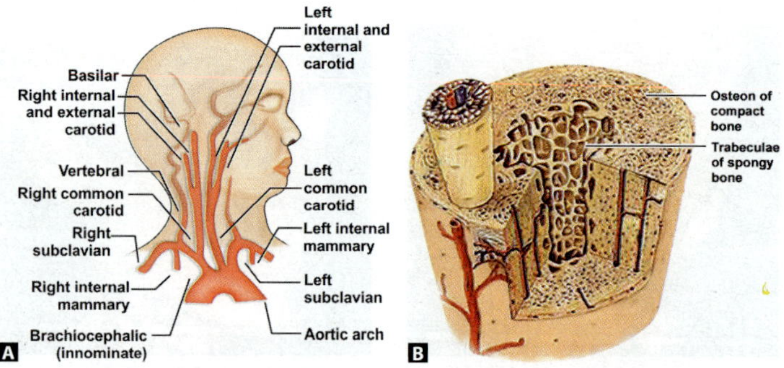

Figs A and B: *Common carotid artery; (B) Compact spongy bone*

membrane associated cell receptors and soluble serum glycoproteins.

Complete radiolucent radiopaque areas: Radiolucent and radiopaque areas may show sun burst appearance. Peak age of incidence is around 25. Jaw lesions have fewer tendencies to metastasize hence better prognosis.

Complex caries refers to lesion involving three or more than surfaces.

Composite faced crowns are also used as long-term provisional restorations. The laboratory grade composite is cured by an intense light and sometimes with additional heat and pressure.

Composite is a tooth colored restorative material. The word "composite" refers to the mixture of filler particles in a liquid resin. Commonly, the resin used is BIS-GMA (bisgammamethylmetacrylate). Filler particles are added to alter the color and wear characteristics. Common filler particles are silica, aluminium, zinc, tin, copper and iron.

Composite resin cements are liners having antibacterial effect with reparative dentin. Calcium hydroxide mixed with resins is initially less irritating but are able to stimulate the formation of reparative dentin. It acts as a contract dressing in the event of exposure of pulp. There is an evidence that these materials breakdown in time and create a gap between the restoration and the cavity wall.

Composite syringe is a device which helps to dispense composite into tooth preparation.

Compound caries refers to lesion involving two surfaces of a tooth.

Compound fracture involves overlying skin and adjacent tissues including bone.

Comprehensive fluoride therapy refers to the use of both systemic and topical fluoride therapies to maintain a caries free oral environment.

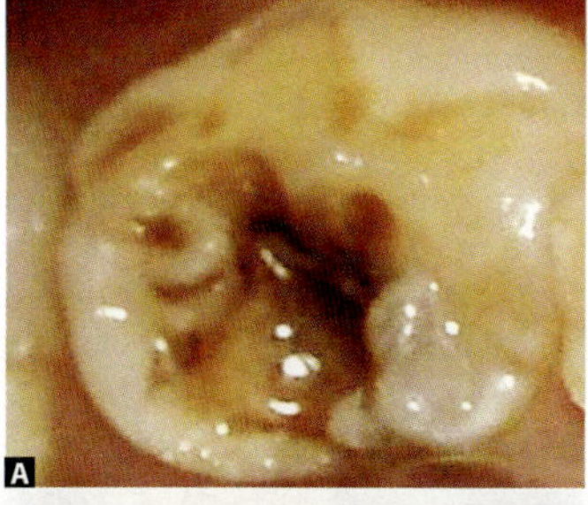

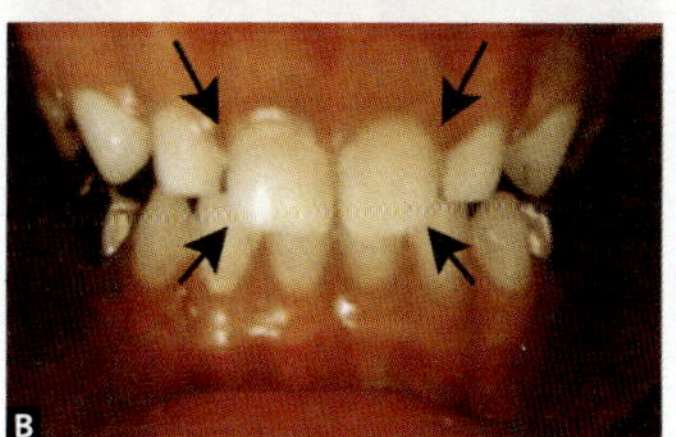

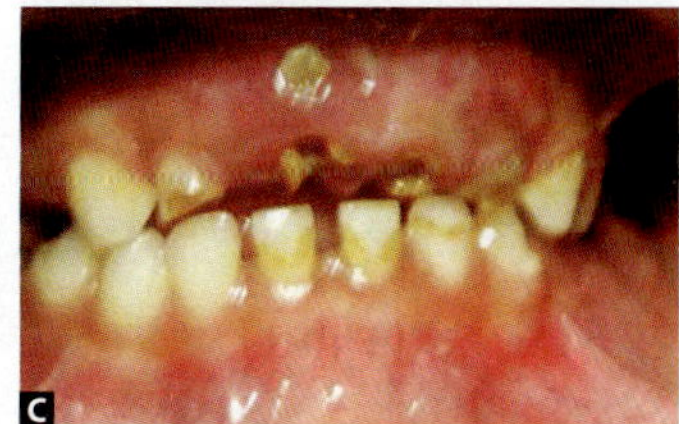

Figs A to C: *(A) Complex caries; (B) Composite faced crown; (C) Compound caries*

Compression plates are plates designed on the same principle, for anatomical reasons, it is only used on convex surface of the mandible towards its lower border. These are applied on the bone surface using screws which engages itself in the inner cortical plate hence it should be placed below the inferior dental canal.

Compton scatter refers to one of the interactions of radiation.

Compudent featuring the WAND handpiece. This has been approved by US Food and Drug Administration. (FDA) as local anesthesia delivery device.

Compulsive eating is an uncontrolled episode of overeating without other signs of eating disorder. Most that compulsively overeat do so in response to stress of feelings of depression.

Compulsive habits are deep-rooted habits that have acquired a fixation in the child to the extent that the child retreats to the habit whenever his security is threatened by events which occur around him. The child tends to suffer increased anxiety when attempts are made to correct the habit.

Concave refers to the curving inward away from the viewer.

Concept is a phenomenon expressed in words sometimes used as a more concrete term than construct.

Conceptualization is the process of developing a mental configuration of a concept.

Concordent refers to a condition where a disease occurs in both twins.

Concrescence is union of two adjacent teeth by cementum alone without union of the underlying dentin. Unlike fusion and gemination, concrescence can be developmental or post-developmental inflammation. More frequent in posterior maxilla. Usually occurs between maxillary second and third molars.

Concurrent disinfection is a measure taken that can keep the patient's environment clean on a daily basis.

Condensation polymerization is a polymerization process in which a by-product such as water or alcohol is formed as chain grows.

Condenser refers to a dental hand instrument used to pack plastic type restorative material into a cavity preparation.

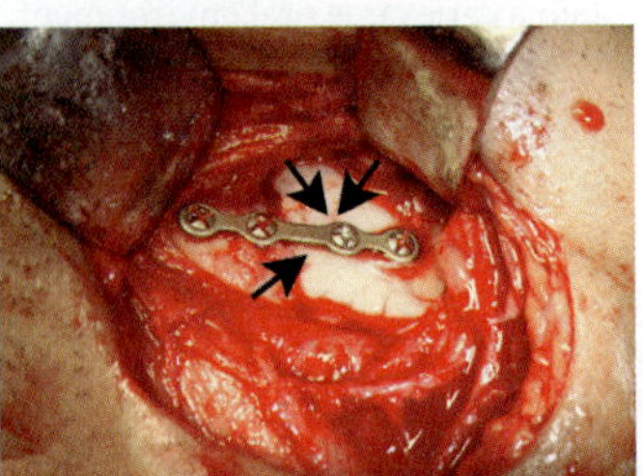

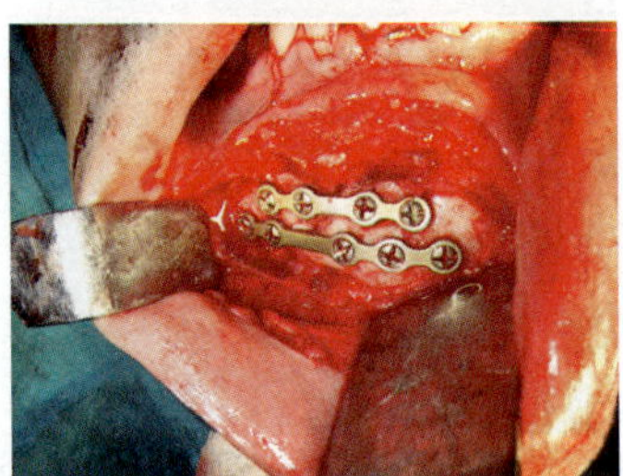

Fig.: *Compression plates*

Condensing osteitis is well-defined radio-opacity below the apex of a non-vital tooth suffering from long-standing pulpitis.

Condiments refer to the agents those besides giving flavors and stimulating the flow of digestive juices. Condiments relieve flatulent distension occurring from the fermentation in the intestines. Black pepper, cloves, chillies and coriander are all used in the preparation of different foods to give color, flavor and taste. Condiments are known as food adjuncts. These should be used in strict moderation. If taken in excess, they tend to irritate and inflame the mucosa of stomach. Vinegar is a well-known antiseptic and preservative. It is used for pickling fish, fruits and vegetables. It also softens hard muscle fibers of meat and cellulose of green vegetables.

Condyle is a rounded projection on a bone.

Condyloma acuminatum is an infectious disease caused by virus (HPV). It is transmissible and auto inoculable viral disease. It presents as soft pink nodules which proliferate and coalesce. These lesions appear as small in size, multiple and white or pink nodular. Surgical excision may be required.

Cone cut is a clear, unexposed area on a dental radiograph that occurs when position indicating that device is misaligned and X-ray beam is not centered over the film.

Cone image shift technique is that as the vertical or horizontal angulations of X-ray tube head change, the object buccal or closest to the tube head moves to opposite side of radiograph when compared to lingual object. In other words, we can say that the cone image shift technique separates and identifies the facial and lingual structures. As the cone position moves from parallel either towards horizontal or vertical, the object on the film shifts away from the direction of cone, i.e. in the direction of central beam.

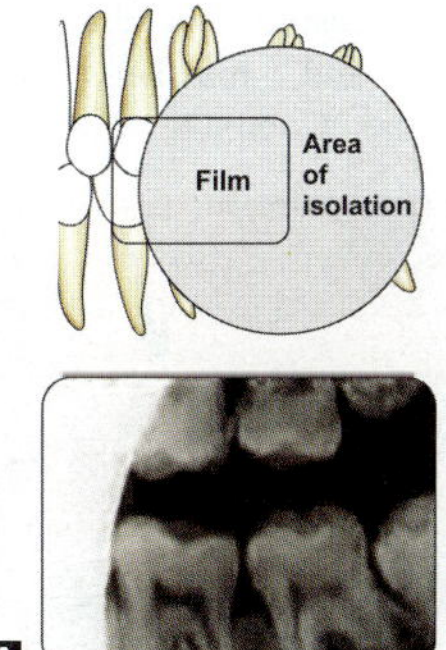

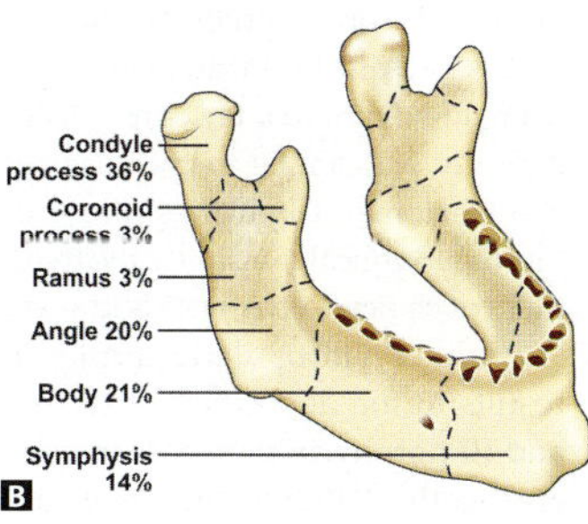

Figs A and B: *(A) Cone-cut; (B) Condyle*

Confabulation is fabrication to cover gaps in memory. It is most commonly seen in alcoholism.

Confidentiality is the ethical requirement to restrict disclosure of client information outside therapy session also.

Confidentiality refers to the right of the patient to have information about his illness remains private.

Conformational epitopes: Brought together in space through folding of polypeptides a polysaccharide chain into a 3D conformation. Lost if AG is denatured and fails to fold properly.

Confusion can result from fluid and electrolyte imbalance or due to lack of oxygen. It may result due to many diseases and may even be irreversible. It is the inability to think quickly and coherently. It is aggravated by stress.

Confusional insanity is characterized by unstable attention and poor perception of present reality, disorientation and inability to act coherently. It results from mental or physical exhaustion and fever.

Congenital epulis protuberant mass of maxilla or mandibular gingiva that is present by birth. Size varies from a few mm to a few cms. Histologically, it is similar to granular cell myoblastoma. Capillaries are numerous. Surgical excision is the treatment of choice. Recurrence is known.

Congenital erythropoietic porphyria results in the deposition of types I and III porphyrin pigments in bone and teeth. Although this is a rare in-born error of metabolism, the dental effects are more pronounced.

Congenital lip pits are pits present on lips congenitally.

Congenital syphilis is contracted in utero from a mother who had treponemal infection, i.e. transmission of infection from untreated mother to fetus. Untreated maternal syphilis can lead to stillbirth, premature birth and neonatal death. A child may be born with syphilitic features. Syphilis produces classic patterns of hypoplastic dysmorphic permanent teeth. Saber shins, rhagades, frontal bossing and saddle nose are common structural anomalies. Congenital syphilis clinically will present with 1) interstitial keratiti; 2) deafness; 3) tooth anomalies (Hutchinson's triad).

Congenitally missing teeth by missing teeth is meant those teeth whose tooth germ did not develop sufficiently to allow the differentiation of the dental tissues. The teeth most frequently found congenitally missing are mandibles, second bicuspids, maxillary lateral incisor, and maxillary second bicuspids. Complete absence of

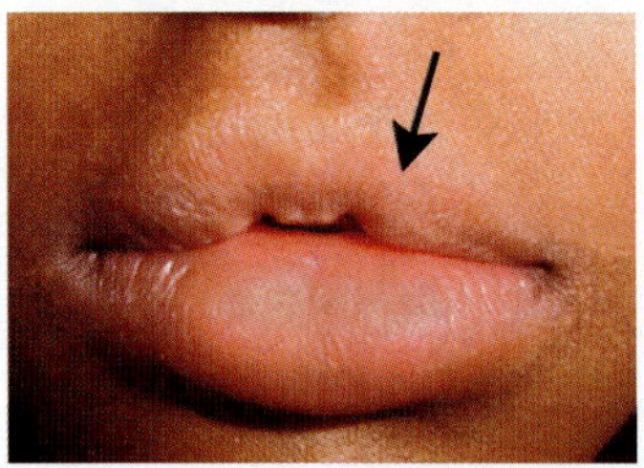

Fig.: *Lip pits*

all teeth called Anodontia (rare) Oligodontia partial presence of teeth.

Connation refers to joined teeth.

Conscious sedation is a minimally depressed level of consciousness. Patient maintains airway and responds to verbal command.

Consensus refers to generally accepted view.

Consent is a patient agreement with a physician doing surgery or certain tests. Consent is valid when patient has been told about implications, side effects of procedure in clear terms. When patient is not fit, consent can be given by near relatives.

Consent of sexual intercourse refers to a woman of and above the age of 18 years is capable of giving consent, to an act of sexual intercourse. But the consent must be conscious free, voluntary and given in full command of senses.

Constrictive pericarditis healed: Pericarditis may cause marked thickening of visceral and parietal layers of the pericardium making thick rigid cage closely developing the heart which hampers the filling of cardiac chambers. Tuberculous pericarditis is the most important cause. Areas of caseation necrosis may be recognized. Pericardial fluid is thick, opaque and consists of fibrin, caseous material and blood. Heart is reduced in size. Stroke volume is low and progressive heart failure results.

Contact angle is an angle formed between the surface of a liquid drop and the solid surface on which it rests.

Contact area refers to that portion of the proximal surface of a tooth that touches the adjacent tooth.

Contact dermatitis can be described as itching or burning sensation at the site of contact develops. Mucosa becomes remarkably inflamed and edematous. Small vesicles may form on rupture areas of erosion and ulceration develops. Certain dental material has been implicated causing contact dermatitis, acrylic when used as a denture material may produce allergy. Treatment includes withdrawal of offending material.

Contact hypersensitivity is characterized clinically by eczema at the site of contact with the allergen seen maximally at 48 hrs. The most common Ag are haptens such as nickel, chromate, chemicals

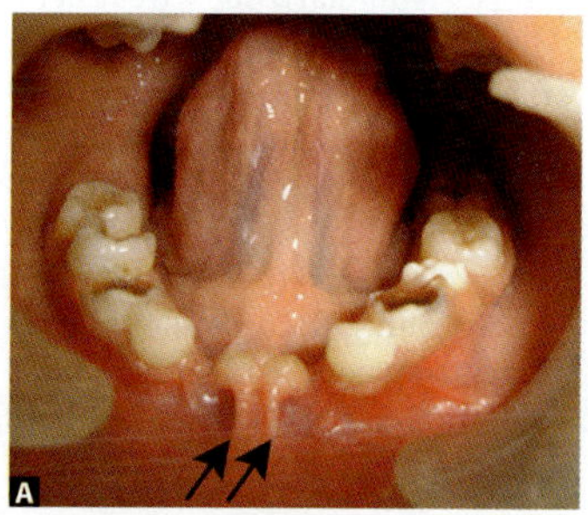

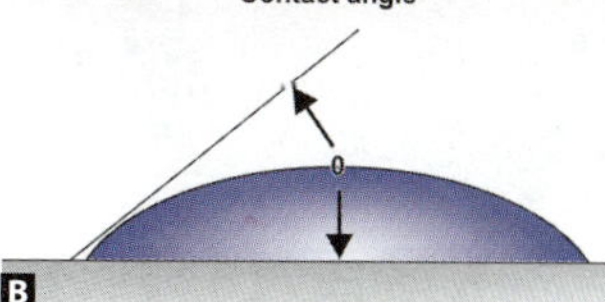

Figs A and B: *(A) Hypodontia and double frenum; (B) Contact angle*

found in rubber, poision ivy and poison oak. It is the major cause of occupational disease. Small haptens which induce hypersensitivity would not by themselves be antigenic, however, these low molecules weight compounds penetration epidermis and become conjugated either covalently or non-covalently to body proteins.

Contact precaution is the measure used to block transmission of pathogens by direct or indirect contact.

Contact stomatitis see stomatitis venenata.

Contagious disease refers to an infective disease that can be transmitted to another person.

Contaminated refers to not sterile.

Contemporaneous records means "Recorded at that time" essential requirement of dated entry summarizing treatment, diagnosis, report, observation, positive signs of symptoms and absence of signs. If you speak to the patient or refer to patient or speak to his/her doctor do remember to write it down and date of entry. Records should be in diary sequence with other dated enteries and no attempt should ever be made to cover one's track by altering or improving an original record card.

Content analysis is a process by which the text of archival record is reduced to quantifiable information.

Continence training is the process of restoring control of urination.

Continuous fever occurs when fever does not fluctuate more than 1°C about 1.5°F during 24 hours but never touches normal.

Continuous suture is a method of suturing, one thread runs from one end to final end and is tied at last.

Continuous variable is a variable that theoretically can be measured to finer degrees.

Continuous wave the laser beam is emitted at one power level continuously as long as the device is activated by pressing the foot switch.

Contracture refers to shortening or distortion. It is a permanent damage due to shrinkage of muscles.

Contralateral refers to opposite extremity.

Contrast film refers to the characteristic of film that influences radiographic contrast.

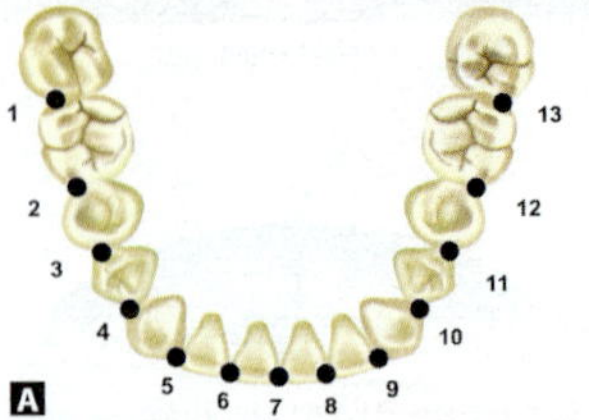

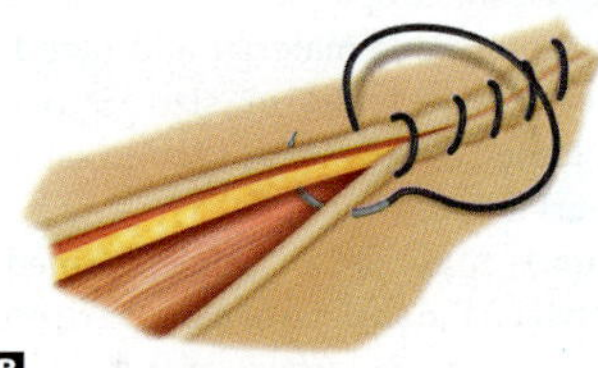

Figs A and B: *(A) Contact area; (B) Continuous sutures*

Contrast refers to comparison of two means specifically multiple comparison tests conducted as part of complex analysis of variance tests.

Contrast medium is the substance that adds density to a body organ such as barium/iodine.

Contrast short scale refers to radiograph with two densities of gray and a black and white. It results from the use of lower kilovoltage range.

Contributory negligence describes a patient's contribution to the harm. He has not taken drugs as advised. In this way patient contributes to the negligence.

Control tooth refers to healthy tooth used as a standard to compare questionable teeth.

Contusion refers to a bruise. It is a superficial injury usually painful is produced by impact without laceration.

Conventional finger rest is a type of rest which is established on tooth surfaces immediately adjacent to the working area.

Conventional hot air oven utilizes radiating dry heat for sterilization as this type of energy does not penetrate materials easily. So long periods of exposure to high temperature are usually required.

Convex refers to curving outward toward the viewer.

Cooley peg is a device used to seat a crown or bridge restoration into tooth preparation.

Coping is a thin metal covering or cap placed over a prepared tooth.

Copper is needed for normal erythropoiesis as well as for absorption of iron. Other metalloenzymes require copper include tyrosinase and lysyl oxidase.

Copper cement was widely used in temporarily filling material in children's teeth. It has strong germicidal property. In human it produces inflammatory cell infiltration, hemorrhage and necrosis with destruction of odontoblasts in pulp. This effect is due to soluble copper ions which are dissolved in acid.

Copper sulphate poisoning is known as 'neela thota'. Symptoms develop within 15-30 minutes. There is a metallic taste in the mouth. There is a sense of burning with abdominal pain. Vomiting and diarrhea develops. Vomited matter is green or blue colored. Convulsions and

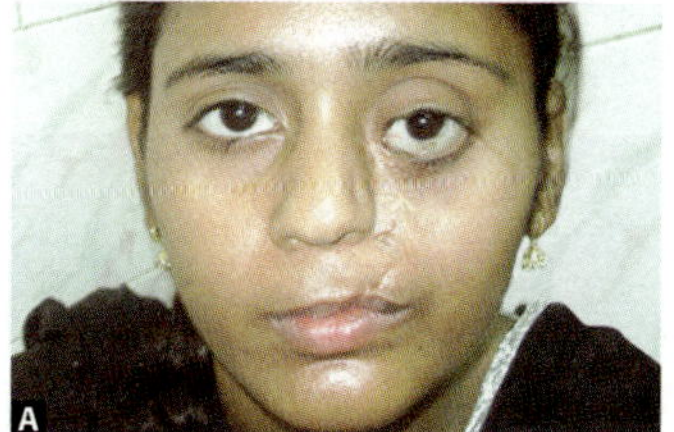

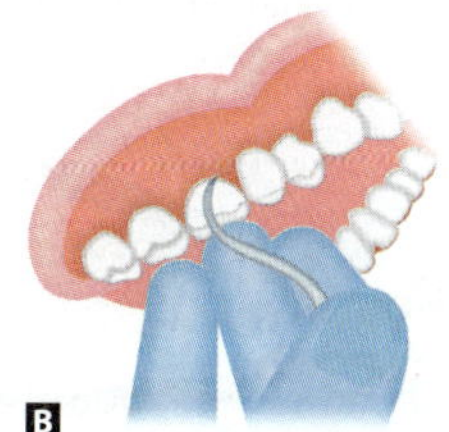

Figs A and B: *(A) Contracture; (B) Conventional finger rest*

coma precede death. 30 gram is fatal dose and person may die within 3-5 days.

Core temperature is the warmth at the center of body.

Cornea refers to the choroid consists of a network of blood vessels supported by connective tissue containing many pigmented cells that give it a dark brown color. It is the dark color of the choroid that darkens the interior of the eyeball. It also prevents reflection of light within the eyeball. Both these factors are necessary for formation of sharp images on the retina. Within the choroid, there is an outer vascular layer made up of small arteries and veins, and an inner capillary layer. Cornea is not exactly circular. As the cornea is more convex than the sclera, the junction of the two is marked, on the exterior of the eyeball, by a groove called the sulcus sclerae. The cornea is made up of five layers.

Corneal abrasion refers to the injury of the cornea. The symptoms include significant eye pain, foreign body sensation, photophobia and tearing. Person will develop edema of eyelid and redness of conjunctiva.

Corneal ulcer: There will be pain in eye, lacrimation, photophobia and blurring of vision. Marked blephobia and blurring of vision. Marked blephrospasm is present. There is rough and yellowish white area on cornea. Surrounding cornea may be hazy. Ciliary congestion is present. Small amount of pus may be visible in lower part of anterior chamber.

Corneal xerosis is due to deficiency of vitamin A. Liquefaction of cornea is a medical emergency. Cornea may become soft. Process is rapid and is an important cause of blindness.

Coronal: It divides the body into anterior and posterior.

Coronal dentin dysplasia is inherited as autosomal dominant type. Primary teeth are translucent with amber color. Primary teeth present normal color and normal crown. Permanent teeth may or may not have pulp stones.

Coronal perforation can occur during access cavity preparation. If the perforation is above the periodontal attachment, leakage of saliva into cavity or sodium hypochlorite in mouth is the main sign. But if perforation occurs into the periodontal ligament, bleeding is the hallmark feature.

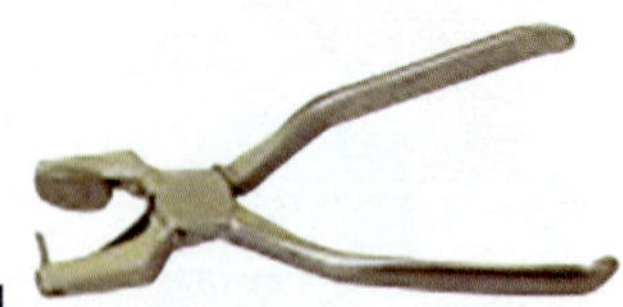

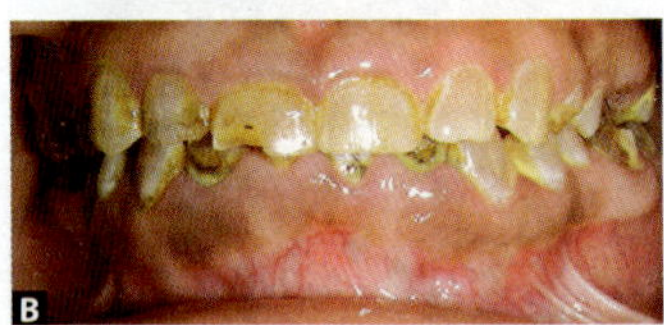

Figs A and B: *(A) Cooley peg; (B) Coronal dentin dysplasia*

Coronary arteries refer to those arteries which carry blood to the muscles of heart. Left and right coronary arteries arise from aorta. In coronary thrombus obstruction and narrowing takes place. This reduces the blood supply to the part which is a major cause of heart disease.

Coronary embolism refers to the blocking of a coronary blood vessel by a clot.

Coronary sinus refers to the area that receives deoxygenated blood from the coronary veins and empties into right atrium.

Corpora arenacea, or 'brains and' are the sections of the pineal gland show aggregations of salts containing calcium. They are by-products of secretory activity.

Corrective orthodontics refers to reduce the severity of an existing malocclusion or to eliminate it.

Corrosives are those substances which cause destruction of the parts with which they come in contact due to protoplasmic coagulation and extraction of water. Corrosives include acids and alkalis. There will be burning pain in mouth and throat. Bowels are constipated. There may be tenesmus; voice becomes hoarse and husky.

Cortical refers to the outer layer of bone appears radio-opaque.

Cortical plate refers to the compact bone covering the alveolar process.

Corticosteroids inhalers are the choice of treatment in bronchial asthma. Oral prednisolone and inhalational steroids like beclomethasone, betamethasome are used in the prophylactic treatment of moderate cases. Exact mechanism is not known but there is stabilization of most cells, inhibitors of release of inflammatory mediators. These reduce edema of submucosal tissues.

Cortisol refers to the steroid secreted by adrenal cortex. It is one of the stress hormones.

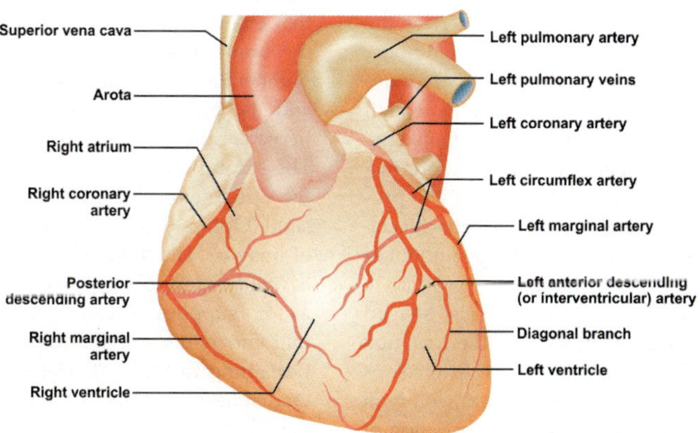

Fig.: *Coronary arteries*

C

Cortisol deficiency can lead to relatively rapid onset of clinical symptoms, including loss of consciousness and possible death. Adrenocortical deficiency is called Addison's disease.

Cosmetic dentistry is the branch of dentistry that deals with the aesthetic improvement of the color and shape of teeth performed by a general dentist.

Cost benefit ratio is the difference between the expense of having a program or not to have a program.

Costen's syndrome is a condition in which severe shooting pain radiates down the cover jaw. Pain may be in temple area on chewing. It is due to malocclusion.

Cough formulas are commercially available preparations of centrally acting cough suppressants, expectorants and mucolytics. These may also be combined with antihistamines, antiadrenergics and bronchodilators like salbutamol.

Cough is a relax action to clear the airways of mucus or foreign body. It may be a symptom of underlying disease. In bronchitis cough contains large amount of phlegm. Brochospasm as in asthma produces dry cough. Pneumonia will produce cough with pain. Bronchiectasis causes morning large amount of foul smelling cough.

Cough lozenges are disc-shaped tablets taken to treat the irritation of pharyngeal mucosa. It develops in diseases like influenza, common cold and pneumonitis. Irritation of mucosa results in cough.

Coupling agent is a chemical attached to the filter surface for the purpose of creating a bond with the resin matrix upon polymerization. It improves strength and wearing resistance.

Cowden's syndrome describes hamartomas involvement of many organs with a potential of neoplastic transformation. It is inherited as autosomal dominant character. Multiple cysts over lips and gingiva are seen. Tongue is also fissured. Hemangiomas and neuromas are also seen.

Cracked tooth syndrome describes development of a crack in a restored or an unrestored tooth due to excessive occlusal forces is one of the main causes. There is sharp pain on biting. Pain is similar to that of trigeminal neuralgia. Radiographs are unable to show cracked tooth.

Cranial refers to towards head.

Cranial nerves are those nerves that emerging from the surface of the brain. They are identified by number (in cranio-caudal sequence) and also bear names—First cranial nerve is called the olfactory nerve. The second cranial nerve is called the optic nerve. It is the nerve of sight (Optics = science of formation of images). The third cranial nerve is called the oculomotor nerve as it supplies several muscles that move the eyeball (Ocular = pertaining to the eye). The fourth cranial nerve is called the trochlear nerve. It is so called because it supplies a muscle (superior oblique) that passes through a pulley (trochlea = pulley). The fifth cranial nerve is called the trigeminal nerve because it has three major divisions; (1)—The ophthalmic division to the orbit; (2)—The maxillary division to the upper jaw; (3)—The mandibular division to the lower jaw. The sixth cranial nerve is called the abducent nerve because it supplies a muscle (lateral rectus) that 'abducts' the eyeball. The seventh cranial nerve is the facial nerve because it supplies the muscles of the face. The eighth cranial nerve is called the vestibulocochlear nerve because it supplies structures in the vestibular and cochlear parts of the internal ear. It is, sometimes, called auditory nerve (auditory = pertaining to hearing) and stato-acoustic nerve (stato = pertaining to equilibrium; acoustic = pertaining to sound or hearing). The ninth cranial nerve is called the glossopharyngeal nerve as it is distributed to the pharynx and to part of the tongue (glossal = pertaining to the tongue). The tenth cranial nerve is called the vagus. It has an extensive course through the neck, the thorax and the abdomen. The eleventh cranial nerve is called the accessory nerve because it appears to be a part of the vagus nerve (or 'accessory' to the vagus). The twelfth cranial nerve is called the hypoglossal nerve (because it runs part of its course below the tongue before supplying the muscles in it (hypo = below; glossal = pertaining to tongue).

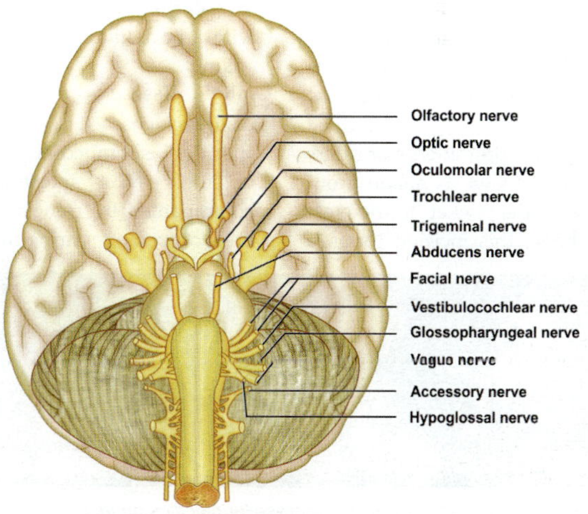

Fig.: *Cranial nerve*

Craniometry is the metric study of cranial dimension in dry skulls.

Craniopharyngioma these arise from hypophyseal duct. Being suprasellar they present with visual loss and hydrocephalus. Size may vary from small rounded nodule to large multilocular cyst. Suprasellar calcification is seen. Cystic tumors require evacuation.

Craniosynostosis is a premature fusion or closure of one or more sutures of skull. It may be primary or secondary. Skull may show silver beaten appearance.

Crede maneuver is the act of bending forward and applying hand pressure over the bladder to stimulate urination.

Cresol is three times potent as phenol and is equally toxic. Lysol is a 50% cresol in linseed oil and is widely used for disinfecting floors. It is fairly an efficient bactericide. It is a popular root canal antiseptic. It is lesser irritant than phenol. It is a popular phenol derived root canal medicine.

Crest refers to a prominence or ridge.

Crevicular incision is made from the base of the pocket, to the crest of the bone, this incision forms a v-shaped wedge ending near the crest of the bone.

Critical instruments are used to penetrate soft tissues and bones are known as critical and are to be used after every use. Such instruments include forceps, scalpels, bone chisel and surgical burs.

Critical pH is the pH at which a solution is just saturated with respect to a particular mineral, such as tooth enamel. If the pH of the solution is above the critical pH, then the solution is supersaturated with respect to the mineral, and more mineral will tend to precipitate out. Conversely, if the pH of the solution is less than the critical ph, the solution is unsaturated, and the mineral will tend to dissolve until the solution becomes saturated. The concept of critical pH is applicable only to solutions that are in contact with a particular mineral, such as enamel.

Crohn's disease is a glaucomatous disorder characterized by non-specific, submucosal alteration of the gasket intestinal tract, accompanied by stenosis, necrotic breakdown and scaring of mucosa.

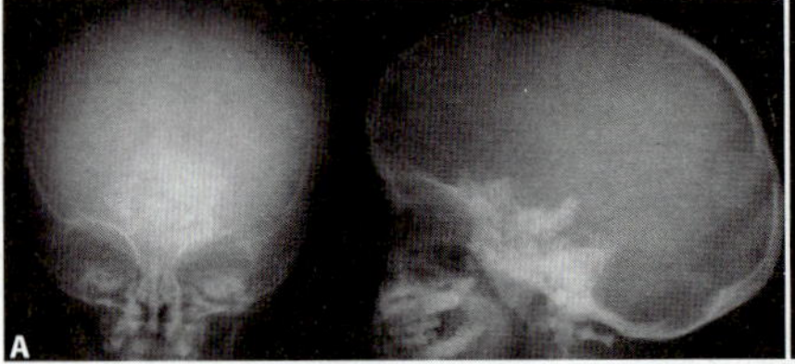

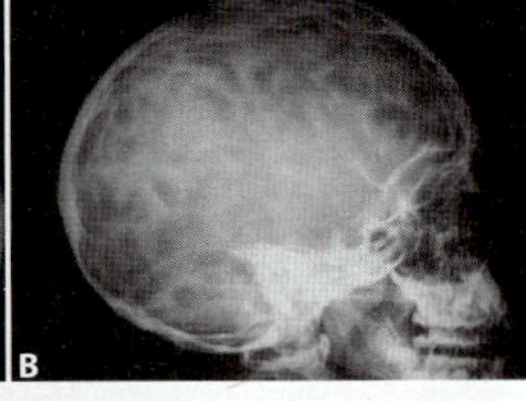

Figs A and B: *(A) Extensive supra-seller calcificaion in a child due to craniopharyngioma; (B) Craniosynostosis*

Oral manifestations: aphthous ulceration most frequent lesion, cobblestone appearance of oral mucosa, confined to buccal mucosa, diffuse erythematous, granular enlargement, gingival lesion are copulated, hypertrophy edematous and fissured, ulceration may be present.

Cross arch finger rest is a type of rest which can be established on the other side of the same arch.

Cross contamination refers to passing of disease indirectly from one patient to another through the use of improper sterilization procedures.

Cross-linked polymer refers to a polymer with a three dimensional network structure.

Cross-sectional study refers to measurements made of different samples and studied at different periods of time.

Crossbite refers to malocclusion in which the facial aspects of the maxillary teeth are located labial to mandibular teeth.

Crowing respiration is slow deep inspiration accompanied by high pitched crowing sound.

Crown is an artificial restoration and replaces at least ¾th of natural crown of tooth. These are made up of various materials. Temporary crowns are used to maintain appearance and avoid pain. Metal crown of aluminium or stainless steel are used on back teeth. Temporary crowns are cemented with an adhesive which can easily be removed and cleaned for fitting of permanent crown.

Crown-cast refers to a cast restoration that covers the entire anatomic crown of the teeth.

Crude death rates are defined as the number of deaths per 100 estimated midyear populations in one year, in a given place.

Crude fibre is that part of a plant which is not broken down by boiling repeatedly in weak acid and weak alkali. It is a part of cellulose and part of lignin which makes wood harder. Dietary fibre is which passes through the small intestine completely undigested. Bran & whole wheat flour are a good source of it.

Cryosurgery refers to surgery performed with the use of low temperature.

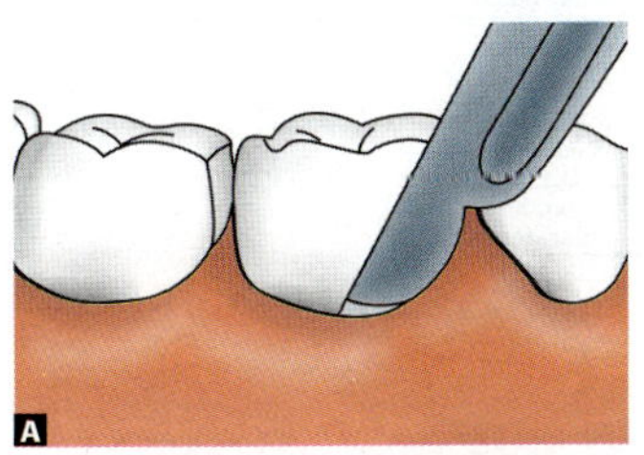

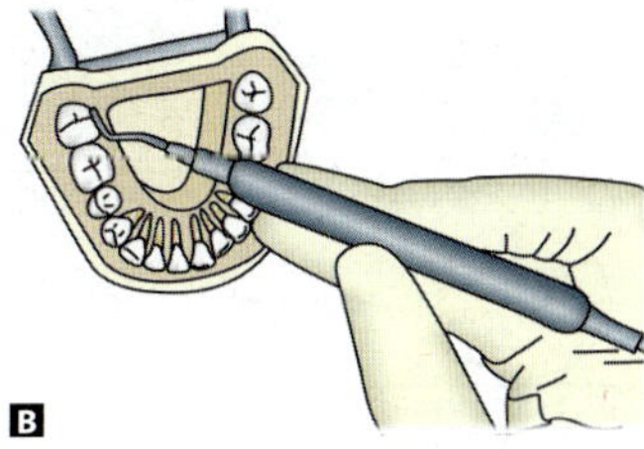

Figs A and B: *(A) Crevicular incision; (B) Cross arch finger rest*

Crystal habit refers to the external geometrical shape of a crystal.

Crystals in urine are seen in normal as well as in abnormal urine. Calcium oxalate crystals are small, colorless resembling envelops seen in chronic renal disease. Uric acid and urate crystals are four sided yellow or brownish seen in gout. Phosphate crystals are colorless 3 to 6 sided prisms having little clinical significance.

Cullen's sign includes are irregular, bluish hemorrhagic pitch on the skin around the umbilicus and occasionally around abdominal scars. It may be due to trauma or hemorrhage.

Cumulative index is an index that measures all the evidence of a condition, past and present, e.g. DMF index for dental caries.

Cumulative trauma disorder is the term used to identify the group of musculoskeletal disorders involving injuries to to tendon, bones and muscles.

Cure stage is a stage at which an impression material hardness and may give off heat.

Cure-dual is a process where hardening of restorative material is brought about by both self-curing and light curing.

Curettage refers to scraping of epithelial lining of the periodontal pocket to separate diseased soft tissue.

Curettes are the fine instruments used for subgingival scaling, root planning and removal of soft tissue lining of the periodontal pocket. The instrument has a cutting edge on both the sides with a rounded toe. The instrument is finer than the sickle scaler and therefore easy to use in deep pockets.

Curing refers to the act of polymerization of a chemical compound.

Curve of Wilson refers to the cross arch curvature of posterior occlusal plane.

Cushing's syndrome results from glucocorticoids when this excess

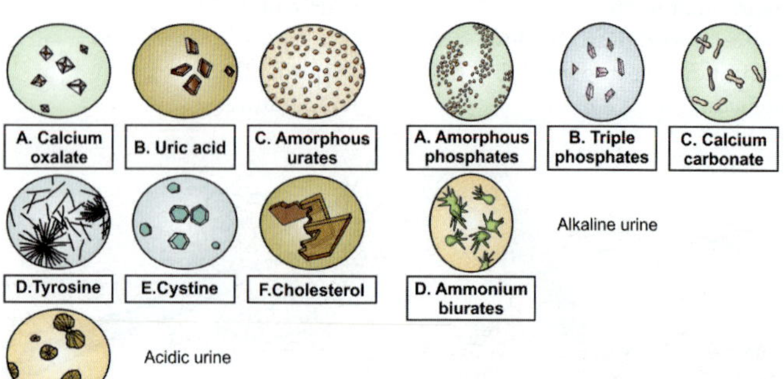

Fig.: *Crystals in urine*

is secondary to ACTH producing primary tumor it is called Cushing's disease. In practice one of the commonest causes is exogenous administration of corticosteroids. Clinical features include obesity, amenorrhea, muscular weakness and fatigue ability and symptoms of depression. Polyuria, headache and hyperpigmentation may develop. Face becomes round, like full moon. Osteoporosis may be severe to cause vertebral collapse. Pathological fractures are common.

Cushing's syndrome adrenal hyperactivity is seen. Patient may be hypertensive and hypoglycemic and show moon face. Gingiva, palate and buccal mucosa may be blotchy due to melanin granules.

Cusp refers to the elevated projection on the crown of a tooth that makes up a divisional portion of occlusal surface.

Cusp of carabelli the most common example of this phenomenon is the cusp of carabelli located on the palatal surface of mesiolingual cusp of a maxillary molar. It is most obvious on first molar.

Cuspid refers to the third tooth from the center of the mouth towards the back, also known as canines.

Cuticle is a thin edge of skin at the base of nail.

Cutting end of burrs are made of different shapes. Round shape is used for reaching to cavities at low speed. Pear shape is used for outlining the cavity.

Cyanocobalamine (Vitamin B_{12}) is a red crystalline substance containing the metal cobalt, it is necessary for the synthesis of DNA. It is not present in food of vegetable origin. It is only available in food of animal origin. It is synthesized by bacteria in human colon but is not being able to absorb. This is relatively heat stable and little is lost in cooking. Daily requirement is 0.5 to 2 microgram.

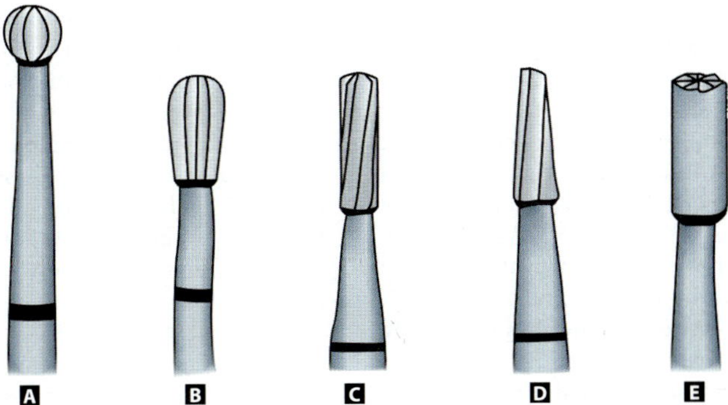

Figs A to E: *Bur (A) Round; (B) Pear; (C) Fissure; (D) Tapered fissures; (E) End-cutting*

C

Generally its deficiency is not seen except in malabsorption syndrome, post-gastrectomy or Crohn's disease. It develops neurological symptoms in 10% of cases of pernicious anemia. Subacute degeneration of spinal cord may occur. Deficiency of it may lead to sore tongue with or without depapillation.

Cyanosis is bluish discoloration of the skin and mucous membrane caused by an increased quantity of reduced hemoglobin (>4 g%) in superficial blood vessels. Cyanosis is looked for at lips, nailbeds, malar area, ear lobes and mucous membrane of the oral cavity. Cyanosis is classified into central and peripheral types.

Cyclamate is another sucrose substitute about 30 times sweeter than sucrose with a pleasant taste.

Cyclic neutropenia is an unusual form of agranulocytosis with periodic or cyclic diminution in polymorphs. Etiology of disease is not known. Infants and young children suffer more. Symptoms are milder than agranulocytosis. Patient exhibits severe gingivitis, stomatitis and ulceration. Isolated painful ulcers occur that may last for 10-14 days. These heal with scarring. There is mild to severe loss of superficial alveolar bone. For 4 to 5 days patient may show normal blood count. At the peak of disease, neutrophils completely disappear. There is no specific treatment for the disease.

Cyclopropane is the only alternate gas to nitrous oxide. It is stored under pressure. It is inflammable and explosive in both air and oxygen. It tends to cause increased salivation.

Cyclosporine was first isolated in switzerland in 1970 as a Metabolite of the fungus specious talypocladium but has little nature as an antifungal antibiotic. However as a cyclic polypeptide with potent immunes suppressive actions, cyclosporine, a survival of allergenic transplant involving skin, heart, kidney, liver, pancreas, bone marrow and lung. It is also used in the treatment of autoimmune disorders such as behcht diseases, rheumatoid Arthritis, SLE, bullous pemphigoid and pemphigus, Crowns disease and insulin – dependent disables.

Cyelopia is a single or partially divided eye in single orbit; absence of nose or presence of proboscis, severe microcephaly with no division between anterior lobes of brain.

Cylindroma is a malignant tumor of salivary gland origin derived from minor or major salivary glands. It is not capsulated and infiltrates surrounding tissue. Tumor is composed of deeply stained, small uniform epithelial cells. These cells are arranged in oval islands. Complete surgical excision is the remedy.

Cynacobalamine (Vitamin B_{12}) is a red crystalline substance containing the metal cobalt, it is necessary for the synthesis of DNA. It is not present in food of vegetable origin.

It is only available in food of animal origin. It is synthesized by bacteria in human colon but is not being able to absorb. This is relatively heat stable and little is lost in cooking. Daily requirement is 0.5 to 2 microgram. Generally its deficiency is not seen except in malabsorption syndrome, post-gastrectomy or Crohn's disease. It develops neurological symptoms in 10% of cases of pernicious anemia. Subacute degeneration of spinal cord may occur. Deficiency of it may lead to sore tongue with or without depapillation.

Cyst is a closed sac or pouch lines with epithelium containing semisolid or fluid. Fluid may or may not be infectious.

Cystic duct is a duct from gallbladder. It joins the hepatic duct to form the common bile duct.

Cystic fibrosis is an autosomal recessive inherited disease. There develops deficiency of pancreatic enzyme and increased susceptibility to respiratory infections. Sodium content increases in sweat.

Cysticercosis is most common parasitic infection that affects central nervous system. Man is the usual definitive host of Taenia solium. Infection occurs by consuming raw or improperly cooked pork. Cyst contains head and suckers and refractile hooklets. Cysts evoke intense inflammatory reaction which resides after the death of scoleces. Signs and symptoms include seizures, raised intracranial pressure and chronic meningitis. If lodged in brain parenchyma, symptoms may include aphasia, ataxia, sensory loss to motor palsy. Average interval between infection and manifestation is 5 years. MRI shows circular cystic lesions or calcified nodules. Albendazole 15 mg/kg/daily for 30 days are effective calcified cysticerci don't respond to the therapy.

Cytogenetics is an area of biology concerned with chromosomes and their implication in genetics.

Cytokeratins are those filaments which are typically expressed in the epithelium. Ten cytokeratins are specific to 'hard' tissues (e.g. Nail and hair). Approximately 20 cytokeratins are found more generally in epithelial lining internal body cavities.

Cytokines molecules that are released by host cells into the local environment, provide molecular signals to other cells thereby affecting their function.

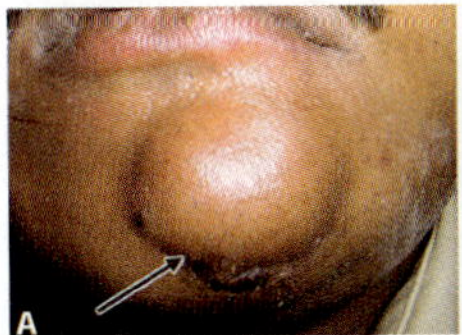

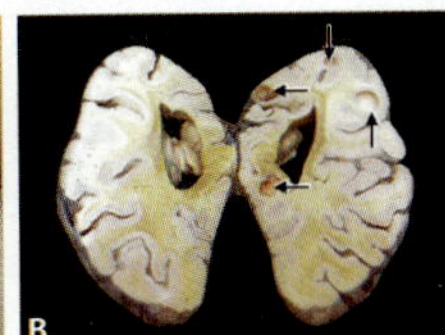

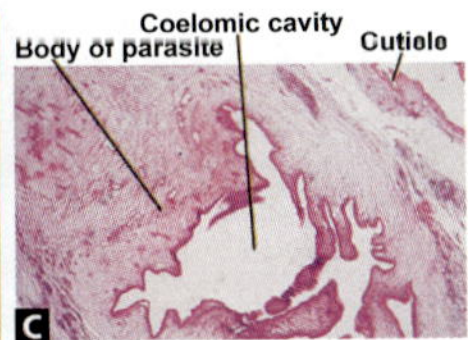

Figs A to C: *(A) Soft tissue cyst; (B and C) Cysticercosis brain*

C

Cytoskeleton is a system of proteins that supports the topography of the cell membrane and organizes the arrangement of the cytoplasmic components into defined areas. The cytoskeleton is composed of three types of filaments: actin (or microfilaments), microtubules, and intermediate filaments. Its major functions are: determining cell shape, organelle anchoring and polarity determination, motility (and migration), anchoring of the cell to external structures, metabolic functions, separating duplicated chromatids and homologous chromosomes into separate cells.

Czechoslovakian caries index: The Czechoslovakian caries index was introduced by Poncova, Novak and Matena in 1956. This index is mainly used to compare caries experience in one group with that of the other groups with a similar population density but living in different environments. In this index, the "variables" seem to be controlled. In all examination studies and tests in which this index is used, the average number of teeth, tooth surfaces and tooth areas and the condition of previously extracted or crowned teeth were considered.

D

Dead space is the part of lung where air is moved in and out but no exchange of gas occurs.

Dean fluorosis index is an index for assessment of dental fluorosis was introduced by Trendley H Dean in 1934 - known as 'Dean's classification system for dental fluorosis or 'Dean's fluorosis index'. Dental fluorosis is shown on a seven-point scale; 'normal', 'questionable', 'very mild', 'mild', 'moderate', moderately severe', and 'severe'. This first description of fluorosis index could be considered an ordinal scale, although no numbers were used. Dean revised version of his fluorosis index in 1942 where he used a six-point scale, i.e., "normal", "mild", "very mild", "moderate" and "severe" where he combined the "moderately severe" and "severe" in 1989.

Death certificate is a legal document confirming a person's death.

Debridement refers to the treatment of a bacterial infection by removing irritants and debris (bacteria, calculus) from the periodontal pocket so as to allow healing of adjacent tissues.

Decalcification refers to loss of calcium salts from enamel. It is the first stage of decay. It causes weakening the teeth and making them more susceptible to decay.

Decayed-missing-field-surface index (DMFS): When the DMFT index is employed to assess each individual surface of each tooth, it is termed as "decayed-missing-filled-surface index" (DMFS index). The only difference here is that the surfaces are examined. Surfaces examined posterior teeth: each tooth has five surfaces examined and recorded; facial, lingual, mesial, distal and occlusal. Anterior teeth: each tooth has four surfaces for evaluation; facial, lingual, mesial and distal.

Decayed-missing-filled teeth index (DMFT index) the decayed-missing-filled index was introduced by Henry Klein, Carrole E. Palmer and Knutson JW. In 1938, DMF index was the most universally employed index for measuring dental caries. This index is based on the facts that the dental hard tissues are not self-healing, established caries leaves a scar of some sort. The tooth either remains decayed, or if treated, it is extracted or it is filled. The DMFT index is, therefore, an irreversible

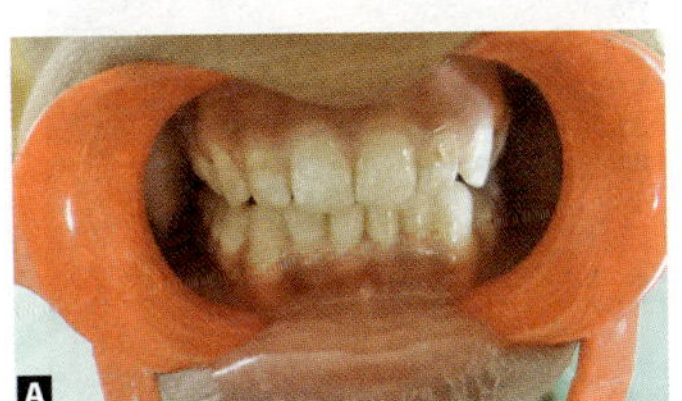
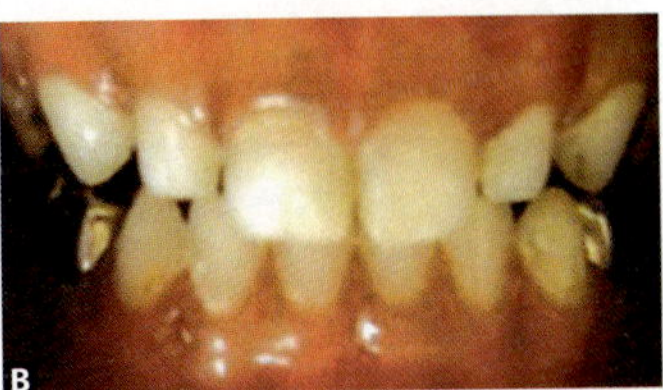

Figs A and B: *(A) Dental fluorosis; (B) Deciduous dentition*

index, meaning that it measures total lifetime caries experience.

Deciduous dentition *see* primary dentition.

Deciduous teeth are the baby teeth; teeth that exfoliate or shed. See primary teeth.

Deep cementopathia is a condition where there is inhibition of continuous cementum formation. It was hypothesized that cementopathia was a disease of eruption and a foreign body response was initiated by the cementum, as a result the host attempted to exfoliate the tooth which consequently results in bone resorption and pocket formation.

Deep dermal burns refer deep partial thickness burns.

Deep partial thickness burns are the one which involve the epidermis and papillary dermis and reticular layer of dermis to varying depths. A few sweat glands and hair follicles are left behind in the reticular dermis from which there is marginal spread of epithelium which gradually covers the wound. This process usually takes more than 6 weeks and the healing takes place by extensive repair which leads to hypertrophic scarring.

Deep sedation refers to a controlled state of depressed consciousness accompanied by partial loss of reflexes. Person is unable to respond to verbal command.

Def' index was described by Gruebbel AO. In 1944, it was used as an equivalent index to DMF index, for measuring dental caries in primary dentition. As defined by Gruebbel, d = decayed teeth, e = indicated for extraction, f = filled teeth. The basic principles and rules for def index are the same as that for dmf index.

Deficiency: Vitamin C deficiency does not cause gingivitis but increases the severity of inflammation in minimal amount of plaque. *Clinical features* appears as gingival enlargement is marginal

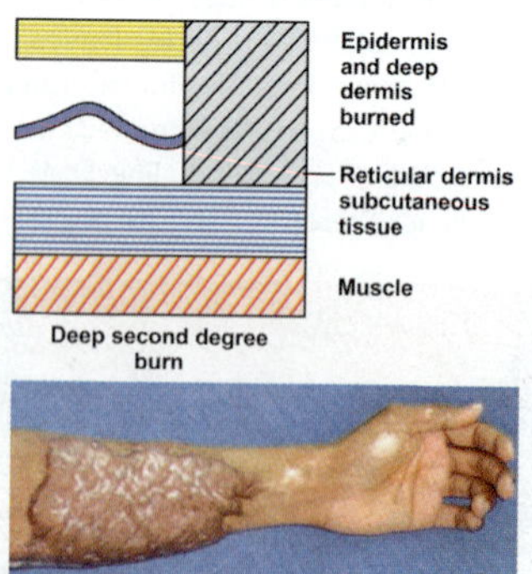

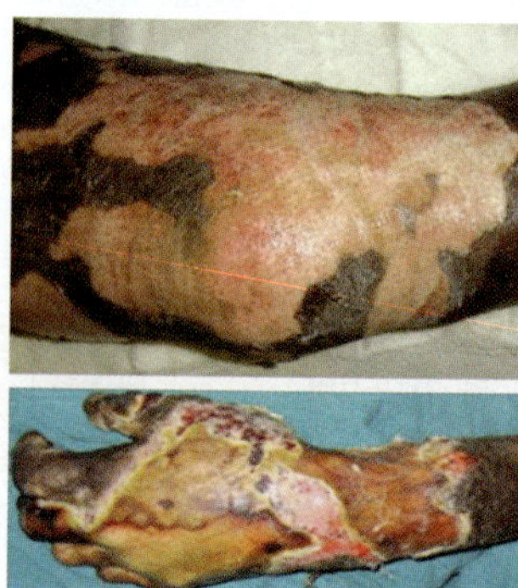

Fig.: *Schematic and clinical presentation of deep partial thickness burn*

appears bluish red in color, tender, grossly swollen and boggy. It is soft and friable in consistency with a smooth and shiny surface. Hemorrhage occurs spontaneously or on slight provocation in long-standing cases. Gingiva develops a purple hue and surface narcosis with pseudomembrane formation is common feature.

Defluoridation refers to the removal of excess fluoride from water.

Deformation refers to an alteration in shape, form or structure of a previously normally formed part, e.g., clubfoot.

Deglutition refers to swallowing.

Dehiscence can be expressed as the denuded areas along with the loss of marginal bone. Such defects are more common on facial surfaces and on anterior teeth.

Delayed eruption of teeth refers to late eruption of teeth not falling within the given time range. It could be due to various reasponses such as in some cases fibromatosis gingiva will not allow eruption due to the presence of connective tissue. Systemic diseases doing so include rickets, cretinism and cleido–cranial dysplasia.

Delayed reaction refers to an allergy causing skin eruptions in response to certain drugs. It is caused by sensitized lymphocytes and not by antibodies.

Delayed union refers to the time taken for a mandibular fracture to unite is delayed beyond the expected time for that particular fracture, it may be assumed that the healing process is disturbed.

Delinquency: Delinquent is one who shows deviation from normal behavior.

Delirium is a disturbance of consciousness or an acute confusional state in which orientation is impaired, the critical faculty is blunted or lost and thought content is relevant or incoherent. Patient becomes restless, uneasy and sleepless. Delusions and, sometimes hallucinations are present. It may develop in high fever, due to overwork, mental stress and drug intoxication. It lasts for a short period and is seen in alcohol abuse, metabolic disorders and high fever.

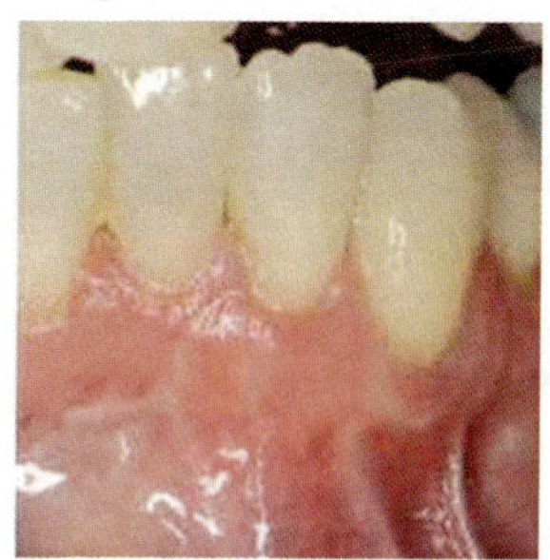

Fig.: *Dehiscence*

Delirium tremens refers to a disorientation of time and place and a peculiar kind of delirium of horrors resulting from hallucination of sight and hearing. Patient imagines insects crawling under the skin. There may be coarse muscular tremors and may develop loss of memory and insomnia. He may commit suicide, homicide or violent assault.

Delta hepatitis is a defective virus that can replicate only in those who are already infected with HBV. Its transmission and epidemiology is similar to HB virus.

Delusion is an exaggerated belief in one's importance, wealth or talent.

Dementia is a clinical syndrome having failing memory and loss of other intellectual functions. There develops behavioral and personality changes also. Loss includes memory, verbal facility, and ability to deal with mathematical symbols. Patient develops lack of initiative, irritability loss of interest and inattentiveness. There is loss of coordination between speech, thought and action. Delusions and hallucinations may occur. Locomotion may fail.

Demianoff's sign is a lumbar pain caused by stretching the sacrolumbalis muscle. Place the patient supine on table and raise the extended leg. Lumbar pain which prevents lifting the leg high enough to form a 10° angle is a positive sign.

Demineralization refers to the loss of mineral from tooth enamel just below the surface in a carious lesion due to acid attack by microorganism or substrate. Usually appearing as a white area on the tooth surface.

Dendrite is the process that conducts impulses toward the cell body of a nerve.

Dendritic cells are accessory cells of the immune system. Similar cells are found in the epidermis and mucous membranes (Langerhan's cells). They increase in number during inflammation and may also play a role in repair processes of the pulp. Dendritic cells are primarily found in lymphoid tissues but they are also widely distributed in connective tissues, including the pulp. These cells are termed antigen presenting cells and are characterized by Dendritic

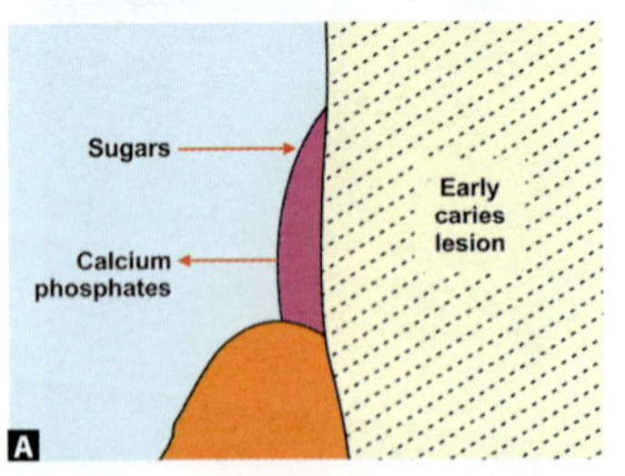

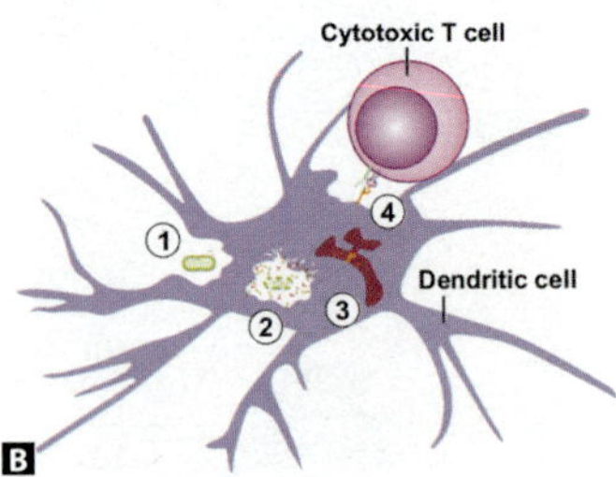

Figs A and B: *(A) Demineralization; (B) Dendritic cells*

cytoplasmic processes and the presence of cell surface class ii antigens. They are known to play a central role in the induction of T cell dependent immunity. They engulf protein antigens and then present an assembly of peptide fragments of the antigens and class ii molecules.

Dens evaginatus can be defined as a tubercle or protuberance from the involved surface of the affected tooth. This is also referred by other terms like occlusal tubercle, Leong's premolar, tuberculated premolar, occlusal enamel pearl. This protuberance has an outer layer of enamel, a core of dentin and may also contain pulp extension into it. Most commonly, it is seen on occlusal surface of premolars and also may occur in the form of a drop, nipple or cylindrical cone. Occurs predominately in people of mongoloid origin. This condition is clinically important because fracture or wear of the tubercle frequently leads to the major complications like pulp necrosis, periapical infection, often before the root completion.

Dens invaginatus/dens in dente/dilated odontome is a deep surface invagination of the crown/root that is lined by enamel. Dens invaginatus can be divided into coronal and radicular type. Coronal type has been further divided into three types (Oehler 1957), type I—invagination confined to the crown, type II—extends to the root portion and ends in a blind sac that may or may not communicate with the adjacent dental pulp, type III—extends through the root and perforates in the apical or lateral root surface without any communication with the pulp. Radicular type is rare. Strip of enamel lined invagination extends into the root surface. In most cases dens invaginatus is detected by chance on radiograph. Clinically an unusual crown morphology in the form of dilated peg-shaped, barrel-shaped crown or deep foramen cecum may be important hint. As maxillary lateral incisors are commonly involved, these teeth should be investigated thoroughly clinically and radiographically,

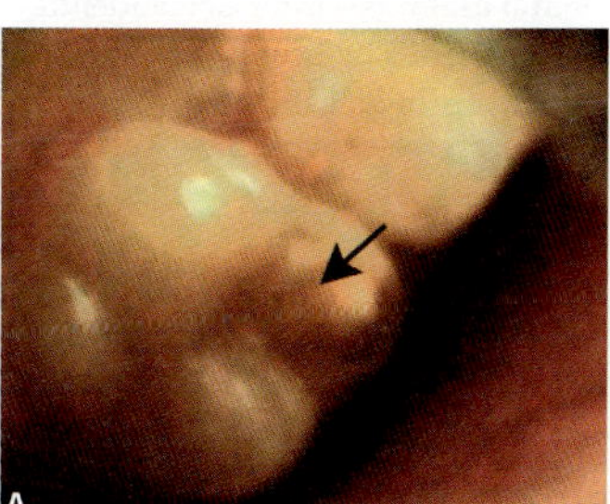

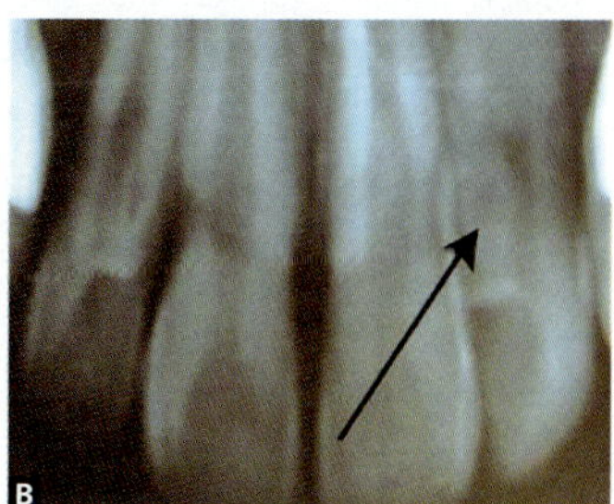

Figs A and B: *(A) Dens evaginatus; (B) Dens invaginatus*

at least in case of deep pit in foramen cecum region. If one tooth is involved contralateral tooth also should be investigated. In case of coronal type, pulpal involvement can occur shortly after the eruption of tooth, early diagnosis is mandatory.

Density of material refers to the amount of mass of a material in a given volume. Common unit of density in grams/cubic centimeters. High density of material makes them heavy.

Dentaire internationale (FDI) numbering system refers to a numbering system that uses a two-digit tooth recording system. The first digit indicates the quadrant and the second indicates the tooth within the quadrant. The numbering is from the midline toward the posterior. The permanent teeth are numbered as follows: maxillary right quadrant is #1, maxillary left quadrant is #2, mandibular left quadrant is #3, and mandibular right quadrant is #4.

Dental amalgam refers to an alloy of a silver tin alloy containing other metals; usually copper and zinc at will be mixed with mercury forming an amalgam.

Dental caries can be defined as a microbial disease of the calcified tissues of the teeth, characterized by demineralization of the inorganic portion and destruction of the organic substances of the tooth resulting in cavitations. Dental caries can occur on any aspect of the tooth but the surfaces which are more prone to the accumulation of plaque and bacteria, are the one which are more susceptible to caries. As this closely knitted plaque has a very complex structure and harbors variety of microorganisms. Formation of cavity requires acid producing bacteria, substrate, plaque, and host susceptibility factor.

Dental caries severity index for primary teeth was introduced by Aubrey Chosack in 1985. This reproducible caries severity index for primary teeth is based on clinical examinations only, which could be used in surveys of dental caries and give information in addition to 'def' figures, especially when investigating preventive measures.

Dental chair refers to the chair which is used by patient to obtain treatment.

Dental composite is a mixture of silicate glass particles with an acrylic monomer that is polymerized during the application.

Dental compound is a wax like material used to stabilize the rubber dam clamp.

Dental diagnosis is the act of identifying diseases or problems for which dentist provides the treatment.

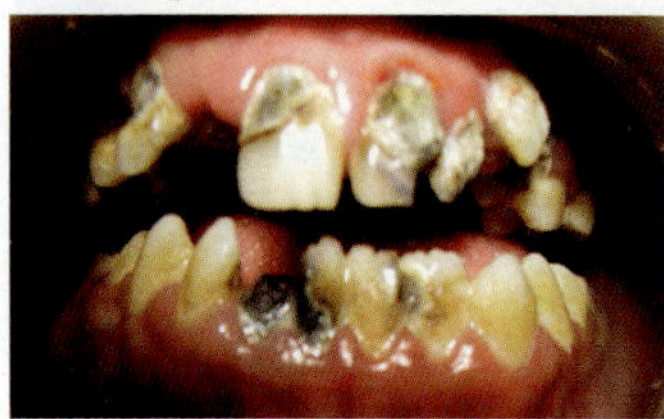

Fig.: *Dental caries*

Dental disability: According to AAPD (2008)—Latest a person should be considered to have a dental disability, if pain infection or lack of functional dentition leads to restriction of nutritional intake adequate for growth and energy needs. Delays or otherwise alters growth and development and inhibits participation in life activities.

Dental discoloration is the term given to the discolored tooth. A tooth presenting with smooth and shiny surface, depicts a healthy tooth. Tooth color varies from individual to individual, i.e. It can range from pearl white to pale yellow. Any deviations from these colors and smooth surface anatomy can be termed as dental stains or dental discoloration.

Dental duplicating materials are used to prepare duplicate casts for prosthetic appliances and orthodontic models. These are used to make an impression of original dental cast. Agar hydrocolloid duplicating materials are used most frequently. Their composition has higher water content.

Dental endoscope is recently introduced system which is used subgingivally in the diagnosis and treatment of periodontal disease. The instrument consists of a 0.99 mm diameter reusable fibreoptic endoscope, over which is fitted a sterile sheath, this fiberoptic endoscope fits on to the periodontal probes designed to accept the system. This device allows clear visualization, deep into the gingival pockets and furcation areas.

Dental fluorosis is a hypoplasia or hypomaturation of tooth enamel or dentin produced by chronic ingestion of excessive amount of fluoride during the period when the teeth are developing. The enamel exhibiting dental fluorosis is called "mottled enamel". GV Black and Fredrick S McKay were the first to coin the term "mottled enamel" in 1916 in Colorado, USA also see Colorado stains.

Dental groove originates in the incisive papilla region and extends backwards to touch the gingival groove in the canine region and then laterally to end in the molar region.

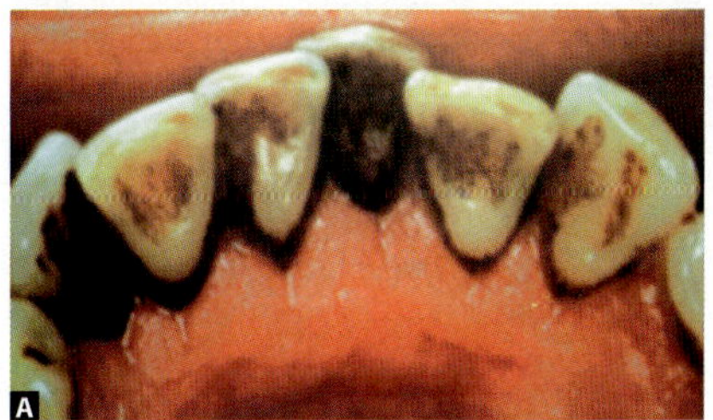

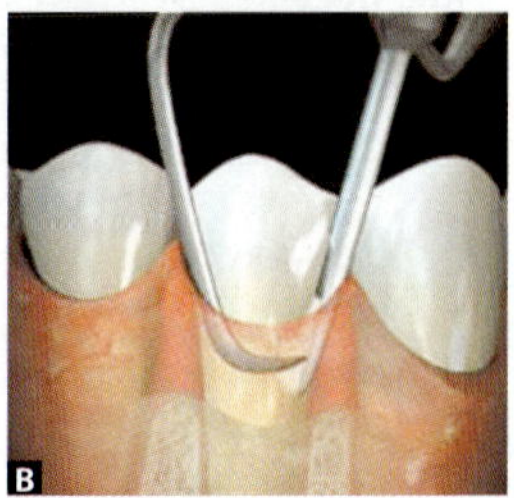

Figs A and B: *(A) Staining of the teeth; (B) Dental endoscope*

D

Dental health index (DHI) was developed by Carpay JJ, Neiman F, Konig KG, Felling AJA and Laminers JGM in 1983. The DHI uses selected teeth for developing the index. Any number of teeth may be examined and the denominator is adjusted accordingly. The DHI was developed to minimize the difference between sound and affected (or extracted) teeth. The sound teeth were given a score of "+1" and the affected (or extracted) teeth were given a score of "-1".

Dental groove originates in the incisive papilla region and extends backwards to touch the gingival groove in the canine region and then laterally to end in the molar region.

Dental home is a place, a source of comprehensive dental care.

Dental hygiene refers to the interventions performed by dental hygienists that are meant for maintaining the oral hygiene.

Dental hygiene clinician refers to the role of dental hygienist, to identify their problems and to help patients to get rid of these.

Dental hygiene research refers to an application of the scientific methods to develop new knowledge and to keep a proper record of it.

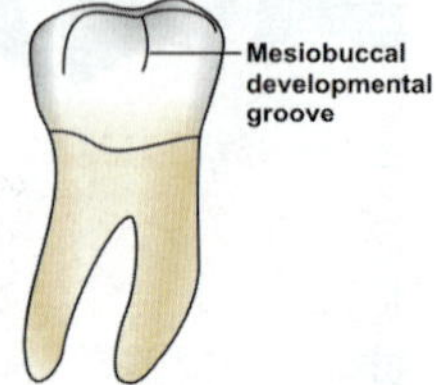

Fig.: *Developmental groove*

Dental hygienist refers to a licensed preventive oral health professional who provides educational, clinical and therapeutic patient service. Dental hygienists are trained for 2 years. Under guidance of a dental surgeon they can do cleaning and polishing teeth, scaling teeth and application of fluorides and fissure sealants.

Dental index (Pamela Zarkowski) is an abbreviated measurement of the amount or condition of disease in a population; a numerical scale with defined upper and lower limits designed by the same criteria and method.

Dental nurse is a professional who is trained in preparing, mixing filling and using impression material. She also helps in suction, illumination and retraction. She keeps the operating field clean and dry.

Dental percussion is generally conducted by gently tapping a tooth with tip of dental mirror handle. There may be tenderness to percussion or dull percussion note. It shows inflammation of periodontal ligament and periodontitis. Greater tenderness to percussion in an apical direction suggests apical periodontitis.

Dental practice act is a law that regulates the practice of dentistry, dental hygiene and individuals.

Dental public health is an art of preventing and controlling dental diseases and promoting oral health and prevention of dental disease including control through organized community efforts where the whole community is treated as patient.

Dental pulp organ can be defined as a firm, cohesive and resilient unit and this is because pulp is composed principally of gelatin-like substance called ground substance, which is reinforced throughout by irregularly arranged and interlaced collagen fibers and fiber bundles embedded in its stroma are cells, blood vessels and nerve fibers that make up loose connective tissue.

Dental record refers to a complete record of health and dental status which will help in diagnosis and treatment planning for the patient and comparing the effect of it.

Dental resin refers to a dental material applied to the tooth which is used in cases of restoring also known as composites.

Dental sclerosis refers to the process of deposition of calcium is not understood. Increased mineralization of tooth decreased conductivity of odontoblastic process.

Dental shade guides refers to the template are used in determining the color of natural teeth so that substitutes restorations will have similar color and esthetics.

Dental tape is a polishing paste used for polishing proximal surfaces that are inaccessible to other polishing instruments; care should be taken to avoid injuring the cementum and the gingiva. The area should be cleansed with warm water to remove the remnants of paste.

Dental technician is highly skilled craftsmen who construct crown, bridges, inlays, splints and orthodontic appliances. In dental lab these are not qualified to carry out any form of dental treatment on the patient.

Dental therapist is an auxiliary dental worker who has completed 2 years course. He can perform non-invasive procedure such as cleaning and polishing teeth, application of fluorides and fissure sealants. He can administer local infiltration analgesia for extractions, fillings and scaling.

Dental unit refers to a control center for the dental hand-pieces, oral evacuator, air water syringe, saliva ejector, ultrasonic scaler and light.

Dental varnish is a fluid used hypersensitivity treatment which, sometimes, contains sodium fluoride; applied to the tooth surface, covering the outer surface of dentin and thus blocking transmission of stimuli to the pulp.

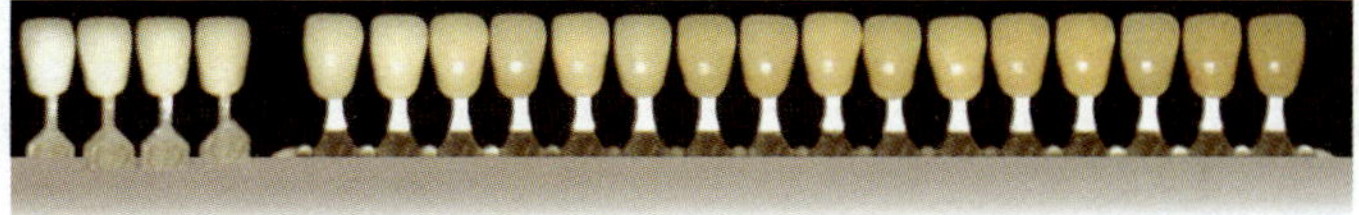

Fig.: *Dental shade guide*

Dentate alveolus fracture is the term which implies fracture of alveolus with associated damage of teeth.

Dentifrice is the substance used with a tooth brush or other applicator to remove bacterial plaque, materia alba and debris from gingiva and teeth for cosmetic and sanitary purposes, and for applying specific agents to the tooth surfaces for preventive and/or therapeutic purposes.

Dentigerous cyst is the most common odontogenic cyst. It has a lumen lined with epithelium. Most commonly affected tooth is mandibular premolar and maxillary third molar. Multiple dentigerous cysts may be accompanied with basal cell nevus syndrome or cleidocranial dysostosis. Cyst varies from 2 cm in diameter to large expansion of jaws. Cysts usually yield a straw colored thin liquid. Cyst is painless and causes delayed eruption of tooth. Painless cyst is indicative of some infection. It generally does not expand so much so that it may press sensory nerve. Pain is localized but may be referred to any part of face. Smaller lesions can be surgically removed.

Dentin bonding is the type of retention that occurs between dental material and the dentin of a tooth. It can include micro-mechanical retention and chemical adhesion.

Dentin dysplasia is a rare disturbance of dentin formation. There is normal enamel with atypical dentin formation with abnormal pulpal morphology. Radicular type appears clinically normal except slight amber translucency. Eruption pattern is normal. Tooth is mobile while type II of coronal type is amorphous and atubular dentin. There is no treatment.

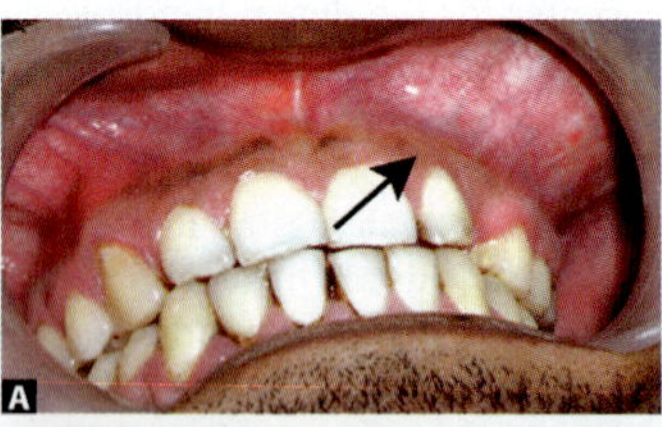

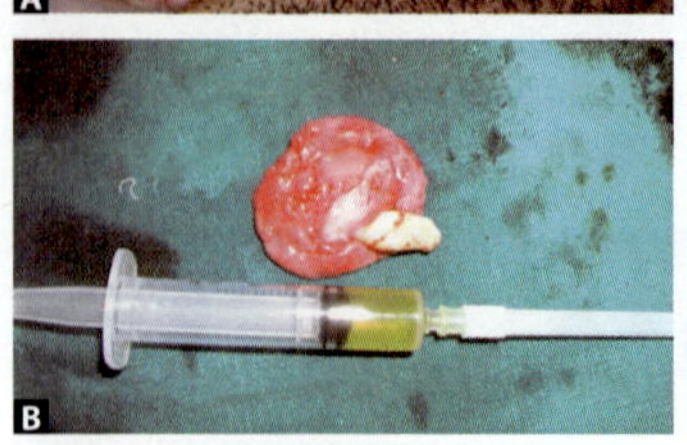

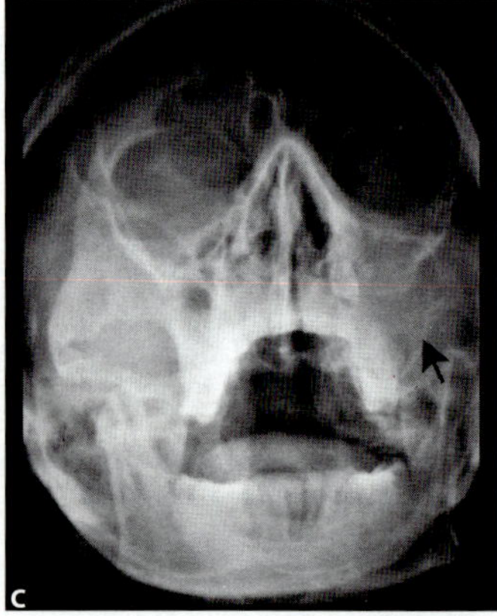

Figs A to C: *(A) Dentigerous cyst with missing canine; (B) Dentigerous cyst with impacted canine and aspirator; (C) Paranasal sinus view showing dentigerous cyst*

Dentin forms the main portion of the tooth which is covered by enamel in the crown region and cementum in the root region. Dentin is hard, dense, calcified tissue similar to the enamel, however, it is softer than enamel and but hardest than the cementum. Dentin is yellow and elastic in nature and capable of forming a new dentin called as secondary dentin. Composition - 70% inorganic substance, 30% organic and water.

Dentin secondary refers to a dentin formed after the eruption of tooth.

Dentinal sensitivity is the mildest form of pulp discomfort. The pain is often characterized as a short, sharp, shock and it is brought on by some stimulating factor such as hot or cold, sweet, sour, acid or touch. It is not pathologic, but is rather, fluid flow in the dentinal tubules which stretches or compresses the nerve endings that pass alongside the tubular extensions of the pulp odontoblasts. Dentinal sensitivity may also develop when dentin is exposed from gingival recession or following periodontal surgery.

Dentinal tubule refers to microscopic canals that run from the outside of the dentin to the nerve inside the tooth.

Dentinogenesis imperfecta is a developmental defect, inherited as an autosomal dominant trait. In this condition the permanent and primary dentitions are involved, enamel appears to be normal, roots are also affected. Post-eruption, and there is a rapid calcification of the pulp chambers and root canals which will lead to the darkening in the color of the clinical crown. Characteristic findings consist of a peculiar opalescent purplish-brown or gray color of the teeth. Rapid attrition of the crowns, and reduction in carious lesions. Enamel, cementum, and periodontal membrane show no microscopic abnormalities, but there are many changes noted in the dentin. The dentinoenamel junction is straight rather than scalloped which probably accounts for the weak attachment of the enamel to the dentin and the tendency for the enamel to chip, leaving

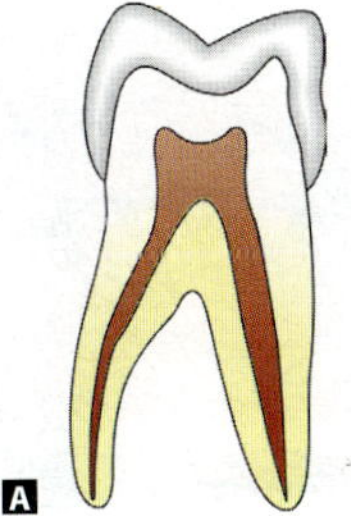

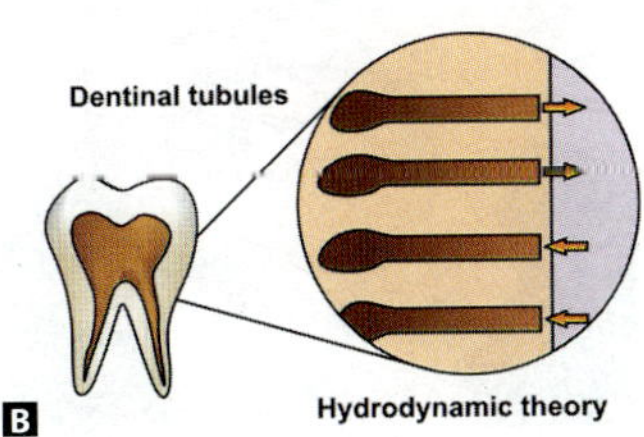

Figs A and B: *(A) Dentin; (B) Dentinal tubules*

exposed dentin. Irregular tubular arrangement can be seen. Smaller number of tubuli, decreasing toward the pulp. Occasional larger diameter of tubuli and cellular inclusion. Numerous branching of the tubuli. Poor calcification of the teeth. The circumpulpal dentin picture resembles irregular secondary dentin formation. The teeth are much smaller than normal, about one-half the dimensions or one-eighth the volume. Enamel appears as a very thin layer, and is quickly worn away in the mouth. Pulp chambers and canals show in the radiographs of deciduous teeth during formation, but are almost completely obliterated in erupted teeth of the permanent set. The teeth are not sensitive to grinding, indicating that the dentin does not contain vital fibrils. Enamel hypoplasia is a disorder affecting the structure of the teeth. It is often seen as one component associated with many syndromes or enamel hypoplasia may be mild enough resulting in a pitting of the enamel surface or a horizontal line across the enamel of the crown.

Dentinoma is a rare tumor. It develops in central mandible in molar area. Radiographic findings are not specific. It is large, solitary, opaque mass. Masses of calcified material are seen. It consists of irregular dentin as there is lack of enamel formation. Surgical excision with thorough curettage helps.

Dentition the entire set of teeth is refered to as dentition. The dentitions consist of the natural teeth in the jaw bones that consist of primary and permanent dentition. The dentition is of three types, i.e. Primary dentition, mixed dentition and primary dentition.

Dentoalveolar anterior cross-bite are the one in which one or more maxillary anterior teeth are in lingual relation to the mandibular anteriors. The cross-bite is generally due to discrepancy and not skeleton. In termed dento-alveolar anterior cross-bite. This is often manifested as single tooth cross-bite and usually occurs due to over-retained deciduous teeth that deflect the erupting permanent teeth into a palatal position. They can be effectively treated using

A

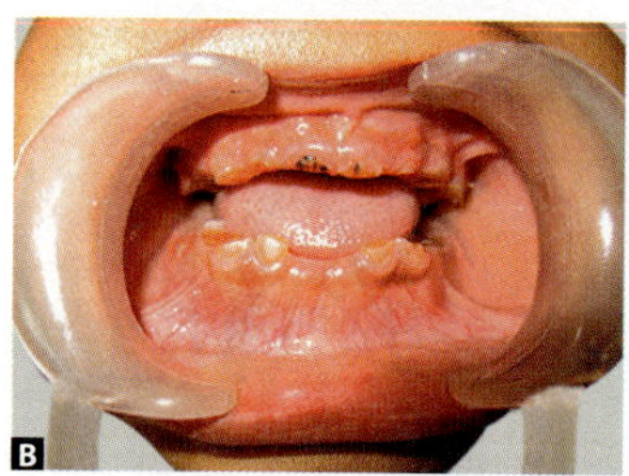

Figs A and B: *Dentinogenesis imperfecta*

tongue blades, Catalans appliance and double cantilever spring with posterior bite plate.

Dentoalveolar fractures are those that involve avulsion, subluxation, displacement or fracture of teeth in conjunction with fracture of the alveolus. They may occur alone or in association with mandible.

Dentulous areas refer to area with teeth.

Denture adhesive is an adjunct to stabilize and retain denture by increasing peripheral seal. It is commonly available in powder and paste form.

Denture base is a material used to contact the oral tissues and support artificial teeth.

Denture hyperplasia is a chronic inflammatory tissue reaction to ill-fitting dentures with overextended or sharp denture border. It develops in 5-10% of elderly denture wearers. It is painful when traumatized and ulcerated. It is seen as single or several folds of pink tissue in the sulcus related to periphery of a denture. Lower jaw is more frequently affected. After adjustment of dentures, the inflammation and edema may subside and produce clinical improvement.

Denture induced fibrous hyperplasia refer denture hyperplasia

Denture porcelain is defined as a white translucent ceramic fired to a glazed state. It has an excellent biocompatibility, natural appearance and high resistance to wear and distortion. Disadvantages include brittleness; require mechanical attachment and produce clicking sound on contact. Higher density increases weight of teeth.

Denture irritation hyperplasia refer denture hyperplasia.

Denture sore mouth is a diffuse inflammation of maxillary denture bearing area. Pain and burning are usually reported during periods of exacerbation although raw area will persist for years till denture is born. Raised antibody titers against C. Albicans are found in saliva and serum. Three clinical varieties are found, a localized simple inflammation or pinpoint hyperemia, a more diffuse erythema granular type.

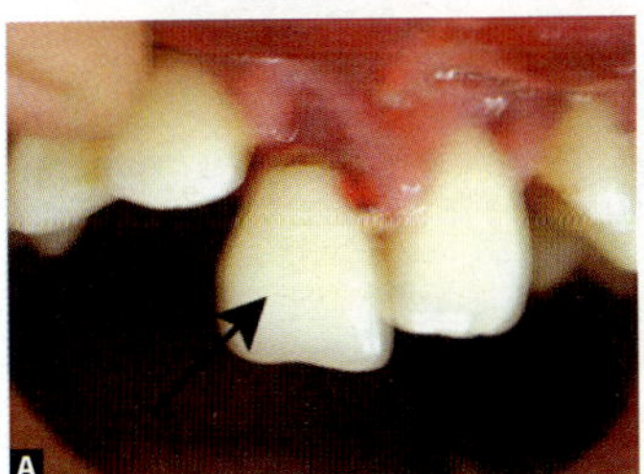

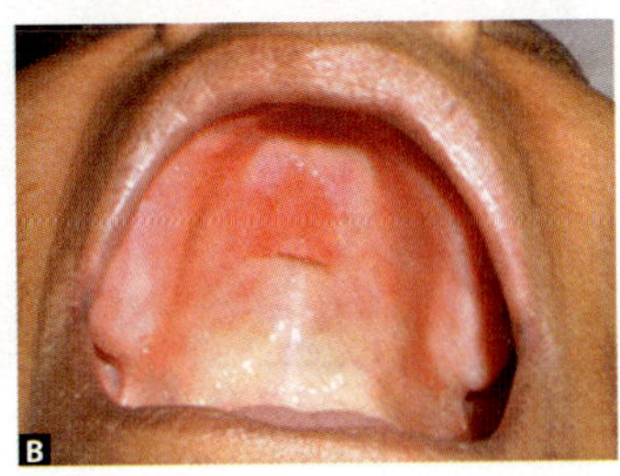

Figs A and B: *(A) Avulsion; (B) Denture hyperplasia*

Denture stomatitis is an inflammation of oral mucosa associated with wearing dentures. It is generally found under maxillary mucosa. Mucosa becomes red and has velvety appearance. There may be burning sensations.

Deontological ethics is an ethical theory that focuses on morality rather the consequences of action.

Deposition refers to a process of laying down of new bone.

Depression is an abnormal psychological state. There develops a low mood, interest and vitality. It differs from normal sadness in the severity of symptoms.

Depressor angularis oris is a facial muscle that arises from oblique line of mandible below and lateral to depressor labii inferioris. It draws the angle of mouth downwards and laterally in opening the mouth and in sadness.

Depressor labii inferioris is a facial muscle. It is quadrilateral and arises from oblique line of mandible. It draws the lower limb downwards and laterally during mastication.

Dermoid cyst is a painless slowly growing swelling at the site of lines of embryonic fusion. It is generally seen above the outer canthus of eye, behind the ear, root of nose and midline of body. Majority of these develop during adulthood. It produces a bulge in mouth causing difficulty in eating. It is smooth, soft and nontender when infection develops, sinus may be formed. Overlying skin remains free but is attached to deeper tissue. Once removed surgically, these don't recur.

Descriptive study is a research that involves describing, analyzing and interpreting data to evaluate a current population event or situation.

Desensitization refers to the blocking of painful stimuli which cause dentinal hypersensitivity.

Desiccate is to make dry; to remove all moisture.

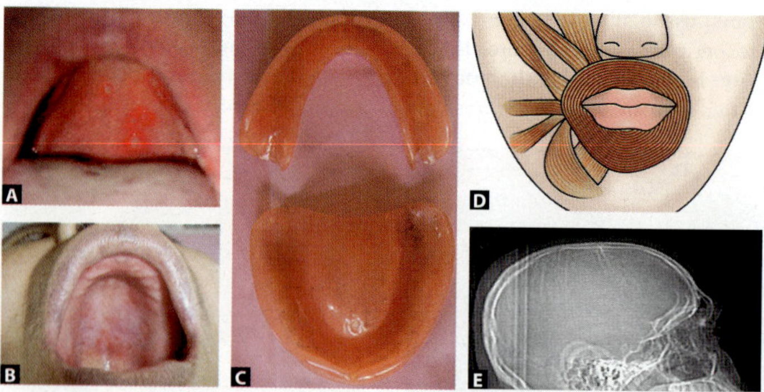

Figs A to E: *(A and B) Denture stomatitis involving palate; (C) Ill Fitting denture surfaces; (D) Depressor angular oris; (E) Dermoid cyst*

Desmin are the filaments that are found predominantly in muscle cells. It forms an interconnecting network perpendicular to the long axis of the cell. Desmin fibers anchor and orientate the z bands in myofibrils, thus generating the striated pattern.

Desmoplastic fibroma is benign neoplasm arising from mesenchymal tissues of jaw bone. It develops in younger age group. Mandible is affected more. *Clinical features:* These are generally asymptomatic neoplasm. Neither teeth nor lesion is tender. Treatment includes local excision and curettage.

Development (Moyers) refers to all naturally occurring unidirectional changes in the life of individual from its existence as a single cell to its elaboration as multifunctional unit terminating in death.

Development (Todd) refers to progress towards maturity.

Developmental anomaly is an abnormality in which a tooth has deviated from its normal form due to aberration in odontogenesis. The dental anomalies have been reported more often in Eskimos, Mongols and Orientals. Such variations can be traced to ancestral times and have been reported to have a genetic basis.

Developmental depression is a concavity in a surface that is formed while the tooth was developing.

Devitalization pulpotomy is a 2-stage procedure and involves the placement of devitalizing paste over the pulp exposure in the first sitting to fix the entire coronal and radicular pulp tissue. The basic technique, first introduced by Witzel in 1898, used a true paraformaldehyde paste.

Dewells method is a three-step extraction procedure. In first step the deciduous canines are extracted to create space for the alignment of the incisors. This step is carried out at 8-9 years of age. A year later the deciduous first molars are extracted so that the eruption of first premolar is accelerated. This is followed where in the first premolars are enucleated at the time of extraction of the first deciduous molars. This is frequently necessary in the mandibular arch where the canines often erupt before the first premolars.

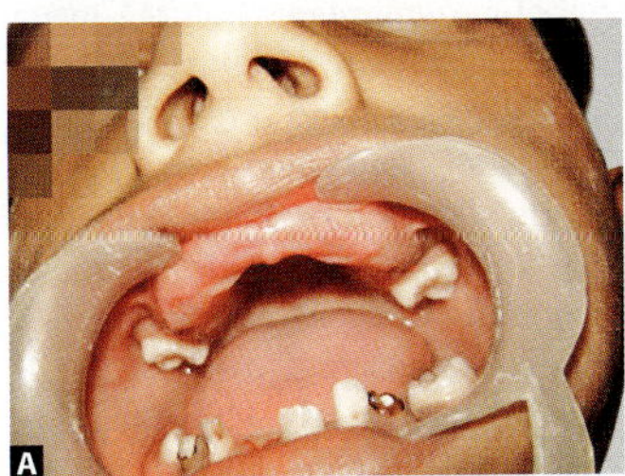

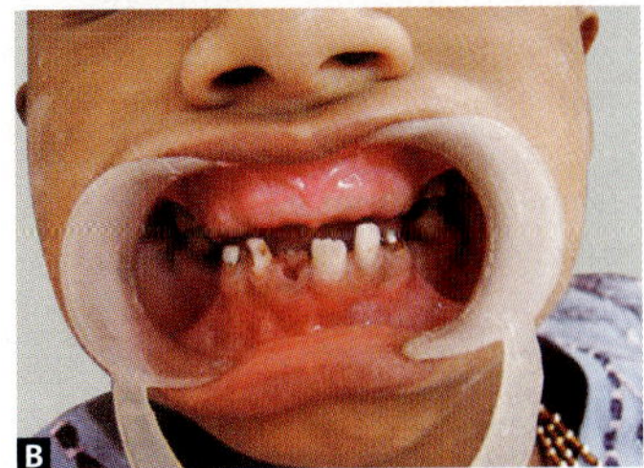

Fig.: Developmental anomaly showing hypodontia of upper jaw

DF index is another method of getting around the exfoliation problem is the 'df' index in which the missing teeth are ignored. This is the method of choice of the World Health Organization in their basic survey technique. The 'df' index can be applied to the whole tooth as the decayed-filled-tooth ('dft' index) or to the individual surfaces as the decayed-filled-surface ('dfs' index).

Dhatura seeds are used to stupefy travellers in railway stations, places of pilgrimage in order to commit theft, robbery and rape. These are mixed with colored food, cereals, vegetables curry etc. An average size fruit contains 400–500 seeds. Seeds are similar to brinjals. Its poisoning results in giddiness, vomiting and staggering gait. Face is flushed, pupils are dilated. Patient makes pill rolling movements. Stomach is to be washed with weak solution of potassium permanganate or 2-4% tannic acid. Emetics are to be given.

Diabetes insipidus is a disease resulting from an inadequate secretion of antidiuretic hormone marked by great thrust and passage of a large volume of urine.

Diabetes mellitus represents a syndrome of disordered glucose metabolism and inappropriate hyperglycemia that results from an absolute deficiency in insulin secretion, a reduction in the biologic effectiveness of insulin or both. Predisposing factors include: genetic disorder, primary destruction of islets of Langerhan's in the pancreas caused by inflammation, cancer or surgery, an endocrine condition, such as hyperpituitarism and hyperthyroidism, administration of steroids, resulting in iatrogenic diabetes. Classification of diabetes mellitus: insulin dependent diabetes mellitus (IDDM) – type 1, noninsulin dependent diabetes mellitus (NIDDM) - type II.

Diabetes mellitus type I is the primary form of diabetes and is genetic. This is a more severe form where circulating insulin is essentially absent, plasma glucagon levels are elevated and pancreatic β-cells do not respond to insulinogenic stimuli. Human lymphocyte antigen (HLA) which is located on 6th human chromosome adjacent to immune response genes are closely associated with development of type I diabetes.

Diabetes mellitus type II describes a heterogeneous group composed of milder forms of diabetes that occurs most frequently in adults and only occasionally in children. Most type II diabetics do not require exogenous insulin therapy to sustain life.

Diabetic gangrene occurs in a diabetic patient of above the age of 50 years who presents pain, ulceration and discharge. Lesion starts with boil or trauma, usually great toe is involved. In moist gangrene affected part is swollen with offensive discharge. It spreads extensively with sloughing of tissues. There is no line of demarcation.

Diabetic kidneys refer to the specific lesions of diabetes include diabetic glomerusclerosis and exudative lesions. Others lead to pyelonephritis. Microalbuminuria is indicative of kidney's involvement. Kidneys are enlarged. External surface may show scars due to hypertension.

Diabetic nephropathy incidence is between 10-20%. All such patients have diabetic neuropathy. There develops proteinuria with progressive renal failure along with enlargement of kidney. Patients of diabetic type I develops more of nephropathy. There should be protein restriction. Curtailment of sodium and potassium. Hypertension is to be controlled along with diabetes.

Diabetic peripheral neuropathy microangiopathy with obliteration of vasa nervorum or poor myoinositol uptake and increased nerve accumulation of serbital and fructose are pathological mechanisms of diabetic neuropathy. It manifests with symmetric paressterias, pain and loss of tendon jerks.

Diabetic retinopathy changes are either simple or proliferative. In background lesions there is microaneurysm formation, venous dilatation, dot hemorrhages. In proliferative form new vessel loss. Senile cataracts develop 10-15 years earlier in diabetics. Snow flake cataracts are characteristics in young diabetics. In proliferative type photocoagulation is the only answer.

Diagnodent is a new method of caries detection; diagnodent introduced by KaVo, Germany in 1999, which is based on the principle of fluorescence. It enables to recognize at an early stage pathological changes that prove difficult or even impossible to detect, initial lesions, demineralization, changes affecting the tooth enamel. The incidence of fissure, approximal and residual caries can be identified. It is also useful in determining the amount of carious involvement/decalcification in different areas of the same tooth.

Diagnosis is an art wherein scientific methods are applied to the

Compressed capillaries
Nodular deposits
Increased mesangial matrix
A

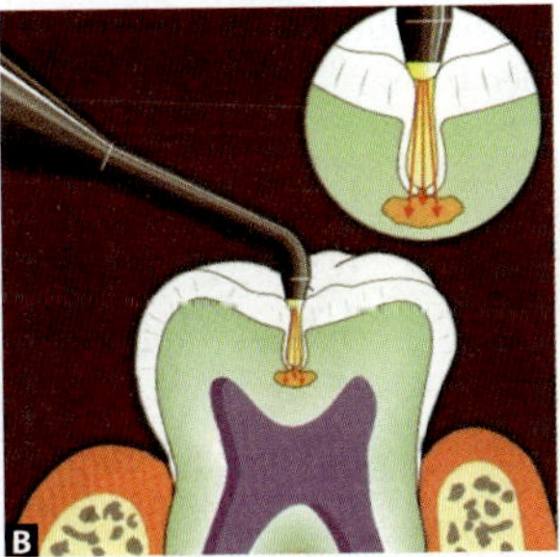

Figs A and B: *(A) Histological section of diabetic nephropathy; (B) Diagnodent*

elucidation of problems presented by a patient. It can be defined as utilization of scientific knowledge for identifying a diseased process and to differentiate from other disease process. The diagnostic process actually consists of four steps; First step— Assemble all the available facts gathered from chief complaints, medical and dental history, diagnostic tests and investigations; Second step—Analyze and interpret the assembled clues to reach the tentative or provisional diagnosis; Third step—Make differential diagnosis of all possible diseases which are consistent with signs, symptoms and test results gathered; Fourth step—Select the closest possible choice also.

Diagnostic refers to the procedures performed by the dentist to identify what's going on in the mouth.

Diagnostic casts are replicas of the tissues of the maxillary and mandibular arches made from impressions.

Dialysis is a process of separating crystalloids from colloids by the difference in their rates of diffusion through a semipermeable membrane.

Diaphragm is a membrane and partition that separates one thing from another. It is a flat muscular sheet that separates chest from abdomen.

Diaphragma sellae is formed by the folded dura mater Superior to the hypophysis.

Diaphragmatic breathing is the breathing that promotes the use of diaphragm rather.

Diarrhea is one of the manifestations of intestinal infection where there is the passage of watery stool.

Diastema is a facial muscle; a space between the teeth. It refers to an abnormal space between two adjacent teeth.

Diastolic dysfunction is an inability of the heart to fill with blood during diastole at a normal filling pressure.

Diazepam is a drug of barbiturate family and was introduced fifty years back for minor insomnia and anxiety. Dose dependent mild cardiovascular depression may occur. Chances of dependence increase if drug is used for longer period. Diazepines are used in the management of mild anxiety and tension. Librium and valium

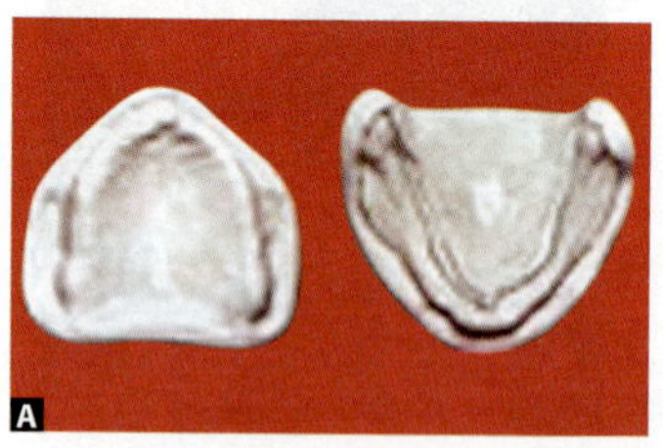

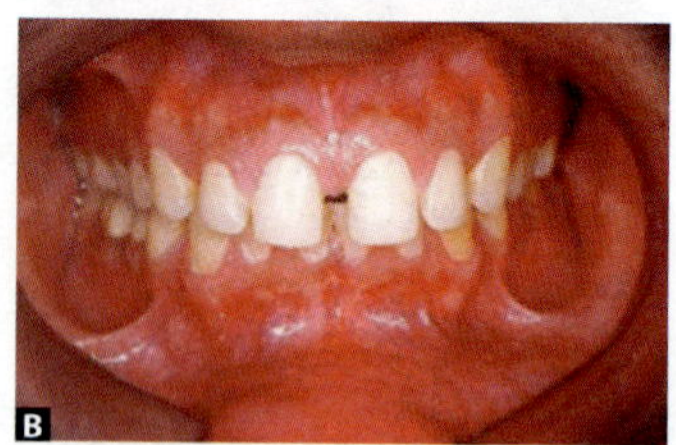

Figs A and B: *(A) Diagnostic casts; (B) Midline diastema*

are commonly used. It is rapidly absorbed and acts for 3–4 hour. Drowsiness, lethargy and ataxia are common. Minor dependence of physical dependence may develop.

Differential diagnosis is an art of distinguishing one disease from another also. It is the process of listing out the various diseases having common signs and symptoms, of which only one could be attributed to patient's suffering.

Differentiation is the change from generalized cells or tissue to more specialized kinds during the development.

Diffuse atrophy of alveolar bone is a periodontal disease reported by Gottlieb in 1923 characterized by loss of collagen fibers in the periodontal ligament and was replaced by loose connective tissue and severe bone resorption leading to widened periodontal space.

Diffuse gingivitis is said to occur when the marginal gingiva, interdental gingiva and attached gingiva all are affected.

Diffuse lesion is said to have occured when the border of lesions are not well-defined and it is not possible to define exact parameters of lesions.

Diffusion refers to spreading, spreading of dissolved particles.

Dilaceration is an abnormal angulation or bend in the root or less frequently the crown of a tooth. It is caused by trauma to the root development. Any tooth may be affected. Dilaceration does not interfere with eruption. Dilacerated tooth erupts into complete occlusion, but follows altered path. Minor dilacerations of normal teeth requires no treatment. If eruption is delayed or abnormal, surgical exposure and orthodontic movement is required. Caution must be exerted during endodontic treatment of dilacerated teeth to avoid perforation of the root.

Dilantin sodium is an anticonvulsant drug used in epileptic seizures. But it causes fibrous hyperplasia of gingiva. Gingival hyperplasia begins as early as 2 weeks after drugs. There is increase in size of gingiva which is painless. Gums may become warty. It has tendency to bleed. Discontinuing drug is best treatment.

Diode lasers have a solid active medium; it is a solid-state semiconductor laser that uses some combination of Al, gallium and arsenide to change electric energy

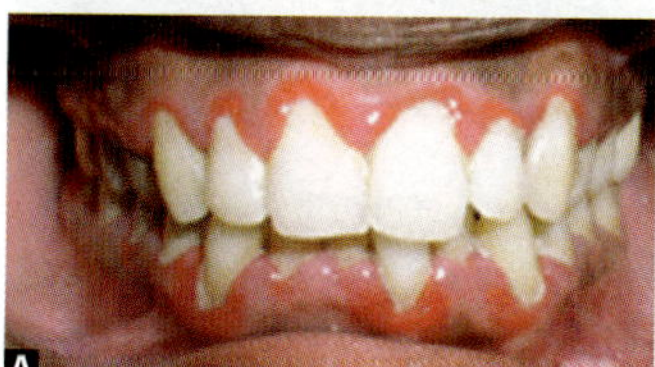

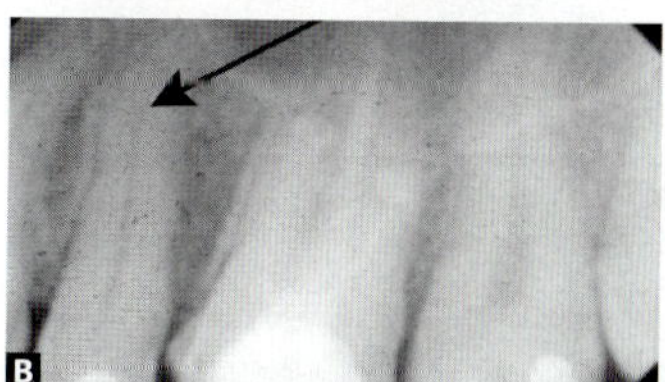

Figs A and B: *(A) Diffuse gingivits; (B) Dilaceration hyperplasia*

into light energy. It has a wavelength range from 800–980 nm. Laser energy is delivered fiberoptically in continuous-wave and gated-pulse mode; used in contact with the tissue. It is poorly absorbed by tooth structure so that soft tissue surgery can be performed safely in close proximity to enamel, dentin and cementum. It is an excellent soft tissue surgical laser indicated for cutting and coagulating gingiva and mucosa and for soft tissue curettage, or sulcular debridement.

Diphtheria is an acute infection caused by corynebacterium diphtheria. It is a disease of childhood. Child becomes restless, headache, fever, sore-throat and mild redness and edema of pharynx may take place. After a short incubation period of 4 days, disease starts with malaise, loss of appetite, sore-throat and fever. Fever may be very high. On examination, one finds uniform greyish or yellowish white membrane covering tonsil. It may extend to pharynx and soft palate. Membrane is adherent to underlying mucosa. Cervical glands are enlarged. In severe case membrane may show hemorrhagic areas and there may be bleeding. Neurological complications include palatal paralysis, ocular paralysis and peripheral neuritis within 6-8 weeks but all three are reversible. Throat swab will confirm the diagnosis. Immunization with anti diptheria serum.

Diphyodont refers to having two successive sets of teeth.

Diplegia refers to a child whose 2 limbs are more compromised as compared to other two the lower extremities are severely involved and the arms are mildly involved in diplegic patients. Fifty percent of children who have spastic cerebral palsy have diplegia. Diplegia is becoming more common as more low-birth-weight babies survive. Intelligence is usually normal, and epilepsy is not common. These children often have visual perceptual deficits and strabismus.

Diplococcic refers to cocci arranged in pairs.

Diplopia is said to have occurred when objects are seen double. This happens when a muscle of the eyeball is weak, and a movement

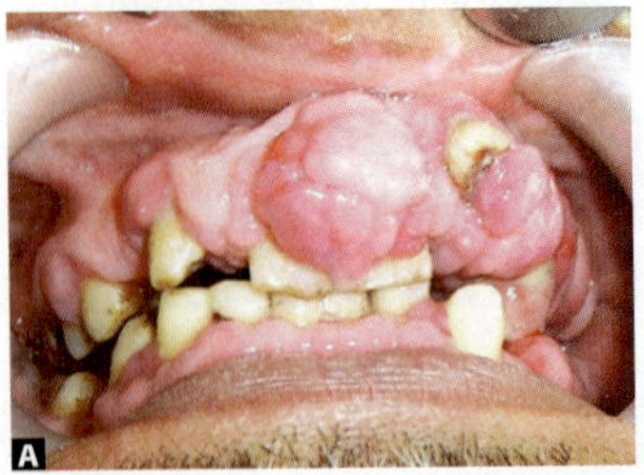

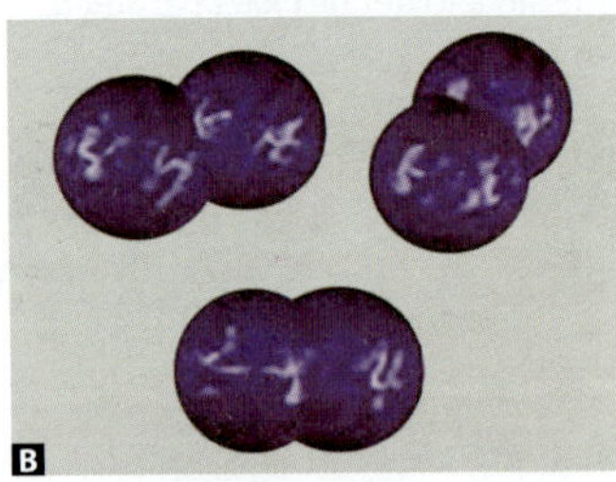

Figs A and B: *(A) Dilantin-induced hyperplasia; (B) Diplococci*

involving that muscle is performed, the movement of the defective eye is slightly less than that of the normal eye. As a result images of the object on the two retinae are not formed at corresponding points but over two points near each other. The brain, therefore, 'sees' two images, one from each retina.

Direct contamination refers to direct contact with impurities or germs.

Direct current refers to current in which electron flows in one direction.

Direct digital imaging is a method of obtaining a digital image in which an intra-oral sensor is exposed to X-rays to capture a radiographic image. It can be viewed on computer monitor.

Direct digital radiography is a technique where currently, digital radiographic images may be obtained by video recording and digitization of a conventional film radiograph or by direct digital radiography. The first digital dental radiograph introduced in dentistry is called radiovisiography (RVG). According to Wenzel (1998), the sensitivities are relatively high for detection of occlusal lesions into dentin with a false-positive fraction between 5% and 10%. The imaging system uses a charge-coupled device (CCD) or storage phosphorus screen.

Direct ground microscopy is a microscopic procedure where specimen is illuminated obliquely by a special condenser organism appears bright as light rays hit them.

Direct suture loop is a type of interdental ligation where the needle is passed from buccal interdental papillae, which then comes out from the lingual aspect of interdental papilla, the two are gently pulled together and conventional knot is given. The knot is generally placed on the labial/buccal aspect for the ease of accessibility.

Direct wiring is a technique where the middle portion of the 6 inch wire

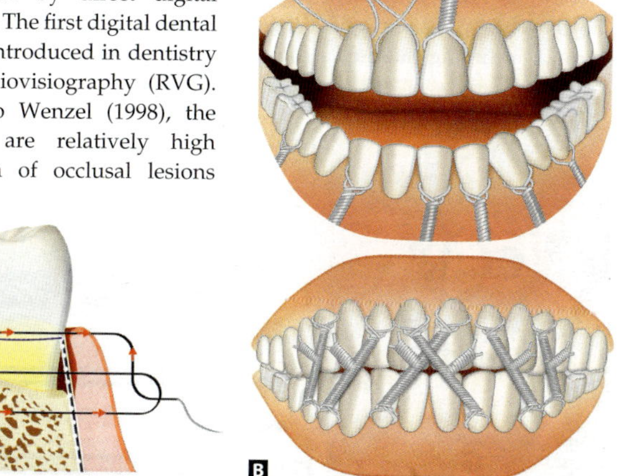

Figs A and B: *(A) Direct suture loop; (B) Direct wiring*

is twisted around a suitable tooth and free ends of wire are twisted together to produce a plaited wire. Similarly, it's done throughout the upper and lower arch, then after the reduction of the fracture the plaited ends of the upper and lower wires are twisted together.

Disability refers to a physical or mental impairment that substantially limits one or more of an individual's major life activities.

Disabled child is one who has a mental, physical, medical or social condition that prevents the child from achieving full potential when compared to other children of the same age. Disabled includes all handicapping conditions or combinations thereof that a health professional might encounter. Defines a handicapped individual as one who, over an appreciable time, is prevented by a physical or mental condition from full participation in the normal activities of his age group, including those of a social, recreational education and vocational nature.

Disaccharide is a carbohydrate composed of two monosaccharides lined together.

Disclosing agent is an erythrosine based solution: Dr Sumter Arnin (1963) introduced disclosing agents into preventive dentistry in the form of 'wafers', which are tablets of erythrosine food dye, termed FDC Red. No. 3 (a 6% solution in water). Other brands are 'ceplac' disclosing tablet, rose pink food dye, red cote solution, c-red solution. *Disadvantages:* indiscriminate staining of lips, cheeks and tongue. Iodine based solution: Talbot's iodine comprises iodine 1.6 g, ki 1.6 g, water 13.4 mld glycerin to make 30 mL. Plaque is stained brown or black.

Discoid is a spoon-shaped dental hand instrument with a cutting edge around the total periphery.

Discoid lupus erythematosis in a mixed red and white lesions are more common. A radiating pattern

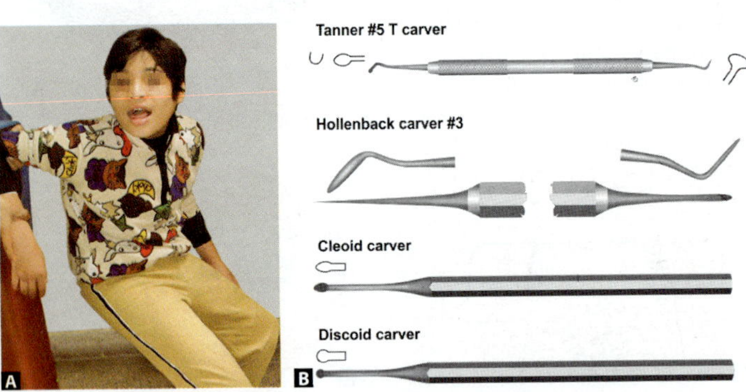

Figs A and B: *(A) Disabled child; (B) Discoid ends of the carvers*

of very delicate white lines is seen. Alternate red, white and red zones provide a characteristic appearance. Histological changes consist of hyperorthokeratosis with keratotic plugs. Most of the intraoral lesions in DLE occur on the cheeks with the gingival tissues and border of lip. Hot and spicy food will produce burning sensation. It responds to cortisone well. White patches on lips and buccal mucosa are adherent. Lesions are symmetrical and no induration is present. Malignant transformation is possible.

Discoloration refers to the change in color of teeth due to various reasons, i.e. yellow is due to heavy plaque build up. Green color is due to poor oral hygiene and is difficult to remove. Black is due to iron compounds from oral fluid. Tobacco stain is rare but develops with chromogenic bacteria.

Disease eradication literally means to 'tear out by roots'. Today smallpox and polio are the diseases, which have been eradicated.

Disease index: The'd (decay) portion of the dmf index best exemplifies a disease index. The indices measuring gingival/sulcular bleeding are essentially symptom indices. This type of index measures the 'number' or 'proportion' of people in a population with or without a specific condition at a specific point in time or interval of time.

Disinfectant refers to a chemical agent used to kill pathogenic microorganisms without sterilizing the material.

Disinfection refers to a cleaning process which destroys the majority of microorganism, but not highly resistant forms such as bacterial and mycotic spores.

Displaced flaps are the ones, when the flap is placed apically, coronally or laterally to their original position.

Displacement is the movement of whole bone away from one another creating space within which enlargement of each of the separate bone takes place.

Disposable refers to items that are not reusable.

Disposable materials refer to materials intended for one—use and discarded, (e.g., gloves, paper gowns, cotton rolls, etc).

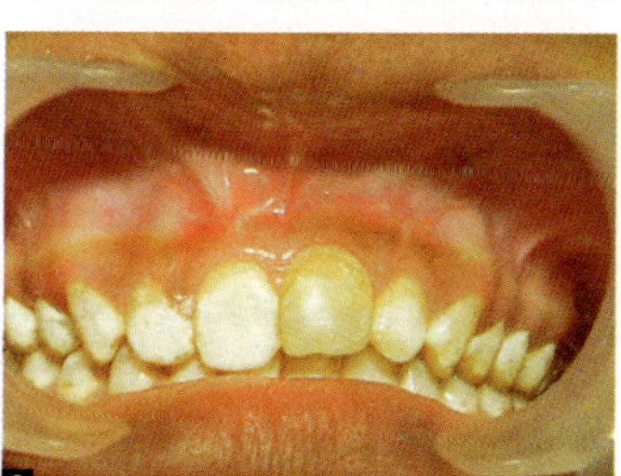

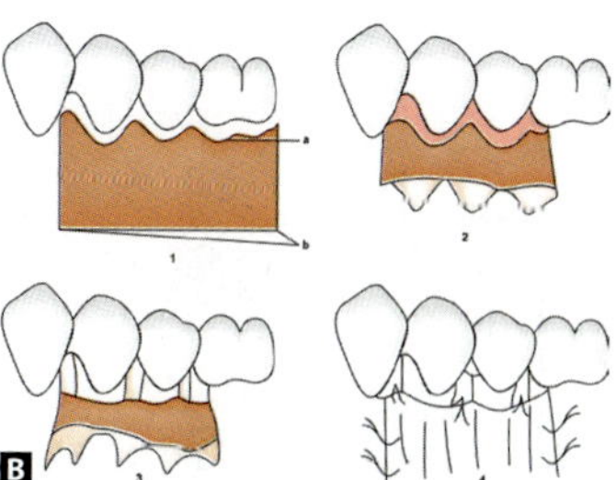

Figs A and B: *(A) Discolored tooth; (B) Apically displaced flap*

D

Dissecting aneurysm refers to term where the blood from lumen of vessel enters the substance of wall and extends along the wall of the vessel resulting in blood filled channel. No true aneurysmal dilatation is present. Onset is sudden and may be fatal.

Distal refers to the surface of the tooth farthest from the midline of the dental arch.

Distal step terminal plane is characterized by the distal surface of the lower second deciduous molar being more distal to that of the upper. Thus the erupting permanent molars may be in Angle's class II occlusion.

Distal wedge procedure is used for deep periodontal pockets distal to last molar.

Distomolar refers to supernumerary teeth.

Distortion geometric is a characteristic that refers to a variation of true size and shape of the object being radiographed. Radiograph distortion is influenced by object film alignment and X-ray beam angulation.

Distraction is intentional diversion of attention.

Distraction osteogenesis is the process of generating new bone by stretching.

Diuretic is a substance which increases urine secretion.

Divergent refers to spread.

Diverticulitis coli colonic diverticula are acquired and are false containing mucosa and submucosa herniated through muscular coats. Lack of fiber in diet, high intraluminal pressure results in diverticula formation. Sigmoid colon is generally affected when inflamed, these produce pain, discomfort and tenderness in left iliac fossa. Diarrhea is a common feature. Bleeding per rectum may be severe. In severe cases may result in intestinal obstruction. Barium enema shows outpouching of colonic mucosa.

DMF index refers to the index used to assess caries in children before ages of exfoliation—for children over 7 years and up to 11 or 12 years, the decayed, missing and filled primary molar and canines, have been used to determine decayed-missing-filled teeth (dmft), or decayed-missing-

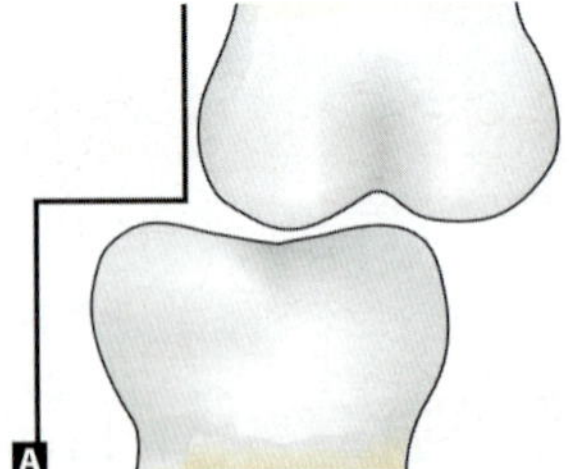

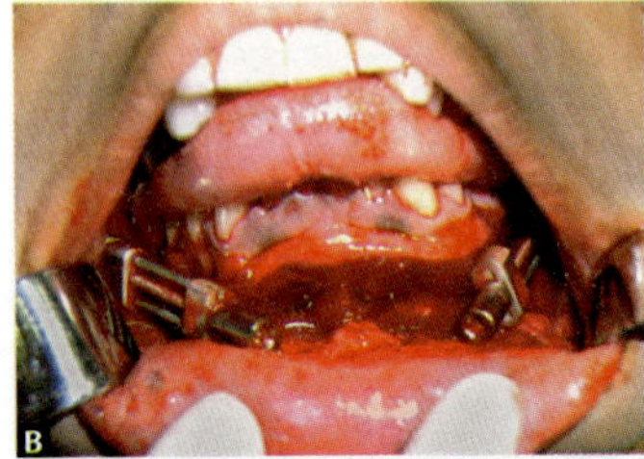

Figs A and B: *(A) Distal step; (B) Intraoral distractor*

filled surfaces (dmfs), when surfaces are counted.

DNA probe is an advanced diagnostic aid that helps to identify the organism associated with periodontal disease. It identifies species-specific sequence of nucleic acids that make up DNA, thereby permitting identification.

Doctor-Nurse relationship refers to a team where doctor role is to diagnose and cure the patient while nursing role lies in the process of care—helping, comforting and guiding.

Doctor-Patient relationship can be referred as where patient enters voluntarily into a contract to agree to follow doctor's advice. Doctor exercises an authoritative role because of being superior in professional knowledge. If doctor communicates well on an emotional plane, on a cultural plane and at intellectual plane he is a successful doctor and patient will develop confidence in him.

Doll's eye reflex is said to have occured when infant holds the fixation of faces, on the movements or changing intensity of light within their visual fields.

Doppler stethoscope is a device that helps in directing sounds by the velocity of blood moving through a blood vessel.

Dorendorl's sign is a fullness of supraclavicular groove. This sign may occur in aneurysm of aortic arch.

Double teeth refers to two conjoined teeth. However, this term should not be applied to teeth joined only through their root cementum. They are referred by other terms like "bifid teeth" *also see fusion*.

Douche is a procedure for cleaning the vaginal wall and cavity.

Down syndrome is also known as trisomy 21 or trisomy G, as it is a condition resulting from an abnormality of human chromosome number 21. It is characterized by mental deficiency and growth retardation. Oral manifestations present are periodontal disease with periodontal pockets, diastema, crowding, high frenal attachment, macroglossia, tooth anomalies.

DPT refers to a vaccine which renders immunity simultaneously against 3 diseases diphtheria, pertussis and tetanus which is an administrative gain. In addition, pertussis component in DPT vaccine enhances the potency of diphtheria toxiod. There are two types of vaccine—plain and adsorbed.

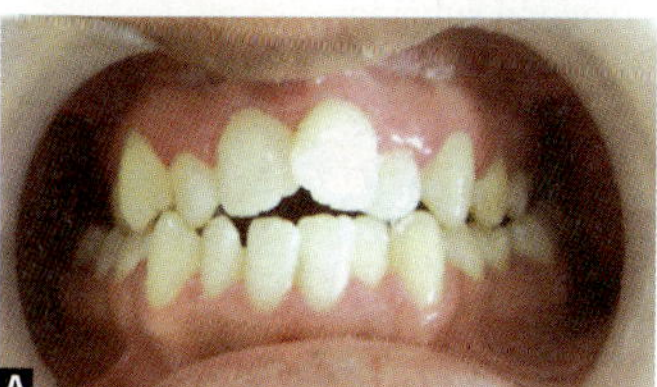

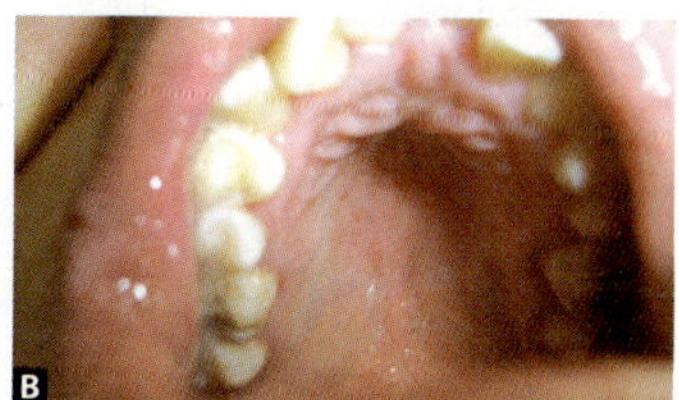

Figs A and B.: *Intraoral manifestations of Down syndrome*

Dracunculiasis is caused by largest viviparous nematode, the dracunculus medinensis popularly known as guinea worm. Larvae liberated by female worms are ingested by an intermediate host cyclops. People consuming the contaminated water with cyclops develop dracunculiasis. The lesions are usually seen in various parts of body, feet, nape of neck and back. During removal of worm, it is broken. The affected part becomes swollen, painful and inflamed. Death of adult female worms results in serious and grave complications. Arthritis, abscess formation and fibrosis of joints develop.

Draping is an art to isolate and drape the planned surgical site to prevent contamination of the prepared field.

Drifting is a change in position of the bone due to continuous resorption and deposition when it happens in relation to teeth it is known as mesial drift.

Drop attack is a clinical manifest and is associated with diffuse brain lesions. Patient may suddenly fall on ground. Attacks may occur many times a day. These are common in old age due to weakness, ataxia and gait disorder. Event is unexpected but consciousness is retained.

Droplet infection occurs by large particle droplets spatter which is transmitted by close contact. Spatter generated during dental procedures may deliver micro-organisms to the dentist.

Drowning is a form of death in which atmospheric air is prevented from entering into lungs by submission of body in water/liquid. Drowning person feels auditory and visual hallucinations. Asphyxia supervenes within 2 minutes after complete submersion and heart stops in 2–5 minutes afterwards. A find white leathery froth is seen at mouth and nostrils. Skin may be goose skin and grass, Gravel's sticks may be found firmly grasped in hands due to cadaveric spasm. On post-mortem, lungs are distended and pit on pressure of fingers. Water cannot get into left side of heart if body is thrown into water after death.

Drug allergy is a hypersensitive adverse reaction towards a drug. Oral reactions include stomatitis medicamentosa. In early reactions vesicles or bullae may be found. Occasionally purpuric spots appear. Involvement of gingiva, palate, lips and tongue are common. On discontinuation of drug, allergic reaction subsides.

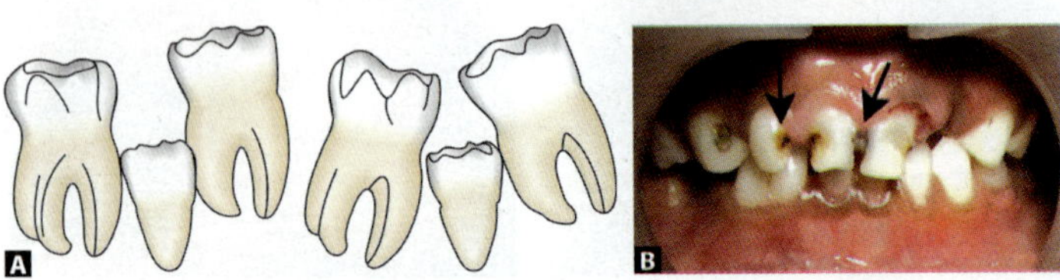

Figs A and B: *Schematic and clinical presentation of mesial drifting*

Drug eruptions are an eruption of skin or mucous membrane after oral or systemic administration of drugs. Drug eruptions vary in severity from a mild rash to toxic epidermal necrolysis. Onset may be sudden or delayed. Lesions may be local or generalized. Well-defined edematous wheels are seen in aspirin reaction. A few small oral vesicles or urticaria lesion to painful oral ulcerations are seen in case of sulfonamides and barbiturates. Fixed drugs are well-circumscribed dusky red or purple lesions on mucous membrane is seen in tetracycline, sulfonamide. Lichen planus like eruptions are seen in antimalarials and chlorpromazine.

Drug tolerance is diminished effect of a drug due to its continuous usage.

Drugs in pregnancy certain drugs can be excreted in milk affecting the infant. We should avoid the use of aspirin, benzodiazepines ciprofloxacin, cytotoxic drugs, corticosteroids, diuretics, lithium, etc.

Dry cough is a clinical manifestation that is produced as a result of stimulation of irritant receptors in the pharyngeal wall. These receptors are distributed throughout the tracheobronchial tree. Character of cough is hacking and it can be disturbing. In some common conditions such as pertussis and tracheobronchitis it may be associated with whoop sound.

Dry gangrene is a clinical condition that generally affects lower limbs and is due to slow occlusive vascular disease such as atherosclerosis and thromboangitis obliterans. Spread is very slow. Affected area becomes cold and clammy. Part becomes black, dry and shrivelled. A well-demarcated line of separation.

Dry heat sterilization refers to a method for sterilization of instruments. This type of sterilization involves heating air which further transfers energy from air to the instruments. In this type of sterilization, higher

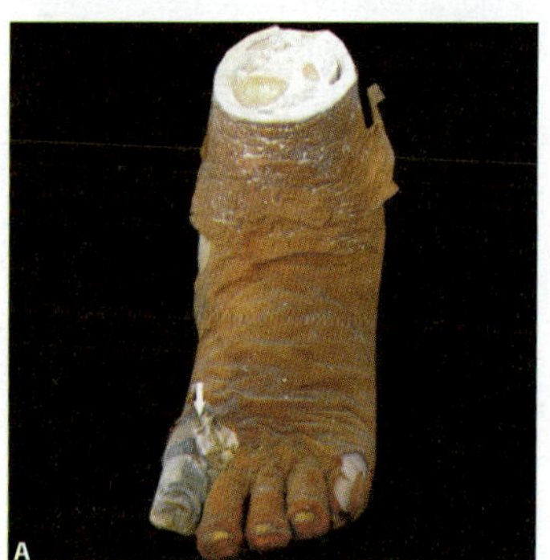

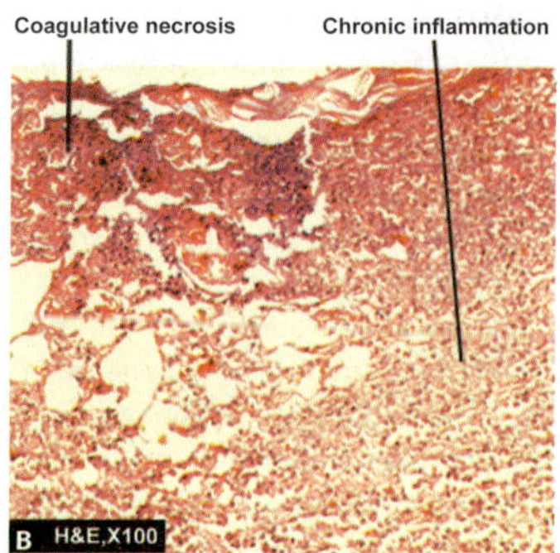

Figs A and B: *Dry gangrene foot (A) Macroscopic; (B) Microscopic*

temperature is required than steam or chemical vapor sterilization. It penetrates less well is less effective than moist heat. It takes 45 minutes to reach 160°C.

Dry socket is a postoperative complication of the extracted tooth. It can develop when infected clot gets the dislodged leaving the socket in an infective state extraction. It generally take place in lower bicuspid and molar socket. Dry socket is extremely painful and is treated by packing of zinc oxide eugenol Healing of such wound is very slow.

D-speed film is an intraoral film. Letter'd' identifies the film speed.

Dual arch tray is an impression tray that takes an impression of the desired upper and lower teeth.

Dual cure bond agent is an adhesive material that can be changed to its final hard state by light curing.

Dual energy X-ray absorptiometry (DEXA) is a body composition analysis used to provide regional estimates of fat mass with minimal radiation. Dexa measures the differential attenuation of two main X-ray photon energies as they pass through the body. Total tissue mass is separated into fat, bone, mineral and lean according to measured X-ray attenuation.

Dual wavelength spectrophotometry (DWLS) is a method independent of a pulsatile circulation. The presence of arterioles rather than arteries in the pulp and its rigid encapsulation by surrounding dentin and enamel make it difficult to detect a pulse in the pulp space. This method measures oxygenation changes in the capillary bed rather than the supply vessels and hence does not depend on a pulsatile blood flow.

Ductless glands are specialized glands that secrete hormones directly into blood.

Due care is a legal term for just, proper and sufficient care. No negligence.

Due cause is to show justifiable reason an action.

Duga sign is a sign of dislocated shoulder. Ask the patient to place affected hand on opposite shoulder and elbow toward the chest. Inability to do so is a sign of shoulder dislocation.

Dunlop beta hypothesis states that best way to break a habit is by its conscious, purposeful repetition. He suggests that the child should be asked to suck his thumb observing himself as he indulges in the habit. This procedure is very effective if the child is asked to do the same at a time when he is involved in an enjoyable activity.

Duodenal ulcer refers to the ulcers in the duodenum and characterized by pain that develops 2-3 hours after meals and is eased by food.

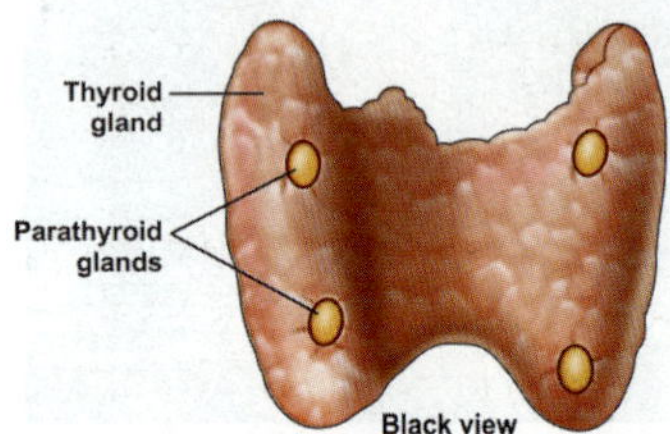

Fig.: *Ductless glands*

Pain generally develops in night during 12-2 am. Pain is aggravated by coarse foods, alcohol, and nervous tension. Antacids give relief. Recurrent nausea and vomiting suggest possibility of duodenal ulcer. There develops deep tenderness over lesion. Superficial tenderness may be present.

Dye lasers use complex organic dyes, such as rhodamine 6 g, in liquid solution or suspension as lasing media. They are tunable over a broad range of wavelengths.

Dysarthria anarthria is a complete loss of speech due to a disorder of neuromuscular lesion. It is rare but dysarthria which is an impaired articulation is common. Speech is slurred and indistinct. Lesion at highest level may cause it.

Dyskeratosis congenital (Zinsser – Engman Cole Syndrome) is a rare X-linked disorder characterized leading to atrophic, leukoplakic oral mucosa. Tongue and cheek are adversely affected. Oral lesions starting before the age of 10 as vesicles and white necrotic patches with candida, ulcerations and erythroplakic changes. Nail changes are the first manifestation of disease. Skin may become atrophic, face starts appearing red. There may be mental retardation, small sella turcica, eyelid infectious and dental abnormalities. There is no possible treatment.

Dyskinetic comprises of 15% of CP cases. Athetoid includes involuntary movement such as arm, legs and hand. Dystonic includes trunk muscles more than limbs that result in fixed or twisted posture of the body.

Dysmenorrhea is the pain and cramps i n back and lower abdomen associated with menstruation.

Dysphoria is an unpleasant emotional state. It is a mixture of sadness with low-grade anxiety and negativity. It is a normal spectrum of human experience.

Dysplasia is an abnormal formation of cells of a particular tissue. Dysplasia is characterized by a proliferation of cells with altered nucleus size and shape. Dysplasia can vary in grade. Not all dysplasias are associated with malignancy.

Dyspnea is an abnormally uncomfortable awareness of breathing.

Dystonia is abnormally increased muscular tone causing fixed

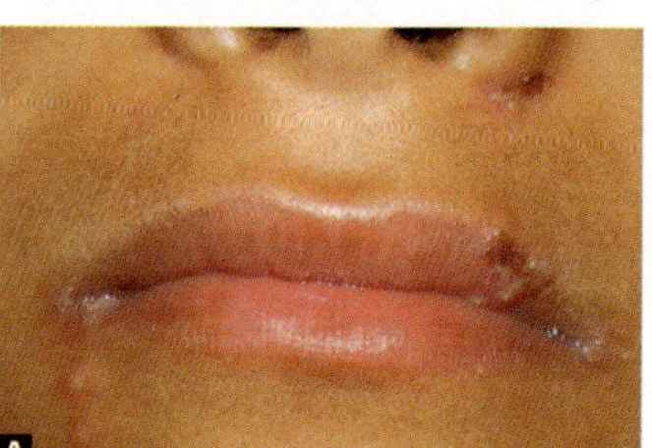

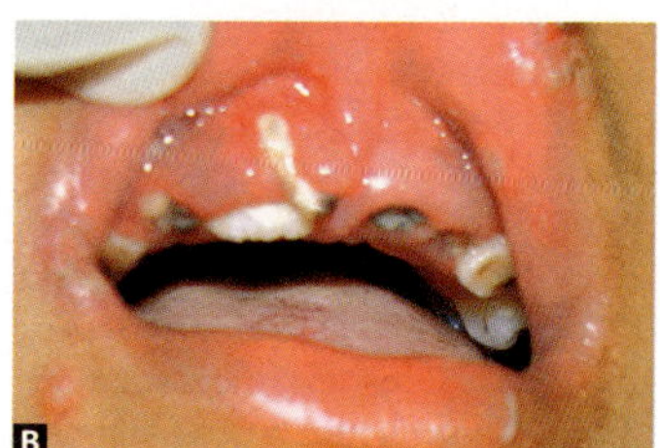

Figs A and B: *Epidermolysis bullosa*

abnormal postures. There is sustained contraction of both agonist and antagonist muscles. Focal dystonia leads to spasmodic torticollis and writer's cramp. Spasms are slower and involve trunk more than limbs that result in fixed or twisted posture of the body. It can be seen in Wilson's disease and Huntington's disease.

Dystrophic refers to disorder developed due to defective or faulty nutrition.

Dystrophic epidermolysis refers to extensive bulla formation and desquamation. Hands, feet, esophagus and oral cavity are involved. Oral mucosa becomes thick, gray and inelastic. Lesions are smooth. Buccal and lingual sulci become obliterated. Scarring develops. Lips may become immobile. Person may be dwarf. There may be associated conjunctival scarring, laryngeal stenosis and hoarseness of voice.

Dysuria is a painful urination is usually associated with inflammation. Pain is referred to the tip of the penis.

E

Early adolescence is a stage of development that includes casting off childhood role and emergence into adolescence. Physically it is characterized by developmental changes and the onset of puberty, initiated and indicated by the growth spurt.

Early onset periodontitis (EOP) *see* Juvenile periodontitis.

Early shift occurs during the early mixed dentition period. The eruptive force of the first permanent molar is sufficient to push the deciduous first and second molars forwards in the arch to close the primate space and thereby establish a Class I molar relationship. Since it occurs early in the mixed dentition period, it is called early shift.

Ebola virus infection is a member of the Filoviridae, causing hemorrhagic fever. It is transmitted from person to person. Virus spreads through blood. Mucosal bleeding is common. Patients die in intractable shock. Patients in high fever become delirious. No antiviral therapy is effective.

Eburnation refers to the term where radiographically bone end appears sclerosed or rounded off. Eburnation can be observed in cases of non-union of fractures.

Eccrine sweat glands are more and widely distributed of sweat glands. These are located throughout body specially palms and soles. Sweat plays an important role in temperature regulation. These function throughout life.

Echinococcosis hydatid disease is caused by Echinococcus granulosus. Dogs and cattle are the definite hosts where man is an accidental host. The cyst contains hydatid fluid which is colorless with a specific gravity of 1005 to 1010. The fluid is antigenic, toxic and can cause severe allergic reactions. Most common sites are liver, lung spleen and brain. Development of hydatid is slow.

Echocardiography (ECG) is a diagnostic test which provides measurement of left ventricular size, function and thickness. Size of all four chambers can be determined. Morphology of heart values can be examined. Hypertrophic cardiomyopathy, pericardial effusion, mitral valve prolapsed can be diagnosed.

Ecchymosis is erythrocyte extravasation into submucosals common on lips and face, the lesion will appear of brown color, i.e. when hemoglobin is degraded to hemosiderin. Patients on anti-coagulant therapy may present it commonly.

Ecologic plaque hypothesis (Marsh PD (1994) refers to a theory that proposes that the organisms associated with disease may also be present at sound sites, but at levels too low to be clinically relevant. Disease is a result of a shift in the balance of the resident microflora drives by a change in local environmental conditions. The bacterial composition of plaque remains relatively stable despite regular exposure to minor environmental perturbations. This microbial homeostasis is due to a dynamic balance of both synergistic and antagonisticmicrobial interactions. However, homeostasis can break down, leading to shifts in the balance of the micro flora, thereby predisposing sites to disease.

Ectoderm is the outermost layer of three germ layers of an embryo.

Ectopic lingual thyroid nodule is a small mass of thyroid tissue located at tongue. Clinically, it appears as a smooth nodular mass at the base of tongue. It may be asymptomatic causing feeling of fullness in throat or difficulty as feeling of fullness in throat or difficulty in swallowing. Sometimes it may require surgical removal.

Eczema is a superficial skin inflammation characterized by vesicles, redness, oozing, crusting, scaling and itching. Scratching or rubbing may lead to lichenification.

Edema is the presence of an excess of fluid in interstitial space causing swelling of the tissues. Edema may be localized or generalized. Generalized edema is known as anasarca, in which the fluid may also accumulate in the pleural cavity (hydrothorax) and peritoneal cavity (ascites). Edema over feet is known as pedal edema. Edema may be of the pitting or non-pitting type.

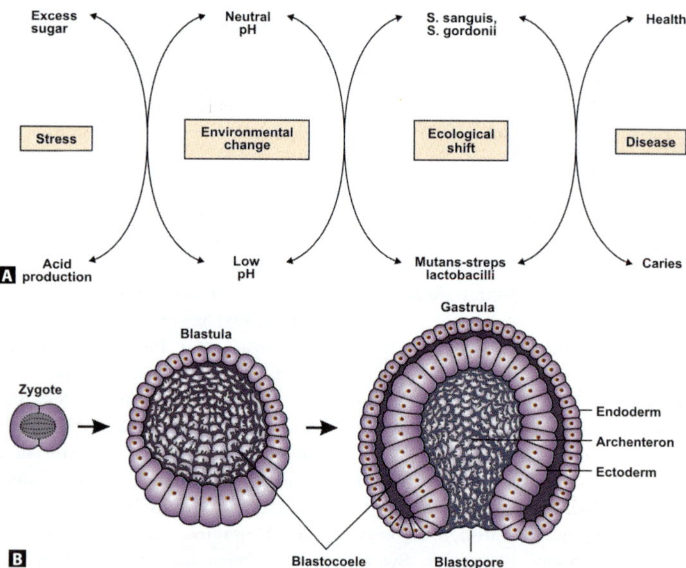

Figs A and B: *(A) Ecological plaque hypothesis; (B) Ectoderm*

Edentulous refers to area bearing no teeth.

EDTA is most commonly used chelating agent. It was introduced in dentistry by Nygaard-Ostby for cleaning and shaping of the canals. It contains four acetic acid groups attached to ethylenediamine. EDTA is relatively nontoxic and slightly irritating in weak solutions. The effect of EDTA on dentin depends on the concentration of EDTA solution and length of time, it is in contact with dentin. Serper and Calt in their study observed that EDTA was more effective at a neutral pH than at a pH 9.0. They showed that for optimal cleaning and shaping of canals EDTA should be used at neutral pH and with lower concentrations.

Educational neglect is a condition where parents fail to provide education, which leads to failure of cognitive and intellectual development of child. Failure to educate the child. Making them work at home instead of providing education. In a country like India where a girl child education is discontinued in order to take care of younger brother/sibling is the most common form of education neglect. Educational neglect can cause lack of confidence that can seriously impact the normal psychological growth and development. Not educating special child/child with learning disability can be categorized as a form of educational neglect.

Effector cells are the unique cells specialized to secrete large amount of Ig proteins into surrounding. Secreted Ig retains the ability to bind the specific ligand and then referred to as antibodies which constitutes 7-26g/L in adult and 25% of total serum protein. In human approximately 109 B-cells are generated each day. Plasma cells are oval or egg shaped with abundant cytoplasm and an eccentrically placed round nucleus. Clumps of dark staining chromatin are distributed around inner aspect of membrane giving the nucleus a characteristic 'Pin wheel/Clock face' appearance. Protein secretory organelles include Golgi apparatus. Ig is not present on surface of plasma cell but produced in copious amount in cytoplasm and

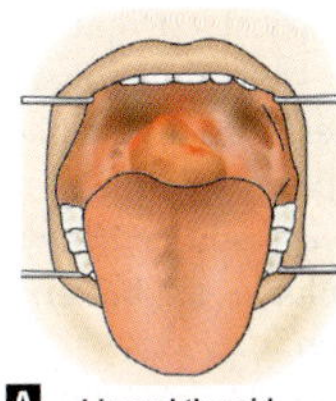

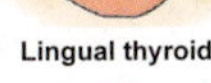

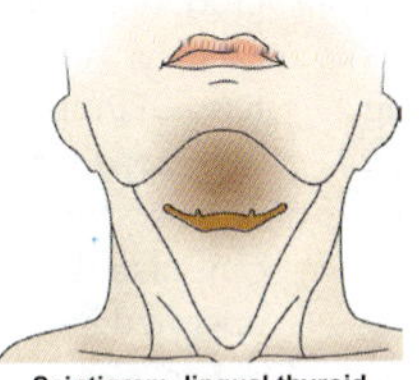

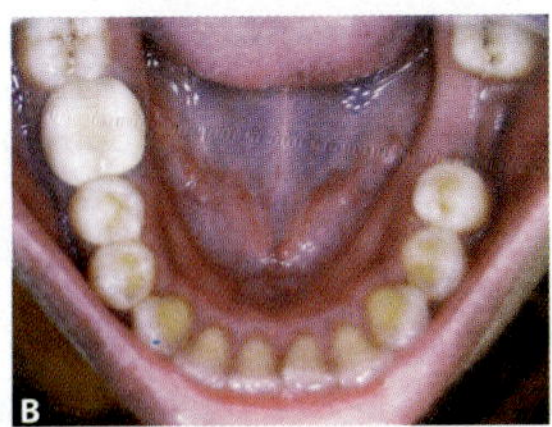

Figs A and B: *(A) Ectopic lingual thyroid (B) Edentulous space*

secreted into extracellular space. Plasma cells are terminally differen-tiated and have a short life-span of days to weeks.

Efferent refers to the nerves that carry motor messages away from the brain or central point.

Efficacy refers biological effects of treatment delivered carefully controlled conditions usually determined by randomized controlled trial.

Ego is a part of psychosexual theory. In Latin meaning 'I', it develops out of Id in 2nd and to 6th month of life when infant earns to differentiate between itself and outside world Mediation between Id superego, unlike Id, Ego is governed by the reality concerned with memory and judgment develops after birth, expands with age and it delays, modifies and controls Id impulses on realistic level.

Ehlers-Danlos syndrome is a group of hereditary disorder of connective tissue. There is hyper-elasticity of skin, hyper-extensibility of joint and fragility of skin and blood vessels. Oral mucosa gets bruised easily and is excessively fragile. Gingival tissues appear fragile and bleed after tooth brushing. Tooth mobility is not increased. There will be hypermobility of temporomandibular joint causing repeated dislocation of jaw. Hypoplastic changes in enamel have been noted. There is no known treatment.

Ejaculation is a subjective response to emission.

Elastic refers to the capability of sustaining deformities, without permanent change in size or shape.

Elastic modulus is the measure of rigidity or stiffness of a material at stresses below its elastic limit.

Elastomers are the impression material. The advantage of this material is their elasticity which makes it suitable for all types of denture. It is stronger than alginate and less subject to change in dimension on standing.

Electra complex is said to have occurred when the young girls develop an attraction towards their father and they resent mother being close to the father. Freud has reported that little girls have a comparable Electra complex to resolve this.

Electric heating pads are available of various sizes. Heating is by conduction so effect is superficial.

Electric pulp test is a diagnostic test which uses electric current to stimulate nerve fibers in the pulp to test vitality.

Electric pulp tester is a diagnostic tool device used for evaluation of condition of the pulp by electrical excitations of neural elements within the pulp. The pulp tester is an instrument which uses the gradations of electrical current to excite a response from the pulpal tissue. Pulp testers are available with cord which plugs into electric outlets for power source they can also be available as battery operated instrument.

Electric shock refers to the shock that results from passing current through the entire body. It usually does not produce cutaneous burns but has more severe effects on central nervous system cardiovascular system and other systems of the body. The patient usually suffers from trembling, sweating and, pallor. Intracranial pressure may be raised and patient may become unconscious because of cerebral edema. There may be temporary deafness, auditory hallucinations, paralysis, and stiffness of limbs, sudden blindness from retinal detachment or cataract occurs at a later stage. Delayed neurological effects are rare. Apnea or cardiac arrest is the most severe presentation which requires immediate manual cardio-pulmonary resuscitation (CPR).

Electric tooth brush is a powered tooth brush which uses electricity to simulate the brushing action of a patient.

Electrical flash burns are the electrical burns that result from fire or resulting from electrical sparks or flash. Degree of damage depends upon the time duration of exposure to the flash or the proximity of the patient to the actual flash.

Electrosurgery is a surgical method which uses a tiny arch of electric current to make the incision in the gingiva.

Electrothermal burns are the electrical burns that result from accidental contact with elements of electrical instruments. These are specially seen amongst children.

Electrocoagulation is a procedure performed to obtain hemorrhage control by using electrocoagulation current with the help of fine tungsten wire used for electrosection.

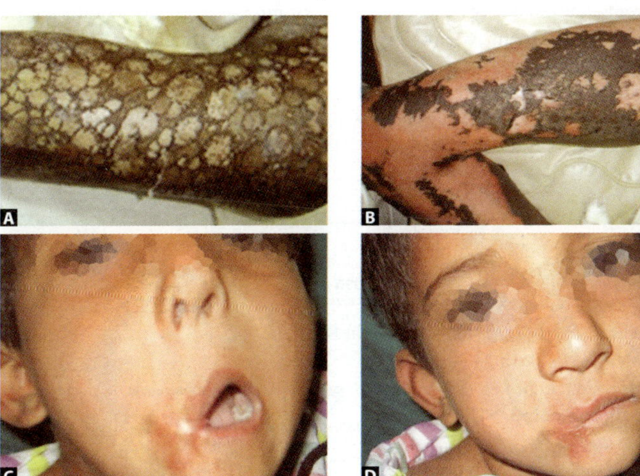

Figs A to D: *(A and B) Electrical flash burns; (C and D) Electrothermal burns*

Electroencephalogram is a recording of the electrical activity in the cerebral cortex that is sometimes, used as an index of arousal or anxiety. Electrodes are placed over scalp. Arousal and agitation is associated with rapid, irregular, low amplitude impulses. While relaxation is associated with slow, steady, high amplitude impulses.

Electroencephalography involves the detection, amplification, filtering, storage and analysis of small changes in electrical potential produced by brain, the underlying cortex. Recordings are made with electrodes in specific scalp locations. Accuracy of EEG diagnosis is overrated.

Electrogustometry refers to a procedure where taste bud fields can be stimulated by low voltage anodal and cathodal currents applied by means of battery. Instrument is known as electrogustometer.

Electrolyte refers to a substance that ionizes in solution rendering the solution of conducting a current.

Electromyogram is a recording of electrical activity of a muscle that sometimes, is used as an index of tension and anxiety. Mostly electrodes are placed over skin.

Electromyography is a study of voluntary and spontaneous electrical activity of muscle. The potentials generated by stimulation of motor unit are recorded by concentric needles. In neuropathy axons are lost then surviving axons sprou.t and take over nearby denervated muscle fibers resulting in larger and longer EMG record while in myopathy some fibers cannot be activated and recorded muscle potential is smaller. Electromyography is one of the major criteria in diagnosing myofascial pain. Electromyography finds out the changes in muscle activity and knowing the process of muscle pain and monitoring the effect of treatment.

Electron microscopy is a microscopic procedure where light waves are replaced by a beam of electrons which allows resolution of

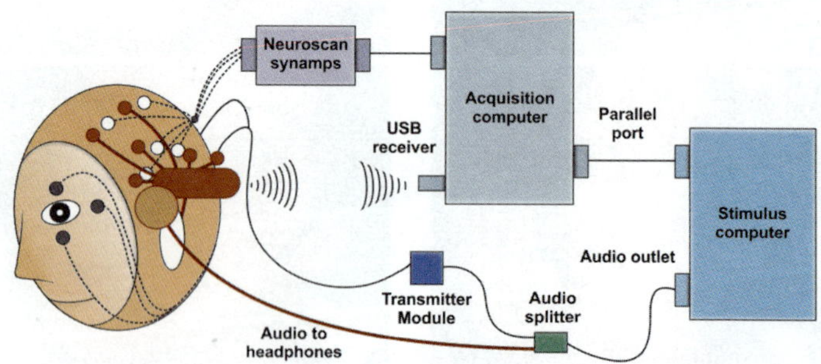

Fig.: *Schematic presentation for electroencephalography*

extremely small organism such as several of 0.001 micro millimeter size.

Electronic apex locator is the process to determine the location of the apex of the tooth.

Electroplating is the process of depositing metal from solution onto the surface of an impression using an electric current.

Electrosection is the term used for incisions, excisions and tissue planning with the help of single wired active electrodes that can be bent or adapted to perform any kind of cutting procedures.

Electrosurgery is a surgical technique performed on soft tissue using controlled high frequency electrical currents.

Elephantiasis is an infectious disease that starts below the malleolus and then spreads to involve foot but thigh is rarely involved. Swelling pits on pressure to start with but later on overlying skin may become rough and thickened.

Elevators are the surgical hand instruments that are designed to elevate a periosteum, a retained root, impacted tooth, or a fractured root out of the bony socket. Many types of elevators are available such as periosteal elevator, cryers elevator, straight and universal elevators.

E-line (Esthetic plane): A line drawn from also tip to chin. Normally the upper lip is about 2 mm behind E-line while the lower lip lies on that plane.

ELISA (Enzyme-linked immunosorbent assay) is as a screening test and used commonly in commercial laboratories when performed properly. Currently licensed enzyme immune assays have a specificity and sensitivity exceeding 98 to 99%, the ultimate reliability depends on the setting in which they are used.

Elongated styloid process associated with it is known as Wagle's syndrome. There is a unilateral pain extending from ear to neck.

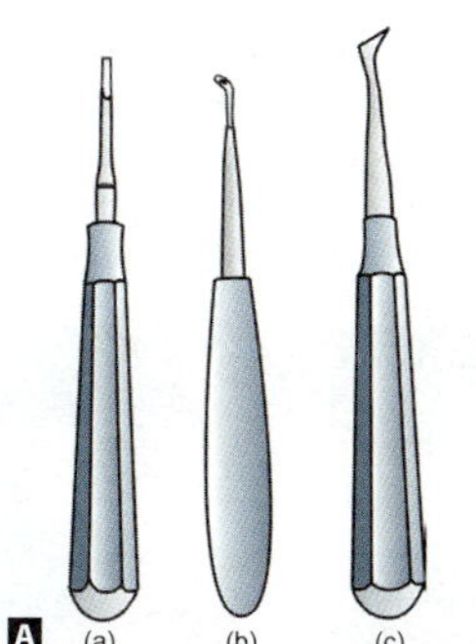

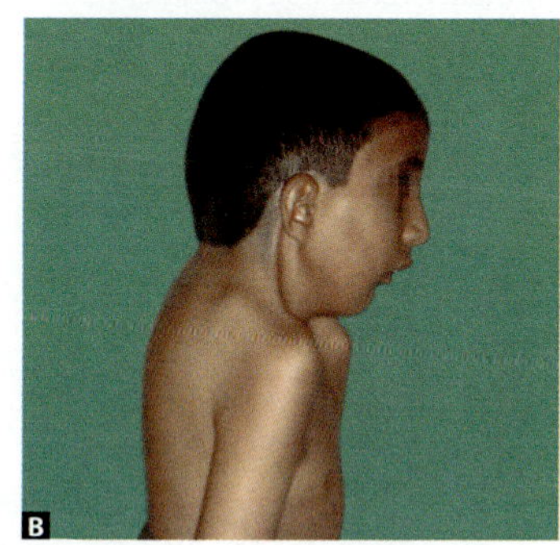

Figs A and B: *(A) Elevators [(a) Coupland; (b) Warwick James; (c) Cryer]; (B) Elongated styloid process*

Persons develop a feeling of foreign body in throat.

Embedded denticles refer to large pulpal calcification that embedded in dentin. Such calcifications are more commonly seen in aged pulp due to dense cross-linking between collagen.

Embedded teeth refer to those teeth that don't erupt on its own, owing to a lack of eruptive force.

Emboli are the moving clot.

Embrasure refers to the space between two teeth created by the sloping away of the mesial and distal surfaces.

Embrittlement refers to render susceptible to breakage under slight bending.

Embryo is the earliest stages of development, the first 8 weeks.

Embryology is a study of the development of an individual from conception to birth.

Emesis basin is a kidney-shaped basin for receiving expectorated or vomited material.

Eminence refers to a prominence.

Emission of electron: Once an electron moves to a higher energy orbit, it eventually wants to return to the ground state. When it does, it releases its energy as a photon—a particle of light. This phenomenon is termed spontaneous emission of radiation.

Emotion is a complex reaction by the whole organism, often to an abrupt shift in social circumstances, involving widespread bodily change in visceral function such as heart beat, breathing and glandular secretion and characterized mentally by strong feelings, excitement, agitation and turmoil. Emotion is a state of mental excitement characterized by physiological, behavioral changes and alterations of feelings.

Emotional abuse is said to have occurred when a child's parent or caregiver repeatedly rejects the child or uses threats to frighten the child.

Empirical therapy: Theory prescribed without the benefit of laboratory test getting done.

Empty habits are those habits that are not associated with any deep-rooted psychological problems.

Emulsion is the suspension of very small droplet of one immiscible liquid in another.

Enamel hypocalcification is a developmental anomaly that results in a disturbance of maturation of enamel matrix. It appears as a localized white chalky spot on the

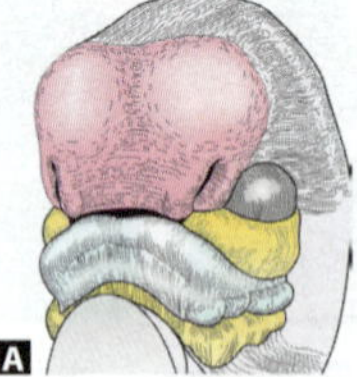

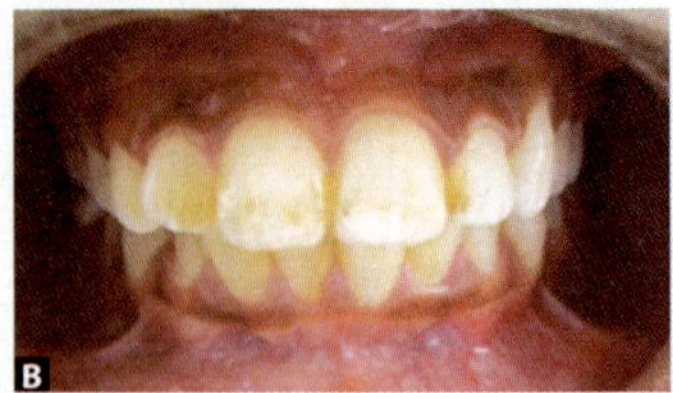

Figs A and B: *(A) Embryo; (B) Enamel hypoplasia*

middle third of smooth crowns. Underlying enamel may be soft and susceptible to caries. Remedy improves aesthetic appearance.

Enamel hypoplasia is the incomplete formation of enamel resulting in alteration of tooth form or color. It results due to damage to ameloblasts during enamel matrix formation. Due to tetany hypoplasia is pitting. Due to infection there may be any type of hypoplasia from a mild brownish discoloration to a severe pitting irregularity. When single tooth is involved it is known as Turner's tooth.

Enamel pearl is small, spherically-shaped enamel located on a root surface. It develops due to abnormal displacement of ameloblasts during tooth formation. It is usually found on maxillary molars. It does not require any treatment.

Enamel refers to the outermost surface of the anatomical crown. It is thickest at the top of the crown and becomes thinner and ends in a knife edge at the cervical line. The color of the enamel varies with its thickness and mineralization. The color varies from yellowish white to grayish white. Enamel appears whiter if it is thicker. The more mineralized enamel shows more translucency. The translucency gives yellowish color to the tooth. Enamel is densely mineralized, hardest and highly polished in the human body. This dense mineralization gives the enamel ability to resist wear and tear of the crown. Composition-Inorganic content 96%-97% by weight (Calcium, Magnesium, Po_4, Na, Co_3) Organic content soluble proteins, insoluble proteins, peptides, citric acid and water.

Encephalitis refers to the inflammation involving cerebral hemispheres, brain stem and cerebellum. Viral encephalitis is more common. Viral encephalitis may be primary, para or post-infections. Onset is abrupt with lethargy, drowsiness confusion and behavioral abnormality. It may progress to stupor or coma. Cerebral hemispheres when

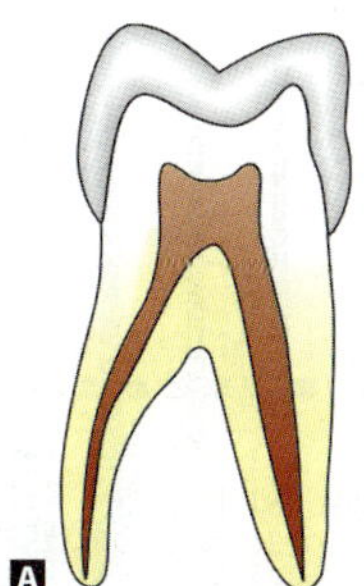

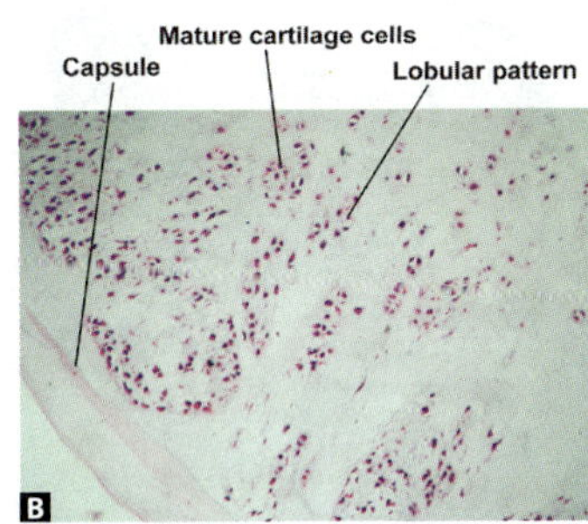

Figs A and B: *(A) Enamel; (B) Enchondroma*

involved cause aphasia and sensory loss.

Enchondroma is a benign bone tumor of residual islands of cartilage specially of bones of hand. It is painless developing between 10-30 years. X-ray presents areas of radiolucency that expands and deforms bone. Margins are well defined. Cortex remain intact. Stippled or punctate calcification may be found.

Endemic is a disease present in a community or among a group of people, the continuing prevalence of a disease as distinguished from an epidemic.

Endoactivator system refers to an ultrasonic irrigation device which works on the principles of vibration to remove the smear layer, debris and clumps from the root canals.

Endocranium is a fibrous membrane (similar to periosteum) lining the inside of the cranial cavity.

Endocrine system consists of a series of ductless glands found in body. These glands which then produce hormones to regulate the rate of metabolism, growth and sexual development. Hormones are secreted directly into blood. Glands include thyroid, parathyroid, ovaries, testes, pituitary, pancreas and adrenal medulla.

Endocrine therapy is the treatment with hormones with drugs to interfere with hormone production. There may be surgical removal of endocrine glands.

Endodontia refers to within a tooth.

Endodontic emergency is defined as the condition associated with pain and/or swelling which requires immediate diagnosis and treatment. The main causative factors responsible for occurrence of endodontic emergencies are—Pathosis in pulp and periradicular tissues, traumatic injuries.

Endodontic file is a hand instrument used to smooth, shape and enlarge root canal.

Endodontics is the branch of clinical dentistry associated with the prevention, diagnosis and treatment of pathosis of the dental pulp and their sequelae

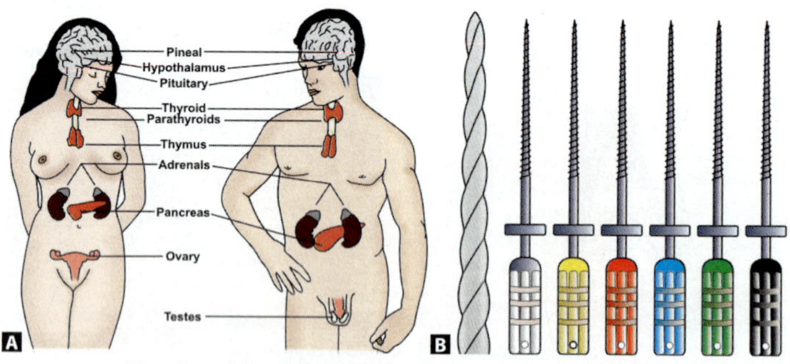

Figs A and B: *(A) Endocrine system; (B) Endodontic file*

that all forms of root canal therapy including root filling, pulpotomy, pulp capping and apicoectomy. Aim of treatment is to remove the inflamed pulp and replace it with permanent root filling.

Endodontist is a specialist dentist who has undergone a special training in diagnosing and treating the problems associated with the pulp space of the tooth.

Endo-extractor refers to the kit used to retrieve the broken instruments or silver pound from the obstructed canals. Here cyanoacrylate adhesive is place on it so as to lock the object into the extractor. Technique for removal is same as that for Masserann extractor.

Endogenous intrinsic stains refer to those stains that get incorporated within the tooth structures that have occurred to take place during the development of the tooth and are more suggestive of developmental anomalies of tooth. As the name suggests these teeth cannot be removed by regular prophylactic procedures.

Endogenous malodor *see* true oral malodor.

Endorphins are a chemical in CNS that influences pain perception—a natural pain killer.

Endoscopic method for caries detection is potentially sensitive diagnostic tools, which involve the use of endoscopic methods. These give a magnified image of the carious lesion to be viewed. Initial studies on the potential benefits of endoscopic examination, either with white light (VMV) or with filtered fluorescence excited by a blue curing light (VFF), have been performed by Longbottom and Pitts (1990). They suggested that it may detect a greater number of carious lesions than do conventional methods. One advantage of endoscopy is a 5-to-10 fold magnification of the sites. Disadvantages include meticulous drying and isolation of teeth taking about 5 to 10 mins for an examination, as compared with 3 to 5 min. for conventional methods.

Endosteum can be described as tissue lining the internal bone cavities. Unlike periosteum, the endosteum is composed of single layer of osteoblasts and, sometimes a small portion of connective tissue.

Endotoxins are cell wall lipopolysaccharide of Gram negative cocci and bacilli and are not actively released from cell. These cause fever, shock and other symptoms.

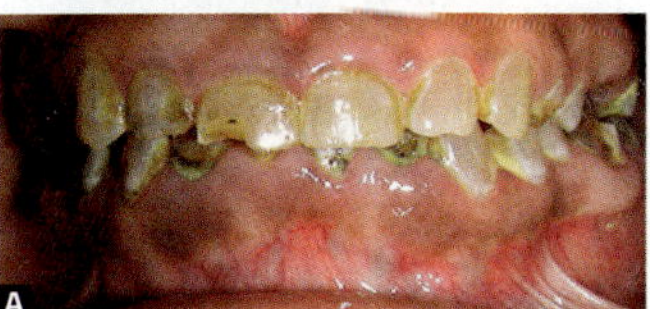

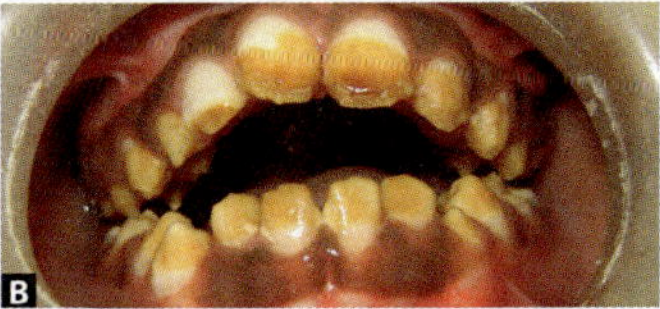

Figs A and B.: *Endogenous intrinsic stain due to: (A) Dentin dysplasia; (B) Amelogenesis imperfecta*

Energy refers to capacity for doing work.

Enlargement due to puberty refers to gingival enlargement may be seen in males and females during puberty, in area of plaque accumulation. Enlargement is usually confined to marginal gingival with bulbous inter-proximal papilla seen more frequently on facial aspect than the lingual aspect. Features of inflammatory enlargement are seen and it undergoes spontaneous reduction after puberty if plaque and calculus is removed.

Enlargement due to vitamin C.

Enteric fever is a systemic disease caused by *Salmonella typhi* and *Salmonella paratyphi*. Humans are the only host for *S. typhi* and *S. paratyphi*. In most, the infection results from consumption of contaminated food or water. The source of infection is acutely infected patients or chronic carriers. Incubation period is 5-14 days.

Eosinophils are white blood cells that comprise 1-3% of all blood leukocytes. These are weak phagocytes. The function of these is to detoxify the proteins before they can damage the body. These help in dissolution of old clots. Eosinophils collect at the site of antigen antibody reaction. In trichinosis large number of eosinophils develops.

Eosinophilia is a condition in which eosinophil count increased beyond 450/μl in peripheral blood.

Eosinophilic enteritis is a condition where blood shows eosinophilia with eosinophilic infiltration of gut wall. Some may show steatorohea with malabsorption, hypoalbuminemia or intestinal obstruction and some with ascites with eosinophilia. Corticosteroids help. Barium study may show mucosal edema, nodular masses, sawtootheal mucosal pattern. Parasite infertation should be excluded.

Eosinophilic granuloma is a solitary non-neoplastic proliferation of histiocytes. Also known as pulmonary histiocytosis X(PHX)/langer-hans cell histiocytosis (LCH) was introduced by Lichenstein and Jaffe in 1940. There may not be any symptoms. Patient may develop local pain and swelling. On X-ray, lesion appears as irregular radiolucent area involving superficial alveolar bone. Cortex is destroyed, pathological fracture may

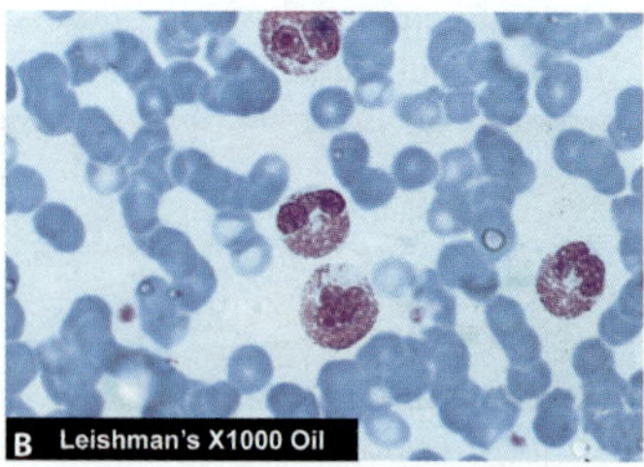

Figs A and B: *(A) Gingival enlargement due to puberty; (B) Eosinophil*

develop. Once the lesion matures, fibrosis occurs. Prognosis is good.

Esophageal varices are tortuous and dilated veins at the junction of lower end of esophagus and cardia of stomach. These occur in cirrhosis of liver. Rupture and hemorrhage may lead to death.

Ephebodontics is the science of dentistry which deals with the children who are in the process of growing up from childhood to manhood or womanhood. Medically adolescence can be considered as the period beginning with the appearance of the secondary sex characters and terminating with the cessation of somatic growth.

Epidemiologic indices (Irving Glickman) are attempts to quantitate clinical conditions on a graduated scale, thereby facilitating comparison among populations examined by the same criteria and methods.

Epidemiology (Nikki Foruk) has been defined as a study of health and disease states and effects of ecological or extrinsic factors and intrinsic factors on these states also.

Epidemiology can be defined as the frequency and severity of health problems in relation to age, sex, geography, race, economic status, nutrition and diet. This information is obtained from different kind of research epidemiological studies such as mortality rates, morbidity, effects of treatment and prevention.

Epidermal burns refer first degree burn.

Epidermoid cyst is a painless slow growing swelling of skin of insidious onset. It usually occurs over scalp, face, neck and scrotum. Palm and soles are not affected. It is hemispherical in shape. A black dot called punctum may be present on the top of swelling. It is mobile over deeper tissues but fixed to skin. It is not transilluminant. Overlying skin may not have hair.

Epidermolysis bullosa is a genetic skin disease which causes oral ulceration. Ulcers develop

A
Burn epidermis
Dermis
Subcutaneous tissue
Muscle
First degree burn

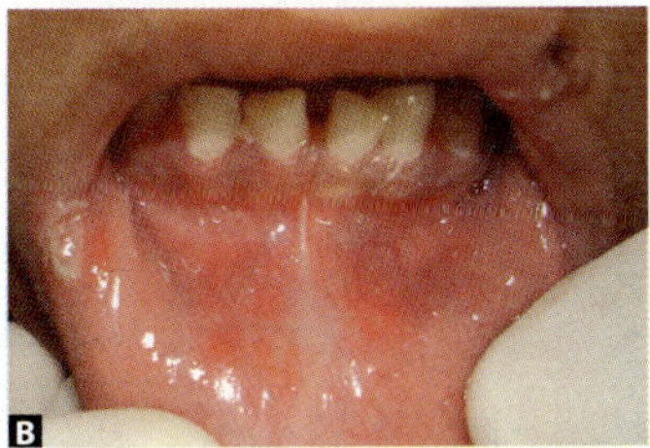

Figs A and B: *(A) Clinical picture and line diagram for epidermal burns; (B) Epidermolysis bullosa*

recurrently. Skin lesions are bullae which rupture to give ulcers. Oral ulcers vary in frequency and severity. Complications include ankyloglossia. These cannot be cured or effectively controlled. Only supportive line of treatment is given.

Epidural hematoma *see* Subdural.

Epiglottis is the cartilaginous appendage overlying the opening of larynx.

Epilepsy is a sudden, transient disturbance of cerebral function due to abnormal, chronic, recurrent and paroxysmal neurological discharge in brain. Each episode of such neurological dysfunction is called a seizure although; (1)—A single seizure cannot be categorized epilepsy; (2)—Epilepsy is derived from the Greek word "epilambanein" meaning to take or to seize. Between 400 BC and 200 AD Hippocrates, Aretaeus, Celsus, and Plinius all provided careful descriptions of major and minor seizures. Hippocrates even recognized that seizures originated in the brain. Epilepsy refers to a pattern of chronic seizures of any type over a long period.

Epinephrine is the substance that causes blood vessels to constrict.

Epinurium refers to tough fibrous sheath covering the whole nerve.

Epiphysis cerebri is a small piriform structure present in relation to the posterior wall of the third ventricle of the brain. It is also called the It is about 8 mm in length, and about 4 cm in width and in thickness. It is situated in the median plane just below the splenium of the corpus callosum, and just above the superior colliculi of the midbrain.

Epistaxis refers to bleeding from the nose.

Epithelial adaptation is the close approximation of the gingival epithelium to the tooth surface without the complete obliteration of the pocket.

Epithelial rests of Malassez are the remnants of Epithelial Hertwig's root sheath ie after the formation of radicular portion as the tooth elongates, the root sheath breaks up and begins to partially disappear and the remaining

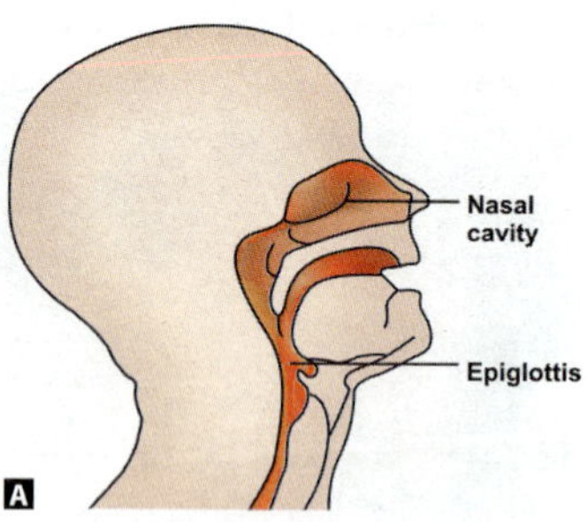

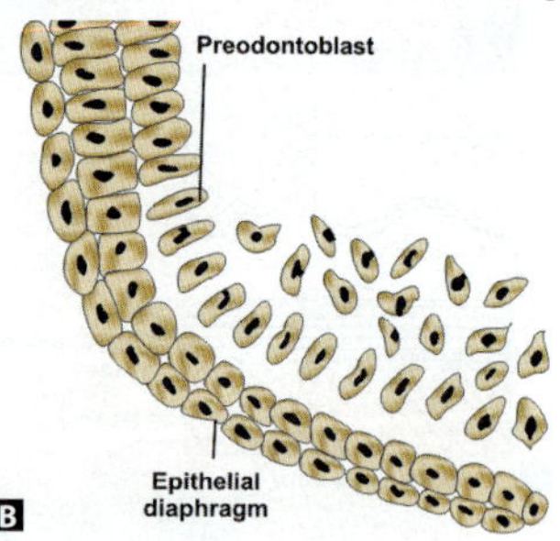

Figs A and B: *(A) Epiglottis; (B) Epithelial rests of Malassez*

portion is termed as epithelial rests of Malassez.

Equine gait steps is a neuropathic gait ie due to paralysis of pretibial and peroneal muscles. There develops a slapping noise as foot strikes the floor seen patients with foot drop.

Er, Cr:YSGG (2790 nm) are solid state lasers that have an active medium of a solid crystal of yttrium-scandium-gallium-garnet that is doped with erbium and chromium.

Er:YAG (2940 nm) has an active medium of a solid crystal of yttrium-Al-garnet that is doped with erbium. Both are delivered fiber optically in the free running pulsed mode. The fibers are air-cooled and have a larger diameter than the other lasers mentioned, making the delivery system somewhat less flexible. They have the highest absorption in water of any dental wavelength and have a high affinity for hydroxyapatite. These lasers are ideal for caries removal and tooth preparation when used with a water spray.

ERB's palsy is a paralysis of arm due to the damage to cervical nerve roots 5 and 6 of brachial plexus.

Erben's reflex is a slowing of pulse when head and trunk are forcibly bent forward. It shows vagal excitability.

ERG refers to unit of energy equivalent to 10^{-7} joules or 2.4×10^{-8} calories.

Ergonomics is the study of person's environment, his abilities and limitations.

Erogenous zones are different external areas of body which are exceptionally sensitive to sexual stimulation including breasts, buttocks, thighs, ear lobules, etc.

Erosion is the term often used for breaches of the epithelium in which there is little damage to the underlying lamina propria. Such lesions, if penetrating the epithelium only partially, usually have a red or red and yellow appearance. If they penetrate the full thickness of the epithelium, however, they are typically covered by a fibrinous exudate and may then have a yellowish appearance.

Erosion in relevance to dentistry is a loss of tooth substance by a chemical process. There is no bacterial erosion. Smooth lesions

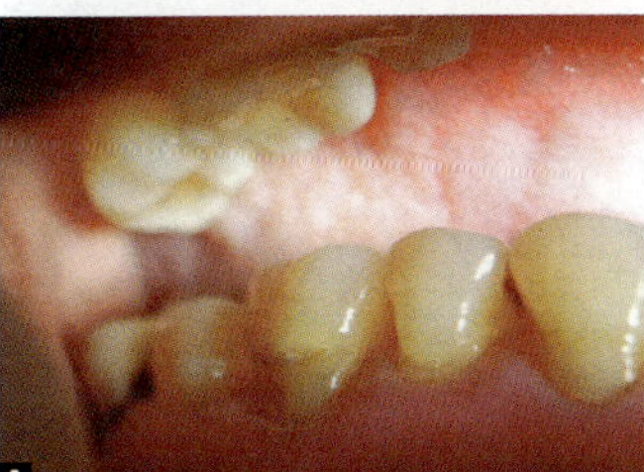

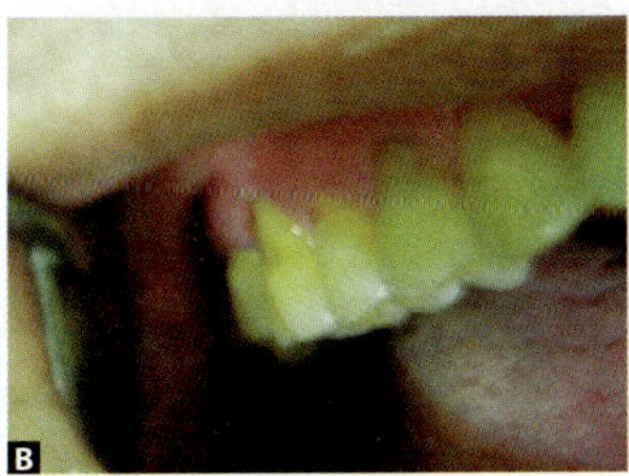

Figs A and B: *Dental erosion*

with no chalkiness appear on labial and buccal surface of teeth. Proximal surfaces may also be eroded. It may affect the labial surfaces of anterior teeth; erosion may also involve the dentin. It may occur due to decalcification of tooth.

Erosive lichen planus is an erosive bullous lesion of lichen planus occurs in severe form. It has been associated with drug therapy and reaction to dental restorations. The association between erosive lichen planus and squamous cell carcinoma remains controversial. It will start as vesicles or bullae. There is formation of vesicles, bullae, irregular shallow ulcers of oral mucosa. Biopsy is needed for correct diagnosis. Treatment of choice is of tropical ointment.

Euthanasia *see* mercy killing.

Eruption cyst is a soft tissue lesion fiound around the crown of an erupting tooth.

Eruption refers to migration of tooth into functional position.

Eruption sequestrum is a tiny irregular sequel of bone overlying the crown of an erupting permanent molar just following eruption of tips of the cusps. On X-ray, it appears as tiny irregular opacity which lies over central occlusal fossa.

Erythema induratum is a type of panniculitis. Lesions appear as erythematous, slightly tender nodules. Skin over nodule ulcerates. Caseation necrosis is to identify lesion. Granuloma is observed in the septae. Gradually fibrosis sets in.

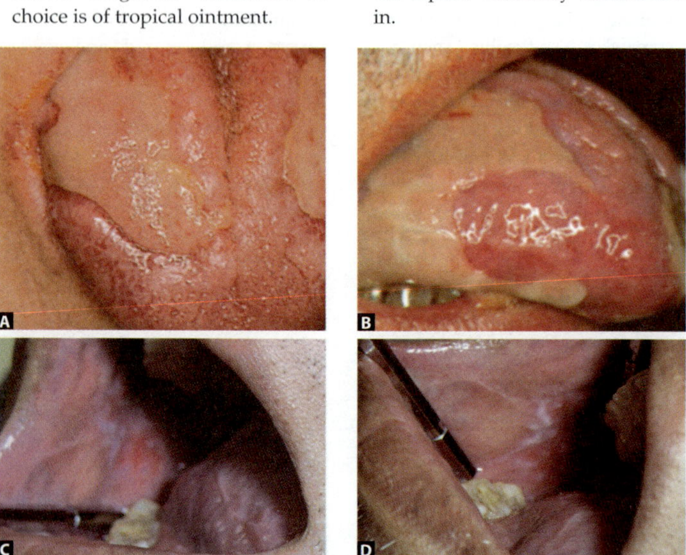

Fig.: *Erosive lichen planus*

Erythema multiforme is an acute dermatitis of unknown etiology. It is a nonviral condition. It can affect skin and submucosa separately or in combination. It occurs chiefly in young adults. Individual symptoms vary in size. In skin central vesicle is surrounded by concentric erythematous skin colored rings. Ulcers are painful and most commonly located on lips, tongue and buccal mucosa. A concentric ring-like appearance of lesions looks like bull's eyes. The hyperemic macular, papules or vesicles may become eroded or ulcerated and bleed freely.

Erythematous candidiasis is a poorly understood condition associated with corticosteroids, topic or systemic broad spectrum or HIV disease. It is generally seen on the dorsum of tongue, palate or buccal mucosa. There may be associated or angular candidiasis.

Erythroblastosis fetalis is a clinical condition where Rh incompatibility occurs due to destruction of fetal blood that results in congenital hemolytic anemia. Some infants may be stillborn. Jaundice, edema and compensatory erythropoiesis may develop. Blood pigment may be seen in the enamel and dentin of developing teeth. One can see green, blue or brown line. Strain is intrinsic. Enamel hypoplasia, defect in tooth crowns also known as Rh hump.

Erythromelalgia is a paroxysmal bilateral vasodilatory disorder of unknown etiology. Symptoms include erythema, warmth and bilateral burning pain lasting minutes to hours on feet and palms. Relief may be got by cooling and elevating the part.

Erythromycin is a potent antibiotic which is active against Gram-positive organisms. Gram-negative bacteria except hemophilus influenza all are resistant. Clindamycin is better tolerated. Better it is used in upper respiratory tract infections.

Erythroplakia is a lesion of oral mucosa presenting as bright red,

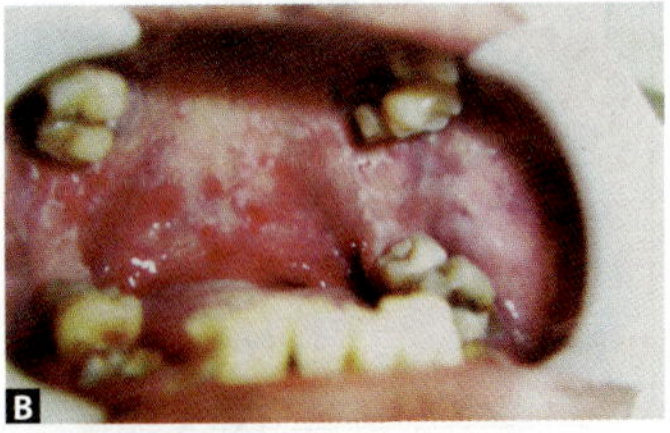

Figs A and B: *(A) Eruption sequence; (B) Erythematous candidiasis*

velvety plaque which cannot be classified as any other disease. It is less common than white lesion leukoplakia. Several clinical variants have been described. It develops in elderly age group. Biopsy is needed. After removing the irritant Toluidine blue staining should be done. A lesion that stains is likely to be precancerous in nature.

Eschar refers to a slough produced by burning or corrosive application.

Escharotics are the corrosive which can produce sloughing.

Esophagitis refers to inflammation of the esophagus. It may be acute or chronic in nature. Symptoms include odynophagia, dysphagia, chest pain, heart burn, fever and abdominal pain. Anorexia, fever and white lesions on tongue will develop.

Essential fatty acids refer to the fatty acids that are essential for human body but cannot be synthesized within the body. They are selective in promotion of growth as well as the maintenance of dermal integrity, i.e. linoleic, linolenic and arachidonic acid. These are present in vegetable oils in large quantities than in animal fats.

Esthetic refers to appearance.

Etch refers to treating enamel with phosphoric acid to provide retention for resin sealants.

Etchant refers to acid solution to etch tooth structure.

Etched porcelain veneers are esthetic porcelain facings that are placed on anterior teeth.

Etching process involves the use of 30 to 50% phosphoric acid which is applied to pits and fissures to seal. Acid removes inorganic materials and creates tiny crevices or micropores into which sealant material can flow. Mechanical bonding is the force which holds the sealant to the enamel.

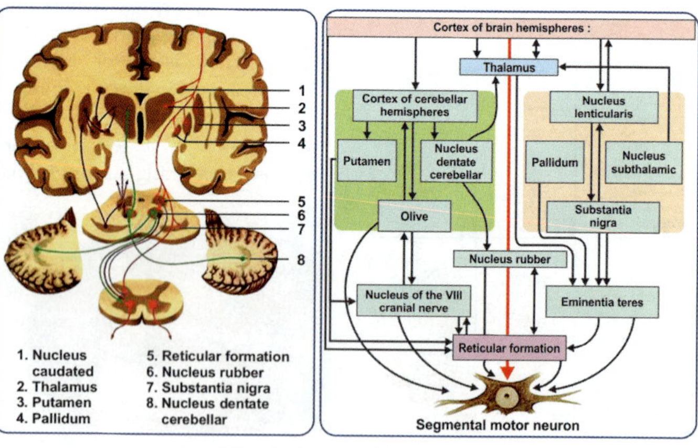

Fig. : *Extrapyramidal system*

Ethical dilemma is a choice between two undesirable alternatives. It is a situation that includes two or more important opposing ethical principles.

Ethics: Rules of morals, moral principles, rules governing standards.

Ethmoidal air sinuses are located within the lateral part (or labyrinth) of the ethmoid bone. They can be divided into anterior, middle and posterior groups. Each labyrinth (right or left) is bounded medially by the medial plate and laterally by the orbital plate of the ethmoid bone. The ethmoidal air sinuses lie between these plates. They are seen in coronal section in which their close relationship to the orbit can be appreciated.

Ethnographic research refers to the type of research whose purpose is to develop an indepth picture of the culture of a group.

Ethyl alcohol is an antiseptic that is used on skin and kills vegetative forms of bacteria. It is ineffective against spores. It is effective in concentration of 50 to 70% by weight. In higher concentrations, it is less effective.

Ethylene oxide is a room temperature gas used to sterilized instruments and equipment.

Ethylene oxide sterilization (ETOX) refers to sterilization method that is best used for sterilizing complex instruments and delicate materials. Ethylene oxide is highly penetrative, noncorrosive gas above 10.8°C with a cidal action against bacteria, spores and viruses.

European System (Conservative) systems, that is used for diagnosing pit and fissure caries, which consists of certain conservative criteria, was described by Backer-Dirks O, Houwink B, and Kwant CW, in 1961. Description of the system: In upper molars, the mesio-occlusal and disto-occlusal-palative fissures are assessed

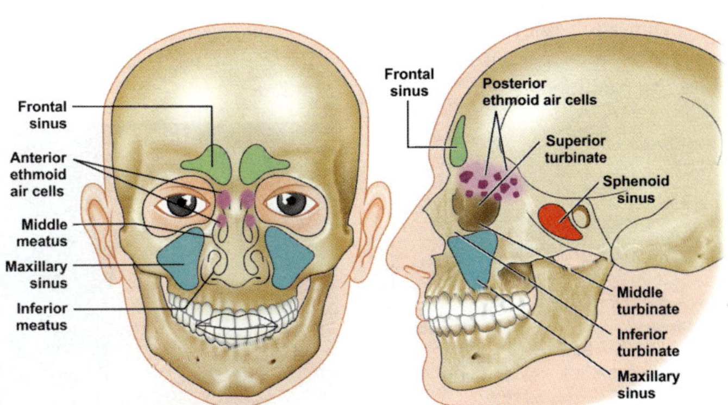

Figs A and B: *Sinuses: (A) Coronal view; (B) Lateral view*

E

separatively. In lower molars, the occlusal fissures and the buccal pits are assessed separately. Teeth are dried, sharp new explorer are used for assessment. Caries is diagnosed in four categories: C. I—Minute black line at base of fissure, C. II— In addition, a white zone along margins of fissure [dark in transmitted light), C. III—The smallest perceptible break in the continuity of the enamel, C. IV—Large cavity more than 3 mm wide.

Eustachian tube is the tube extending from inside the ear to the throat to equalize air pressure.

Eutectic is an alloy or solution whose components are proportioned to the melting point which is the lowest possible for those components.

EVA system is the most efficient system used for the correction of overhanging and overcontoured proximal alloy and resin restoration.

Evidenced-based dentistry is an oral health care that requires judicious integration of systemic assessment of clinically relevant scientific evidence about patient's oral and medical condition.

Ewing's sarcoma is a malignant neoplasm with destructive lesion of bone. Tumor may arise from undifferentiated cells of reticulo-endothelial system. *Clinical fea-tures:* It develops between 5 to 25 years. Mandible is affected more than maxilla. Person develops fever, leukocytosis, ESR is raised. Jaw bone is expanded. Mobility of tooth is a common feature. Neoplasm develops surface ulcer. *Radiological features:* Expansion, distortion of cortical bones. There is radiolucent area with ill-defined margins. Periosteum shows lamellar layering. Facial neuralgia, lip paresthesiaz and low-grade fever are present too. X-ray shows formation of layers of new bone giving an onion peel appearance. Osteophyte formation may be seen. Some cases may show sunray appearance. Neoplasm is radiosensitive. Radiotherapy and chemotherapy is the line of treatment.

Excavators are sharp double-ended hand instruments. These are used to remove carious dentin. Spoon-like cutting edges are having oval outline.

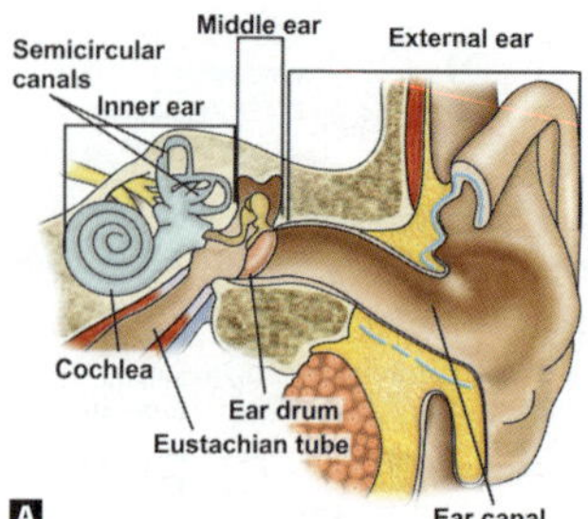

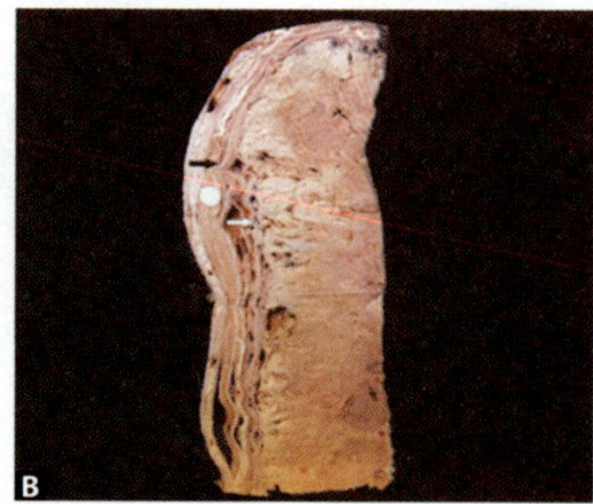

Figs A and B: *(A) Eustachian tube; (B) Ewing's sarcoma*

Excimer lasers (the name is derived from the terms excited and dimers) use reactive gases, such as chlorine and fluorine, mixed with inert gases such as argon, krypton or xenon. When electrically stimulated, a pseudomolecule (dimer) is produced. When lased, the dimer produces light in the ultraviolet range.

Excisional biopsy refers to the removal of entire lesion plus some adjacent normal tissue.

Excisional new attachment procedure (ENAP) is a technique developed by US Naval Dental Corps and is a definitive subgingival curettage procedure performed with a knife.

Excoriation is a chemical skin injury.

Excursive movement refers to any movement away from intracuspal position.

Exercise electrocardiography is done to confirm diagnosis of angina and to determine severity of limitation of activity due to angina. It is useful to evaluate response of therapy. It may also be used to screen asymptomatic population for silent coronary disease also know as stress test or treadmill test.

Exercise tests is the measure of the performance of a controlled physical task with increasing workload physical task with increasing workload to examine a person's maximal physical capacity.

Exfoliate refers to shed.

Exfoliative cytology is a type of biopsy procedure that is widely used for the diagnosis of carcinoma of uterine cervix. These days for oral cancer, cytology is done because it is quick, simple, painless and bloodless procedure. It helps to confirm false negative biopsies or where biopsy is not desirable.

Exhaustion psychosis is a condition that results from exhaustion of nervous system in older people. Insomnia, dyspepsia, anorexia, loss of physical activity irritability altered power of hearing occurs. Patient loses self-interest. Self-control and memory deteriorates. Later on mental confusion and depression occurs.

Exhumation is a lawful digging out of a buried body from the grave. It is necessary to identify the dead body or to determine the cause of death in a doubtful case. Only a magistrate can issue order for this.

Exocrine glands are the glands that secrete their products into ducts that empty onto a surface or into a cavity.

Exodontics is the science and practice of removing teeth.

Exogenous intrinsic stains refer to those stains present within the tooth substance but come from an outside source and not from within the tooth itself, such stains present themselves as exogenous intrinsic stain.

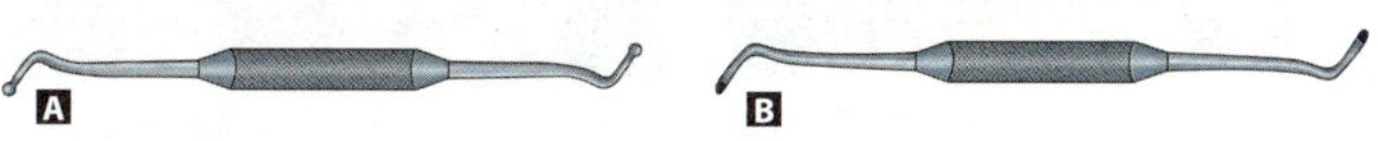

Figs A and B.: *Excavators*

E

Exogenous malodor refers to halitosis at other times of the day is often the consequence of eating various foods such as garlic, onion or spices (in curries), durian, cabbage, brussels sprouts, cauliflower, radish or habits such as smoking or drinking alcohol. Avoidance of these foods and habits is the best means of prevention.

Exostoses are the outgrowths of bone of varied size and shape. They can appear as small nodule, large nodule, sharp ridges, spike like projections or any combination of above.

Exothermic refers to heat releasing.

Exotoxins are both Gram positive and Gram negative bacteria that secrete exotoxins. Exotoxins are polypeptides. These are highly toxic. These are good antigens and induce synthesis of antitoxin useful in disease like tetanus.

Expansion appliance refers to the type of fixed or removable appliance that is used for the expansion of the constricted arch.

Experimental epidemiology refers to the study of epidemics among colonies of experimental animals such as rat/mice.

Experimental research in which at least one independent variable is subject to controlled manipulation.

Experimental study research in which officer controls the condition.

Explanatory theory refers to the one which examines the why and how questions that undergrid a problem.

Exploratory stroke is a vertical motion performed by probes and explorer to detect calculus, pocket depth, caries and the general contour of tooth surfaces.

Explorer refers to a hand instruments used to locate caries as well as hard deposits. These are available in various sizes and shapes for the variety of uses.

Exposure refers to a measure of ionization produced by radiation in air.

Exposure button is a component of dental X-ray machine control panel, activates the dental X-ray machine to produce X-rays.

Exposure light is a component of dental X-ray machine control panel providing a visible signal when X-rays are produced.

Exposure time refers to the time interval during which X-rays are produced.

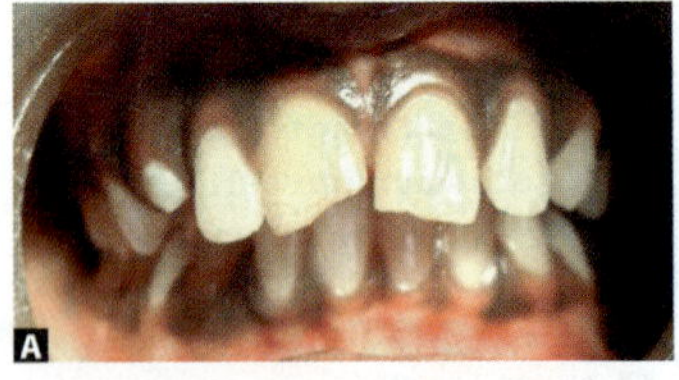

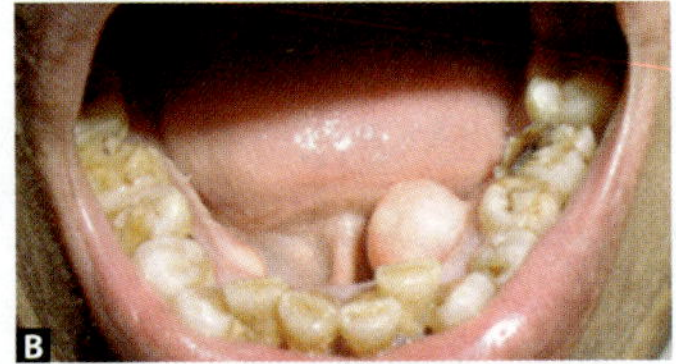

Figs A and B: *(A) Exogenous intrinsic stains due to use of obturating material; (B) Exostoses*

Expressed consent refers to the permission given in written or verbal form.

Extended shank curettes are the modification of standard Gracey curettes. The terminal shank is 3 mm longer which allows the deeper penetration into deep periodontal pockets. The blades are also comparatively smoother and thinner to allow easy subgingival insertion.

External acoustic meatus is a tube passing medially from the bottom of the concha of the auricle. It is closed medially by the tympanic membrane. The total length of the tube is approximately 24 mm. Of this, the wall of the outer 8 mm is cartilaginous, while that of the inner 16 mm is bony.

External ear is formed together with the auricle and external acoustic meatus.

External jugular vein is formed by union of the posterior division of the retromandibular vein with the posterior auricular vein. The origin lies within the lower part of the parotid gland or just below it. The level corresponds to the angle of the mandible.

External nares are the external openings of the nasal cavities and are on the inferior aspect of the nose. They are bounded laterally by the alae nasi and medially by the lowest part of the nasal septum.

External pin fixation is a method of achieving immobilization where extensive communication of the whole or the large part of mandible is required. The stainless steel or the titanium pins are inserted into each major bone fragment which diverge from each other but are connected by a cross bar which are attached to each pin by the mean of universal joints. They are mainly

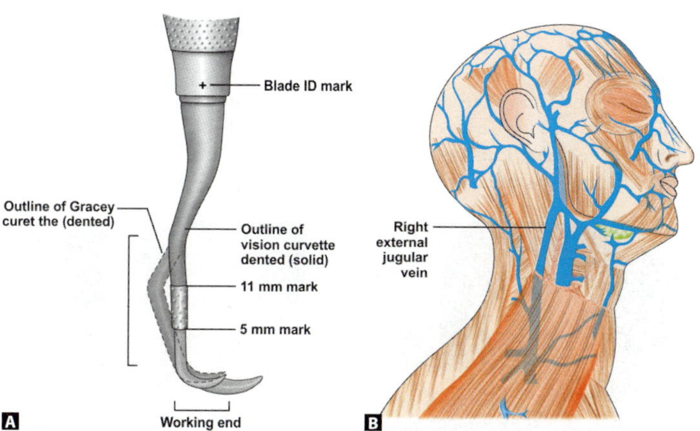

Figs A and B: *(A) Dental explorer; (B) External jugular vein*

indicated for infected fracture line, for extensively comminuted fractures and for the treatment for bimaxillary fractures.

External root resorption is a condition associated with either physiologic or a pathologic process that results in loss of substance from a tissue-like dentin, cementum or alveolar bone. In external root resorption, root resorption affect the cementum or dentin of the root. It can be—Apical root resorption, lateral root resorption and cervical root resorption.

Exteroceptors are the pain receptors which are stimulated by the immediate external environment; with most of the impulses being sensed at conscious level, e.g., free nerve ending – tactile and superficial pain. Krause's corpuscles are cold receptor, Meissner's corpuscles are tactile skin receptors. Merkel's corpuscles are tactile receptor in the oral mucosa and submucosa of the tongue. Ruffini's corpuscles are pressure and warmth receptors.

Extirpation refers to complete removal or eradication of pulp from the pulp chamber or root.

Extraoral film refers to type of dental X-ray film that is placed outside the mouth during X-ray exposure. These are used to examine large areas of skull or jaws.

Extrachromosomal are the structures that are not part of chromosomes. DNA units in the cytoplasm control cytoplasmic inheritance.

Extraction elevators are lever like instrument used for luxation of a tooth from its socket.

Extraoral refers to outside the mouth.

Extrapyramidal system is a neural network that takes care of the involuntary movements and coordination. Movement and posture disturbances resulting from disorders of basal ganglia and cerebellum. It includes ataxia, athetosis, dysarthria, dystonia and muscle rigidity and spasticity.

Extrusion is a term given to migration of teeth in an incisal or occlusal direction.

Exudates is the accumulation of material in a body cavity or on a body surface.

Eye strain headache refers to uncontrolled visual refractive error is present. Pain is relieved by proper spectacles.

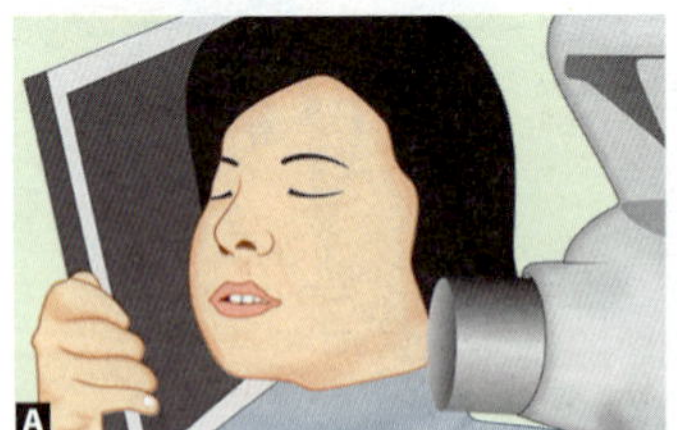

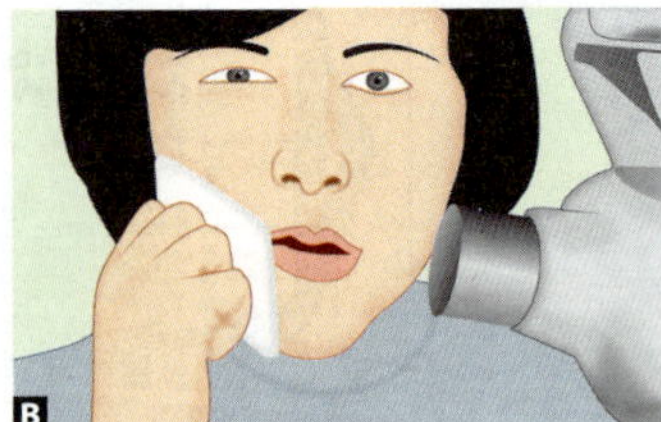

Figs A and B: *Extraoral films and radiography*

Fabricated wounds refer to those types of wounds that are produced by a person on his body or by another person with his consent. These are called fictitious, forged or inverted wounds. Intention of these is to charge enemy with assault or attempted murder. Woman may inflict on her reproductive organs to bring a charge of rape.

Facemask is the disposable or non-disposable item designed to protect the face from microorganisms. Although these masks are permeable to microorganisms, mask should ideally have at least 95% infiltration efficiency for particles 3 to 5 micromillimeter and should be changed for each patient. When dealing with TB, patient mask with greater filtration capacity should be worn.

Facial hemiatrophy is a progressive atrophy of some or all tissues on one side of face. Exact cause is not known but it may be due to atrophic function of cervical sympathetic nervous system, trauma and hereditary. There may be hollowing of cheek and eyes may be depressed. Loss of facial hair is common. Hemiatrophy of lips and tongue is also reported.

Facial hemihypertrophy is a rare congenital anomaly where there is a unilateral over-development of the affected part of the face. The defect is apparent at birth and becomes obvious with advancing age. Also known as hemifacial hypertrophy or congenital hemifacial hyperplasia exact etiology is not known but may be due to hormonal imbalance, incomplete turning and chromosomal abnormality. Familial occurrence has been reported in a few cases. Dentition of hypertrophic side is abnormal in regard to crown and root size and rate of development. On the developed side permanent teeth erupt before their counterpart. Tongue may be enlarged.

Facial nerve (VII cranial nerve) arises from the pons, passes through the facial canal and exits from the skull through stylomastoid foramina. It then passes through the parotid gland and subsequently divides into branches. It provides motor innervation to all muscles of the facial ex-

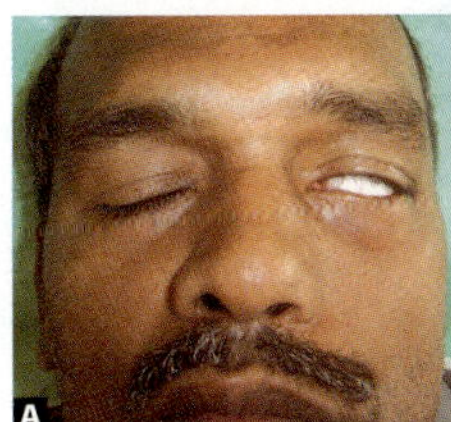

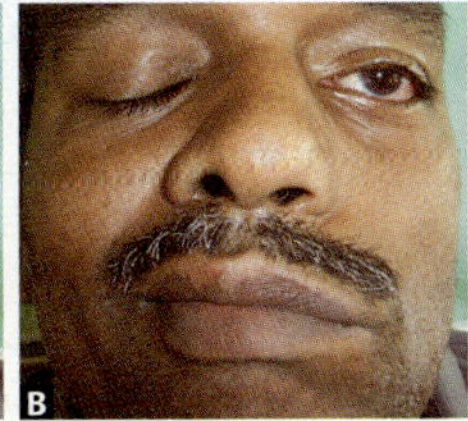

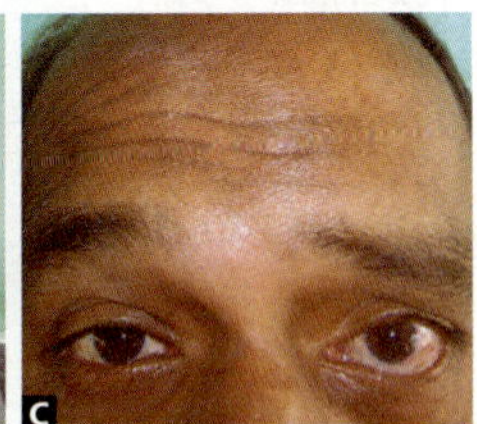

Figs A to C: *Facial neuritis*

pression and the stapedius. Through its branch, the chorda tympani, it carries taste sensation from the anterior two-thirds of the tongue. It also carries cutaneous impulses from the anterior wall of the external auditory canal. Motor root supplies muscles of face, scalp and auricle.

Facial neuritis (Bell's palsy) results from the inflammation of facial nerve. Location is usually but not necessarily within facial canal. Taste aberration may also be seen. Angioneurotic edema may also put pressure on the nerve in facial canal to cause pain.

Facial pain may occur due to maxillary sinusitis, neoplasia of maxilla, caries, dental abscess, atypical facial neuralgia, trigeminal etc. Pain provoked by cold and hot is of dental origin.

Facial refers to the surface next to the face; the outer surface of a tooth resting against the cheeks or lips.

Facial vein is a continuation of the angular vein and is commonly known as anterior vein of the face that begins near the medial angle of the eye by the union of two superficial veins of the forehead, i.e. supratrochlear and supraorbital

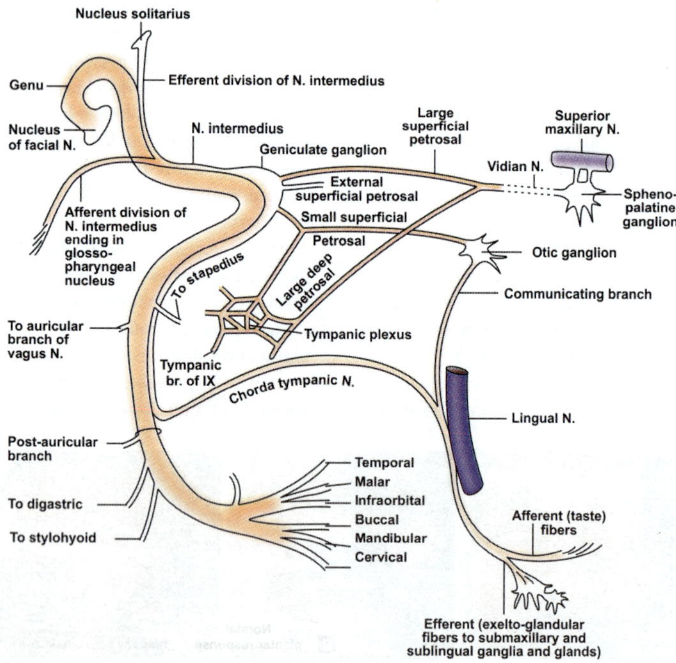

Fig.: *Facial nerve*

veins. The vein run downwards and backwards across the face and terminate by joining the anterior branch of the retromandibular vein to form the common facial vein that ends in the internal jugular vein.

Factor analysis is a multivariate correlational technique used to reduce a large number of variables into a smaller number of factors clustering related variables.

Facultative anaerobes are the organisms that can grow in the presence or absence of oxygen, e.g. *Staphylococcus*. Microaerophilic grow in an oxygen environment but derive their energy only from fermentative pathways that occur in absence of oxygen, e.g. *Streptococcus*, etc.

Fainting is actually a loss of consciousness caused by reduced blood supply to the brain. It is known as syncope too. In most of the dental patients, cause is psychological or due to fear of bleeding and pain.

False denticles refer to the pulp stone that are laid as concentric layers of calcified tissue. These appear within bundles of collagen fibers. They may arise around vessels. Calcification of thrombi in blood vessels called phleboliths, may also serve as nidi for false denticles. All denticles begin as small nodules but increase in size by incremental growth on their surface.

Familial fibromatosis is a kind of enlargement generally characterized by slowly progressive, non-hemorrhagic enlargement of the maxillary and mandibular gingiva or may be localized to either jaw. Enlargement may be bilateral, thus the name, symmetrical gingival fibromatosis has been suggested by Wiktop, 1971, but since, the enlargement is not always symmetrical, the name was given a focal gingival fibromatosis. Gingiva are grossly enlarged and pink color, firm, lathery in consistency and a minutely rebelled surface. Secondary inflammatory changes may be present.

Fan sign is a component of Babinski's reflex. This sign refers to the spreading apart of patient's toes after his foot is firmly stroked.

Fastidious bacterium is a bacterium that is difficult to isolate or grow in the laboratory owing to its complex nutritional requirement.

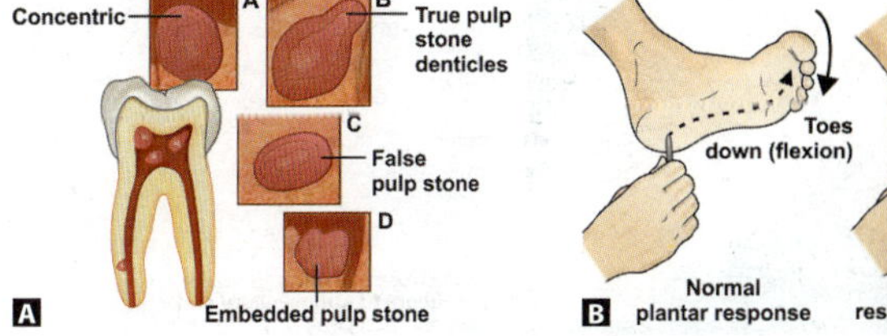

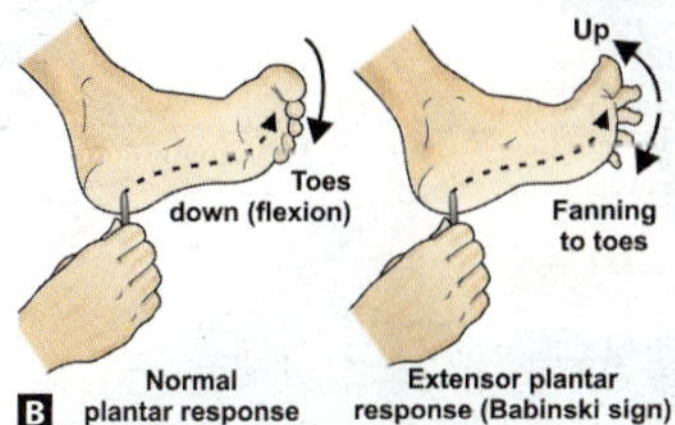

Figs A and B: *(A) False denticles; (B) Fan sign*

Fat soluble vitamins are not excreted when consumed in excess; rather these are stored in liver and adipose tissue. These can be toxic when consumed in large doses over a long time specially vitamin A and vitamin D. Deficiency of fat-soluble vitamins occurs in malabsorption syndromes, pancreatic and biliary diseases. Fat-soluble vitamins include vitamin A, D, E and K.

Fatal dose of snake venom—12 mg of dried Cobra venom and 15 mg of Daboi venom is fatal for human being. Average dry weight of lyophilized venom in one bite was 0.2 gm from a cobra, 0.15 gm from a russel viper, 0.022 gm from krait and 0.0046 gm from echis carinatus.

Fatigue is defined as transient loss of sensorium due to decreased cerebral blood flow. There is generally a spontaneous recovery.

Fats contain carbon, hydrogen and oxygen padding around the organs and keep them in place. It protects nerve. Fat insulates body avoiding rapid change of body temperature. It carries vitamins A, D, E and K. Fats are concentrated source of calories each gram giving 9 calories.

Fatty acids are of two types. Saturated fatty acids are palmitic acid, stearic acid and cholic acid. While unsaturated fatty acids are oleic acid, linoleic acid, linolenic acid and arachidonic acid. Saturated fatty acids are harmful to heart.

Fatty liver is a mild injury due to changes in metabolic activity of hepatocytes. It is seen more on occasional drinking. Liver is enlarged, pale or yellowish in color. Microscopically central and mid zones are involved more. Variable fatty change of hepatocytes gives vacuolated appearance.

Favorable fractures are the one where the vertical fracture or the horizontal fracture lines are unopposed by the action of the muscle around them. However, these types of fractures are easier to reduce and stabilize.

F-distribution is a distribution of squared t statistics, the basis of analysis of variance.

Febrile refers to pertaining to fever.

Febrile seizure refers to the type of seizure, those occurring after the

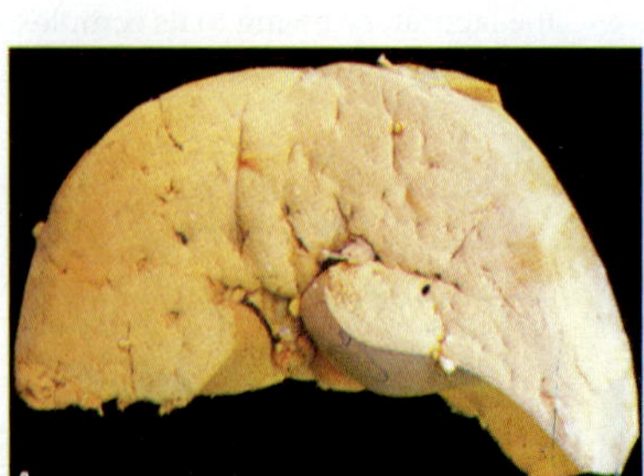

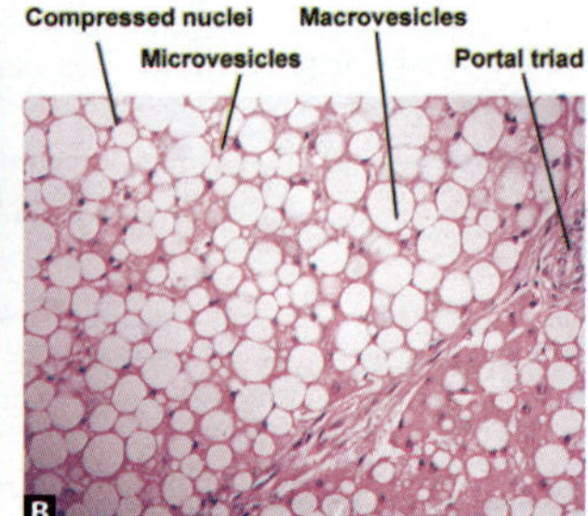

Fig.: *Macroscopic and microscopic presentation of fatty liver*

age of one month these are associated with a febrile illness not caused by CNS infection. These occur without previous unprovoked or neonatal seizures. These may be generalized or partial.

Feeble mindedness refers to those kind of people who are better than imbecile but are still incapable of protecting themselves, hence require care and supervision. They don't show any physical defect. They are frequently impulsive as regards sexual acts, murders and assaults.

Female ejaculation is not a correct term used for secretion of lubricating fluid by glands adjacent to vagina during sexual stimulation. As sexual stimulation and excitement build up the flow of lubricating fluid increases. In certain cases sudden contraction of vaginal wall causes fluid to spurt which is commonly mistaken as female discharge.

Fenestration can be described as the isolated areas in which the root is denuded of bone and the root surface is only covered by periosteum and overlying gingiva along with the intact marginal bone.

Fergusson gag is an adjustable prop used to force open the mouth and keep the jaws apart.

Fermentation refers to an anaerobic biochemical pathway in which substances are broken down and energy and reduced compounds are produced. Such as procedures like making curd out of milk. Here microorganisms multiply with great rapidity. Enzymes act in the starch present producing carbon dioxide. The oxygen does not participate in the process.

Festinating gait is a type of gait that is peculiar to Parkinsonism. Arms are flexed in front of the body. Legs are stiff and bent at hips and knees. Steps are short and shuffling. The upper part of body advances ahead of lower part. Patient can run better than walking.

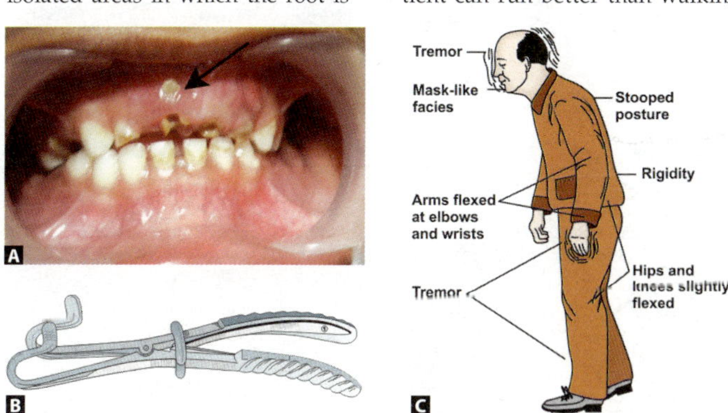

Figs A to C: *(A) Fenestration; (B) Fergusson gag; (C) Festinating gait seen in Parkinsonism*

Patient bends forwards and advances with rapid, short and shuffling gait. Arms don't swing. When pulled, he may walk backwards.

Fetishism is a psychosexual disorder in which sexual gratification is repeatedly or exclusively achieved through fondling, kissing or licking inanimate objects such as women's bra, hair, undergarments etc. Handling these objects is often accompanied by sexual fantasies and masturbation.

Fever hypoplasia refers to a linear alteration of enamel that may be manifested as the result of a febrile episode during the chronological point in tooth development such that the distribution of enamel changes will vary between teeth at different stages of crown formation. Some studies have indicated that the exanthematous diseases, including measles, chicken pox and scarlet fever are etiological factors. In general, it might be stated that any systemic disease is potentially capable of producing enamel hypoplasia, since the ameloblasts are one of the most sensitive groups of cells in the body in terms of metabolic function. The type of hypoplasia occurring from these disease states is usually of the pitting variety. Clinical studies indicate that most cases of enamel hypoplasia involve those teeth that form within the first year after birth.

Fiber refers to the thread-like structure. The walls of every cell are composed of Fiber. It is more abundant on outer sides of seeds, fruits, peas and beans. Daily requirement of Fiber is 6 gram.

Fiberfill is a new methacrylate resin-based endodontic sealer.

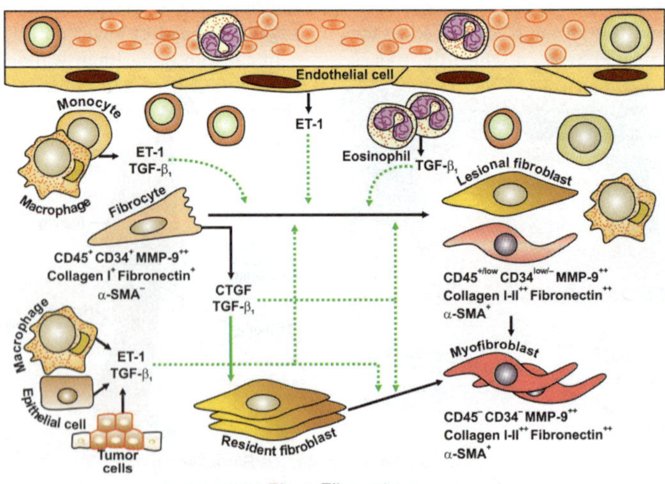

Fig.: *Fibrocytes*

Fiberfill root canal sealant is used in combination with a self-curing primer (Fiberfill primers A and B). Its composition resembles to that of dentin bonding agents.

Fiber reinforced denture base material is a material used for fabricating dentures. It has high stiffness, very good impact strength and good fatigue life. It gives good surface finish. Disadvantage is of poor color and poor surface.

Fiber optic transillumination (FOTI) is an advanced diagnostic aid that has been designed for the detection of approximal caries by Freidman and Marcus in 1970. The principle of transillumination is that there is a different index of light transmission for decayed and sound tooth structure. Illumination is delivered by means of Fiber optics from the light source to the tooth structure. The resultant changes in light distribution as the light traverses the tooth are then recorded as an image for analysis. Since tooth decay has a lower index of light transmission than the sound tooth structure, an area of decay shows up as a darkened shadow that follows the decay along the path of dentinal tubules.

Fibrin is the main fibrous protein in a blood clot.

Fibrinolytic system is activated by Hageman factor which causes activation of plasminogen. This results in release of fibrinopeptides and fibrin degradation products which cause increase in vascular permeability and leukocytic chemotaxis.

Fibrocytes are the mature form of fibroblasts. Their quantity increases with maturity of the pulp and their primary function is the maintenance of collagen Fibers.

Fibroadenoma breast is a common benign neoplasm of younger age. It is a round or ovoid rubbery, discrete, movable nontender mass 1-5 cm in diameter. It does not occur after menopause. Excision helps.

Fibroma is the most common benign soft tissue neoplasm. It is an elevated lesion of normal color. It is well-circumscribed, smooth and pedunculated about 1-2 cm in diameter. It may be firm and nodular and might be soft in

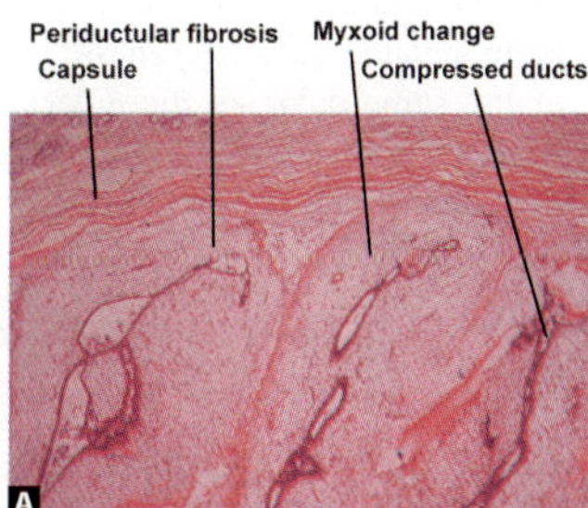

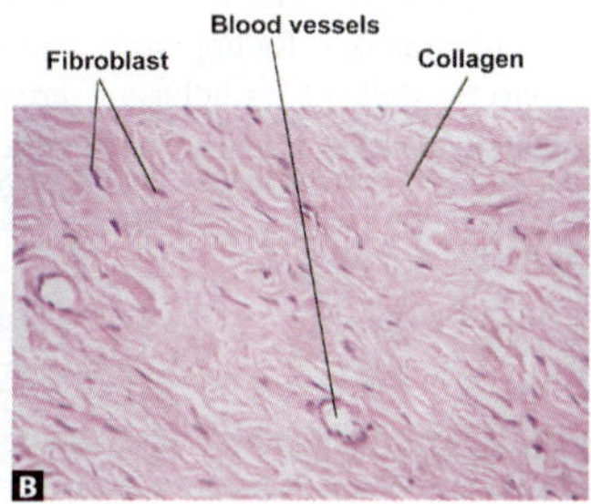

Figs A and B: *(A) Fibroadenoma breast; (B) Fibroma*

nature, when infected superficial ulceration may be seen. Soft fibromas are spongy otherwise may be hard fibroma. Conservative surgical excision may help.

Fibromatosis gingiva is a diffuse fibrous overgrowth of gingival tissues. It is dense, diffuse, smooth or nodular overgrowth of gingival. Tissues are not inflamed. As there is no inflammation, hemorrhage takes place. Crowns of teeth look hidden. It may require surgical correction due to cosmetic purpose.

Fibromyalgia affects about 2% adults and is a condition causing increased sensitivity to pain in many parts of body. These are especially sensitive to touch and pressure. Other symptoms include fatigue, sleep disturbance, stiffness depression and anxiety.

Fibrosarcoma develops from fibroblast cells. *Clinical features:* It commonly arises from cheek, tongue, gingival and floor of mouth. Among the jaw lesions, mandible is most commonly involved. To start, it is asymptomatic. Soon it enlarges into a large, painful fleshy mass. Lesion is firm and indurated. These are not capsulated tumors. Radiographs show sharply defined radiolucent area. Radical surgery chemotherapy is the treatment of choice.

Fibrosseous integration can be described as relationship between endosseous implants and bone in which soft tissue such as fibers or the cells are interposed between the two surfaces.

Fibrotic pocket wall is said to have occurred where there is relative predominance of newly formed connective tissue cells and fibers and the pocket wall is more firm and pink.

Fibrous dysplasia is a lesion of bone developed as a result of abnormal proliferation of fibrous tissue. As lesion matures, it destroys trabaculae. Radiographs in early stage will show radiolucent lesion. Intermediate lesion will be smoky, mottled or hazy pattern. Intense aggregations will be distributed throughout lesion. In mature stage, picture will be of salt and pepper type, ground glass or orange peel appearance. It may result in irregularity of bone without pain. There may also be malocclusion.

Fibrous epulis is a pain-free swelling on the gum. There is a firm, pedunculated or sessile mass. It is of the same color as the adjacent

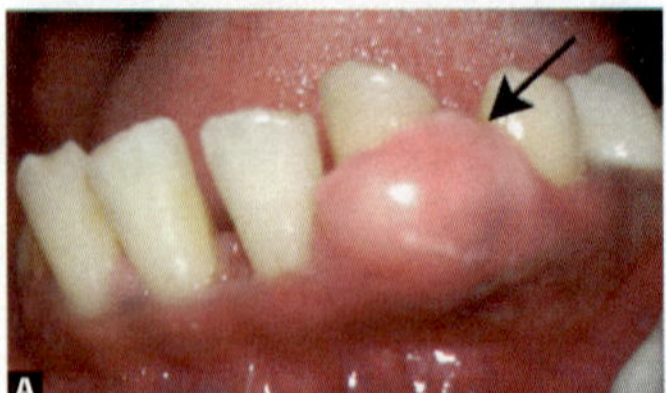

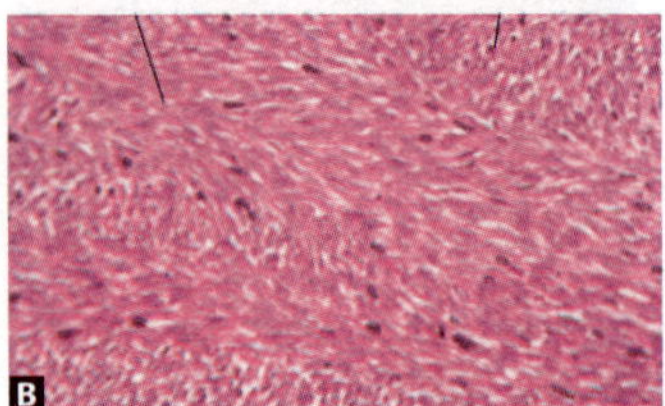

Figs A and B: *(A) Fibromatosis gingivae; (B) Fibrosarcoma*

gingiva. Biopsy confirms the diagnosis.

Fibrous gingival hyperplasia refers to gingival enlargement where often single papilla or several papillae will be enlarged. Sometimes inflammatory changes are superimposed on the fibrous hyperplasia. Chronic low-grade irritation of gingival tissue can result in localized hyperplasia of fibrous tissue. Treatment includes removal of local irritation.

Fibrous hyperplasia is the commonest tissue reaction to chronically-ill fitting denture. There is development of elongated rolls of tissue in the mucobuccal fold. It is slow in development. Inflammatory fibrous hyperplasia is to be surgically excised.

Fibrous nodule refer Fibroma.

Field block is a method of obtaining anesthesia by injecting the anesthetic agent solution close to large terminal nerve branches. More circumscribed, most often involving one tooth and the tissues surrounding it.

Fifth branchial arch refers to the fifth arch which is a transitory structure that disappears, almost as soon as it forms and bequeaths no permanent structural elements.

Fifth pharyngeal pouch appears as a diverticulum of the fourth pouch. The endoderm of the fifth pouch forms the ultimobranchial body. The calcitonin secreting cells of this structure, however, are derived from neural crest tissue and are eventually incorporated into the thyroid gland. The laryngeal ventricles could present the remnants of fifth pharyngeal pouch.

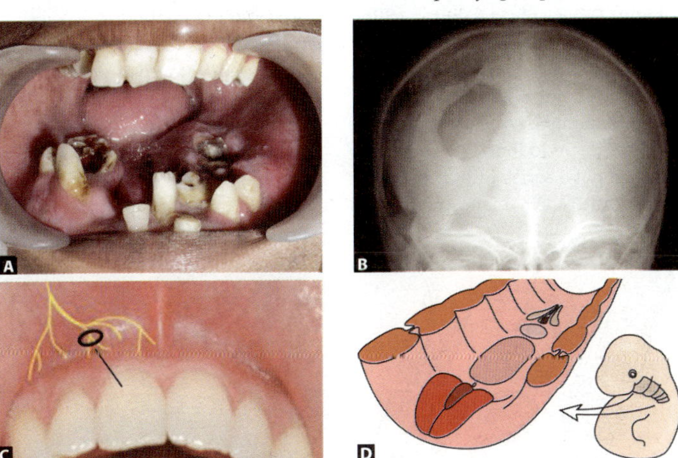

Figs A to D: *(A) Intraoral view of fibrous dysplasia showing displacement of teeth causing malocclusion; (B) Radiograph showing polyostotic lesions of fibrous dysplasia of skull; (C) Field block; (D) Fifth pharyngeal arch and pouch*

Figure eight suture is also a type of interdental ligation where the suture given is in the shape of eight hence the name and is indicated the two flaps are not in close apposition to each other.

Filament circuit is the circuit that regulates the flow of electric current to the filament of X-ray tube.

Filariasis is caused by two species *Wuchereria bancrofti* and Brugia malayi. Microfilariae mature in lymph nodes and rarely produce visible damage. Lymphadenopathy is characteristic but not diagnostic. Scrotal swelling is due to *Wuchereria bancrofti*. Allergic manifestations are due to toxic metabolites released by worm. Incubation period is one year. Acute stage shows fever with inflammation of lymphatic vessels and swelling of affecting part of body. Fever subsides but swelling persists. In chronic stage typical elephantiasis develops. Swollen part becomes thick and rugose/papillomatous.

Files are periodontal instruments which have series of blades on the base and their main purpose is to fracture or crush the tenacious calculus. As files can gouge easily and roughen the root surface if used improperly, therefore, these are not the ideal instruments for fine scaling.

Filing: The term filing indicates push-pull motion of an instrument. This method is commonly used for canal preparation. But this active insertion of instrument with cutting force is a combination of both resistance to bend and apically directed hand pressure. This may lead to canal ledging, perforation and other procedural errors.

Filling refers to a restoration placed on a tooth to restore its function and appearance.

Film badge is a device to measure and monitor radiation exposure worn by persons frequently exposed to radiation.

Film hanger is a stainless steel device equipped with clips used to hold films during manual processing.

Film mount refers to a cardboard, plastic or vinyl holder used to support and arrange dental radiographs in anatomic order.

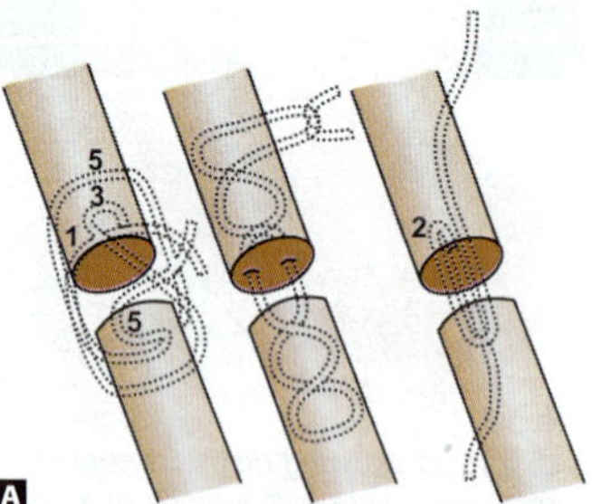

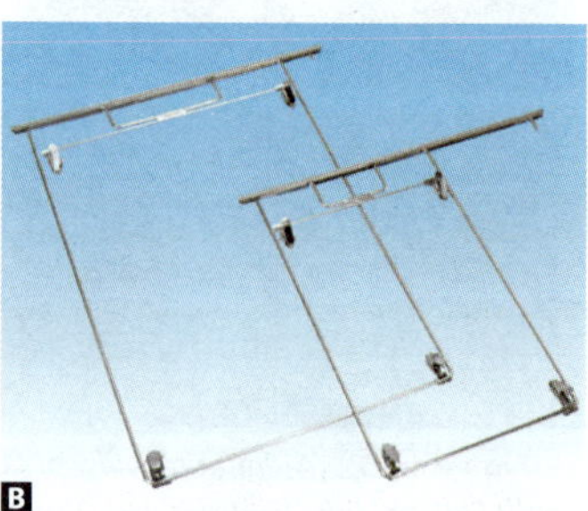

Figs A and B: *(A) Figure eight suturing; (B) Film hanger*

Film overexposed is an exposure error resulting in dark film due to excessive exposure to X-ray time, kilovoltage or milliamperage or a combination of these.

Film speed is the sensitivity of film to radiation exposure.

Final diagnosis is a diagnosis-based on clinical laboratory data.

Fine needle aspiration cytology (FNAC) is a convenient and expeditious means of differentiating cyst from solid tumors and getting cytological specimen. It is performed with a 21-gauge needle fitted to a 10 mL syringe.

Fine particle composite resins contain fine sized filler particles of 0.5 to 3 micro mm. It is more polishable than micro-filled composites.

Finger nail artifact is a film handling error, a black fingerprint when the film has been touched by fingers contaminated with developer.

Finger pluggers is a finger instrument that is used for vertical compaction of gutta-percha. They apply controlled pressure while compaction, and have more tactile sensitivity than hand plugger. Care should be taken with spreaders and pluggers while compacting the gutta-percha in canals. They should be cleaned prior to their insertion into the canal; otherwise the set sealer from previous insertion may roughen their surface and may pull the cone outside the canal rather than packing it. Also one should discard the instrument when it has become bent or screwed to avoid instrument separation while compaction.

Fingerprints and ridges: The surface of the palms, fingers, soles, and toes are marked by series of ridges and grooves. They appear either as straight lines or as a pattern or loops and whorls, as on the tips of the digits. These epidermal ridges develop during the third and fourth fetal months as the epidermis conforms to the contours of the underlying dermal papillae of the papillary region. The ridges increase the surface area of the epidermis and thus function to increase the grip of the hand or foot by increasing friction. Because the ducts of sweat pores, the sweat and ridges from

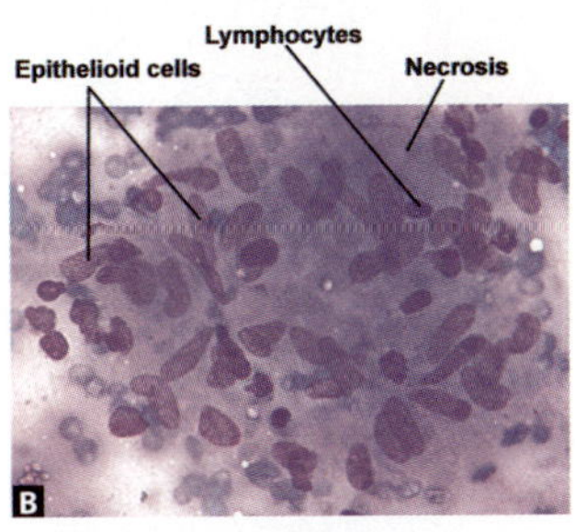

Figs A and B: *Fine needle aspiration cytology (FNAC)*

fingerprints (or footprints) when a smooth object is touched. The ridge pattern is genetically determined and is unique for each individual. Normally, the ridge pattern does not change during life, except to enlarge, and thus can serve as the basis for identification through fingerprints or footprints. Comparisons of the structural features of the papillary and reticular region of the dermis.

Finger rest stabilizes the hand and the instrument by providing a firm fulcrum as movements are made to activate the instrument, this helps in preventing injury and laceration to the gingiva occurring due to poorly controlled movements. The fourth/ring finger is most commonly used as rest. The finger rest is of two types: the intraoral rest and the extraoral rest.

Finger sweep is an insertion of index finger into mouth along the inside of the check and deep into throat to the base of the tongue.

Finger-on-finger rest is established on the index finger or thumb of the nonoperating hand.

Finishing disks are small abrasive disks of sand paper used to contour and polish various restorations.

First appraisal the first dental appointment is very important and can set the stage for subsequent appointment. By scheduling the patient early in the day and by allowing sufficient time to talk with the parents and the patient before initiating any dental care, a practitioner can establish a good relationship with them. It is necessary to make appointments short and stress free for patients having poor stress tolerance and easy fatigability.

First branchial arch is the first mandibular pair of branchial arches is the precursor of the jaws, both maxillary and mandibular and appropriately bound the lateral aspects of the stomodeum which, at this stage, is merely a depression in the early facial region. The maxilla is derived from a small maxillary prominence extending cranioventrally from the much larger mandibular prominence

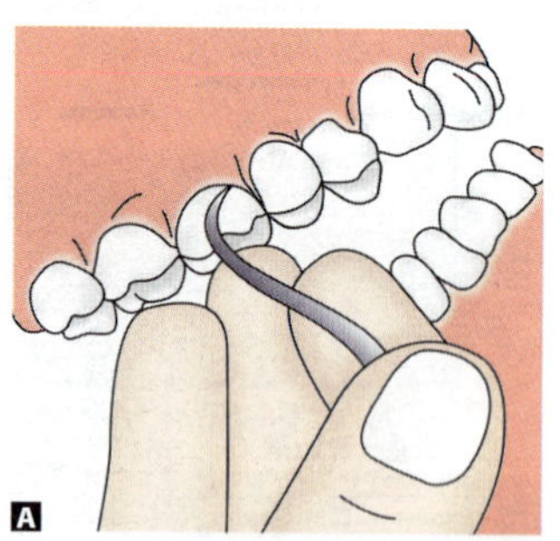

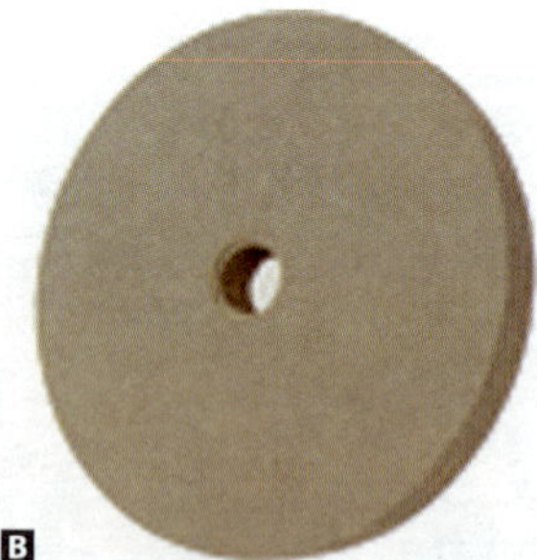

Figs A and B: *(A) Finger rest; (B) Finishing disk*

derived from the first arch. The cartilage skeleton of the first arch known as Meckel's cartilage, which arises at the 41st to 45th day providing a template for subsequent development of the mandible but most of its cartilage substance disappears in the formed mandible. The mental ossicler is the only potion of the mandible derived from market cartilage by endochondral ossification. Persisting portions of Meckel's cartilage from the basis of major portions of two ear ossicles, the head and neck of the malleus and the body and short crus of the incus and two ligaments. The anterior ligament of the malleus, sphenomandibular ligament. The musculature of the mandibular arch subdivided and migrates to form: The muscles of mastication, mylohyoid muscle, anterior belly of the digastric, Tensor tympani, tensor veli palatini muscles all of which are innervated by the nerve of the first arch, i.e. the mandibular division of the 5th cranial or trigeminal nerve.

First degree burns are limited only to the most superficial layers of epidermis and heal spontaneously within 7 days because of abundance of epithelial cells which regenerate very fast. So this healing is by regeneration only and does not leave any scars.

First pharyngeal pouch: The ventral portion of this pouch is obliterated by the developing tongue. The dorsal diverticulum deepens laterally as the tubotympanic recess to form the auditory tube, widening at its end into the tympanum or middle ear cavity separated from the first branchial groove by the tympanic membrane. The tympanium occupied by the dorsal ends of the cartilages of the first and second branchial arches develop into the ear ossicles. The tympanum maintains contact with the pharynx via the auditory tube throughout life. The proximal portion of the expanding and elongating auditory tube becomes lined with respiratory mucous membrane and fibrous tissue and cartilage form in its walls. Chondrification occurs in the 4th month of influence. From four centres in the adjacent mesoderm growth of the cartilaginous portion of the tube is greatest between 16 and 28 weeks intrauterine. These, after increase in tubal length, is primarily in the osseous portion of the tube. The

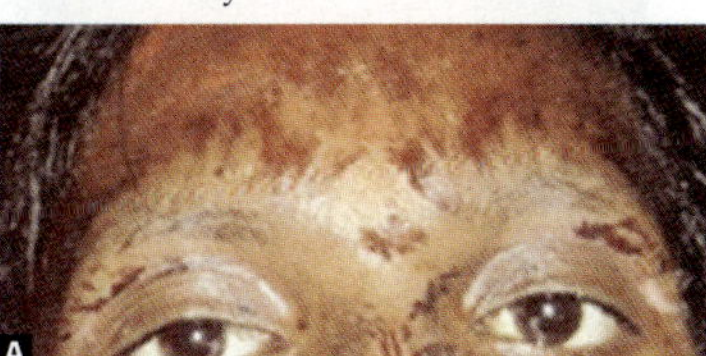

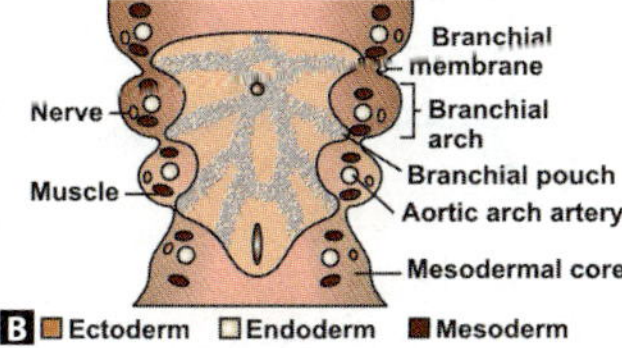

Figs A and B: *(A) First-degree burn; (B) Branchial arch and pouch*

changing location of the opening of the auditory tube reflects the growth of the nasopharynx. The tubal orifice is inferior to the hard palate in the fetus, is in level with it at birth, and well above the hard palate in the adult.

First transitional period is characterized by the emergence of the first permanent molars and the exchange of the deciduous incisors with the permanent incisors.

Fissure refers to deep clefts between adjoining cusps. They provide area for retention of caries producing agents. These defects occur on occlusal surfaces of the molars and premolars, with tortuous configuration that are difficult to assess from the surfaces. These areas are impossible to keep clean and highly susceptible to advancement of the carious lesion (Orbans, 1990).

Fissure sealant is a material that is placed in the pits and fissures of teeth in order to prevent or arrest the development of dental caries. These are defined whereby pits and fissures that occur principally on the occlusal surfaces of the molar and premolar teeth are occluded by application of fluid materials, which are then polymerized. (Bali RK, Batra R, Tandon S, (2001).

Fissure sealing is a procedure done to seal the occlusal fissures. Occlusal fissures are natural stagnation areas where caries occurs. In the past fissure filling was done using amalgam. In it one has to cut a cavity in sound enamel. But new glass ionomer cement allows fissure sealing to be done without any cavity preparation.

Fissured tongue *see* scrotal tongue.

Fistula refers to an abnormal passage formed in the gum tissue through which an abscessed tooth drains.

Fixation of film is a procedure done to fix a film, i.e. when fixer solution removes the unexposed underdeveloped silver halide crystals from the film emulsion.

Fixed drug eruption is the lesion which appears in same site each time a drug is taken. Reaction subsides when the drug is discontinued. Reaction causes vasculitis and subsequent damage to the vessel wall giving rise to erythema and edema of superficial layers of skin and mucosa.

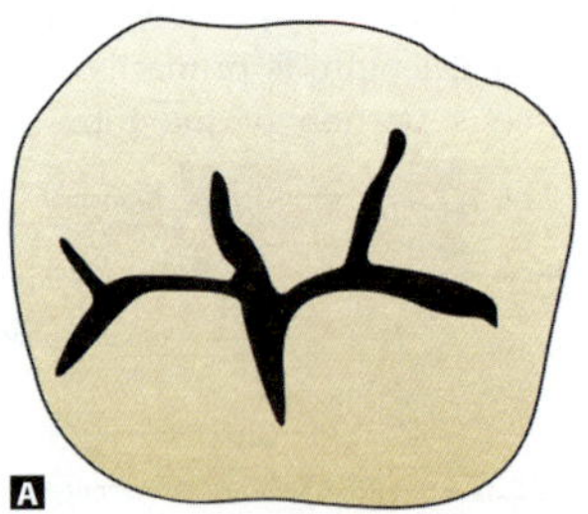

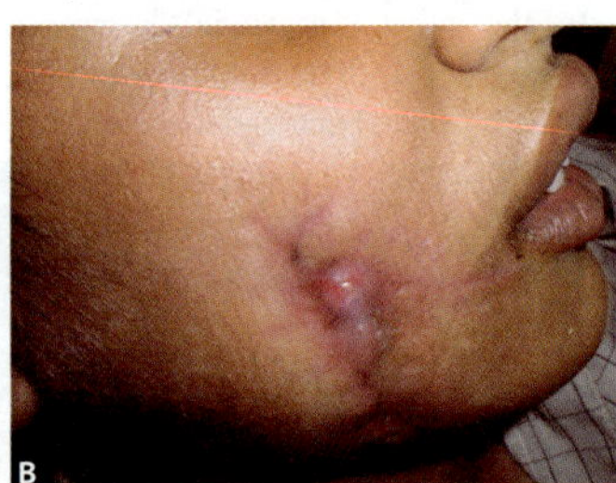

Figs A and B: *(A) Fissure; (B) Parotid fistula*

Fixed functional appliances are those appliances that are fitted on the teeth by the operator and cannot be removed by the patients.

Fixed habit breakers are the fixed appliance that helps in breaking the deleterious habit of the child. Heavy gauge stainless steel wires are designed to form a frame that is soldered to bands on the molars.

Fixers spots refer to a chemical contamination error white spots appear on film as a result of fixer solution contacting the film before processing.

Flap surgery is a procedure used for deep periodontal pockets to remove the diseased lining of the periodontal pocket and the marginal gingiva.

Flare-up is described as the occurrence of pain, swelling or the combination of these during the course of root canal therapy, which results in unscheduled visits by patient. Pain may occur soon after initiating endodontic treatment for an asymptomatic tooth or shortly after the initial emergency treatment or during the course of treatment. American Association of Endodontics (AAE) defines a flare-up "as an acute exacerbation of periradicular pathosis after initiation or in continuation of root canal treatment."

Flash refers to the excess material that extrudes beyond the intended margins of a restoration.

Flat foot in the young child the foot appears to be flat because of the pressure of a large amount of subcutaneous fat on the sole. Otherwise medial margin of foot from heal to the first metatarsal head is arched above the ground because of medial longitudinal arch. Medial longitudinal arch consists of calcaneum, the talus navicular bone and three cuneiform bones and the first three metatarsal. Flat foot person is not able to run fast and for long.

Flatus is a gas which is formed in the intestine and released from rectum.

Flexo file is similar to the K-flex file except that it has triangular cross-section. This feature provides more flexibility and thus ability to resist fracture.

Flexogates are modified Gates-Glid-dens. They are made up of NiTi

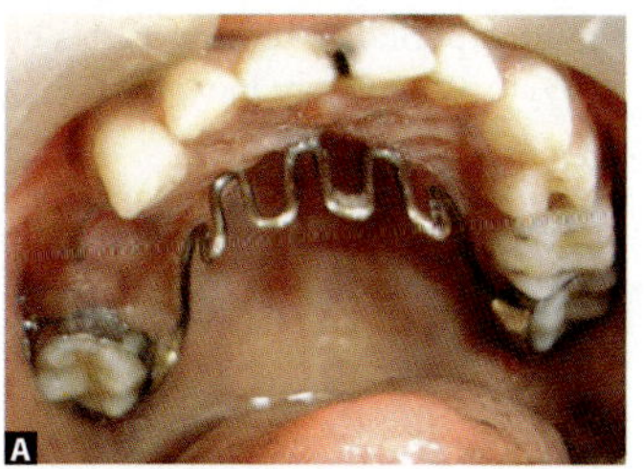

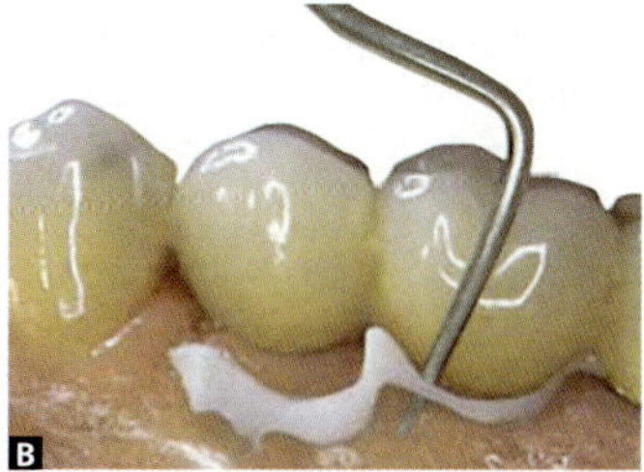

Figs A and B: *(A) Fixed habit breaking appliance with palatal crib; (B) Flash*

and have noncutting tip. They are more flexible and used for apical preparation. Flexogates can be rotated continuously in a handpiece through 360°. These instruments have many advantages over the traditional instruments in that they allow increased debris removal because of continuous rotation, smoother and faster canal preparation with less clinician fatigue.

F

Flex-R-file is made by removing the sharp cutting edges from the tip of instrument. The noncutting tip enables the instrument to traverse along the canal rather than gouge into it. This design reduces the ledge formation, canal transportation and other procedural accidents when used with balanced force technique. Another feature of flex-R file is presence of triangular cross-section which provides it flexibility to be used in curved canals. It is made up of NiTi and cuts during anticlockwise rotary motion.

Florescence refers to emit visible light in the blue or green spectrum.

Florid osseous dysplasia is a disease of disordered cementum and bone development. Radiopaque masses may involve multiple quadrants. Cause is not known. No treatment is indicated.

Floss refers to a thread/tape goes in between teeth for cleaning.

Flow is a plastic deformation that occurs while the material is setting and in the process of developing its final strength.

Fluorescence is the emission of light by an object at different wavelengths. Dental porcelains are also fluorescent under ultraviolet light.

Fluorescence microscopy is used in immunology. It employs the principles of emission of a different wavelength of light of one wavelength strikes a fluorescent object.

Fluoride refers to topical application of a gel or liquid that prevents decay.

Fluoride electrode coupled with standard pH meter is the most recent and universally acceptable fluoride estimation method. Fluoride electrodes with difference make such as Orion (Model 94-09). Radiometers (Model F 1052 F fluoride electrode) are available. This method allows fluoride in aqueous solutions to be measured quickly simply, economically and accurately.

Fluoride mouth rinse is done weekly rather than monthly, some recommended on daily basis for limited period. It reduces caries by 20% to 30% and are inexpensive.

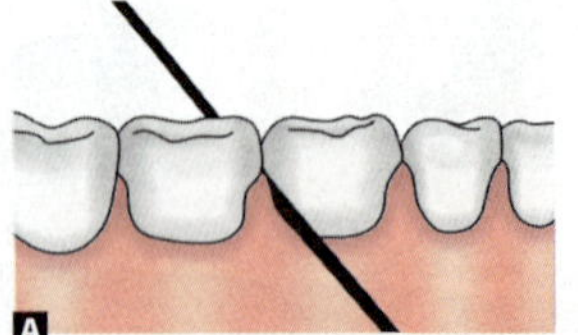

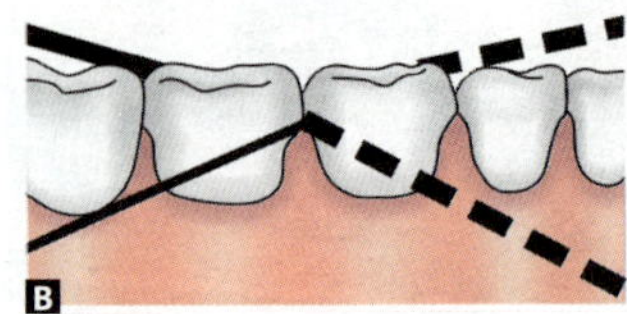

Figs A and B.: *Flossing technique*

Fluoride probe is a computerized periodontal probe consisting of a probe, handpiece, a digital readout, a foot switch and a computer. It is used to measure the pocket depth and has a high degree of accuracy.

Fluoride tablets are effective means of fluoridation that act both systematically and topically at different times of tooth eruption. Guidelines for their use have been laid down by Joyston-Bactal with the recommended dosage being: 6 months to 2 yrs–0.25 mg, 3 Yrs to 4 yrs–0.50 mg, Above 4 yrs–1.0 mg.

Fluoride toothpaste is a method of topical fluoridation. Most of the tooth pastes nowadays contain fluoride to prevent caries. Only a pea-sized amount of tooth paste is used but it has to be kept in mouth. It should not be rinsed out immediately after brushing.

Fluoride varnish is a preventive procedure in which highly concentrated varnish is painted over teeth. Semiannual application is sufficient.

Fluorides topical are the ones where fluorides applied in direct contact of teeth through mouth rinses and tropical fluoride application.

Fluorine is an essential element, about 95% of fluoride in the body is found in bones and teeth. It is essential for formation of dental enamel. Drinking water contains 0.5 mg/L but in endemic areas of fluorosis water contains 3 to 12 mg of fluoride. Sea fish, cheese and tea are rich in fluorides. 0.5 to 0.8/L in water is considered safe limit in our country. Deficiency of it leads to dental caries.

Fluoroscopy is a form of radiography in which image is displayed in real time.

Fluorosis refers to discoloration of the enamel due to excessive fluoride absorption (greater than one part per million) into the bloodstream, also called enamel mottling. It is a permanent damage to the enamel, which consists of white or brown spots that appear on the children's teeth. When fluoride reaches the cells, which make enamel, ameloblasts, become poisoned. As they degenerate they lay down irregular enamel. Instead of the regular hydroxyapatite,

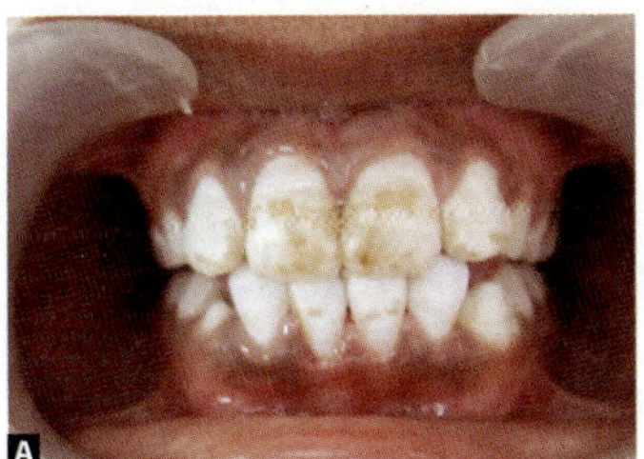

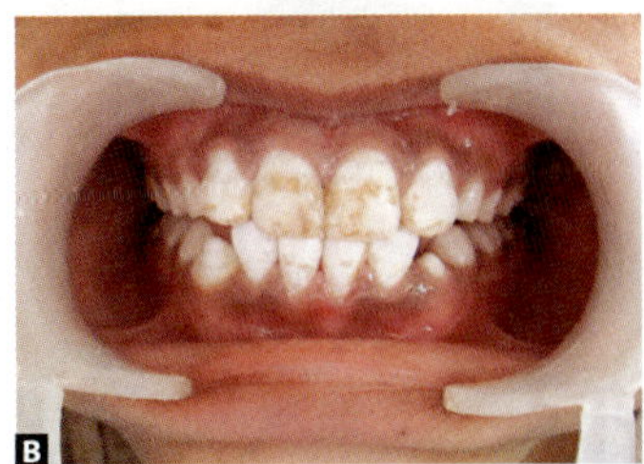

Figs A and B.: *Fluorosis*

they will produce mottled, porous and thin enamel. As the poisoning worsens the enamel may even be absent. At the same time the enamel is being mottled and other hard and ligament tissues are being affected as well.

Fluorosis risk index (FRI) was introduced by David G Fendrys, in 1990. The FRI is designed to permit a more accurate identification of associations between age-specific exposures is fluoride sources and the development of enamel fluorosis. The FRI divides the enamel surfaces of the permanent dentition into two developmentally related groups surface zones, designated either as having begun - (I) formation during the first year of life ("Classification I") or (ii) formation during the third through sixth year of life ("Classification II).

Flush terminal plane is the mesio-distal relation between the distal surface of the upper and a lower second deciduous molar is called the terminal plane. A normal feature of deciduous dentition is to find a flush terminal plane where the distal surface of the upper and lower second deciduous molars are same in the same vertical plane.

Flushing is sudden redness of skin.

Flute is groove present on the working area of file. It collects debris as the file cuts the tooth surface.

Flux is a substance that promotes the flow of solder over the metal parts by cleaning the surfaces and removing oxides during welding.

Focal dermal hypoplasia syndrome is an autosomal dominant disease. There is focal absence of dermis with herniation of subcutaneous fat into defects, skin atrophy and streaky pigmentation. Mental retardation is present. Papilloma of lip is a striking feature. Teeth are defective in size. Microdontia is common, cleft/lip/cleft palate may be seen.

Focal epithelial hyperplasia is a condition where lesion occurs primarily in lips and check. It is 0.1 to 0.4 cms. Flat, raised, whitish plaques are seen. Histologically local acanthosis is seen. Dyskeratosis is not present. Lesions may regress suddenly.

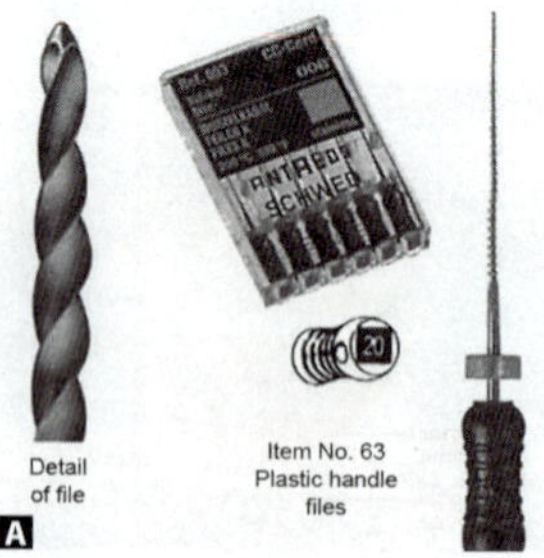

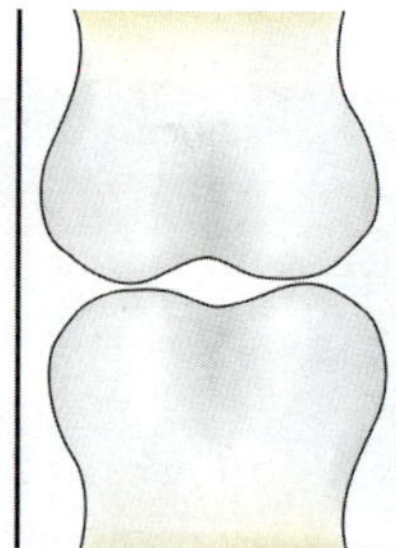

Figs A and B: *(A) Flute; (B) Flush terminal plane*

Focal infection is localized or general infection caused by the dissemination of microorganisms or toxic products from a focus of infection.

Focus of infection refers to a circumscribed area of tissue, which is infected with exogenous pathogenic microorganisms and is usually located near a mucous or cutaneous surface.

Fogged film is a processing error. It appears gray and lacks detail and contrast. Improper safelight in dark room may result in it.

Folic acid was discovered in 1941. Word comes from folium means leaf. Folates are essential for synthesis of DNA. Richest sources are liver, eggs and leafy vegetables. Commonest cause of nutritional anemia is folate deficiency especially in pregnancy hence 500 microgram of folic acid is given to pregnant woman. Deficiency of it causes irritability, forgetfulness and mental sluggishness. 90% alcoholics are said to suffer from it.

Fontanels are the cartilages that bridge the gap between the bones. They are made up of dura mater, primitive periosteum and the aponeurosis from inside outwards. fontanels present at birth are anterior fontanel: between the two parietal bones and the frontal bone, posterior fontanel: between the two parietal bones and the occipital bone, sphenoid fontanel: between the fontal, parietal, temporal and the sphenoid bone, mastoid fontanel: between the parietal, occipital, temporal bone. The anterior fontanel lies at the junction of the sagittal, coronal and frontal sutures. The posterior fontanel is triangular. It lies at the junction of the sagittal and lambdoid sutures. The anterolateral fontanel is present in relation to the anteroinferior angle of the parietal bone. The mastoid fontanel posterolateral is present in relation to the posteroinferior angle of the parietal bone.

Foot and mouth disease is a viral infection. Transmission is through

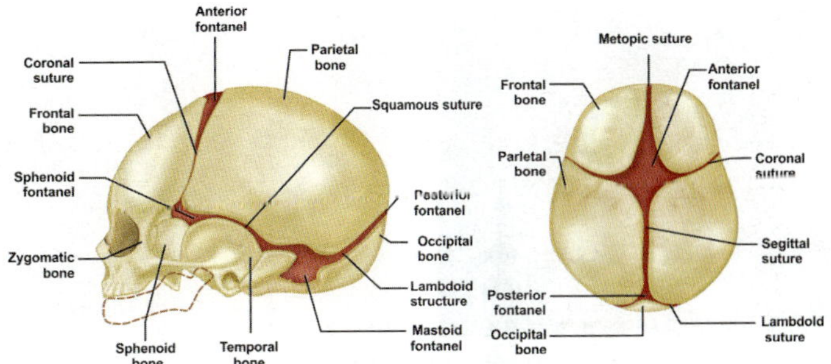

Fig.: *Fontanelles*

contact. Person develops fever, nausea, vomiting and ulcerative lesions of oral mucosa. Lesions of oral mucosa may develop anywhere. Lesions begin as small vesicles which rapidly rupture and heal within 14 days.

Foramen refers to an opening in bone.

Force refers to change of state of rest or motion of a substance.

Force delivery refers to the force produced by an orthodontic wire against a tooth.

Forced expiratory volume (FEV1) is the amount of gas exhaled in the first second on forced expiration. It is 80 percent of the FVC in normal subjects.

Fordyces granules normal oral mucosa contains many tubuloacinar sebaceous glands in vermilion border of lip and buccal mucosa. Histologically these are similar with sebaceous glands except hair follicle as they contain lipase secretion. Function of Fordyces granules is not known. They appear small, white submucosal plaques.

Forensic dentistry is that branch of dentistry that relates and applies dental facts to legal problems, dental identification, malpractice, litigation and dental licensure.

Formaldehyde is a highly toxic irritant gas which precipitates and destroys protein. It is effective against vegetable bacteria, fungi and viruses. It is used to disinfect rooms. In addition, it can be needed to disinfect blankets, beds, books and other articles which cannot be boiled.

Forward decay refers to a type of lesion where the caries starts in the enamel and then it involves the dentin, i.e. wherever the caries in enamel is larger than in dentin.

Fossa refers to a shallow depression on the lingual (tongue) surfaces of some front teeth.

Foster miller probe is a diagnostic probe that determines pocket depth along with detection of CEJ from where level of clinical attachment level is automatically detected.

Four handed dentistry is the delivery of the dental treatment by the

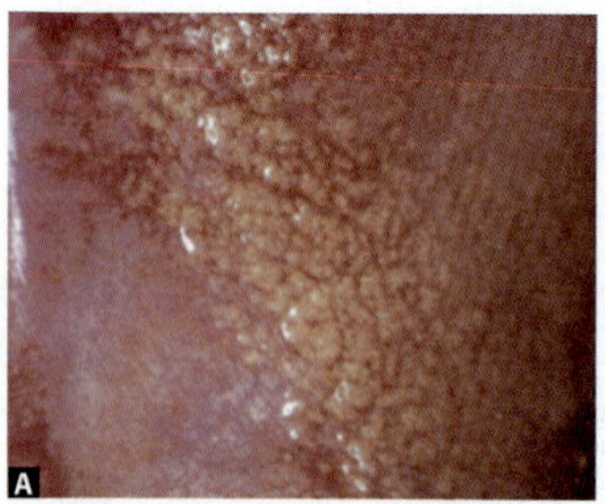

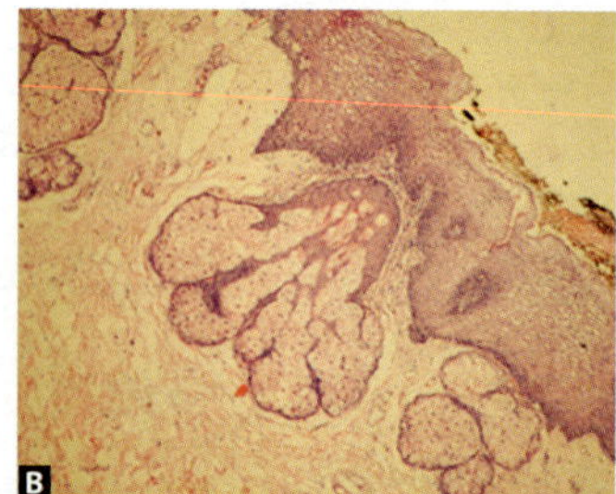

Figs A and B: *(A) Fordyces granules of buccal mucosa; (B) Histological view of Fordyces granules*

dentist and assistant working together at chair side.

Fourth branchial arch the cartilage of this arch probably forms the thyroid cartilage. The arch muscles develop into the cricothyroid and constrictors of the pharynx, the palatoglossus muscle of the muscles of the soft palate and the palatoglossus muscle of tongue. The nerve of the fourth arch is superior laryngeal branch of the vagus (Xth cranial nerve, which innervates these muscles. The fourth arch artery of the left side forms the arch of the aorta, that of the right side contributes to the right subclavian and brachiocephalic arteries. The para-aortic bodies of chromaffin cells that secrete noradrenaline arise from the ectomesenchyme of the fourth and sixth branchial arches.

Fourth degree burns refer to a type of burn where the damage extends beyond the skin till muscle, fascia or bone. However, this is not a universally accepted term and is not used.

Fourth pharyngeal pouch the fate of the endoderm of the ventral diverticulum is uncertain; the lining membrane may contribute to thymus or thyroid tissue.

Fracture refers to the breach in continuity.

Fracture of teeth is a cause of sudden severe trauma such as fall, blow or road accident. There are several classifications of fractured teeth. If crown is fractured but pulp is maintained, the teeth remains alive.

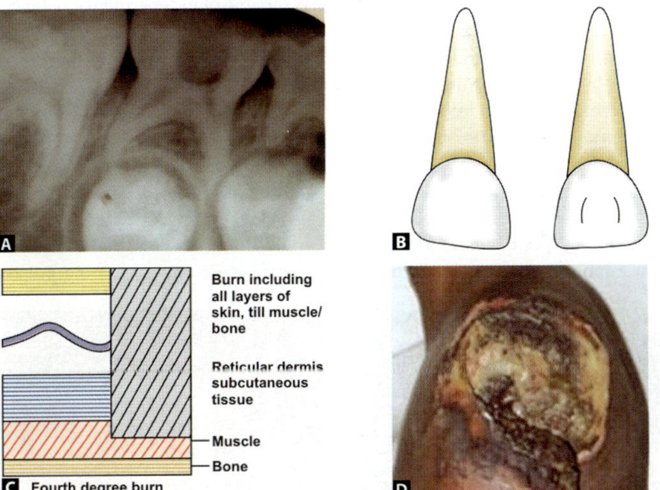

Figs A to D: *(A) Forward decay; (B) Lingual fossa; (C) Line diagram of fourth degree burn; (D) Clinical picture of fourth degree burn*

There may not be severe pain. Tooth may be sore and slightly loose. Fractured crown exposing pulp is more serious. Pulpotomy or pulpectomy may be required.

Fracture stress strength is a limit of applied force which a material can withstand without fracture. It is the strength of material. The stress at fracture is normally used to characterize the strength of a material.

Fracture toughness is a measure when crack is present.

Fragile X syndrome is a genetic disorder that is passed down from the mother's side of the family. Boys are more often affected, although both genders may be. Physical characteristics of those with Fragile X syndrome include a long, narrow face, prominent ears, jaw, chin and forehead, macro-orchidism (enlarged testicles), hyper-extended finger joints, double jointed thumbs and an excessive growth rate into the early childhood years. The individual may experience an intellectual disability, autistic-like behaviors, strabismus (cross-eyed), enlarged head, slanted eyes, poor muscle tone and coordination, as well as many other characteristics. 15 to 20% of people affected with Fragile X syndrome experience seizures.

Frankel's sign: In tabes dorsalis the excessive range of passive motion at the hip joint. It takes place due to decreased tone of foot and ankle.

Free (uncapsulated) receptors are the predominant form of nociceptors, especially in the cutaneous tissues, oral mucosa and periodontal tissues.

Free flowing solder refers to a solder that flows readily over clean metal surfaces and penetrates small openings and joints by capillary action.

Free graft refers to a tissue for grafting is completely removed from its donor site.

Free radical is any atom (e.g. oxygen, nitrogen) with at least one unpaired electron in the outer-most shell, and is capable of independent existence. Free radicals are highly reactive due to the presence of unpaired electrons.

Free running pulsed mode is unique in that large peak energies of laser light are emitted for an extremely short time span, usually in microseconds, followed by a relatively long time in which the laser is off. For example, a free running pulsed

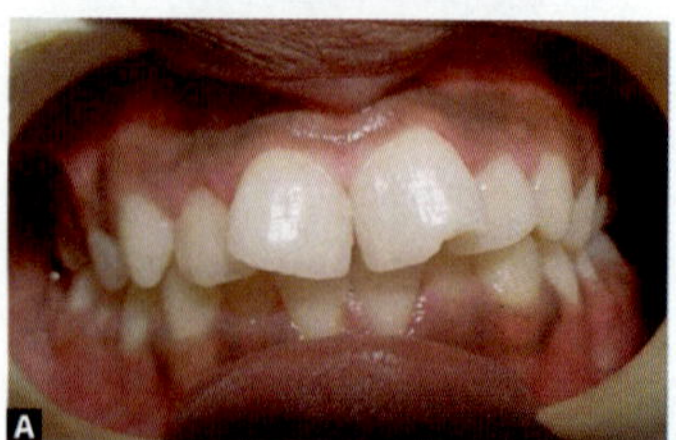

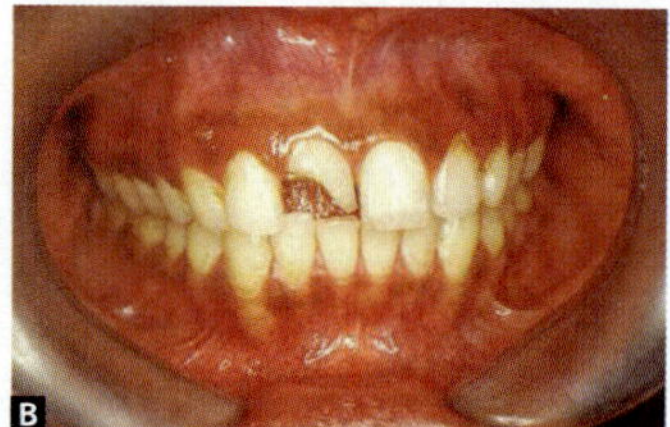

Figs A and B: *(A) Ellis class I tooth fracture; (B) Ellis class III tooth fracture*

laser with pulse duration of 100 μs with pulses delivered at 10 pulses per second would mean that the energy at the surgical site is only present for 1/1000 of a second and absent for the remaining 99.999% of that second.

Frenectomy refers to complete removal of a frenum.

Frenulum lingua is part of the tongue that is attached to the floor by a median fold of mucosa.

Frenum refers to a fold of mucous membrane attaching the cheeks and lips to upper and lower arches.

Frequency distribution refers to tally of number of times each individual score is represented in a data set. It can be presented visually as a histogram of a stem and leaf plot.

Fresh whole blood transfusion: The advantage of it is simultaneous presence of red blood cells, plasma and fresh platelets. It is used in cardiac surgery and massive hemorrhage when more than 10 units of blood is required in 24 hours.

Friable refers to easily breakable.

Friction blister occurs due to excessive friction. Epidermis separates from dermis and plasma oozes in for example blister of ill-fitting shoes.

Frictional keratosis is an isolated area of thickened whitish oral mucosa which can be identified to local irritant. It occurs due to some local irritant an isolated area of thickened whitish oral mucosa develops. Histological studies show various degrees of hyperkeratosis, parakeratosis and acanthosis. Within 2 weeks of treatment, lesion will start reducing in size.

Frigidity is the inability to initiate or maintain the sexual pattern.

Front teeth *see* anterior teeth.

Frontal lobe tumor develops slowness of comprehension, memory disorder, childish behavior and impaired judgement. Tumor or medial surface of frontal lobe may cause urinary urgency. Ataxic gait and profound mental changes appear. With the left frontal lesion intelligence is reduced. Motor aphasia develops.

Frontal sinuses are spaces that are present in the frontal bone. Each sinus lies deep to a triangular area the angles of which lie at a point about 3 cm above the nasion.

Frostbite symptoms of frostbite develop when skin temperature drops from 20 to 14°F. It may be

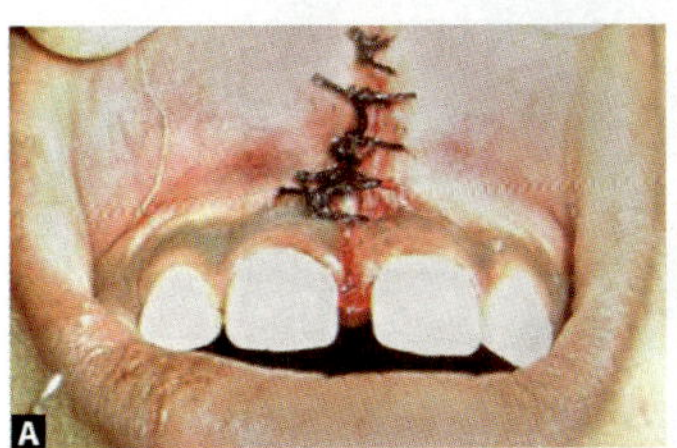

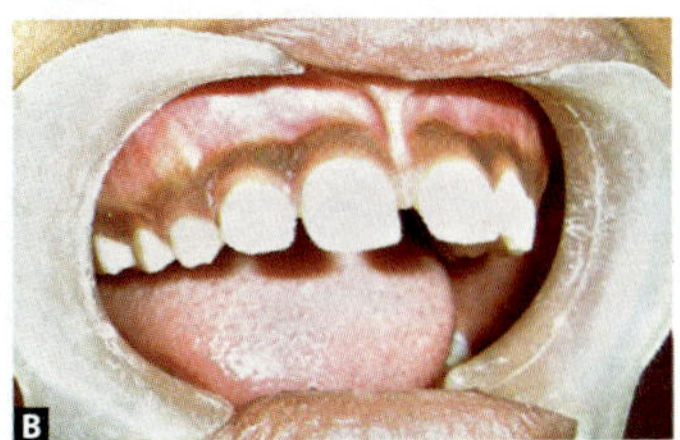

Figs A and B: *(A) Frenectomy; (B) High frenum attachment*

due to impaired circulation, injury or shock. Blisters form within 24-36 hours and become hard and black in two weeks. Tissues up to bones may be involved. There may be discoloration from blue to violet.

Frozen blood: RBCs can be frozen and stored for up to 3 years but the technique is costlier. It is to maintain a supply of rare blood type. In it plasma components are being removed.

Full mouth indices are those indices that measure the patient's entire periodontium or dentition. e.g: Russel's periodontal Index (PI).

Full mouth X-rays refer to those X-rays showing all the teeth. It includes 14 periapicals and 4 bitewings, also known as a complete series.

Full thickness flap refers to the flap where all the soft tissue including the periosteum is reflected to expose the soft tissue.

Fumigation theory is given by Guy de Cahuliac (1300-1368), was the greatest surgeon of Middle Ages believed that worms caused dental decay. He advocated fumigation with seeds of leek, onion and hyoscyamus as a cure for dental caries. The fumigation was also used in earlier times by Chinese and Egyptians.

Function of spinal cord: Each nerve is attached to spinal cord by two roots. Dorsal roots consist of sensory pathways and anterior root the motor pathways. Spinal cord provide a pathway for sensory information travelling from periphery to brain. It also provides a pathway for motor information coming from brain and going to periphery. In addition, spinal cord acts as a major reflex center.

Functional anterior crossbite: This type of crossbite is seen in pseudo, class II malocclusion where the mandible is compelled to close in a position forward of its true centric relation. It occurs as a result of occlusal prematurities that cause the deflection of the mandible into a forward position during closure. These can be treated by eliminating the occlusal prematurities.

Functional matrix theory refers Moss hypothesis.

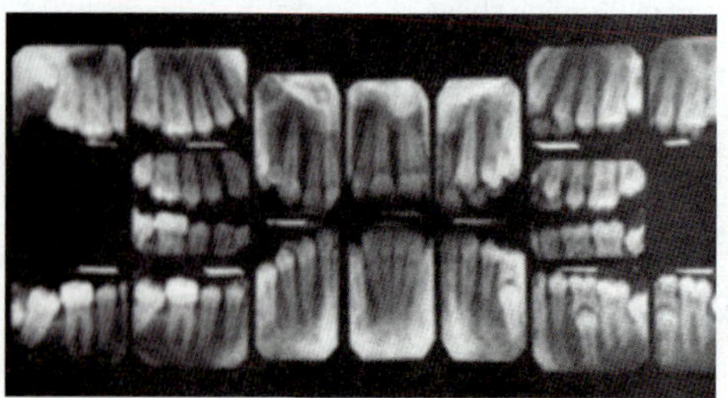

Fig.: *Anterior tooth full mouth X-rays*

Functional measure index (FMI) was proposed by Sheiham A, Maizels J, and Maizels A in 1987, as one of the two alternative indices, which were modifications of the DMFT index. In FMI, the 'Filled and the Sound' teeth are weighted equally, while, the 'Decayed and Missing' teeth are given zero weight. The FMI is calculated by adding the filled and sound teeth and then dividing by total number of teeth present.

Functional tongue thrust is said to be present when the tongue thrust mechanism is an adaptive behavior developed to achieve an oral seal, it can be grouped as functional.

Functions of Proteins: These provide material for growth, wear and tear of tissue. These provide energy and stimulate metabolism. These are source of enzyme needed for digestion. Antibodies which are defence against infections are protein in nature. These maintain acid-base balance.

Fundal height and gestation: Fundal height is just above symphysis pubis at 12 weeks gestation, at umbilicus at 22 weeks and at xiphisternum at 36 weeks.

Fungal infection of lung is generally opportunistic infections. They develop in patients with suppression of immune status. It develops in chronic congestion and edema where fungi get comfortable environment. Histoplasmosis, aspergillosis, cryptococcosis are common diseases.

Furcation refers to the areas between the roots of teeth where the root trunk divides the separate roots.

Furcation involvement is the term given when there is invasion or bony destruction of bifurcation or trifurcation of multirooted tooth due to periodontal disease. The bone loss around each tooth may be horizontal and angular; furcation involvement is a stage progressive periodontal disease.

Furrow refers to a groove.

Fusion refers to union of two separate tooth germs during their formation. They may be joined only by enamel and/or dentin. Pulps may also be fused. Extent of union depends on the stage of development of teeth at the time of fusion. Fused teeth appear broader. They also frequently

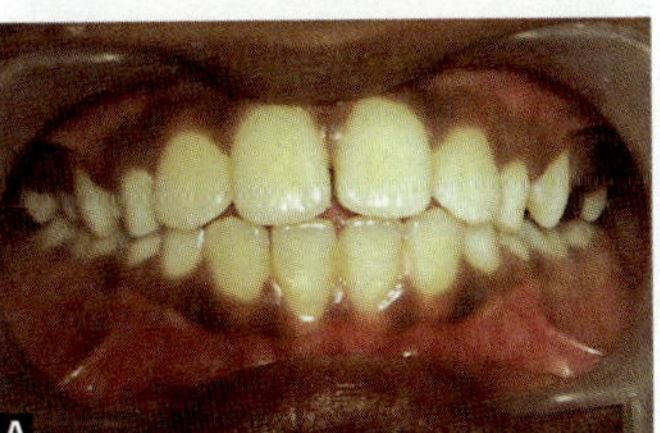

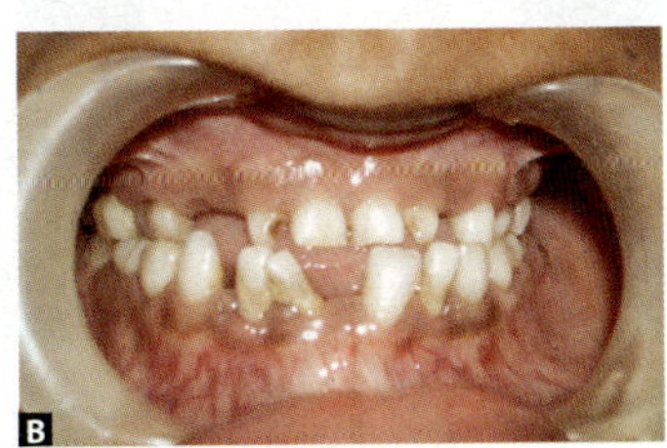

Figs A and B: *Functional tongue thrust*

exhibit incisal notch or grove which may continue onto the root surface. Whereas fusion takes place at an angle causing crooked appearance. Pulpal anatomy: fused teeth tend to have double pulpal space and. However, in both gemination and fusion, the pulp spaces may or may not be separated. *Location in the jaw:* Double teeth in the mandible would almost exclusively represent fusion crowding: fused teeth occupy less space than separate teeth would, causing spacing in the arch. *Number of teeth:* In case of fusion there will be reduction in tooth number.

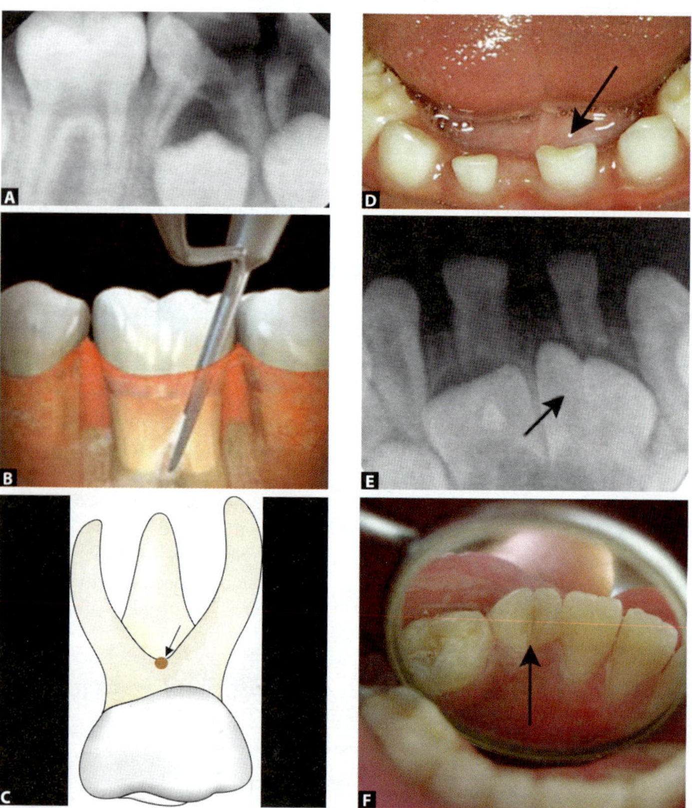

Figs A to F: *(A to C) Showing furcation points and furcation involvement; (D to F) Clinical view of fusion; Radiographic view of fusion; Fusion of teeth (lingual view)*

G

G (Glabella) is the most prominent anterior point in the midsagittal plane of the forehead.

Gabapentin is a drug that is used in the treatment of partial seizures. It is a GABA analogue. Its mechanism of action occurs at calcium channel. It is generally well-tolerated. It is well-absorbed after oral administration and is eliminated by renal excretion. Average half-life is 5-7 hours.

Gag reflex is seen at 18 1/2 week of IU life. In the buccal cavity and pharynx, the ectoderm/endoderm zone is towards the posterior third of the tongue. Touching here elicits a gag reflex, a protective reflex.

Gait is the period between successive points at which the heel of the same foot strikes the ground. 60-65% time of one cycle foot remains in touch to the ground. Gait has four components, antigravity support of body, stepping, maintenance of equilibrium and means of propulsion.

Galactorrhea refers to the bilateral, spontaneous, milky type of discharge from multiple ducts in child-bearing age. It is caused by increased production of prolactin and is most commonly seen after pregnancy. Normal levels of prolactin range from 1–22 mg per mL.

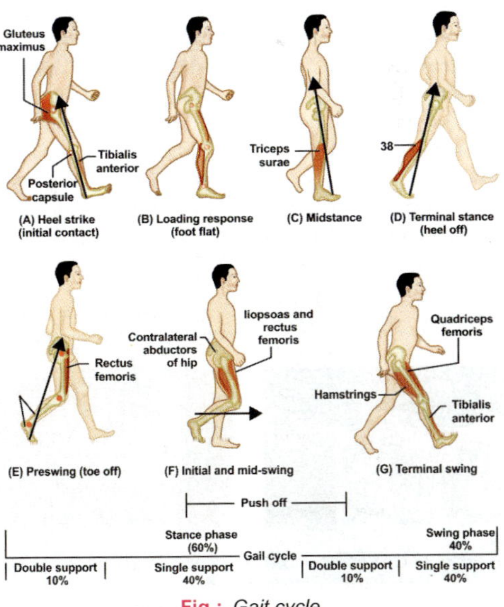

Fig.: *Gait cycle*

Galactosemia is an inability to metabolize galactose. It leads to high blood and tissue galactose level and galactosuria. Each one of the three types develops due to deficiency of specific enzyme. Classical galactosemia is due to galactose –1 phosphate uridyl transferase deficiency. Manifestations include cataract, cirrhosis and mental retardation.

Gallium amalgam is a product formed by the reaction of an alloy powder, silver-tin-copper with a gallium-based liquid alloy, i.e. gallium-indium-tin.

Galvanic current refers to a current of electricity produced by chemical action between two metals suspended in liquid.

Gardner's syndrome is carcinomatous transformation of adenomatous intestinal polyps. There may be osteomas of jaw and accompanying cysts are indictors of Gardner's syndrome and bowel should be examined.

Gas gangrene is caused by C. perfringens, C. histolyticum. Onset is sudden with pain and swelling in affected area, tachycardia and hypovolemic shock. There develops foul smelling blood tinged discharge from wound. Red fluid filled vesicles develop around wound. Palpable crepitus shows gas formation at the site. Hemolytic jaundice and renal failure are common. X-ray may show gas.

Gas lasers (Helium and Helium-Neon, HeNe, are the most common gas lasers) have a primary output of visible red light. CO_2 lasers emit energy in the far infrared, and are used for cutting hard materials.

Gastrointestinal bleeding is the most common cause includes gastric ulcer, gastric erosion duodenal ulcer and esophagitis. Red or coffee ground hematemesis with or without melena indicates upper GI bleeding. Bright red rectal bleeding may be due to lower GI bleeding. Signs include hematemesis, gross on occult blood in stool. Hypotension occurs in late cases. Tachycardia develops earlier.

Gate control theory of pain is the most accepted mechanistic theory of pain. It was devised by Melzack and Wall. According to

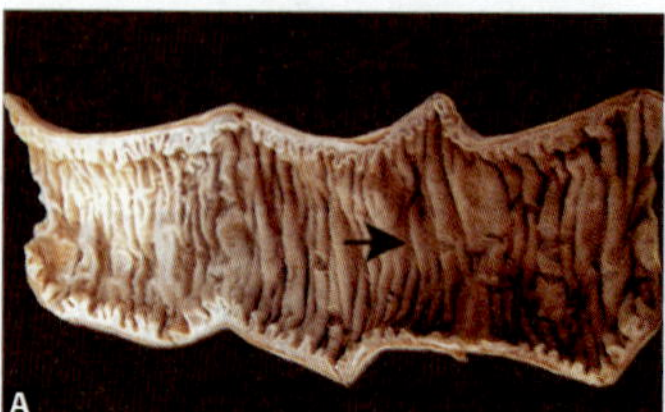

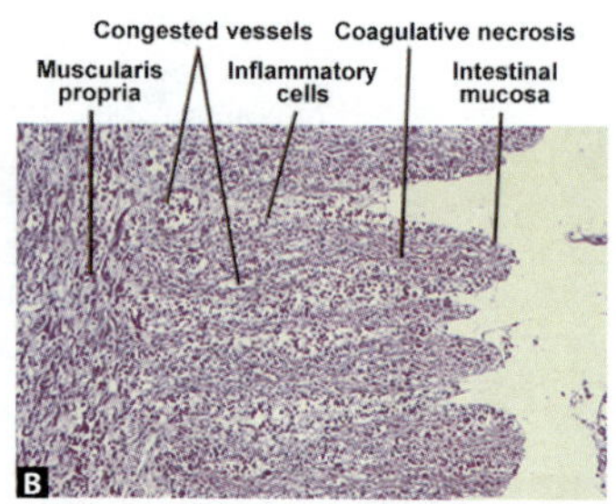

Figs A and B: *Gas gangrene*

this theory noxious stimulation of the Substantia Gelatinosa (SG) functions as a gate control system that modulates the afferent pathways before they influence the transmission cells. The afferent patterns in the dorsal column system therefore function in part as a control trigger which activates selective brain process that influences the modulating properties of the gate control system.

Gated pulse mode there are periodic alterations of the laser energy being on and off, similar to a blinking light. This mode is achieved by the opening and closing of a mechanical shutter in front of the beam path of a continuous wave emission. Duration of on and off times normally is as small as a few milliseconds.

Gates-Glidden bur is a traditional engine-driven instrument includes Gates-Glidden drills which have flame-shaped cutting point mounted on long thin shaft attached to a latch type shank. The flame head cuts laterally. So, used with gentle, apically directed pressure. It has saft tip to guard against perforations. Gates-Glidden are available in a set from 1 to 6 with the diameters from 0.5 to 1.5 mm. Due to their design, Gates-Glidden drills are side-cutting instruments with safety tips. They should be used at the speed of 750 to 1500 rpm, in brushing strokes. These are used to retrieve broken instruments and preparation of post in endodontic procedures.

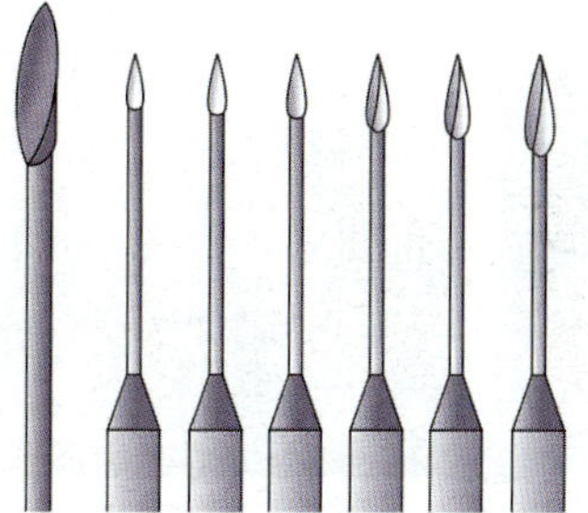

Fig.: *Gates Glidden burs*

Gaucher's disease is the most common lysosomal storage disorder (incidence 1 in 25, 000 live-births). Inheritance is autosomal recessive, with a high incidence seen in Ashkenazi Jews, who have a carrier frequency of 1 in 60. There is a deficiency of glucosidase, resulting in accumulation of its substrate glucocerebroside. The enzyme is encoded on chromosome. There are three types of Gaucher's disease. Type I—adult type, non-neuronopathic. Type II—severe infantile, rare, neurological signs seen at 3 months, die by 2 years of age. Type III—subacute, neuropathic, variable presentation from childhood to 70 years of age.

Gel is a colloidal system in which the solid and liquid are continuous phases. Gel is usually flexible.

Gelatine is a sponge. It can be left adherent to the bleeding surface. It will be completely absorbed in 1–2 weeks. It can be used in treatment of bleeding tooth sockets.

Gemination refers to a double teeth originated from one tooth bud.

This is the result of incomplete splitting. Morphology: In case of gemination, fused crowns exhibit mirror image. Pulpal anatomy geminated teeth usually have an undivided pulp: geminations are more common in maxilla. Gemination results in extra tooth hence requires more space thereby likely to cause crowding but fusion of normal tooth bud with a supernumerary would result in crowding. Hence neither crowding nor diastema seems decisive. Gemination does not reduce the tooth number.

G

Gene therapy is a treatment of inherited diseases by introducing wild type copies of defective genes causing the disorder into the cells of affected individuals.

General anesthetics are the drugs these have the capability to depress excitable tissue at all levels of CNS. There are four stages of anesthesia analgesia and respiratory paralysis. Course of general anesthesia includes three stages, induction of anesthesia which is the period in which concentration of anesthetic agent in blood tissue increases. During maintenance of anesthesia operation is performed. Anesthesia is controlled to maintain constant depth of anesthesia. Third stage is emergence from anesthesia, cessation of anesthetic agent ending with complete recovery of reflexes.

General anesthesia is a procedure done by giving an inhalation drug before a surgical procedure to relieve the sensation of pain.

General somatic afferent fibers are those that carry sensations of touch, pain and temperature from the skin (exteroceptive sensations) and proprioceptive impulses arising in muscles, joints and tendons. These convey information regarding movement and position of joints.

General visceral afferent fibers carry sensations, e.g., pain from viscera (visceroceptive sensations).

General visceral efferent fibers supply smooth muscle and glands.

General visceral efferent nuclei give origin to preganglionic fibers that end in peripheral ganglia. Postganglionic fibers arising in these ganglia supply smooth muscle or glands. These neurons,

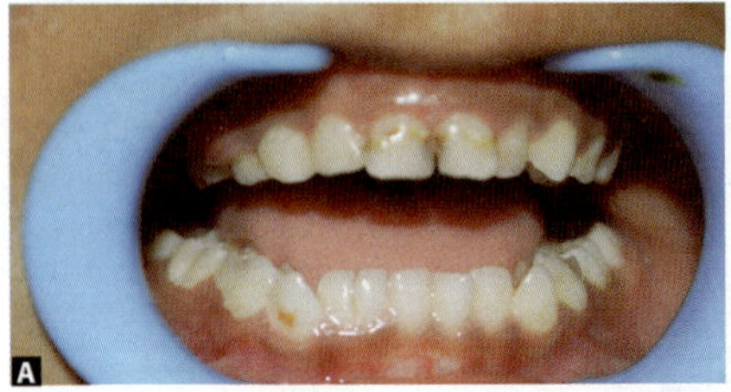

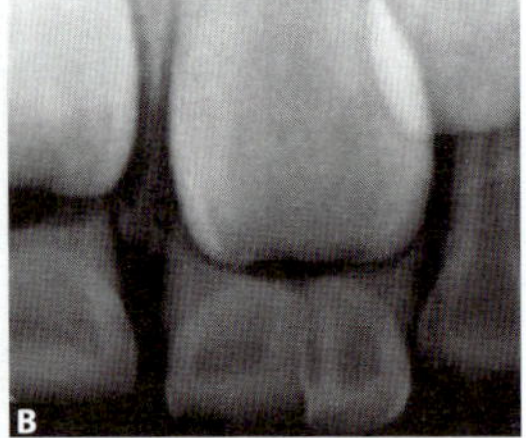

Figs A and B: *Clinical and radiological picture of gemination*

preganglionic and postganglionic, form part of the parasympathetic nervous system.

Generalized diffuse gingivitis involves the entire gingiva.

Generalized aggressive periodontitis usually occurs in the individuals of below the age group of thirty. Clinically there is generalized interproximal attachment loss affecting three permanent teeth other than first molars and incisors. The destruction occurs is episodic in nature with the period of advanced destruction followed by the variable stages of remission.

Generalized gingivitis is said to occur where inflammation involves the entire mouth.

Generalized infection is an infection that has spread throughout the body.

Generalized marginal gingivitis involves the gingival margins in relation to all the teeth.

Generalized periodontitis is said to have occurred when more than thirty percent of the areas assessed in mouth demonstrate the bone loss and loss of attachment.

Generalized seizures are the seizures involving the whole body. Grand mal epilepsy also known as tonic clonic seizure and is the most common form of seizures disorder. This is produced by idiopathic neurologic disorders or may develop in a neurologically sound brain secondary to a systemic, metabolic or toxic disturbance. Causes include drug withdrawal, menstruation, fatigue, falling asleep or awakening. Neurologically induced generalized tonic clonic seizure usually lasts about 2-3 minutes and seldom more than 5 minutes, the entire seizure lasts 5-15 minutes.

Genetic theory is one of the earliest concepts of growth and development and put forward by Brodie as that gene determines all.

Genetics is the history of individual and biological and temperamental effects given in birth and development. It can also be defined as the science of heredity and variation or the science that studies inheritance and expression of inhe-rited traits.

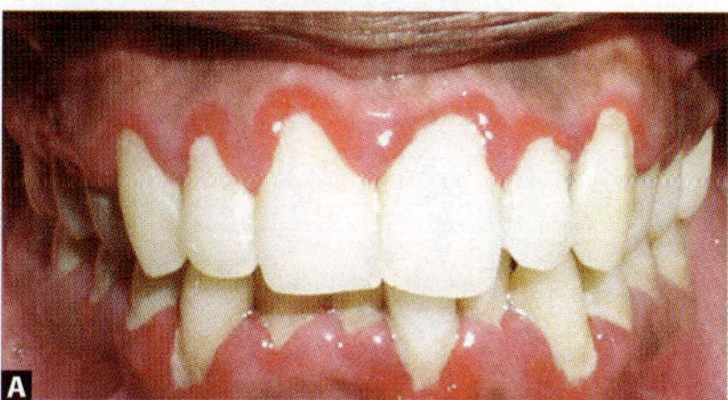

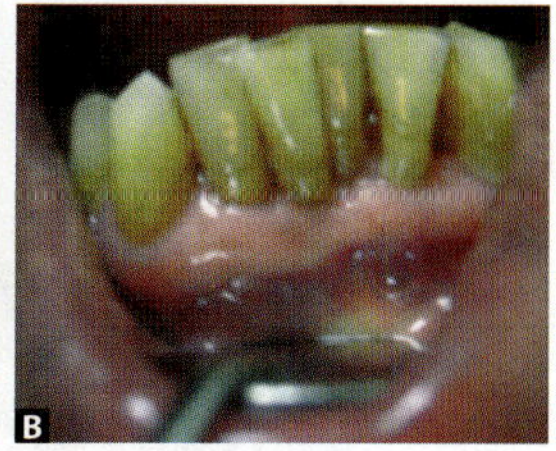

Figs A and B: *(A) Generalized gingivitis; (B) Severe gingival recession with generalized peridontitis*

Geniculate neuralgia is characterized by pain in ear and anterior tongue. Location of pain is similar to sensory distribution of the nerve, i.e. external auditory canal, posterior auricular region and the soft palate. If motor root is also involved, then facial palsy may develop. Pain is not too severe. Short course of high dose steroid therapy is beneficial.

Genital tubercles are the tiny bumps of bone in the anterior region of mandible that serve as attachment sites for genioglossus and geniohyoid muscles. These appear as radio- opaque.

Geographic tongue is also known as migratory glossitis. It refers to irregularly shaped, reddish areas of depapillation. There will be thinning of dorsal tongue epithelium. There is spontaneous development and regeneration of affected area. There may be associated fissured tongue. Etiology of geographic tongue is not clear. An immunologic reaction is suggested. No inheritance pattern is noted. The disease is asymptomatic but some may complain of burning, pain and stinging. Clinically irregularly shaped red patches with white patterns look like a map. Red patches are smaller to start surrounded by a white rim. Red patches go on enlarging and regressing and pattern goes on changing every week.

Geometric teeth refer to non-anatomic posterior teeth.

Geotrichosis is a fungal disease caused by Geotrichum species. Oral lesions are similar to candidiasis or thrush. It is a white, velvety covering of the oral mucosa. It may be isolated or diffuse organisms are

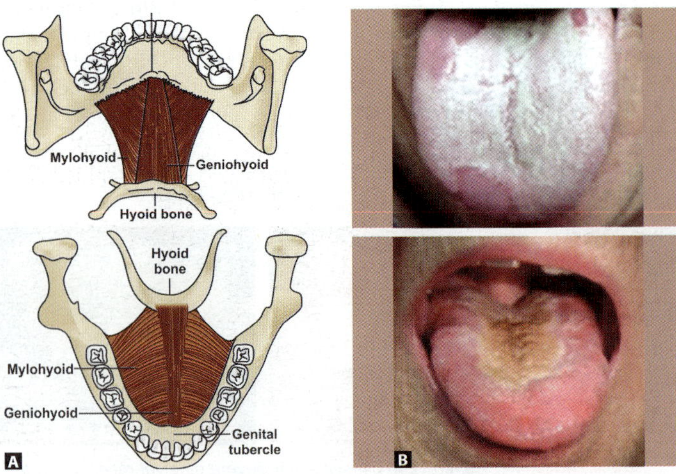

Figs A and B: *(A) Genital tubercles; (B) Geographic tongue*

small rectangular shaped spores 4 to 8 microns.

Gerber space regainer is a space regaining appliance where a seamless orthodontic band or a crown is selected for the tooth to be distalized. This space regainer consists of 'U' shaped tubing and a 'U' shaped rod that enters the tubing. The rod is soldered or welded on the mesial aspect of the first molar to be moved distally. The 'U' shaped wire or rod is fitted into the tube, in such a way that the base of 'U' rod contacts the tooth mesial to the edentulous area. Open coil springs of adequate length are placed around the free ends of the 'U' shaped rod and inserted into the tubing assembly. The forces generated by the compressed open coil springs bring about a distal movement of the first molar.

German measles is an acute specific fever characterized by suboccipital and posterior cervical glandular enlargement. Macular rash starts on first day. Fever is moderate, with malaise. Rash consists of small, pink, discrete macule. Occasionally patient may complain of joint pain. There is typical enlargement of lymph gland and mild coryza.

Germicides refer to anything that destroys bacteria.

Gerontology is the scientific study of factors affecting the normal aging process and the effects of aging.

Gerstmann's syndrome is a combination of right-left disorientation finger agnosia and constructional apraxia. Acalculia and dyslexia are common.

Gomphoses joint movements are minimal. Example includes teeth and jaw.

Ghost teeth are an unusual developmental problem in which one or several teeth in the same quadrant show marked reduction in radiodensity. Very thin enamel and dentin are present. Such teeth if erupt are malformed and non-functional.

Giant cell fibroma develops from fibrous connective tissue, mandibular or maxillary gingiva is mostly affected. Clinical features: Lesion is pedunculated. It has papillary or warty surface. Some may be painless, smooth nodular growth. Histologically multiple multinucleated giant cells are seen. Nuclei are large of giant cells. Numerous small capillaries are noted. Surgical excisiosn is the line of treatment. It may develop at any age.

Giardiasis is protozoal infection of small intestine caused by flagellate Giardia lamblia. Cysts are transmitted as a fecal contamination

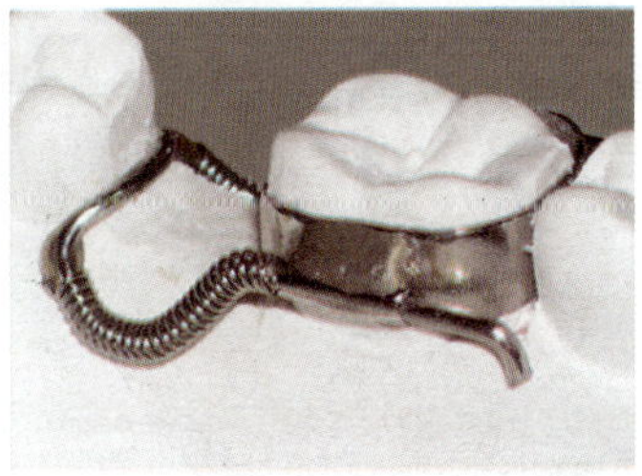

Fig.: *Gerber space regainer*

of water or food by person to person contact. It may result in acute diarrhea and malabsorption. Incubation period is 1-3 weeks. There may be marked weight loss. Single dose Tinidazole is effective in 90% cases.

Gifford sign is a resistance to everting the upper eyelid.

Gingiva is a masticatory type of oral mucosal membrane that forces the covering of the teeth. It is divided into three zones for descriptive purpose.

Gingival abscess is a localized purulent infection involving marginal gingiva or interdental papilla. It is a localized, painful rapidly expanding lesion that is usually of sudden onset. It is generally limited to marginal gingiva or interdental papilla. In early stages, it appears as a red swelling with a smooth, shiny surface. Within 24 hr to 48 hr, the lesion usually becomes fluctuant and pointed and forms a surface orifice from which purulent exudates may be expressed.

Gingival crevicular fluid (GCF) is the fluid which is present in gingival sulcus. The fluid seeps from the gingival tissue through the sulcular epithelium. The main functions which are thought to be performed by this fluid are the cleansing action, antimicrobial action, antibody activity to defend gingiva.

Gingival cyst develops either in free or attached gingiva. It may develop at any age. It is a soft tissue lesion and does not show on radiographs when bigger in size it may bulge the cortical plate of bone. Otherwise it presents a small well-circumscribed painless swelling of gingiva. It resembles a superficial mucocele. Surgical excision is the remedy.

Gingival fibers are the connective tissues of marginal gingiva which are densely collagenous in nature and mainly composed of type I collagen. Their main function is to hold the marginal gingiva firmly, to provide rigidity so that the tooth can withstand masticatory forces and to unite marginal gingiva with the cementum of the root and adjacent attached gingiva.

Gingival fluid (Sulcular fluid) contains a fluid that seeps into it

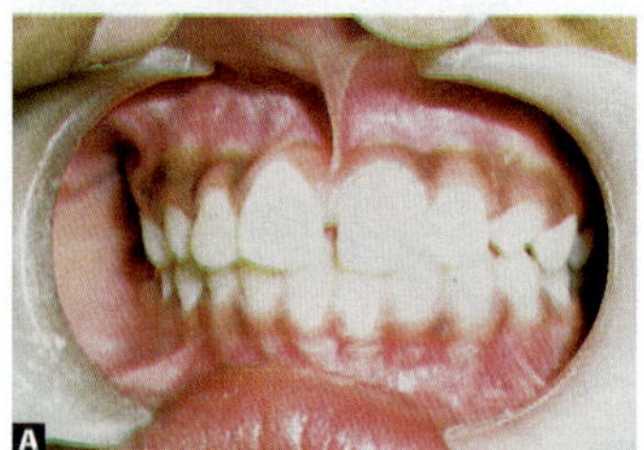

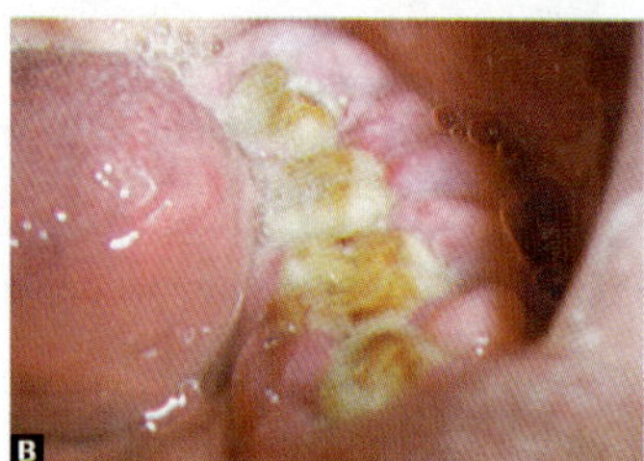

Figs A and B: *(A) Healthy gingiva; (B) Gingival hypoplasia*

from the gingival connective tissue through the thin sulcular wall. The gingival fluid is believed to cleanse material from the sulcus, contain plasma proteins that may improve adhesion of the epithelium to the tooth, possess antimicrobial properties, exerts antibody activity in defense of the gingiva.

Gingival graft is a surgical procedure that removes gingival tissue from one area of the mouth to place it in another area of the mouth which is deficient in gingiva.

Gingival groove is the groove separating the gum pad from the palate.

Gingival hyperplasia is an increase in size of gingiva and soft tissue overfills the interproximal spaces. Hyperplasia may be inflammatory, noninflammatory or mixed. In inflammatory hyperplasia the enlarged gingiva are soft, edematous and sensitive to touch. While noninflammatory is hard, firm, dense and paler. Drugs like calcium channel blocker may cause it. Tooth brush trauma may cause localized thickened gingiva with a more linear appearance. Chronic inflammation can cause firm, rolled and fibrotic. Poor oral hygiene can lead to chronic inflammation and thickened gingiva.

Gingival margin trimmer (GMT) is a dental hand instrument designed to bevel the cervical cavosurface walls of the cavity preparation.

Gingival pocket usually occurs due to enlargement of gingival tissue without any underlying destruction of periodontal tissues.

Gingival recession is the reduction of the height of the marginal gingiva.

Gingival sulcus is the shallow crevice or space around the tooth bounded by the surface of

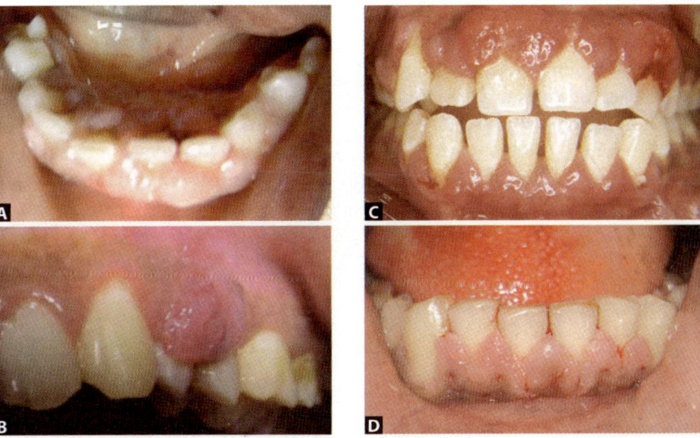

Figs A to D: *Different types of drug-induced gingival hyperplasia*

G

the tooth on one side, and the epithelium linking the free margin of the gingival on the other. The clinical determination of the depth of the gingival sulcus is an important diagnostic parameter. The so-called probing depth of a clinically normal gingival sulcus in humans is 2 to 3 mm. The sulcus depth around the primary teeth is comparatively greater than those that found around the permanent teeth. The mean values range from 1.4 mm to 2.1 mm.

Gingivectomy refers to the excision of the gingiva.

Gingivitis refers to inflammation of gingiva and may occur in acute or subacute form. Plaque or plaque derived endotoxins act as irritants. Food impaction and general oral neglect may result in gingivitis. Gingiva becomes deeper pink to red due to hyperemia and inflammatory infiltrates. Swelling takes place. Inflammatory swelling produces a bulbous appearance. In chronic gingivitis, pus may be expressed on pressure. Irritants are to be removed.

Gingivodental fibers are those present on the facial, lingual and interproximal surfaces. They are embedded in the cementum just beneath the epithelium at the base of the gingival sulcus.

Gingivoplasty refers to reshaping of the gingiva, to create physiologic gingival contours. The procedure is performed with the help of periodontal knife, scalpel, rotary diamond stones or electrodes.

Gland of Blandin and Nuhn is the anterior lingual gland lies close to inferior surface and tip of tongue. Five to seven of its ducts open on small protuberances of mucous membrane under the tongue.

Glandular cheilitis is not very common and lower lip becomes enlarged, everted and firm. Use of tobacco and constant exposure of sun may result in it. Emotional disturbance may also result in glandular cheilitis. There are three types: Simple - these are multiple, pin-headed and painless lesions. Superficial suppurative type - there will be painless swelling, crusting, induration and superficial ulceration of lip. Deep suppurative type—there is deep seated infection with abscess and

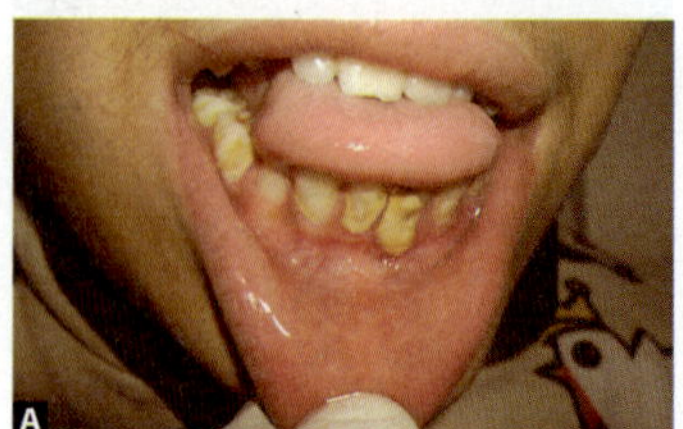

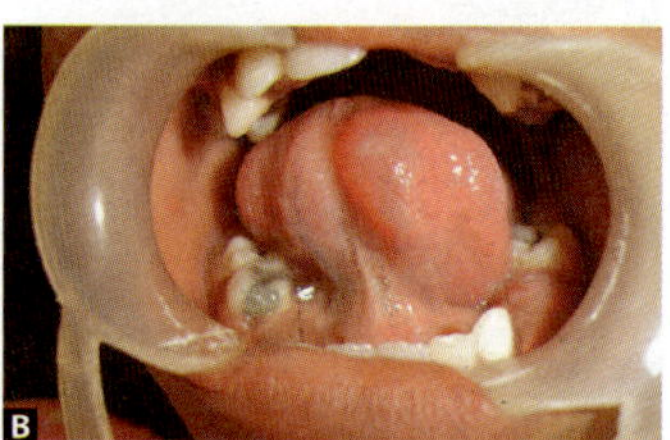

Figs A and B: *(A) Gingival sulcus; (B) Gland of Blandin and Nuhn*

fistula. Clinical Features: It is more common in adults. Lower lip is more involved. Mucosal surface shows numerous dilated salivary duct orifices surrounded by a red macular area. Person notes a mucus secretion at the orifice of duct. In severe form, lip is considerably and permanently enlarged and develops pain and tenderness. Volkmann's cheilitis is a severe form and epidermoid carcinoma may be associated. Vermilionectomy is the line of treatment.

Glandular fever is caused by Epstein Barr virus. Chiefly young people are affected. Deep kissing may transmit it. Person develops fever, sore-throat, headache and lymphadenopathy. Cervical glands enlarge to start with. Pharyngitis and tonsillitis are common. Some cases may be symptomless. Oral lesion includes gingivitis and stomatitis. There may be occasional oral ulcers and palatal petechiae. Some may develop hemorrhagic tendency. Blood may show atypical lymphocytes. Abnormal forms may be oval, horseshoe shaped. Nuclei may be indented and irregular. Thrombocytopenia may be present. There is no specific treatment of this disease.

Glasgow coma scale (GCS) was first described by Teasdale and Jennett in 1974. This scale relates the clinical observation under the three categories: motor response, verbal performance, eye opening allowing any changes over a period of time to be appreciated.

Glass bead sterilizer is rapid method of sterilization which is used for sterilization of instruments It uses table salt which consists approximately of 1 percent sodium silico-aluminate, sodium carbonate or magnesium carbonate. So it can be poured more readily and does not fuse under heat. Salt can be

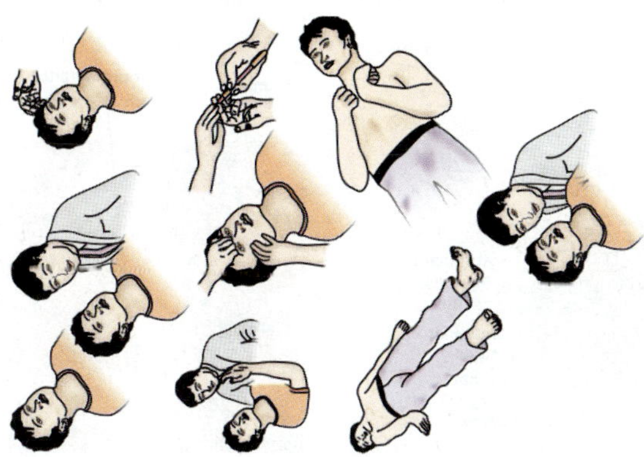

Fig.: *Glasgow coma scale*

replaced by glass beads provided the beads are smaller than 1 mm in diameter because larger beads are not efficient in transferring the heat to endodontic instruments due to presence of large air spaces between the beads. The instruments can be sterilized in 5 to 15 seconds at a temperature of 437 to 465°F (260°C) even when inoculated with spores. It is the term used for destruction of all pathogenic organisms, such as, vegetative forms of bacteria, mycobacteria, fungi and viruses, but not bacterial endospores.

Glass blowers' white patch is a variant of traumatic keratosis affecting cheek and lip. Histologically, it resembles cheek and lip bite.

Glass ionomer cements (GICs) are the one that consist of a basic glass and an acidic water-soluble powder that set by an acid-base reaction between the two components. These cements bond chemically to tooth and possess anticariogenic properties. Non-irritant to the tissue, low thermal diffusivity and biocompatible.

Glenoid fossa is a concave depressed area of the temporal bone, of which mandibular condyle rests.

Glial fibrillary acidic protein (GFAP) is a type of filament found in glial cells surrounding neurons.

Gliomas are very common measuring 50% intracranial neoplasms of brain. There may develop symptoms of increased intracranial pressure. There may be intellectual decline, personality changes, emotional liability, seizures and headache. Clinical manifestations depend on the site of lesion.

Globulin zinc insulin is most active in 8 hour following subcutaneous injection and action fades out by 18 hours.

Globulomaxillary cyst is a well-defined pear-shaped radiolucency found between the roots of maxillary lateral incisor and

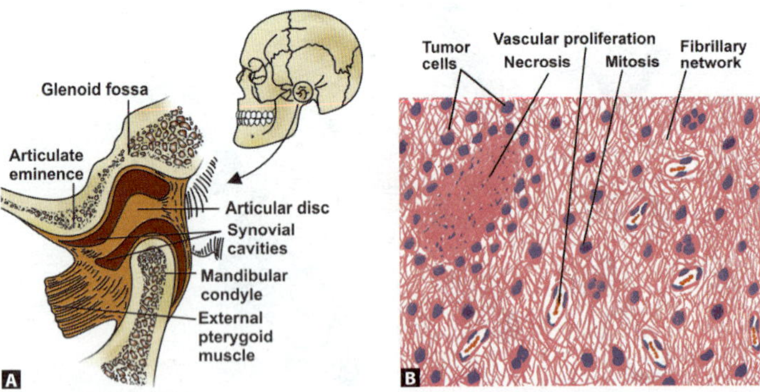

Figs A and B: *(A) Glenoid fossa; (B) Glioma*

cuspid. These are found within the bone at the junction of globular portion of medial nasal process and maxillary process. It is found accidentally being symptom free. Radiographically, it appears as inverted pear shaped.

Glomerulonephritis results in hematuria, dysmorphic red cells, casts and mild proteinuria. Edema is found in periorbital and scrotal lesions. Hypertension may develop.

Gloss is the optical property that produces a lustrous appearance. Luster is the proportion of specular reflection to diffuse reflection. When the incident beam is scattered by the object, there is decrease in gloss. Gloss is an important appearance property of dental restorative material.

Glossopharyngeal nerve (IX cranial nerve) supplies taste sensation to the posterior one-third of the tongue and sensation to the posterior pharynx (along with X nerve). It is attached to the lateral side of the upper part of the medulla (between the olive and the inferior cerebellar peduncle) by three or four roots. The tympanic branch arises from the inferior ganglion. The lesser petrosal nerve leaves the tympanic cavity through a canal that opens on the anterior surface of the petrous temporal bone (lateral to the greater petrosal nerve). The carotid branch arises soon after the glossopharyngeal nerve emerges on the base of the skull. It supplies the carotid sinus and carotid body. Pharyngeal branches are given off to the mucous membrane of the pharynx. Their fibers pass through the pharyngeal plexus. Tonsilar branches supply the palatine tonsil and the soft palate. The lingual branches supply the part of the tongue (mucous membrane) behind the sulcus terminalis.

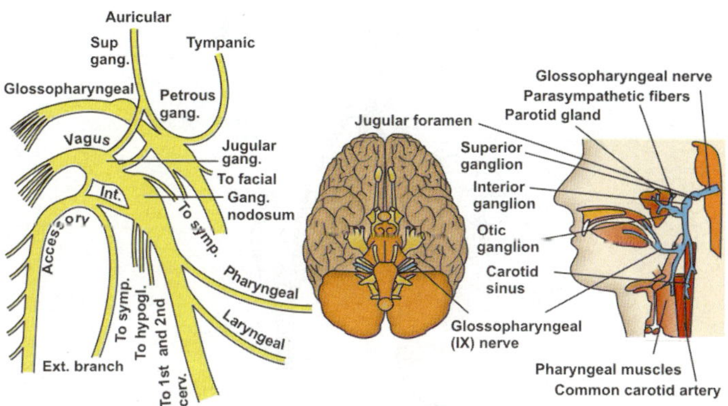

Fig.: *Glossopharyngeal nerve*

Glossopharyngeal neuralgia is a neuralgic pain of glossopharyngeal cranial nerve. Its pain is paroxysmal but less severe than trigeminal nerve pain. Location of trigger zone and pain sensation follows distribution of the nerve. Pain is felt in pharynx, ear and infra-auricular and post-mandibular area. It is triggered by swallowing, talking and chewing. Pain develops in periodic bouts and is brief and lancinating. It occurs in tonsillar fossa, back of throat and larynx. It includes posterior tongue, phar-ynx and infraauricular area. Surgical exploration of posterior fossa with release of division of affected nerve is curative. It occurs frequently in conjunction with trigeminal neuralgia. Sometimes, it may be associated with vagal symptoms. Intra or extracranial tumors may compress cranial nerve. Treatment is similar to trigeminal neuralgia. Such ear pain may be excruciating. Glossopharyngeal neuralgia is neuralgia of 9th cranial nerve. Pain is triggered by chewing and swallowing because all this stimulates pharyngeal mucosa.

Glossy polymer is an amorphous polymer that behaves as a brittle solid.

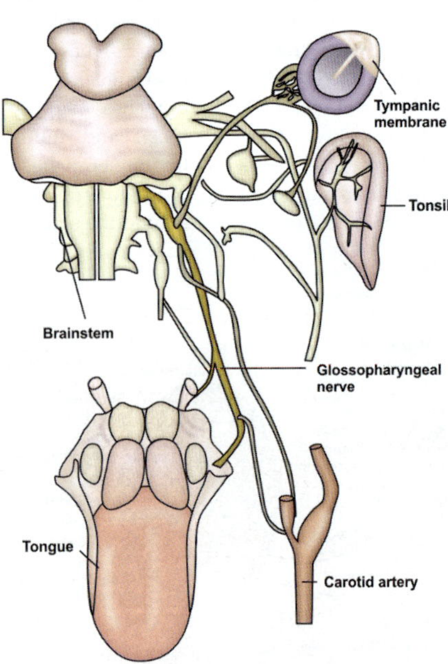

Fig.: *Glossopharyngeal neuralgia*

Gloves are a disposable item that gives protection to health care worker through cuts and abrasions. Gloves should be changed for each patient. Surgical gloves are not to be washed before or after being used.

Glucometer is a small instrument that measures the amount of glucose in capillary blood.

Glutaraldehyde is a high level disinfectant. 20 minutes immersion in 2% alkaline. Glutaraldehyde solution for disinfection and 6-10 hours immersion for sterilization of instruments is recommended. It has a pungent odor, irritating to eyes.

Glycerol: Three carbon carbohydrate which combines with fatty acids to form triglycerides.

Glycogen is also known as animal starch. It is highly branched polysaccharide similar to plant starch. Glucose is stored in human body as glycogen. When blood sugar lowers down, the glycogen is converted in the liver to glucose. Glucose released in blood restores normal blood sugar levels.

Goiter is an enlargement of thyroid occurring due to deficiency of iodine leads to goiter which is marked by swelling of the neck with the enlargement of thyroid gland. Babies born to these mothers may be physically/mentally deformed. Endemic goiter is a public health problem. Common salt fortified with small quantities of sodium and potassium iodate has been widely used in reducing the prevalence of goiter. A simple goiter secretes low levels of thyroid hormones. Other types of goiter hypersecrete thyroid hormones and are known as toxic goiter.

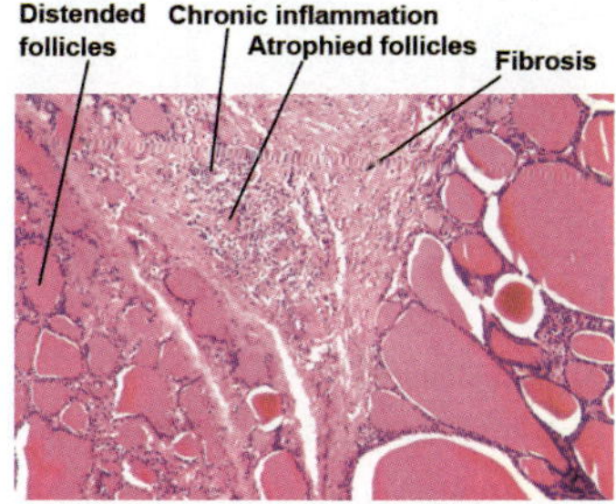

Fig.: *Nodular goiter*

Gold is used as the restorative material. The pulp reaction to case gold crown is a result of type of cement used to retain the restoration. The condensation of cohesive gold is a factor in pulp response. Mild to severe response is seen in 10-20 days. There are no irreversible changes and use of cohesive gold may be found biologically sound. Gold foil shows the least marginal leakage.

Gold filling makes an excellent filling material. It is most malleable so can be directly inserted and adopted to cavity wall. It brings hardness to cavity. It is insoluble in oral fluids and will not tarnish or corrode. It maintains high polish.

Gold inlays are used to amalgam fillings. These are used when teeth have lost cusps or otherwise are too weak. Advantage of gold is that is does not tarnish and has great strength.

Golden proportion refers to the guidelines which dentists use in determining the most esthetic appearance of a particular tooth (teeth need to maintain a certain height to width ratio to look their best).

Gold-palladium alloys were introduced in 1970 and were developed to avoid color change due to silver. The only disadvantage of the gold palladium group is thermal expansion incompatibility with some of higher expansion porcelains. Otherwise rigidity is increased and corrosion resistance becomes excellent.

Gonial angle (A-Go-Me) is the angle formed by the tangents to the body of the mandible and posterior border of the ramus. This not only expresses the form of the mandible but also gives information on mandibular growth direction. If this angle is acute, the growth is horizontal. This is favorable condition for anterior positioning of the mandible with an activator. In skeletally derived malocclusion, a casual type of treatment is possible only by channeling basal growth pattern to provide the morphologic and functional changes needed to establish a normal structural and functional pattern.

Gonorrhea is a venereal disease generally affecting genitourinary parts. Oral-genital sex affects oral cavity. Lips may develop acute painful ulceration. Gingiva may become erythematous with or without necrosis. Gonococcal pharyngitis and tonsillitis are well-recognized lesions.

Good cholesterol: Where the HDL is capable of transporting cholesterol back to liver where it is disposed. It is called good cholesterol and their elevated levels are helpful to heart.

Gout may be primary or secondary. Primary is inherited metabolic disorder. There is hyperuricemia resulting from overproduction or under excretion of uric acid. Depostis of urate crystals can occur in subcutaneous tissues, joints and kidneys. Secondary gout results due to drugs, i.e. thiazides, frusamide or diseases like

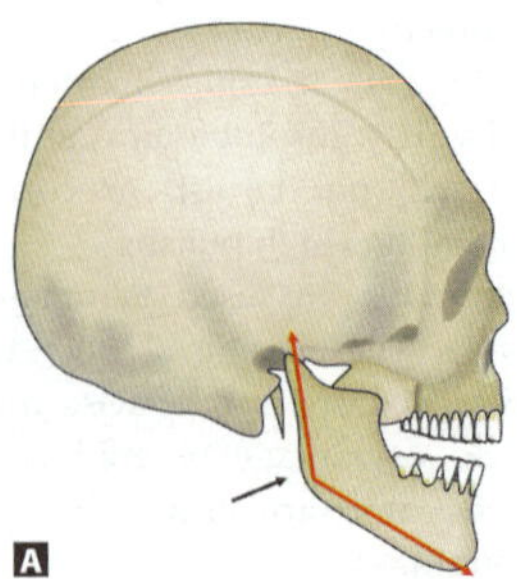

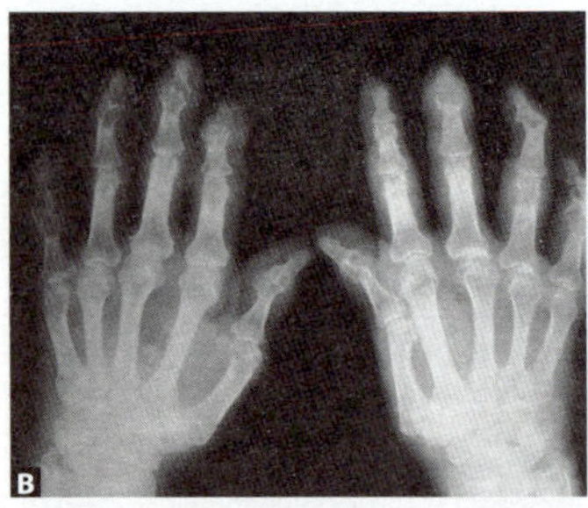

Figs A and B: *(A) Gonial angle; (B) Multiple, punched-out lesions of phalanges in gout*

lymphoma. Colchicines are most effective agent when given within 24 hours of acute attack.

Gracey curettes are the representatives of area specific curettes and can be used only in specific areas of the dentition; they are available as double ended as well as single ended curettes. It is a periodontal instruments that consists a set of four mini-bladed curettes; the sub 0 and number 1-2 are used for anteriors and premolars, number 11-12 are used for posterior mesial surface and number 13-14 are used for posterior distal surface. The length of blade is nearly half of the conventional Gracey curette and is slightly curved upwards which helps in adapting the instrument more closely to the tooth surface.

Grandmal seizures are a type of epileptic seizures involving whole body. There is no aura but sudden loss of consciousness with falling to the ground is there. Cry may be heard due to forced expiration. Finally the muscles are relaxed but patient remains unconscious for some time. Tongue biting and urinary incontinence is not rare. Headache and drowsiness may remain for a few days.

Granulocytes are the precursor and mature form of leukocytes characterized by neutrophilic, eosinophilic or basophilic granulocytes in their cytoplasm.

Granuloma is described a type of nodule which contains granulation tissue. On gingiva, it occurs as a swollen mass.

Granuloma gravidarum is a gingival lesions associated with pregnancy. 30 to 40% women show mild gingival enlargement. Post-delivery enlargement subsides on its own.

Granuloma inguinale is caused by Donovania granualomatosis. It is considered to be a venereal disease. External genitalia are affected more. Papule/nodule ulcerates soon. Lips, buccal mucosa or palate are affected. Painful ulcerated lesions sometimes bleed. Mucous membrane is

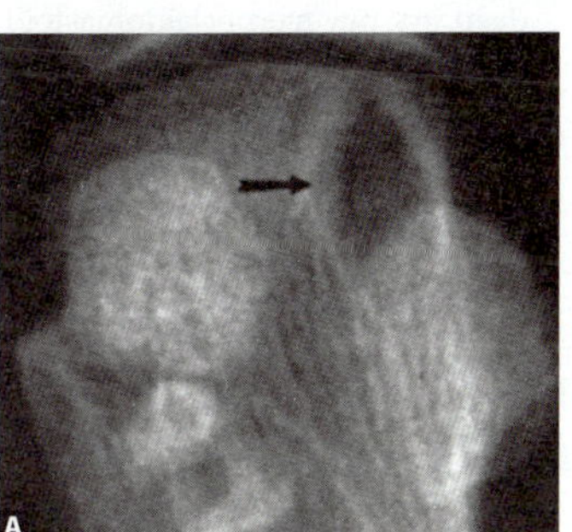

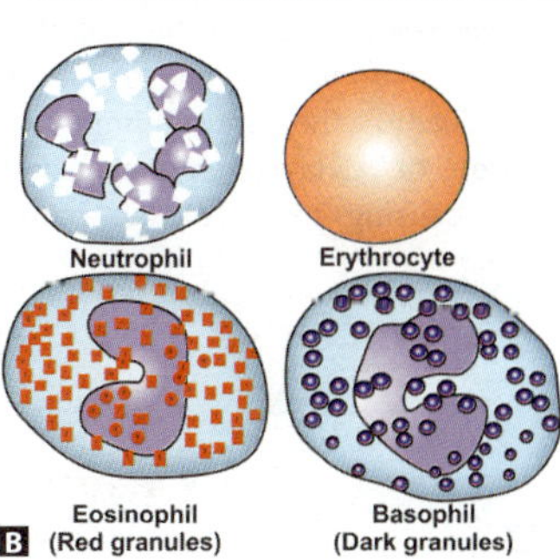

Figs A and B: *(A) Gout; (B) Granulocytes*

inflamed and edematous. Fibrous scar formation may be extensive.

Granulomatous cheilitis is also known as Miescher's syndrome of unknown etiology. Young females are more involved. Histologically, there is focal noncaseating granuloma formation. There will be epithelioid cells with Langhans type of giant cells. Clinical features: Lower lip is diffusely swelled up. There may be fever, headache and visual disturbances. Some may develop scales, fissures and pustules. Swelling is nonpitting. Swelling may be hard as rubber. Regional lymph nodes may be enlarged. It may be associated with Melkerson Rosenthal syndrome consisting of fissured tongue and facial paralysis. Differential diagnosis includes angioedema and sarcoidosis. Angioedema appears suddenly. History of recurrence is there. Sarcoidosis will be excluded by absence of any other manifestation and by a negative Kveim test. It is managed by repeated injection of corticosteroid every few weeks and cheiloplasty.

Granulomatous hypersensitivity: Clinically, the most important form of delayed hypersensitivity, causing many of the pathological effects in diseases, which involve, T-cell mediated immunity. It results from the presence within macrophages of a persistent agent usually a microorganism, which the cell is unable to destroy. May also be due to presence of immune complexes, which results in 'Epithelioid cell granuloma' formation.

Grasp is a precise control of movements during the instrumentation or performing any other dental procedure.

Grasp reflex: When the boy's palms are stimulated, the hand closes. This is also a corresponding plantar reflex. But movements disappeared by 24 months.

Gray lesions are not due to biologic pigment but due to the deposition of foreign material in connective tissue. It may be localized or diffuse. Color may be due to amalgam particles encountered in oral mucosa. Diffuse gray pigmentation is seen in silver, lead and bismuth.

Greater auricular nerve arises from the ventral rami of the second and third cervical nerve. Its origin lies deep to the sternocleidomastoid. Winding around the posterior border of the sternocleidomastoid muscle, it reaches its superficial surface. It pierces the deep fascia

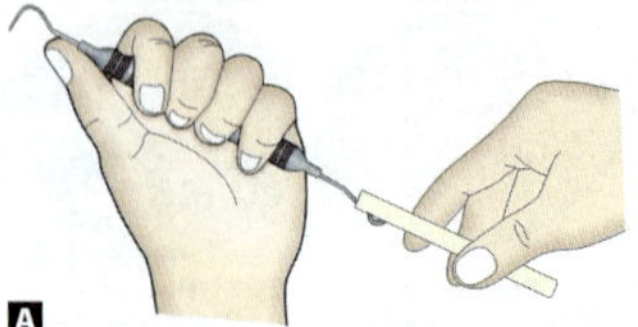

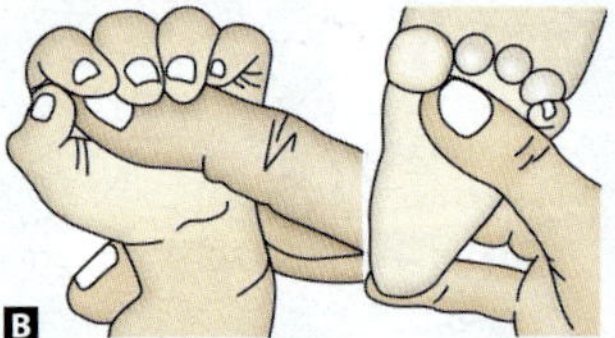

Figs A and B: *(A) Pen grasp; (B) Grasp reflex*

and runs upwards and somewhat forwards over the surface of the sternocleidomastoid muscle. Here it is accompanied by the external jugular vein.

Greater palatine nerve block is used for anesthetizing greater palatine nerve. It is given for anesthetizing posterior portion of hard palate and its overlying soft tissue, up to the first bicuspid.

Green stain: The appearance of these stains varies from light or yellowish green to very dark green. These stains are generally embedded in the bacterial plaque extending from facial to proximal. Generally facial one-third of the maxillary anterior teeth are involved. These stains appear to be soft and are difficult to remove stain of long-standing may cover a decalcified area of enamel. No microorganism has been identified to stain green.

Greenspan's syndrome is a triad of lichen planus, diabetes mellitus and hypertension. It may predispose to squamous cell carcinoma.

Grit size is a numerical grading of particle size. Larger numbers denote five particles; small numbers denote coarse particles.

Groove refers to a long, narrow depression.

Ground nut is known as poor man's dry fruit. It contains about 25% proteins and 40% fat. It does not contain vitamin C but contain high quantity of thiamine and nicotinic acid. In humid area it may develop aflatoxin which is harmful to body.

Ground substance (sol-gel colloidal system) is an amorphous matrix in which the connective tissue cells and fibers of the pulp are embedded. It is generally regarded as a gel rather than a sol and, therefore is considered to differ from tissue fluids. Because of its content of polyelectric polysaccharides, the extracellular matrix is responsible for the water-holding properties of connective tissues. It occupies the space between formed elements.

Growth curve is a graphic representation of the change in size of a bacterial population over a period of time, including a phase of log phase, a stationary phase and a death phase.

Growth field can be explained as follows, i.e. the bone doesn't grow by generalized uniform deposition of new bone on all outside surfaces with corresponding resorption from all inside surface because of the topographically complex nature of each bone's shape. The bone must have a differential mode of enlargement. Some of its parts

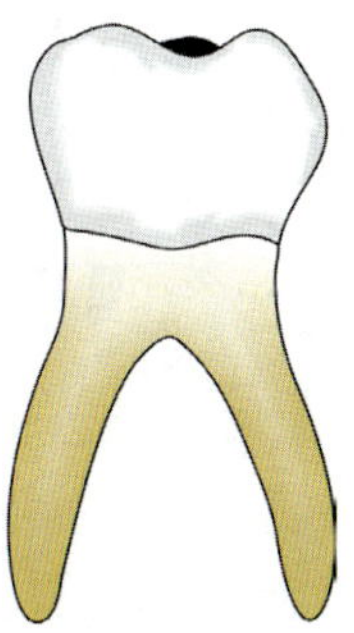

Fig.: *Groove*

G

and areas grow much faster and to greater extent.

Growth (JS Huxley) refers to selfmultiplication of living substance.

Growth (Krogman) refers to increase in size, change in proportion and progressive complexity.

Growth (Meredith) refers to entire series of sequential anatomic and physiological changes taking place from the beginning prenatal life to senility.

Growth (Moss) refers to change in any morphological parameter which is measurable.

Growth (Moyers) refers to quantitative aspect of biological development per unit of time.

Growth site refers to fields that have some special significance or noteworthy role in growth process are often called.

Growth spurts refer to the periods when sudden acceleration of growth occurs. This sudden increase in growth is termed as growth spurts. The growth spurts in the prenatal period and the infantile period involves the division of the cells. On the other hand, the physiological alteration in the hormonal secretion is believed to be the cause of pubertal growth spurts. The timing of growth spurts differs in boys and girls.

Growth (Todd) refers to an increase in size.

Gubernacular canal refers to the holes noted in a dry skull noted lingual to primary teeth in jaws that represent openings of gubernacular cord.

Gubernacular cord refers to the connective tissue overlying a successional tooth that connects with the lamina propria of the oral mucosa by means of a strand of fibrous connective tissue that contains remnants of dental lamina.

Gubernacular foramina are the small openings in maxilla are evidence of eruption pathways of permanent teeth. Gubernacular foramina are sites for gubernacular cords.

Guillain Barre syndrome is caused by progressive demyelinating neuropathy. It is an autoimmune following a nonspecific disease. Impaired swallowing or paresthesia of mouth and face is the early sign. There may be ascending anesthesia and paralysis of legs and trunk. In severe case, respiration is compromised.

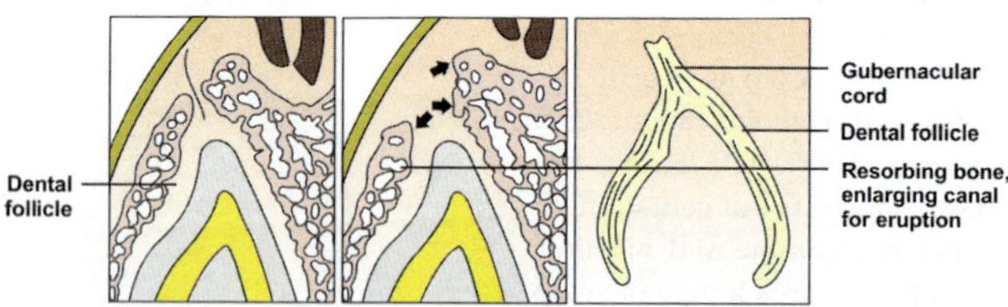

Fig.: *Gubernacular cords*

Gulland's sign is a quick, flexion of hips and knee in response to pinching of the contralateral quadriceps's muscle. It indicates meningeal irritation.

Gum: The mucous membrane over the alveolar processes of the jaws is firmly attached to underlying bone and is referred to as the gingivae.

Gunning type splint is a type of intermaxillary fixation introduced by Gunning in 1866 where the vulcanite overlay of the natural teeth which he used as a splint for fractured dentate mandible. Properly constructed gunning splint should hold jaws in a slightly over-closed relationship as the fractures of mandible are effectively used in this position. The splints are constructed in acrylic resin and the fitting surface is lined by black gutta percha.

Gustatory sense refers to sense of taste, therefore, called gustatory sense and taste are special organs of taste. Taste receptors are located on tongue and are known as chemoreceptors. Basic taste sensations are sweat, salty, sour and bitter.

Gutta percha clay like material used in the filling of root canals. The material used due to its stability and easy manipulation. Material is inert so action is not chemical one. Because it is put after being heated, injury may be thermal. It provides a poor seal of the cavity margins hence saliva may leak and irritate the pulp.

H

Habit (DSM III-R) (1987) is a mental disorder which is non-goal directed, repetitive and intentional behavior often performed rhythmically, that are of sufficient severity to cause physical injury to or to interfere markedly with the normal activities of the child, adolescent or adult.

Habit can be defined as the tendency towards an act that has become a repeated performance, relatively fixed, consistent and easy to perform by an individual or Habit according to *Buttersworth (1961)* is a frequent, constant practice or an acquired tendency which has been fixed by frequent repetition. Habit according to *Finn* is an act, which is socially unacceptable. Habit according to *Hogem Boom (1953)* was also defined as the methodical way in which mind and body act as a result of the frequent repetition of certain definite set of nervous impulses. Habit according to *William James (1972)* is an acquired habit from a psychological point of view, is nothing but a new pathway of discharge formed in the brain by which certain incoming currents tend to escape. Habit according to *Boucher (1982)* was also defined as a tendency towards an act that has become a repeated performance relatively fixed, easy to perform and almost automatic.

Habitual cheek biting refers to a more of a superficial lesion produced due to constant trauma by rubbing, sucking or chewing movements which abrade the area of lip cheek. It does not produce ulceration. These are poorly macerated and reddened areas. It is a subconscious nervous habit.

Habitual mouth breathing refers to a condition where oral breathing persists as habit even after the removal of the nasal obstruction or any other underlying etiology. Interceptive procedures should involve identification and removal of the cause. Persistence of habitual oral breathing is an indication to use a vestibular screen to intercept the habit.

Habitual tongue thrust refers to a condition where the tongue thrust swallow is present as a habit even after the cessation of the malocclusion.

Hemophilia is a fatal inherited bleeding disorder. There is

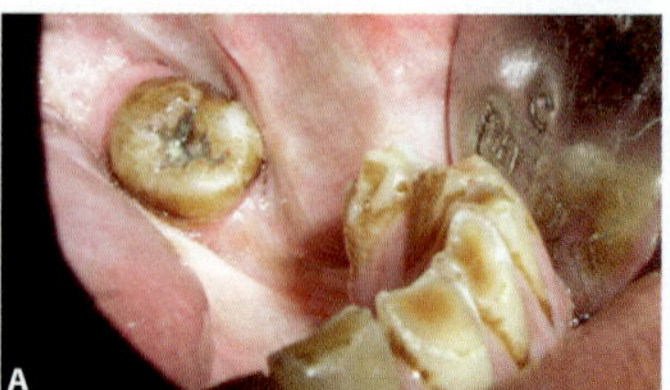

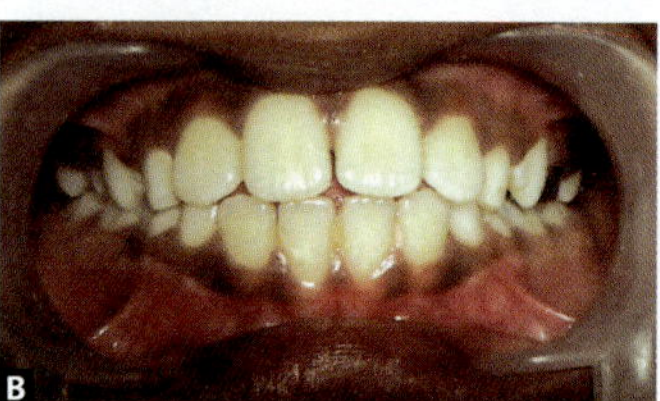

Figs A and B: *(A) Habitual cheek biting; (B) Habitual mouth breather*

reduction in clotting factor. It is a sex-linked recessive trait. It is of two types: Hemophilia A, classic Hemophilia, Hemophilia B, Christmas type. In Hemophilia A, factor VIII is missing and in Hemophilia B, factor IX is missing. *Clinical Features:* Serious bleeding may occur from umbilical cord. Easy bruising and prolonged bleeding. Spontaneous bleeding in subcutaneous tissue. Fatal epistaxis may develop rarely. Gastric bleeding from ulcer may develop. Spontaneous intracranial hemorrhage may develop. *Oral manifestations:* Gingival tissue may bleed after extraction, recurrent subperiosteal hematoma of jaw may develop, high caries index, severe periodontal disease. Dental extraction remains problematic and should be done with a lot of caution.

Hemorrhoids refers to piles is varicosities of the hemorrhoidal venous plexuses. Commonest place to occur is anal sphincter. These may be caused in anal sphincter. These may be caused by increased intrabdominal pressure as in pregnancy, rectal tumors and constipation.

Hair papilla refers to a small, cap-shaped cluster of cells located at the base of follicle where hair growth begins.

Hair source: Hair from head is usually long and soft and taper gradually. Hair from female head is thinner. Hair from beard and moustache are usually thicker than those from any part of the body. Hair from chest, axilla and pubic region are short and thicker. Pubic hair and from axilla show split ends. Hair from eyebrows, eyelashes and nostrils are stiff, thick and bristly. Hair from body surface is fine, short and flexible. They don't show pigment cells in cortex. Medullary canal is small. The fine downy hair of newborn infant has no medullary canal or pigment cells.

Hairy leukoplakia is highly indicative of HIV infection.

Hairy tongue is an unusual condition characterized by hypertrophy of filliform papillae of tongue. Normally keratinized surface layers of filliform papillae are continuously desquamated due to friction of food and anterior upper teeth. These are replaced by new epithelial cells from below. When tongue movements

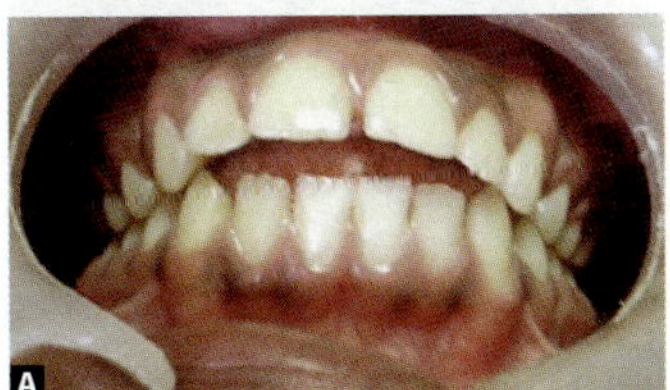

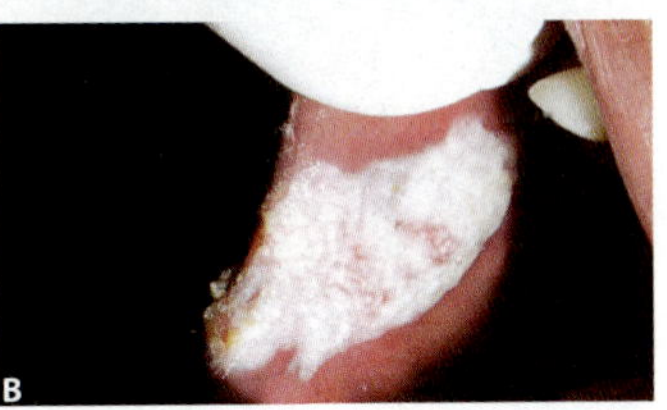

Figs A and B: *(A) Habitual tongue thrust; (B) Hariy leukoplakia*

become restricted during illness, the papilla enlarges and becomes heavily coated. The color of papilla varies from yellowish white, brown, black depending upon the type of stains, the tongue is exposed to. Longer papilla entangles food particles of different colors. Tobacco smoke colors it black. Mid-dorsum is first to be affected. Dehydration and terminally-ill patients also develop thick coatings. Nicotinamide deficiency may produce black hairy tongue in experimental animals. Excessive exposure of radiation to head and neck area and systemic antibiotics may also produce hairy tongue. Because the condition is benign, the treatment is also empirical, in such cases, thorough scrapping and cleaning of tongue is advised to promote desquamation and removal of debris.

Halitosis, in general, means bad breath, and is also known as oral malodor. The term halitosis originated from the Latin word halitus, breath, and the Greek-osis, meaning abnormal condition. Oral malodor is a common complaint that may periodically affect people of all age groups. Oral bacterial decay of food and residual debris causes formation of volatile sulfur compounds which are responsible for bad breath. If no bad breath is detectable and the patient is complaining of it, pseudo-halitosis may be considered. It may be due to halitophobia and may occur in psychiatric diseases.

Halothane is a non-irritating, potent anesthetic agent which can produce profound anesthesia without hypoxia. Its induction and recovery is quick. It is a poor analgesic but is used in dentistry with 70% N_2O/30% O_2 concentration. Skeletal muscle is relaxed. Uterine contractions are depressed. In dental practice it relaxes the masseter muscle and inhibits salivation. Laryngospasm is inhibited and classical signs of anesthesia are lacking.

Hamartomas are tumor-like malformations. These are usually congenital. Once these have achieved adult dimensions, these don't increase in size.

Hand plugger is a hand instrument that has diameter larger than spreader and has blunt end. It is used to compact the warm gutta-

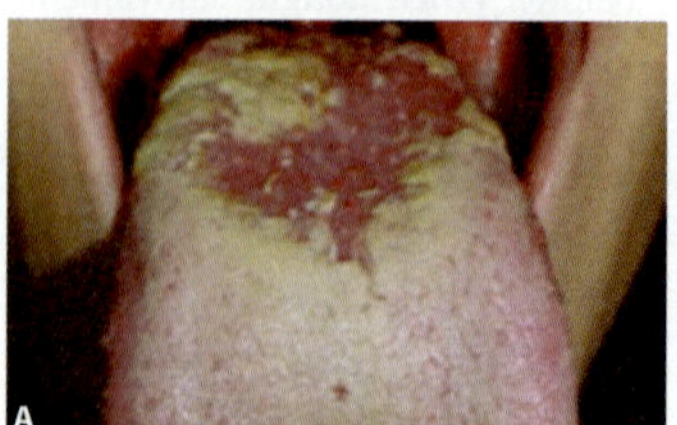

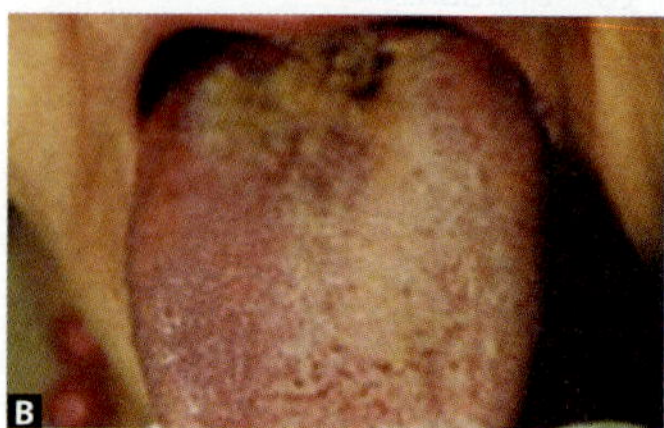

Figs A and B: *Hairy tongue*

percha vertically and laterally into the root canal. It is also used to carry small segments of gutta-percha into the canal during sectional filling technique. Calcium hydroxide or MTA-like materials may also be packed into the canals using hand plugger.

Hand Schuller Christian disease occurs in early life. Oral manifestations are often nonspecific. It includes sore mouth, gingivitis and suppuration. There develops an unpleasant taste. Lesions in skull are sharply outlined. Leukopenia and thrombocytopenia is often found. Prognosis is good.

Hand, foot and mouth disease is an endemic disease of very young children. There is formation of maculo-papular, exanthematous and vesicular lesions of skin. Low grade fever, lymphadenopathy, diarrhea and vomiting develop. Oral manifestation includes small, multiple vesicular and ulcerative oral lesions. Hard palate, lips and gingiva are involved. Intracytoplasmic viral inclusions can be shown in vesicular scrapings. No specific treatment is needed.

Handpiece is an instrument to hold burs, endodontic instruments or oral hygiene scaling tips that connect them to the power source. Actual speed of cutting depends on type of hand-pieces. Low-speed hand-pieces up to 4000 revolutions a minute are driven by a miniature compressed air. Contrangle hand-piece is used because it provides access to every tooth. Air turbine hand-pieces are driven at a speed of 40,0000 revolutions a minute. These are contrangled and are used with a built-in water spray to counteract the heat generated by high speed cutting. There is absence of vibration. Disadvantage is of high-pitched whistling noise.

Hanging is a form of asphyxial death produced by suspending body with a ligature around the neck; the constricting force is the weight of the body. It takes a few seconds when knot is over cricoid cartilage

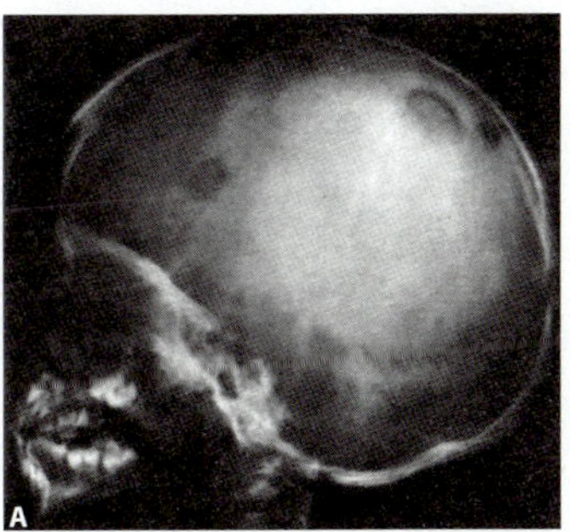

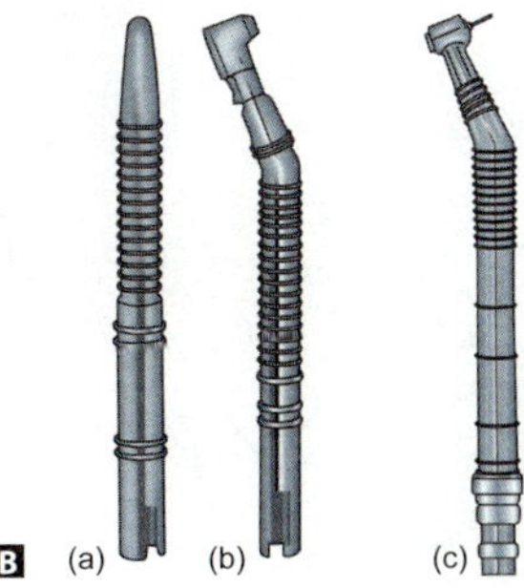

Figs A and B: *(A) Hand Schuller Christian disease; (B) Handpieces, [(a) Straight; (b) Contra-angle; (c) Air turbine]*

and 1–2 minutes when it is over larynx. Neck is found stretched and elongated. Head is always inclined to opposite side of the knot. Face is pale but may be swollen. Tongue is caught between teeth, protruded and bitten. Bloody froth may be seen at mouth or nostrils. Hands are often clenched. Escape of urine or faces is often found.

Hard lasers (High-level energy) refer to thermal lasers emitted at wavelength in the visible infrared and UV range. Example: Er: YAG laser; Nd: YAG laser.

Hard palate is the anterior portion of roof of mouth.

Hardness refers to a material's resistance to penetration when indented by a hard material. The hardness of dental material is reported in Knoop hardness number. Larger the indentation, smaller will be the hardness number. Enamel and porcelain are two of the hardest materials and have highest numbers. Hardness of certain material is enamel 350, dentin 60, acrylic resin 20, dental amalgam 100, porcelain 450, alloys 420.

Harmful habits refer to those habits that have a deleterious effect on the teeth and their supporting structures, such as thumb-sucking, mouth-breathing, tongue-thrusting etc.

Harmonal sialadenosis is associated with menarche, menses and pregnancy. Hypogenitalism, gynecomastia and menopause may also cause it. Diabetes results in retromandibular enlargement of parotid.

Haversian canal refers to a canal in bone tissue containing nerve and blood vessels surrounded by concentric layers of calcified bone tissue.

Headache is produced by stimulation of pain sensitive structures within the cranium or the extra-cranial tissues. Cranial bones

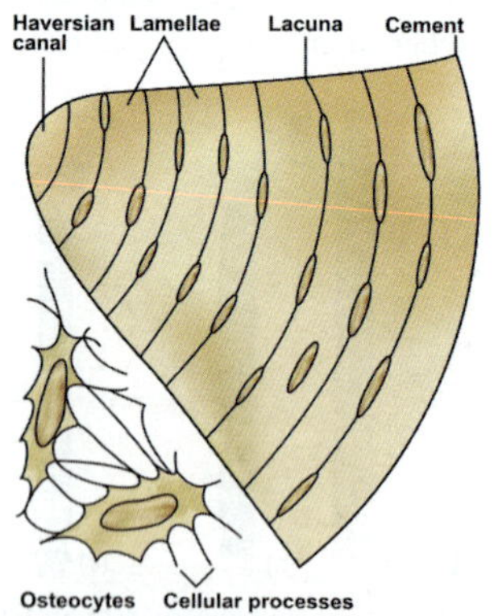

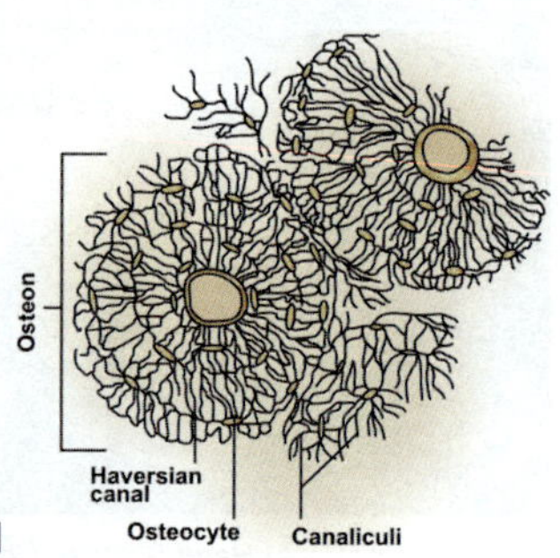

Figs A and B.: *Haversian canal*

are insensitive. Within the skull, sensitive areas are meninges, walls of venous sinuses, large arteries. Most of the cerebral substance itself is insensitive to stimuli which are painful.

Headache of intracranial origin is due to inflammation, compression and distortion of or traction upon the pain sensitive meninges and blood vessels within skull.

Healing of fracture refers to formation of blood clot formed due to damaged blood vessels in medulla, cortex and periosteum. Within 24 hours the hematoma is converted into vascular, fibroblastic granulation tissue. After about 7 days cartilage and osteoid tissues are laid down by osteoblasts. It forms callus. Provisional callus is converted into normal vein. After a period of time bone is moulded by osteoclasts and osteoblasts.

Health history is a structured format and must be recorded as it is.

Health promotion is the science of art of helping the lifestyle of individuals and society to attain optimal health.

Health refers to state of complete physical, mental and social well-being not merely the absence of disease.

Health education is a communication activity aimed at enabling individuals to achieve positive health.

Hearing acquity is the ability to hear and identify the sound.

Hearing impairment hard of hearing or deafness refers to conditions in which individuals are fully or partially unable to detect or perceive at least some frequencies of sound which can typically be heard by members of their species. Hearing loss when applied to humans, the term impaired is rejected, wherein the terms deaf and hard of hearing are preferred.

Heart attack is expressed by sudden onset of a severe crushing pain

H

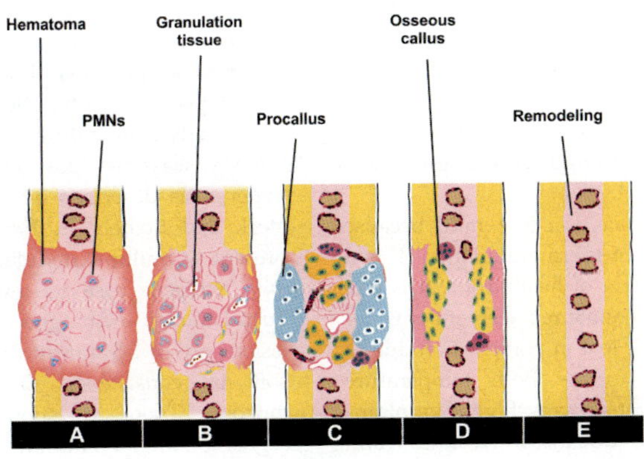

Fig.: *Healing of fracture*

across the chest pain; may radiate to shoulder, left arm and jaw. It is caused by coronary heart disease.

Heart block is a blockage of impulse conduction from atria to ventricles so that the heart beats at a slower rate than normal.

Heat capacity is the amount of energy it takes to raise the temperature of that object by 1°C. Some metals require more energy than others.

H

Heat cramps develop in those who are doing heavy muscular work in high temperature and humidity. There are painful and spasmodic contractions of calf muscles. Sodium chloride level in blood goes down.

Heat cure silicone is the dental material. Advantages include adequate bond strength to acrylic resiliency and more resistant to aqueous environment. Disadvantages include low tear strength and poor resistance abrasion.

Heat cured acrylic denture base is the denture base material used for fabricating denture. It has a good appearance with high glass transition temperature, easy fabrication, low capital cost and good surface finish. But it has low impact strength and fatigue life is too short.

Heat exhaustion is a mild because failure of thermoregulation. It is a mild form of heat stroke. It is due to inadequate replacement of water and salt lost in perspiration due to thermal stress. Body temperature does not go very high. Symptoms include dizziness, weakness and fatigue.

Heat of fusion is the amount of energy required to melt a material.

Heat of vaporization is the amount of energy required to boil a material.

Heat sterilizing refers to the use of an autoclave or dry-heat sterilizer to kill all potential disease-causing agents that remain following patient treatment. Any instrument that is not heat stable and cannot tolerate high temperatures should be thoroughly cleaned and soaked in disinfectant chemicals.

Heat stroke is said to have occurred when there is feeling of heat, headache confusion, disorientation, emotional bursts, giddiness and vomiting develop. Excessive thirst may be fect. Temperature of body may arise up to 106°F. Face will be flushed and pupils dilated. When in shock, hypotension, tachycardia and hurried respiration will set in. Urine becomes scanty. Heat cramps occur due to loss of sodium chloride.

Heat syncope is a mild effect of hot environment. Person standing in sun becomes pale, his BP falls and he collapses suddenly. There is no rise in body temperature.

Heck's disease is focal epithelial hyperplasia described by Archard Heck and Stanely in 1965. It is present as multiple nodular lesion with a sessile base on lower lip, buccal mucosa and tongue. Nodular lesions are of 1-5 mm in diameter, soft in consistency of buccal mucosa. There is spontaneous regression after 4-6 months. It does not require any treatment.

Hedstroem file (H-file) is a root shaping instrument that has flutes which resemble successively triangles set one on another. It is made by cutting the spiral grooves into round, tapered steel wire in the same manner as wood screws are made. This results in formation of a sharp edge which cuts on removing strokes only. Hedstroem file cuts only when instrument is withdrawn because its edges face the handle of the instrument. When used in torquing motion, its edges can engage in the dentin of root canal wall, causing H-files to fracture. Rake angle and distance between the flutes are two main features which determine working of the file. H-file has positive rake angle, i.e. its cutting edge is turned in the same direction in which the force is applied which makes it to dig the dentin, thus more aggressive in cutting. Hedstroem file should be used to machine the straight canal because it is strong and aggressive cutter. Since it lacks the flexibility and is fragile in nature, the H-file tends to fracture when used in torquing action.

Helix angle is the angle formed by cutting edge with the long axis of the tooth.

Helper t-cells refer to CD4.

Hemangioendothelioma is a malignant angiomatous neoplasm of mesenchymal tissue. It is more common in younger age group. Oral lesions are not very common. *Clinical features:* It is a fast enlarging. There is presence of localized, nodular, painful swelling. Surface ulceration is present. Teeth become mobile and bleed on pressure. Jaw shows destruction. Lesion is expansible with cortical expansion. Surgical excision and radiotherapy helps.

Hemangioma is proliferative lesions of vascular tissue. It may be by birth. In oral cavity, these frequently occur. *Clinical features:* These are raised, red/blue/purple lesions. Lesions are raised, but are easily blanched on pressure. These are soft and pulsatile. Capillary hemangioma are characterized by small, numerous, endothelial lined pyogenic granuloma. Cavernous hemangioma reveals large, irregularly shaped, dilated

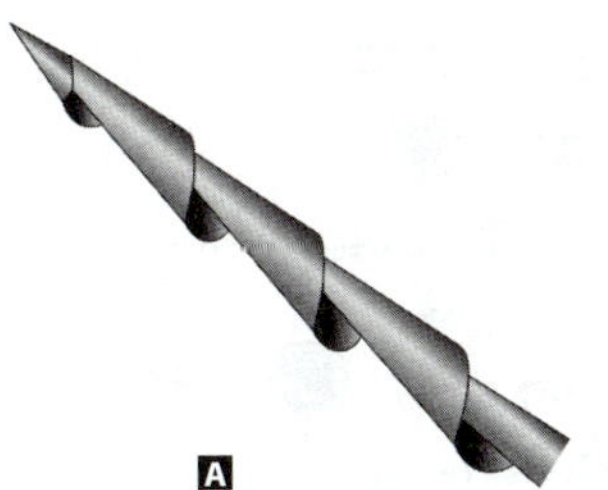

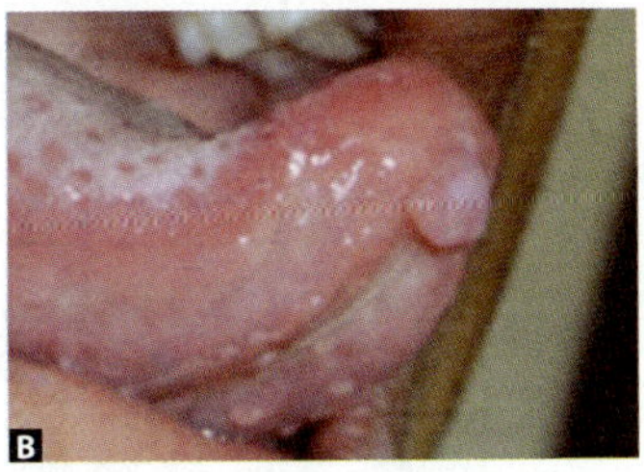

Figs A and B: *(A) H-file; (B) Lingual hemangioma*

endothelial lined sinuses. Such blood pooled sinuses are communicating with each other. These lack muscular coat. Local excision is the treatment. In case of large lesion, sclerosing agents may be given earlier to reduce the size.

Hemangioma of tongue is a painless and slowly growing swelling of tongue. It is diffuse and bluish in color. It is compressible extending into floor of mouth and check.

Hematoma refers to a collection or pooling of blood.

Hematopoiesis is the process by which blood cells grow, divide and differentiate in bone marrow. There are three general classes of blood cells derived from a pool of pluripotent hematopoietic stem cells (HSC), which reside in the marrow and have the unique ability to give rise to all of the different mature blood cell types: RBC, Platelets and WBC.

Hematopoietic stem cells (HSC) are defined by their abilities to self-renew throughout life and give rise to committed progenitors that can differentiate along all of the possible hematopoietic lineages. HSCs are self-renewing cells; when they proliferate, some of their daughter cells remain as HSC, so they are not depleted. HSC daughter cells can commit to any of several alternative differentiation pathways that lead to production of one or more of types of blood cells. Progression along these pathways is coupled to cell division. The more mature forms greatly outnumber the less differentiated precursors. Most types of hematopoietic cells lose

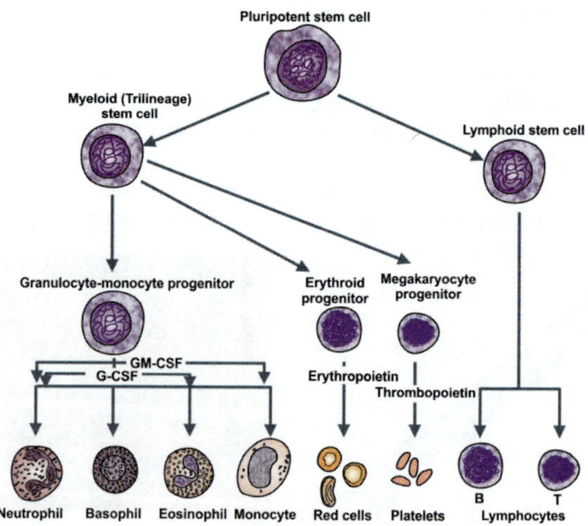

Fig.: *Hematopoietic stem cells*

their replicative capacity altogether, by the time they are fully mature and are said to be terminally differentiated. Progressively HSC initially commit to one of three main alterative different pathways or lineages. The most primitive cell in each lineage called 'Lineage committed progenitors.'

Hematospermia is the presence of blood in the ejaculate resulting from inflammation of prostate or seminal vesicle. Blood in initial portion of ejaculate suggests involvement of prostate while terminal hematospermia implies seminal vesicle origin.

Hemiplegia refers to the involvement in one side of the body, with the upper extremity generally more affected than the lower. Twenty percent of children who have spastic cerebral palsy have hemiplegia. In many cases, the cause is a focal traumatic, vascular, or infectious lesion. A unilateral brain infarct is apparent on MRI. All hemiplegic children walk independently by the age of 3 years.

Hemiplegic gait is a spastic gait in which only one leg is involved. Spasticity does not allow leg to flex freely at hip, knee and ankle. Leg rotates outwards and makes a semicircle. Each leg is advanced slowly. Scissors gait is noted. It is the manifestation of cerebral diplegia, ischemic brain damage and compressive myelopathy.

Hemisection is the splitting of two rooted tooth into two separate portions.

Hemiseptum can be described as one wall bony defect.

Hemochromatosis is an iron storage disease and is of two types. One is idiopathic and secondary form. Normal body contains 2 to 4 gram of iron when it reaches 15-40 gram clinical signs and symptoms of hemochromatosis appear. There is slow progressive enlargement of liver with fibrosis and ending up in cirrhosis. Hemosiderin deposit in skin gives slate gray color. Cardiac arrhythmia and heart failure may develop. Serum ferritin may go > 300 g/L.

Hemolysin is a substance that causes destruction of red blood cells in such a manner that hemoglobin is released.

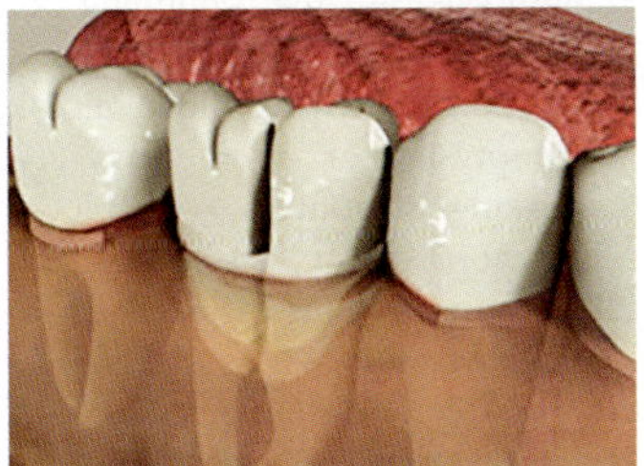

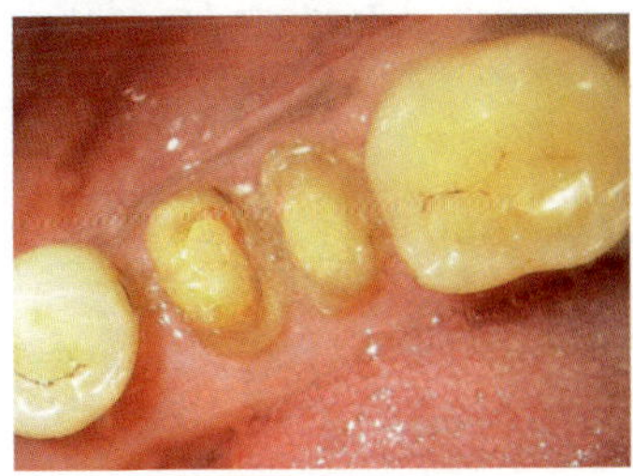

Fig.: *Schematic and clinical presentation of hemisectioned tooth*

Hemolysis can be described as breakage of RBC membrane. Hemolysis can be caused by infection acidosis or drug abuse. Symptoms include fatigue, weakness, light headedness, dyspnea on exertion, upper abdomen pain and nocturnal hemoglobinuria. Person will develop pallor, jaundice and splenomegaly.

Hemolytic anemia is a group of disorder in which red blood cell survival is reduced. Destruction may be episodic or continuous. Reticulocysis is a clue to disorder. Hemolysis increases the indirect bilirubin. Serum LDH levels are strikly elevated. It occurs due to increased hemolysis in body and becomes difficult by bone marrow to compensate. Hereditary causes include thalassemia, hereditary spherocytosis, sickle cell anemia, acquired autoimmune hemolysis and erythroblastosis fetalis. Certain chemical agents can also damage to RBCs. *Clinical features* include: Pallor, weakness and fatigability, jaundice, dyspnea may also occur. *Oral Manifestations:* Pallor of oral mucosa, discoloration of teeth in the event of erythroblastosis. Blood hemoglobin level goes down to 10 mg/dL and average survival of RBC comes down to 12 days instead of 120 days. Reticulocyte count is raised. Treatment includes blood transfusion in severe cases, splenectomy in cases of spherocytosis and administration of folic acid.

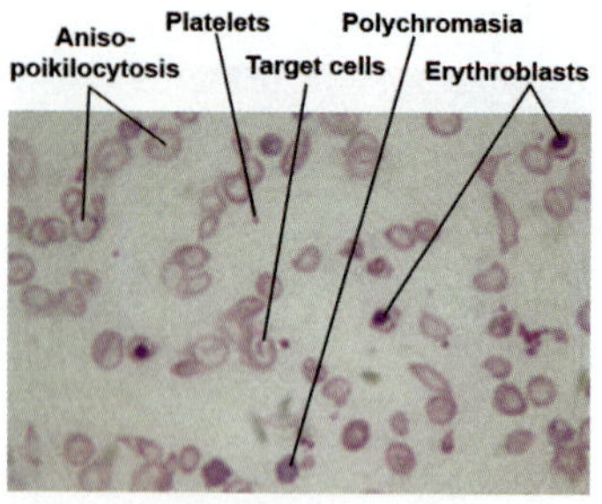

Fig.: *Hemolytic anemia*

Hemolytic uremic syndrome is a condition that results from abnormal premature destruction of RBCs, renal failure and low platelet count. Clinically it can be manifested as vomiting diarrhea, purpuric rash, malaise, fatigue and cremia.

Hemopericardium refers to the presence of blood and blood-stained fluid in the pericardial sac. Causes include transmural myocardial infarct, ruptured aneurysm of aorta and penetrating injuries. When bleeding is rapid, death may take place. Treated pericardium may produce thickening of pericardium and adhesions.

Hemoptysis is the coughing of blood in the sputum. The blood may be coughed up alone (Frank hemoptysis) or there may be streaking of sputum with blood. Expectoration of 200 to 600 mL blood in 24 hours is defined as massive hemoptysis.

Hemostasis is arrest of bleeding.

Hemostat refers to a small surgical clamp.

Hepadnaviruses are small, spherical DNA viruses causing hepatitis, chronic liver infections and liver cancer. Their mode of transmission along with blood is via saliva too.

Heparin is found in large amount in mast cells of liver and lung. It is a strongest organic acid in body. It is released with histamine in anaphylactic shock. It prevents the conversion of prothrombin to thrombin. It may also decrease the conversion of fibrinogen to fibrin.

Hepatic encephalopathy is a life-threatening disorder. It causes mild personality changes and slight tremor. Person becomes lethargic with aberrant behavior. Lastly patient becomes stuporous and hyperventilation sets in. there may develop bradycardia, Decreased respiration and seizures.

Hepatitis A virus is nonenveloped 27 nm RNA virus enterovirus group. It is excreted in feces and transmission is by feco-oral route. The antibody to HVA is detected during first week of infection and IgM type. Incubation period varies from 2-6 weeks. Nausea, vomiting, loss of appetite precedes 1-2 weeks. Dark urine and stool may be noticed. Liver is enlarged and becomes soft. During recovery appetite improves. Management includes restrictions of fat and increased glucose intake. B-complex supplements help.

Hepatitis B is a 42 nm DNA virus with 3 antigenically distinct components. HBsAg can be detected in blood during prodrome and remains during the entire icteric phase. The spread is by infected blood, blood products, and breast milk. Incubation period lasts six weeks to six months.

Hepatitis C 90% cases of post-transfusion hepatitis. Hepatitis C virus is a single-stranded RNA virus. It has properties similar to flavivirus. No vaccine is available. Treatment of HCV is with low-dose alpha interferon with 30-50% success over 3-12 months. After treatment relapse is very common.

Hepatitis G is closely related to HCV and is transmitted through blood. Blood donors suffer the most 1-3%. Not much is known about it because it does not cause any specific disease.

Hepatocellular carcinoma arises from parenchymal cells. It is associated with cirrhosis in general and hepatitis B and C in particular. Liver becomes tender with palpable mass. Friction rub over tumor may be heared. There will be anemia with leukocytosis.

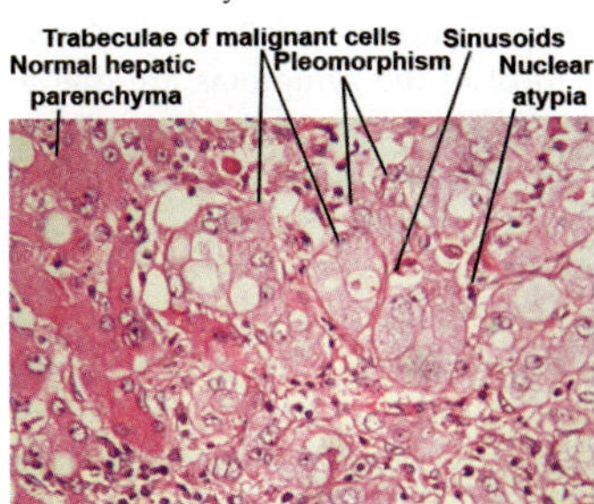

Fig.: *Hepatocellular carcinoma*

Hereditary benign intraepithelial dyskeratosis is also known as Wit-Kop-Von Sallman syndrome. It is an autosomal dominant trait. Appear as white, spongy macerated lesions of buccal mucosa. These are present on floor of mouth, tongue gingiva and palate. There may be white plaques overlaying the cornea producing blindness. Buccal mucosa exhibits thickening of epithelium with pronounced hydropic degeneration. Histologically peculiar intraepithelial dyskeratosis, in addition to acanthosis, is seen. Cell with in cell phenomenon occurs.

Hereditary fructose intolerance (HFI) is caused by remarkably reduced levels of hepatic fructose-1-phosphate aldolase, which splits fructose-1-phosphate into two 3-carbon fragments for further metabolism. Persons affected with this rare metabolic disorder have learned to avoid any food that contains fructose or sucrose, because the ingestion of these foods can cause nausea, vomiting, malaise, tremor, excessive sweating, and coma due to fructosemia. Most of the symptoms are due to a secondary hypoglycemia. These persons live quite comfortably on other foods (glucose, galactose, and lactose-containing foods like milk, bread, dairy products, rice, and noodles). Although there have been only a limited number of cases reported in the literature, the dental caries prevalence in these subjects has been extremely low.

Hereditary hemorrhagic telangiectasia are characterized by multiple round of oval purple papules. The size is below 0.5 cms in diameter. Number may even be one hundred. Purple papules are seen on lips, tongue and buccal mucosa.

Hereditary mucoepithelial dysplasia is an autosomal dominant disorder. Whole of the oral mucosa is involved and oral lesion is a fiery red. Gingival and hard palate are commonly involved. Fissured tongue is seen.

Herpe's zoster is an acute infectious viral disease. It is very painful and of incapacitating nature. Virus causing it is similar to chicken pox. General malaise, pain and tenderness along with the involved sensory nerve are the symptoms. Often trunk is affected. Patient has a linear popular or vesicular eruption of the skin or mucosa supplied by affected nerves. It is unilateral and dermatomic in distribution. It may affect face due to infection of Trigeminal nerve. Extremely painful buccal mucosal lesions occur. Antiviral drugs are to be continued.

Herpangina is a viral disease of summer caused by coxsackie group of virus. Symptoms are mild and of short duration. It includes sore-throat, headache, vomiting and abdominal pain. Small ulcer shows greyish base and inflamed periphery. There may develop fever, pain and enlargement of lymph glands. Lymphocytosis is constant. Disease spreads from one person to another. No treatment is needed as the lesion is self-limiting.

Herpes labialis may be caused by common cold and febrile injection. Prodromal paresthesia, burning sensation and then erythema develops. Vesicles form after an hour or two. Vesicles enlarge, coalesce and weep exudates. After 2 days, these rupture and coalesce. Aciclovir cream helps.

Herpes simplex virus infection AIDS patients, patients on immune suppressed drugs are most likely to develop chronic oral ulcers. On these response of T lymphocytes changes. There is formation of small, round, symmetric lesions associated with recurrent herpes infection. Lesions last from weeks to months. Larger lesions have raised white borders of small vesicles.

Herpetic conjunctivitis is a serious disease because it may cause blindness.

Herpetic Whitlow can be transmitted through saliva or fingers. Incubation period is 2 to 12 days. It causes tingling, fever, chills and general malaise. Infected area becomes red and swollen with severe pain.

Herpetiform aphthae are multiple, painful, recurrent mouth ulcers. Ulcers are multiple; shape is irregular with ill-defined edges. Floor is grey. Size is small up to 1 to 3 mm.

Heterodont refers to different types of teeth within the same dentition, i.e. Incisors, canines, molars.

Heterograft is graft obtained from another species. Usually porcine skin is used. Though used very rarely because it is very expensive.

Hexachlorophene is an anti-bacterial effect bacteriostatic effect. It is used as presurgical scrub. It has been incorporated in tooth paste.

Hiatus hernia is a sliding type stomach with esophagogastric junction slides upwards through the hiatus into chest. In paraesophageal type esophago-gastric junction is fixed below the diaphragm and a part of stomach herniates through the hiatus besides the esophagus. There will be retrosternal chest pain especially on stooping or lying down soon after meals. Nocturnal regurgitation may cause choking attacks.

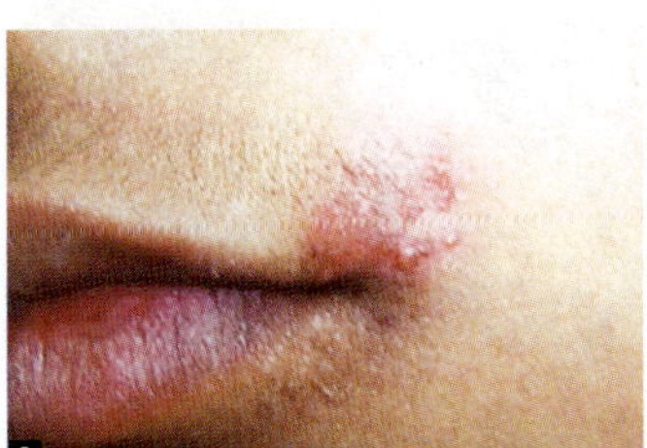

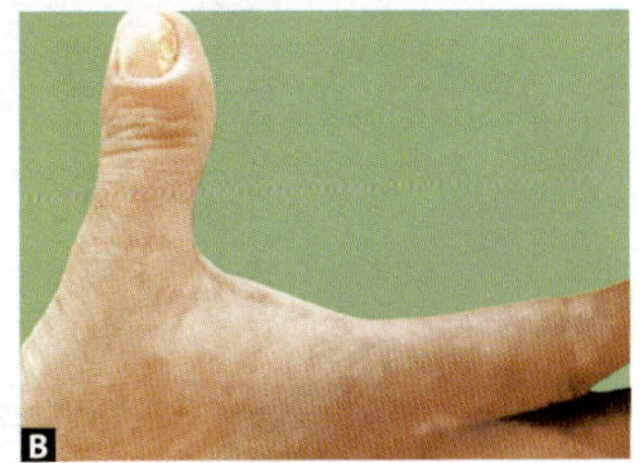

Figs A and B: *(A) Herpes labialis; (B) Herpetic whitlow*

Hierarchy of needs was given by Maslow in the year 1954 believed in self-actualization theory, i.e., the need to understand the totality of a person. The general requirements were arranged in a hierarchy. If one basic requirement is satisfied then next one emerges in the order. The desire for the most basic biologic needs to the more psychological ones becomes them after basic needs have been satisfy. Motivation is constantly required and is a never-ending, fluctuating complex present in almost all organisms. Pain avoidance, tension reduction and pleasure acts as source of motivating behavior.

High copper alloy is a dental alloy with a relatively high copper content by 10% weight. It is corrosion free.

High gold alloys are composed principally of gold and platinum group metals with minor addition of tin, indium and iron. Gold content is 78 to 87% by weight. Tin, indium and iron are added to promote a good porcelain bond to meal oxide. The alloy is light yellow in color. Corrosion resistance is excellent.

High-risk patients are the patients in whom frequency of infectious disease is higher. High-risk patient groups include patients requiring frequent blood transfusions, patients of renal dialysis units and immune deficient individuals. Intravenous drug users are also at risk.

High spots are used in reference to sealant areas with sealant material that interferes with occlusion.

High transverse fracture *see* Lefort III.

High-voltage burns are the electrical burns that are caused by contact with high voltage electric lines ranging from 10,000 to 32,000 volts. The tissues are so extensively and rapidly damaged that they usually involve amputation of a limb either partly or completely. In these cases the damage actually extends into the normal tissues quite proximal to the apparently affected areas. This is to be kept on mind while doing amputation as the level of amputation can be higher than what is planned because

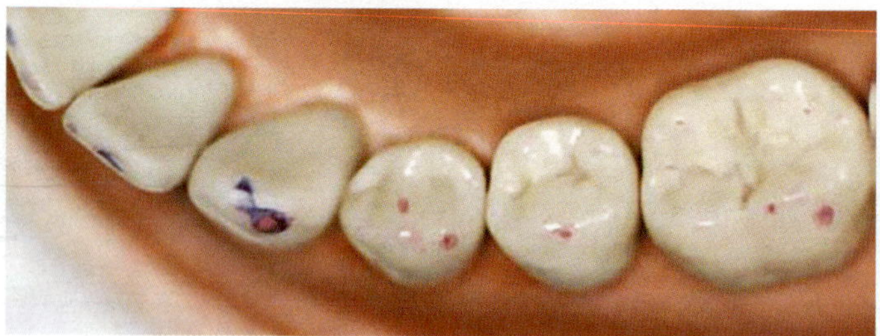

Fig.: *High spots*

of proximally damaged muscles below the normal skin.

High-stepping gait is adopted to avoid tripping from the toes catching the ground. It develops when there is weakness of extensor muscles of feet as in perineal nerve palsy.

Hill's sign: If femoral systolic pulse pressure 60 to 100 mm higher in right leg than right arm, it is indicative of aortic insufficiency.

Hirsutism is a condition where there is growth depending on the testosterone. Cells of hair follicle secrete in enzyme which acts on testosterone and makes it active.

Histamine is a vasoactive amine—acts as a vasodilator, increases permeability of the small blood vessels and functions as a central nervous system neurotransmitter.

Histiocytosis develops due to proliferation of histiocytic cells occurring in bone marrow, spleen and liver. Lesions around jaw are common. Localized destructive lesion occurs. Tooth buds may be destroyed.

Histologic pocket depth *see* biologic pocket depth.

Histoplasmosis is caused by fungus histoplasma capsulatum. It is a demographic fungus. Inhaling infected dust may cause the infection. Person develops low-grade fever, productive cough, lymphadenopathy and enlargement of liver and spleen. Oral lesion develops after pulmonary involvement. Oral manifestations appear as nodular, ulcerative or vegetative lesions. These appear as nodular, ulcerative lesions on buccal mucosa, tongue palate or lips. Ulcerated areas are covered by gray membrane. Organisms may be easily isolated. Nodule may ulcerate and grow slowly. Cervical lymph glands may be enlarged and firm. Culture of infected tissue

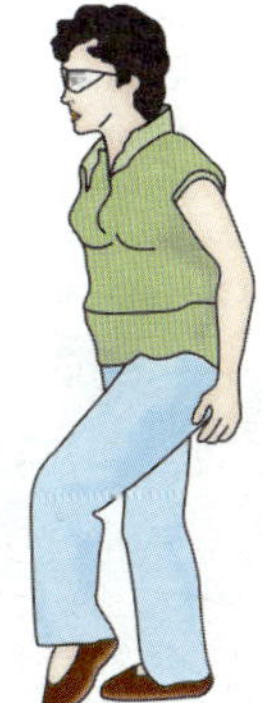

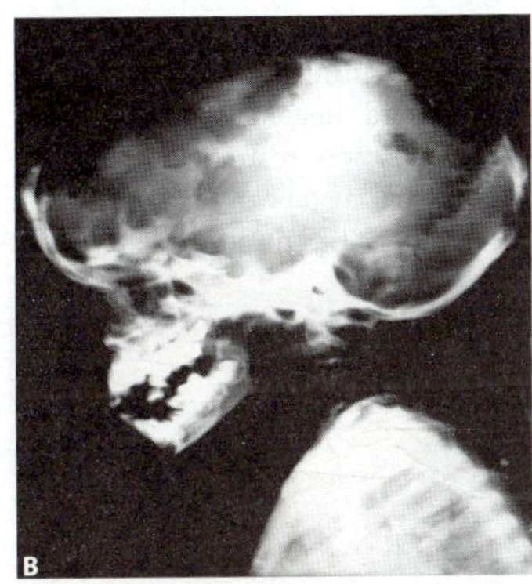

Figs A and B: *(A) High-stepping gait; (B) Punched out lesions in the skull due to histiocytosis*

may give appropriate diagnosis. Treatment includes ketoconazole for 6-12 months.

Historical research is a research in which past events are documented because they are of inherent interest or because they can provide a perspective that can guide decision-making in present.

History is the physician's abstraction of certain facts developed in the course of the patient's interview and arranged in a manner that facilitates diagnosis. Proper history is important for making a correct diagnosis.

HIV-related gingivitis appears as typical redness in gingiva extending into the alveolar mucosa also known as linear gingival erythema.

HIV-related myelopathy usually occurs in AIDS subject. It is less common than encephalopathy. It may develop due to methyl group deficiency and is of 3 types. One is vascular myelopathy in which features are similar to acute combined degeneration. Secondly degeneration restricted to gracile tracts has also been known. Finally HIV specific multinucleate giant cell infiltration is seen in brain in HIV encephalopathy may extend to spinal cord.

HIV-related oral melanosis occurs due to involvement of Addison's disease progressive hyper-pigmentation of skin, nails and mucous membrane may take place, etiology remains undetermined. Buccal mucosa, gingiva tongue and palate may be affected.

Ho YAG: lasers have solid active medium, a crystal of YAG doped with holmium. Fiberoptically delivered in contact with the tissue in free-running pulsed mode. Wavelength is 2120 nm. Ho laser has little affinity for pigmented tissue; its hemostatic ability is decreased because of its lower absorbency into hemoglobin and other similar pigments. Absorbency by tooth structures is low. Frequently used for arthroscopy surgery on the TMJ.

Hoarseness is defined as roughness of voice resulting from variations of periodicity and intensity. To have normal voice, vocal cords should be able to approximate properly, have a proper size and stiffness and be able to vibrate regularly.

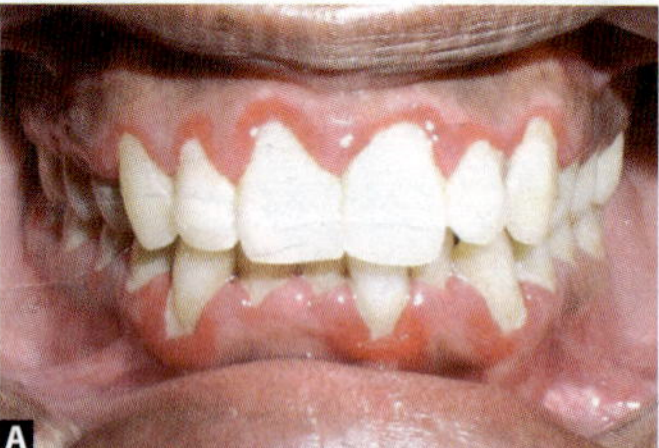

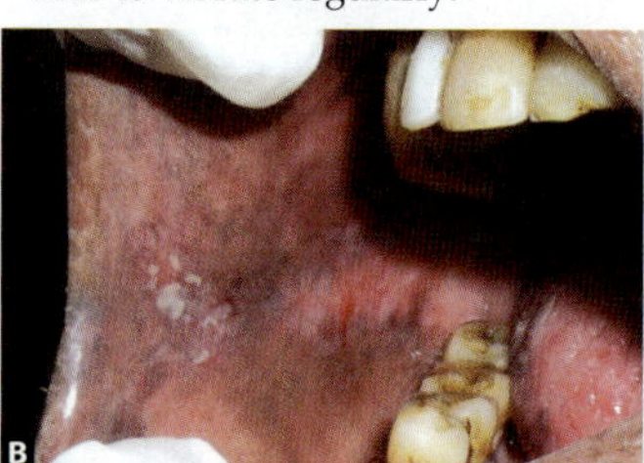

Figs A and B: *(A) HIV-related gingivitis; (B) HIV-related melanosis*

Hodgkin's lymphoma is a malignant histiocytic origin arising from lymph nodes. It is a disease of young adults. Males between the ages of 15-35 years are affected. It may present with asymptomatic lymphadenopathy. Glands are painless, discrete and rubbery. Mediastinal lymph glands or retroperitoneal lymph glands provide clues. There develops, malaise, pyrexia, night sweats, weight loss and pruritus. Lower cervical glands are mostly enlarged with axillary nodes. Nodes are discrete, non-tender, mobile and firm. Feel is like of Indian rubber. Dysphagia and dysphonia may develop. Liver and spleen may be enlarged. Oral lesion includes submucosal swelling with ulceration. Pain is present. Lesion may be fixed to underlying bone. Chemotherapy with radiotherapy helps.

Hoe and chisel are the instruments used to remove tenacious subgingival calculus and altered cementum.

Hoe scalers are the hand instruments used for scaling of ledges or removal of rings of calculus. The blade is bent at 99° angle; thus forming a cutting edge at the junction of flattened terminal surface with the inner aspect of the phase. The blade is slightly bowed so that it can maintain contact at two points on a convex surface.

Holding solution is a disinfecting solution used to cover contaminated instruments before they are processed for sterilization.

Homan's sign: Pain is felt in calf when the foot is pulled upwards. This indicates venous thrombosis.

Homodont refers to the presence of only one type of tooth in the dentition.

Homograft is obtained from any other human being except the patient himself. Usually the patient's own relatives are chosen as donors, i.e. the best donors being siblings followed by the parents. However, fresh cadaveric skin can also be used if prior permission has been taken. In such donors, HIV and HBsAg is tested prior to donation as the contraindications

Hoes

DDP-2953

A

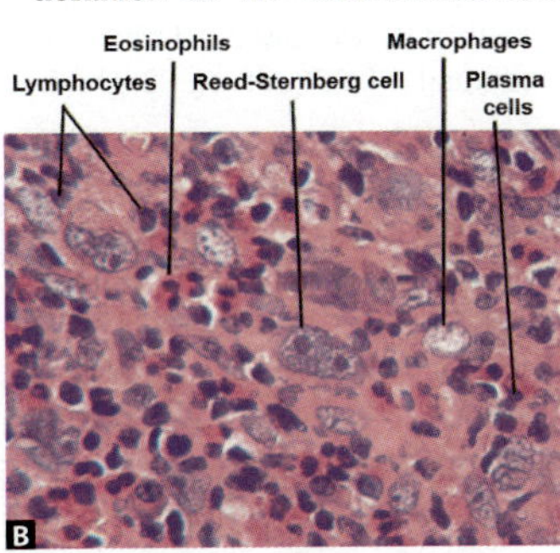

Figs A and B: *(A) Hoe scalers; (B) Hodgkin's lymohoma, mixed cellularity*

for homograft use is hepatitis, AIDS and disseminated fungal infections. Usually fresh skin is used but skin stored for less than 2 weeks can also be used. Older skin can be used in early phases of wound debridement and preparation for autografting. A good 'Take 'of homograft is a good test for wound readiness to accept autograft.

Hopewood House children study was a landmark sugar study done to assess the dental status of childhood between 3 and 14 years of age residing at Hopewood House, Bowral, New South Wales, was studied longitudinally for 10 years. All lived on a strictly institutional diet that, with the exception of an occasional serving of egg yolk, was entirely vegetable in nature and largely raw. Except for weekends between meal, snacks were limited to milk, fruit, and raw vegetables. The dental caries prevalence in young children in Hopewood House was almost negligible in the primary dentition, and approximately one tenth that is seen in the permanent teeth of the average Australian child. A total of 25 out of 82 children remained caries-free over a 5-years study period.

Horizontal bone loss is a bone loss that occurs in a plane parallel to the cementoenamel junction of adjacent teeth.

Horizontal brush scrub is the technique of tooth brushing is commonly used. But unlimited scrubbing motion exerts pressure on the facial tooth prominence. It results in gingival recession and gingival and tooth abrasion.

Horizontal fibers (PDL): These fibers are arranged horizontally emerging from alveolar bone and attached to the root cementum.

Horizontal mattress suture is often used for the interproximal areas of diastema or for wide interdental spaces to properly adapt the interproximal papilla against the bone. The horizontal mattress suture can either be incorporated with continuous, independent sling suture.

Horner's syndrome comprises contraction of pupil of eye, ptosis or drooping of eyelid, anhidrosis and vasodilatation over face. Features depend on the degree of damage of

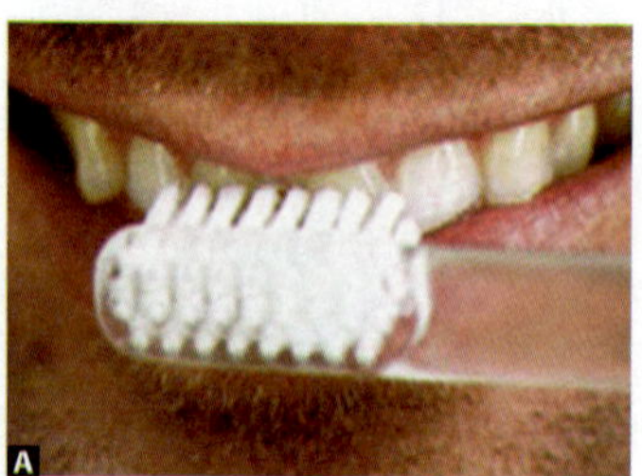

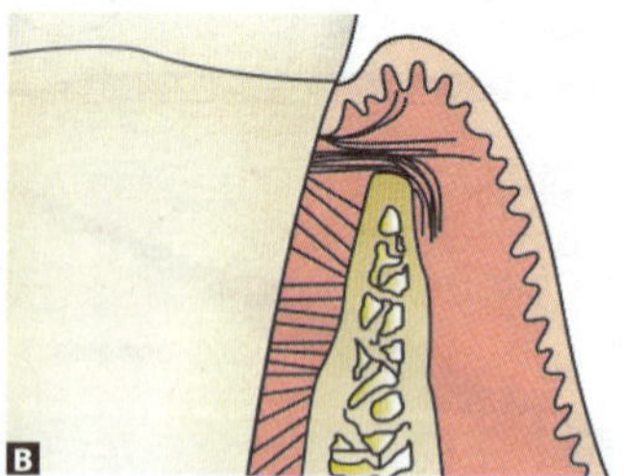

Figs A and B: *(A) Horizontal tooth brushing; (B) Horizontal fibers*

sympathetic path to head and site of the damage.

Horse-shoe kidney is produced by fusion of two ureteric buds. It may remain functionally normal except hydronephrosis or stone may develop.

Host is the organism or in which parasite lives.

Host factors are the factors within an individual host that can influence disease.

Host resistance is the ability of an individual to resist a pathogen or the ability of the person to fight off disease.

Hot air sterilization is done by hot air produced in an electrically heated oven called hot air sterilizer. Contents are kept at 160°C for two hours. It is utilized for sterilizing large batches of instruments overnight. Root canal instruments which are to be kept dry can be sterilized.

Human development index is defined as a composite index combining indicators representing three dimensions, longevity, knowledge and income.

Human fibrin foam is an anti-coagulant used in case of bleeding tooth socket. It can be packed into the socket and sutured if needed. Socket then kept undisturbed.

Humerus is the second largest bone of the body. It is a long bone of arm.

Humidity is always present in atmosphere. It depends on air's temperature. If the air is cooled, excessive moisture precipitates which is known as dew point for that temperature.

Humor's theory: The ancient Greeks considered that a person's physical and mental constitution was determined by the relative proportions of the four elemental fluids of the body—blood, phlegm, black bile, and yellow bile which correspond to the four humors—sanguine, phlegmatic, melancholic and choleric. All diseases, including caries, could be explained by an imbalance of those humors.

Humoral immunity is the one in which antibodies play the predominant role.

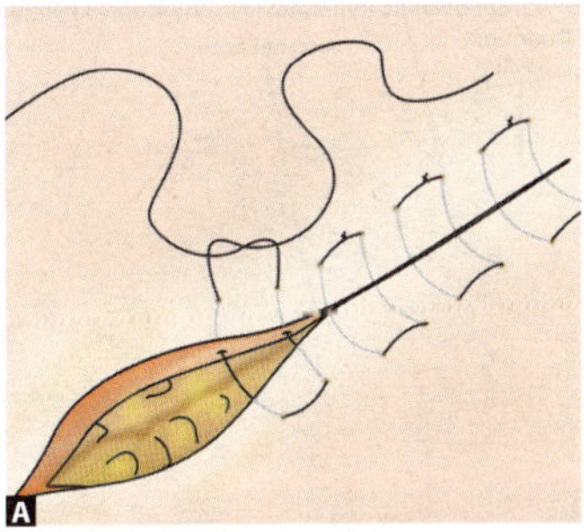

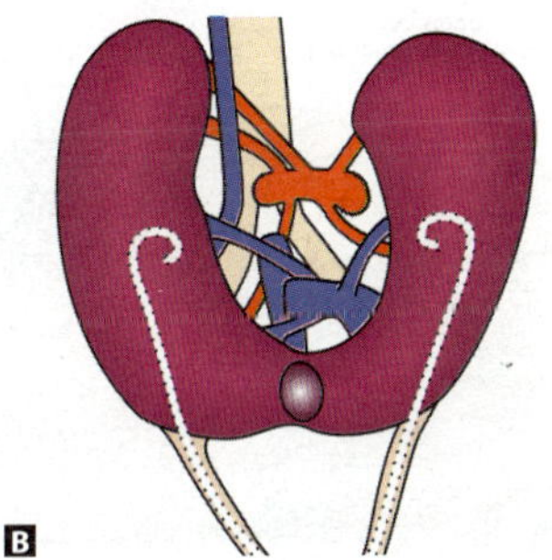

Figs A and B: *(A) Horizontal mattress suture; (B) Horse-shoe kidney*

Huntington's disease is characterized by choreoathetotic moments, personality changes and progressive dementia. Symptoms appear between 35 to 40 years of age. Choreic movements are diagnostic and involve distal as well as axial musculature. Person drops the objects. Walking is associated with more brisk arm and leg movements.

Hurler syndrome is a disturbance of mucopolysacchrides metabolism. Its excretion in urine increases. Symptoms develop within 2 years of life. Head is enlarged, prominent forehead, broad nose and puffy eyelids. There is shortening and broadening of a mandible, thick lips, large tongue. Open mouth and nasal congestion. Short neck and spinal injuries are common. Teeth are small, widely spaced and with altered morphology. Gingival hyperplasia is developed. There is no treatment for the disease.

Hutchinson's wart: The patient is an adult who presents with a warty swelling of tongue. Onset is insidious. It is situated in midline. It is soft and painless.

Hyaline degeneration is a translucent homogeneous material staining pink with eosin. This calcification is common in leiomyoma.

Hybrid composite resins are the type of composites containing colloidal silica of 0.01-0.12 micromillimeter in addition to fine-sized particles.

Hydatid cyst of liver for two species of cystodes echinococcus granulosus and echinococcus mulitlocularis Human being acts as intermediate host. Hydatid cyst of E.granulosus is usually solitary involving right lobe of liver, while E. multilocularis is having germinal membrane which permits formation of new cysts on its outer surface. Renal involvement produces lumbar pain and hematuria. Calcification occurs in 40% cases. Eosinophilia is usual. Complement fixation and indirect hemagglutination tests are positive.

Hydrodensitometry is a method of measuring body composition. Body mass divided by body volume reflects the body's fat content.

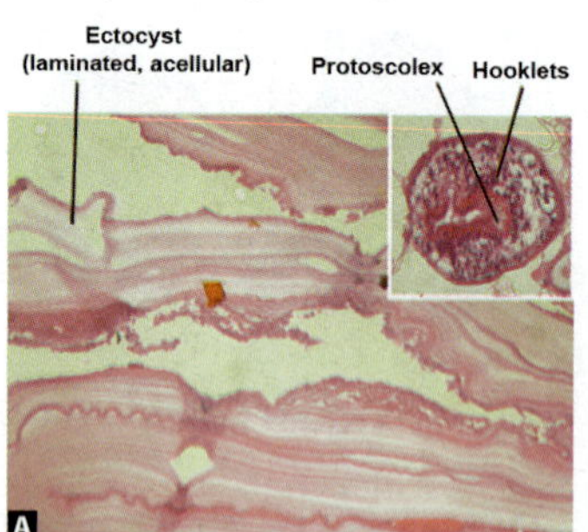

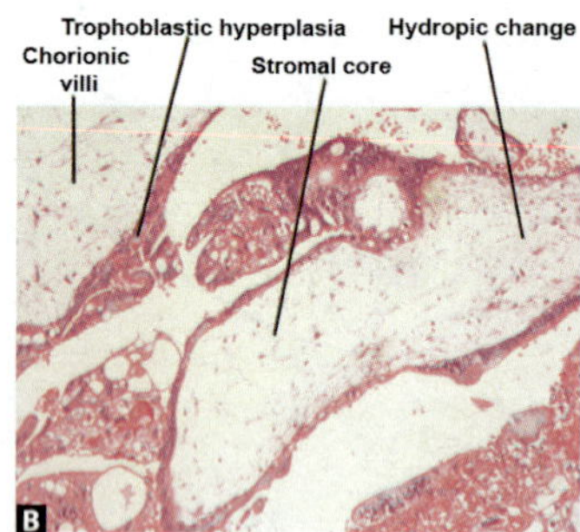

Figs A and B: *(A) Hydatid cyst; (B) Hydatidiform mole*

Body density can be estimated by dividing its mass in air by a volume obtained by weighing a subject both in the air and under the water.

Hydrophosphate cement is an innovation of compounding of zinc phosphate cement is the mixing of dehydrated dihydrogen phosphate of zinc calcium and other materials. These have no marked advantage over the conventional zinc phosphate material.

Hydrogen peroxide is clear, odorless liquid. It is mainly the 3 percent solution which is used as an irrigating agent. It is highly unstable and easily decomposed by heat and light. It rapidly dissociates into H_2O + [O] (water and nascent oxygen). On coming in contact with tissue enzymes catalase and peroxidase, the liberated [O] produces bactericidal effect but this effect is transient and diminishes in presence of organic debris. It causes oxidation of bacterial sulfhydryl group of enzymes and thus interferes with bacterial metabolism. The rapid release of [O] nascent oxygen on contact with organic tissue results in effervescence or bubbling action which is thought to aid in mechanical debridement by dislodging particles of necrotic tissue and dentinal debris and floating them to the surface. It is used as an irrigating solution either alone or alternatively with sodium hypochlorite. The advantage of using alternating solutions of 3% H_2O_2 and 5.2% NaOCl.

Hydron is a rapid setting hydrophilic, plastic material used as a root canal sealer without the use of a core. This was introduced by Wichterle and Lim in 1960. It is available as an injectable root canal filling material. Disadvantages are short working time, very low radiopacity, irritant to periapical tissues, difficult to remove from the canals.

Hydronephrosis refers to the dilatation of renal pelvis and calyces resulting into atrophy of parenchyma. It may be congenital or acquired. It can be unilateral when condition involves the renal pelvis and a ureter, while those involving bladder outlet and urethra hydronephrosis can be bilateral. Bilateral hydronephrosis leads to renal failure and uremia. Kidney may be massively enlarged. One or both ureters may be enlarged depending on level of obstruction.

Hydrophilic liner is a soft liner that is readily wet by water.

Hydrophobic is a water repellent showing a high contact angle.

Hydrostatic pressure is a pressure caused by the weight of a column of water.

Hygiene is the science that deals with the preservation of health.

Hygroscopic is pertaining to the absorbing of water

Hyoid bone is a small U-shaped bone that is present in front of the upper part of the neck. It is not attached to any other bone directly; but is held in place by muscles and ligaments that are attached to it. The bone consists of a central part called the body, and of two cornua on either side.

Hyperimmunoglobulin is the preparation containing specific antibodies used to prevent disease after exposure to a pathogen.

Hyperkinesis refers to excessive motility.

Hyperactive pulpalgia is characterized by short, sharp shock. It is never spontaneous. Pain is of short duration so long irritant is there—may be cold or hot, sweet or sour. Ice-cream excites the nerve in teeth and pain is referred to eyes. Hyperactive pulpalgia is common following the placement of new restoration. Patients also complain this after curettage. It may be associated with caries of tooth. Fractured teeth are more hyperreactive. In maxillary sinusitis, maxillary teeth are involved.

Hypercalcemia refers to the increased levels of calcium in blood. In mild cases, it may be asymptomatic. Person may develop constipation and anorexia. In moderate high person develops polyuria, nocturia and polydipsia. In severe high cases person develops emotional liability, confusion, delirium and psychosis. In late stage, acute renal failure may develop.

Hypercementosis refers to deposition of excessive amount of secondary cementum on root surfaces. It covers the entire root area. It may be caused by accelerated elongation of a tooth inflammation, tooth repair and osteitis deformans. It shows no signs and symptoms. Cemental spikes may be seen. There is no increase or decrease of sensitivity. Radiographically bulging and thickening of rods is noted. No treatment is indicated.

Hyperdontia is the presence of extra teeth beyond the normal complement. Also refer supernumerary teeth.

Hyperemia is an increased blood flow in the pulp. The increased pressure against the sensory nerve endings in the pulp produces the sensation associated with hyperemia. It will explain why the pain appears to be of different intensity and character with application of cold or heat, the

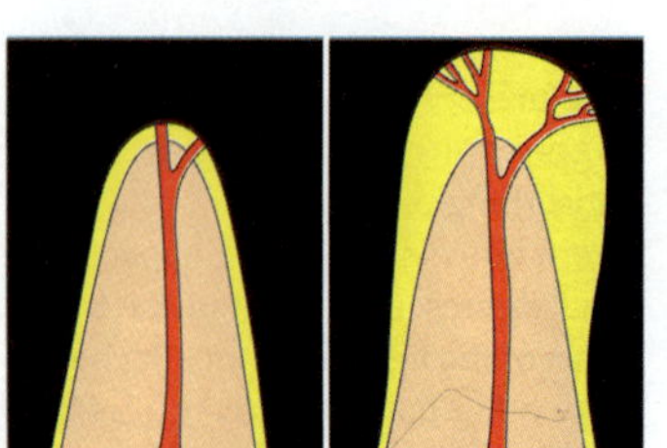

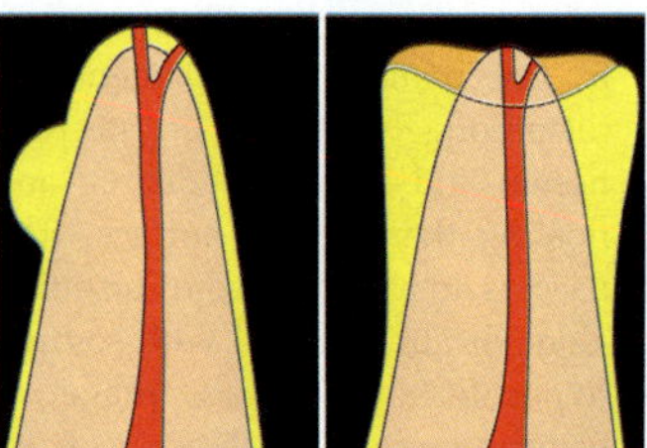

Fig.: *Hypercementosis*

cold producing hypersensitivity response and the heat producing true transient hyperemia.

Hyperkalemia refers to excessive potassium causes it. It may be the result of extensive tissue breakdown, severe dehydration, or excessive amount of potassium. Symptoms include numbness, mental confusion, cold skin and disturbed cardiac rate.

Hypermagnesemia refers to the increased serum levels of magnesium in acute and renal failure. Deep tendon reflexes are lost and necrosis, hypotension, respiratory paralysis occurs with serum level 10 mEq/L. Treatment includes 100-200 mg of calcium.

Hyperparathyroidism refers to excess of circulating parathyroid hormone. Bone and kidney are the target organs. Serum calcium level is elevated. *Clinical Features:* Emotional instability, painful bones and joints, crampy abdomen, bowing of long bones, pigeon chest, collapse vertebra, muscle weakness, fatigue, polyuria and polydipsia. *Radiological Features:* Ground glass appearance, moth-eaten appearance with varying intensity, punctate and nodular calcification may develop in kidney and joints, pepper pot skull due to osteopenia, teeth may become mobile and migrate, loss of lamina dura which may be complete or partial.

Hyperpituitarism results due to hyperfunction of the anterior lobe of pituitary gland producing growth hormone. Before closing of epiphysis, gigantism occurs and after closure, acromegaly. In it, bone overgrowth and thickening of soft tissue causes a coarsening of facial features. Head and feet become large with clubbing of toes and fingers. There will be enlargement of sella turcica, paranasal sinuses and thickening of outer table of skull. Angle between ramus and body of mandible is widened. There is enlargement of inferior dental canal. X-ray will show increased tooth size specially root due to secondary cemental hyperplasia. *Oral manifestations:* Mandibular condylar growth is very prominent, overgrowth of mandible leading to prognathism, lips become thick

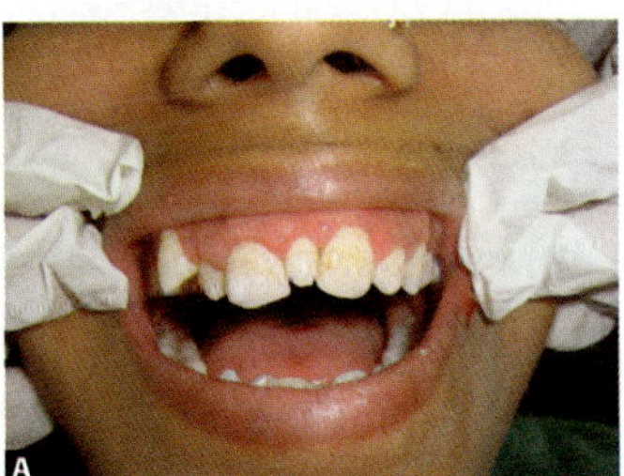

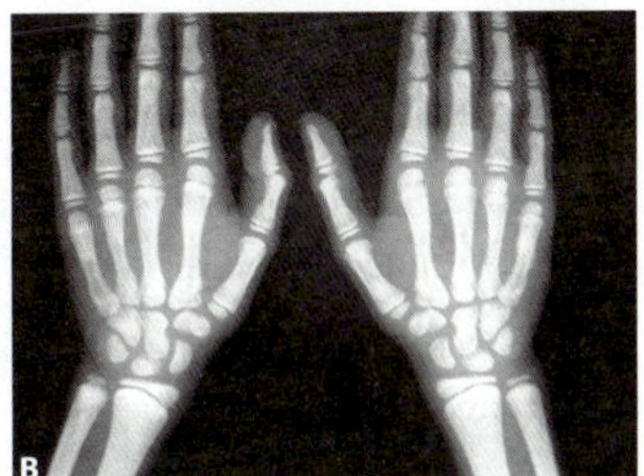

Figs A and B: *(A) Hyperdontia; (B) Hyperparathyroidism*

like Negro's, teeth become more spaced, body and root may be longer than normal.

Hyperplasia is defined as an increase in number of cells in a tissue or organ. Pathological hyperplasia is common in oral cavity. Increase in number of epithelial cells and increased thickness of epithelium due to chronic irritation or abrasion.

Hyperplastic pulp is overgrowth of granulomatous tissue into carious cavity. It results from compressing food against the exposed pulp during mastication. As regards treatment teeth involved in hyperplastic pulpitis are badly decayed, and restoration is virtually very difficult.

Hypersecretion of cortisol leads to increased fat deposition in certain areas, such as face and back, elevates blood pressure, and alters blood cell distribution. Clinically, cortisol hypersecretion is referred to as Cushing's syndrome, a condition usually corrected through surgical removal of part of adrenal gland.

Hypersensitivity is a condition in which there is an exaggerated or inappropriate immune reaction that causes tissue destruction or inflammation.

Hypersensitivity of drug is an unwanted drug reaction related to abnormal individual susceptibility. It is related to genetic factors. Drugs can act as antigens causing immunologically-induced inflammatory response. Topical administration may cause a greater number of reactions than oral and parenteral. However parenteral administration will result in wide-spread reaction. Patients with multiple allergies will have more reaction to drugs.

Hypersensitivity of teeth refers to a sharp, sudden painful reaction in teeth when exposed to hot, cold, chemical, mechanical or osmotic (sweet or salt) stimuli. It is caused by the initiating factors of a hypersensitive pulp and is usually cold food or drink or cold air or stimulation of exposed dentin on the root surface by cold, sweet or sour substances. Fruits and salts may also cause it. The sensation disappears as soon as electrolyte is diluted away or metal is removed. Actually pain can be evoked from dentin by applying to it solutions which exert high osmotic pressure.

Hypersensitivity type II reaction is caused by IgG and IgM antibodies and is capable of causing type III hypersensitivity reaction as well. The main distinction is that type II reactions involve antibodies directed to Ag on the surface of specific cells or tissues whereas type III are due to antibodies against widely distributed antigen or soluble Ag in serum. While damage caused by type II localizes reaction to a particular tissue or cell type, damage caused by type III react affects those organs where Ag-Ab complexes are deposited. These hypersensitive reactions are related to normal immune responses seen against microorganisms and parasites. In the reaction against pathogens, exaggerated immune reaction may be as damaging to the host as the effects of the pathogen itself. These reactions are seen in autoimmune disease and transplantation reactions.

Hypersensitivity type IV reaction is a dela-yed type of reaction. In the original classification by Coomb & Gell in 1968, Delayed hypersensitivity or type IV was used as a general category to describe all those hypersensitivity reactions, which took place more than 12 hrs to develop. DTH cannot be transferred from one to another by serum. It is associated with T-cell protective immunity.

Hypertensive arteriosclerosis shows thickening of arteries in case of hypertension. Medium and large sized arteries show hypertrophy of media due to increased number of smooth muscle cell and elastic fibers. In later stage, hyalinization of vessel wall may occur.

Hypertensive brain hemorrhage are putamen and around internal capsule, thalamus, pons and cerebellum. It generally does not occur in white matter. Putaminal hemorrhage is characterized by contralateral hemiplegia. In bigger hematoma, there may develop bilateral motor palsy, irregular respiration and dilated fixed pupil. Thalamic hemorrhage develops hemisensory defect, unequal pupils. Pontine hemorrhage produces deep coma, pinpoint reactive pupil, quadriplegia and hyperthermia. Cerebellar hemorrhage presents with ataxia, headache and hydrocephalus.

Hyperthyroidism is known as thyrotoxicosis, due to overproduction

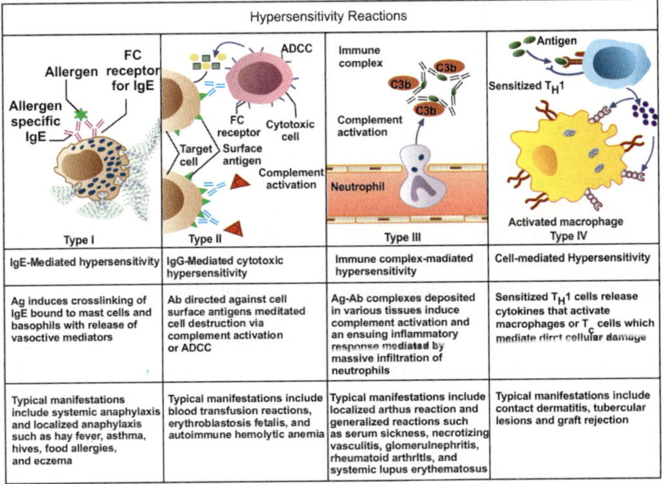

Type I	Type II	Type III	Type IV
IgE-Mediated hypersensitivity	IgG-Mediated cytotoxic hypersensitivity	Immune complex-madiated hypersensitivity	Cell-mediated Hypersensitivity
Ag induces crosslinking of IgE bound to mast cells and basophils with release of vasoctive mediators	Ab directed against cell surface antigens meditated cell destruction via complement activation or ADCC	Ag-Ab complexes deposited in various tissues induce complement activation and an ensuing inflammatory response mediated by massive infiltration of neutrophils	Sensitized T_H1 cells release cytokines that activate macrophages or T_C cells which mediate dirct cellular damage
Typical manifestations include systemic anaphylaxis and localized anaphylaxis such as hay fever, asthma, hives, food allergies, and eczema	Typical manifestations include blood transfusion reactions, erythroblastosis fetalis, and autoimmune hemolytic anemia	Typical manifestations include localized arthus reaction and generalized reactions such as serum sickness, necrotizing vasculitis, glomerulnephritis, rheumatoid arthrltis, and systemic lupus erythematosus	Typical manifestations include contact dermatitis, tubercular lesions and graft rejection

Fig.: *Hypersensitivity reactions*

of thyroxine. It may be caused by Graves' disease. Hyperthyroidism symptoms are due to increased metabolic activity of tissues or body. BMR is increased. *Clinical Features:* Thyroid is enlarged, Enlargement may be asymmetrical and nodular, thyroid may be tender, liver and spleen may be enlarged, nervousness, muscle weakness and fine tremors, cardiac palpitation, irregular heart beat and excessive perspiration, tachycardia, and increased pulse pressure, ankle edema and systolic hypertension, amenorrhea, infertility, decreased libido and impotence. There may be lymphadenopathy and osteoporosis. *Oral Manifestations:* There may be alveolar resorption, trabeculae may be of greater density, faster eruption and premature loss of primary teeth, early eruption of permanent teeth, early jaw development, generalized decrease in bone density, loss of edentulous alveolar bone.

Hypertonic is a solution containing a higher level of salt, i.e. NaCl than is found in living RBC which is 0.9% NaCl.

Hypertrophic lichen planus may occur on oral mucosa as a well-circumscribed elevated white lesion like leukoplakia. Biopsy is required to confirm diagnosis.

Hypertrophy is overgrowth of tissue.

Hyperventilation is a condition caused by rapid respirations leading to acapnia, i.e. carbon dioxide depletion and subsequent respiratory alkalosis. Person develops light headedness, trembling, tingling and numbness. It may be caused by excessive nervousness or hysteria.

Hypervitaminosis is an excess of specific vitamins accumulated in the body to the level of toxicity. Commonest is vitamin A and Vitamin D.

Hypervitaminosis D refers to excess of vitamin D in body. Toxicity has been found to result when daily doses of between 10,000 and 50,000 IU are taken over a prolonged period of time. This vitamin is resistant to heat and cooling process. Being fat-soluble, it is stored in body. Excessive intake of vitamin D results in anorexia, nausea, vomiting, excessive thirst and drowsiness. Cramps and tingling of finger and toes are also noted.

Hypnotics are drugs which are used to induce sleep and drowsiness. They depress the central nervous system acting on central cerebral cortex.

Hypocalcemia refers to where serum calcium falls below 8 mg% is termed as hypocalcemia. It may be due to decreased bone resorption of calcium, decreased intestinal calcium resorption, calcium binding and sequestration. *Clinical features:* Include numbness, cramps, anxiety and tetany followed by convulsions, laryngeal stridor, dystonia and psychosis. 10 ml of 10% calcium gluconate

IV followed by 10-40 ml of 10% calcium gluconate in 5% dextrose gives relief. Oral vitamin D and calcium are needed.

Hypocalcification is the lack or deficiency of initial calcification of organic enamel matrices.

Hypocalcified type of amelogenesis imperfecta is characterized by enamel of normal thickness which is poorly calcified. These are of two types—one is inherited as an autosomal dominant trait and other as autosomal recessive trait. At eruption, teeth present as yellow to orange enamel which is soft and rapidly lost. It leaves exposed dentin on X-ray. Enamel has moth-eaten appearance and is less radiopaque than dentin. Cervical enamel is better calcified.

Hypodontia *see* partial anodontia.

Hypoglossal nerve is a twelth cranial motor nerve. It supplies muscles of tongue controlling its shape and movement. It is purely motor supplying the muscles of the tongue. The hypoglossal nerve arises from the medulla. It leaves the cranial cavity through the hypoglossal canal (or anterior condylar) canal.

Hypoglossal nucleus lies in the medulla. It is an elongated column extending into both the open and closed parts of the medulla. Its upper part lies deep to the hypoglossal triangle in the floor of the fourth ventricle.

H

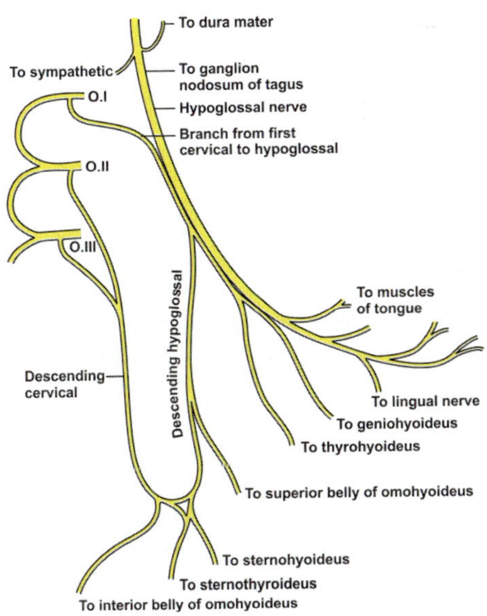

Fig.: *Hypoglossal nerve*

Hypoglycemia is when blood sugar falls below 40 mg %. It occurs when liver glucose output falls below the glucose uptake by peripheral tissues. When brain's requirement is not met, person shows neurological symptoms like psychiatric disorders, fits, epilepsy and cerebrovascular diseases. Patient may feel tired and weak; palpitation, sweating and hunger may develop. Later headache, confusion, visual disturbance, ataxia and personality changes appear. Lastly convulsions and coma may develop. Blood sugar may be very low in polycythemia and leukemia.

Hypoglycemic encephalopathy refers to when blood sugar level falls below 25-30 mg causes confusion, convulsion, hemiparesis and coma. Overdose of insulin may cause it. Initial symptoms are headache, palpitation, anxiety, trembling and profuse sweating. When blood sugar falls below 10 mg/dL, the person develops deep coma, dilated pupils, hypotonia and shallow respiration. Prompt correction of hypoglycemia before the onset of medullary phase reverses the symptoms.

Hypokalemia refers to low level of potassium in the body. Patient becomes listless with slow and slurred speech with intense drowsiness. Tone of muscles is reduced. The reflexes become absent. Patient may develop incontinence of urine. Abdomen is distended and bowel sounds become absent. Pulse may become irregular.

Hypomagnesemia refers to low level of magnesia. In this condition, patient may complaint of anorexia, weakness and apathy. One may feel tremor, ataxia and vertigo along with depression/irritability and psychotic behavior. Hence twice the estimated deficit is to be given.

Hypomaturation can be explained as lack of secondary mineralization or maturation.

Hypoparathyroidism refers to when there is insufficient secretion of parathyroid hormone. It may result from: Autoimmune destruction, surgical damage to parathyroid, parathyroid damage from radioactive iodine I-131. *Clinical Features:* Stiffness in hands, feet and lips, paresthesia around mouth, tingling in fingers and toes, anxiety and depression. Intelligence is lowered. *Oral Manifestations:* Delayed eruption of teeth and hypoplasia of enamel.

Hypophysis cerebri is also called the pituitary gland. Hypophysis cerebri is a small ovoid structure measuring about 13 mm from side to side, about 10 mm front to back, and about 8 mm in vertical diameter. The hypophysis is suspended from the floor of the third ventricle of the brain by a narrow funnel-shaped stalk called the infundibulum. Placed in the cranial cavity, in the floor of the middle cranial fossa. The hypophysis cerebri has, in the past, been usually divided into an anterior part, the pars anterior; an intermediate part, the pars intermedia; and a posterior part, the pars posterior.

Hypopituitarism may be congenital or due to destructive disease. Space occupying lesions like craniopharyngioma, adenomas may result it. *Clinical Features:* There develops symmetrical underdevelopment but in some cases, there may be disproportionate length of long bones. Hypoglycemia may develop due to growth hormone and cortisol deficiency. Onset of puberty is delayed. Person becomes lethargic, fat mass is increased. Skull and facial bones are small. *Oral Manifestations:* Tooth eruption is hampered, dental arch is smaller than normal, so overcrowding of teeth results, eruption of teeth is delayed, and so is the shedding of deciduous teeth.

Hypoplasia of parotid gland is seen with Melkerson-Rosenthal syndrome. It consists of orofacial granuloma, facial paralysis and fissured tongue.

Hypoplasia: Due to congenital syphilis is contracted in utero from a mother who had treponemal infection. Syphilis produces classic patterns of hypoplastic dysmorphic permanent teeth. Saber shins, rhagedes, frontal bossing and saddle nose are common structural anomalies. Congenital syphilis clinically will present with— 1. Interstitial keratosis; 2. Deafness; 3. Tooth anomalies (Hutchinson's triad). The hypoplasia involves the maxillary and mandibular permanent incisors and the first molars. The anterior teeth affected are called "Hutchinson's teeth" while the molars are referred to as "Mulberry Molar" (Moon's molars, Fournier's molars). The upper central incisor is "screw-driver"

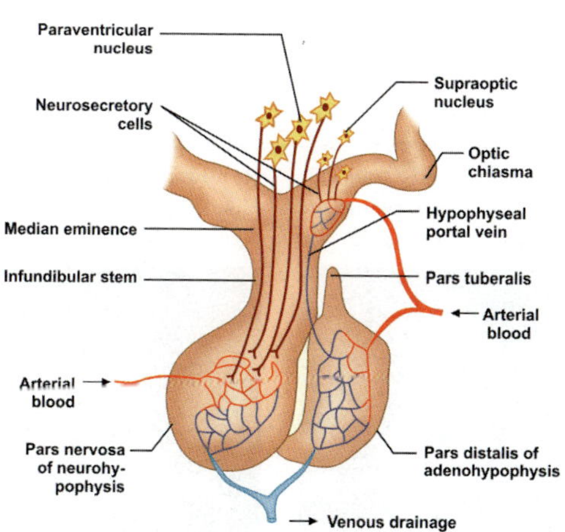

Fig.: *Hypophysis cerebri*

H

shaped, the mesial and distal surfaces of the crown tapering and converging towards the incisal edge of the tooth rather than towards the cervical margin. As a result, diastema is occasionally observed between the central incisors. The cause of the tapering and notching of the maxillary incisor has been explained on the basis of the absence of the central tubercle or calcification center. The crowns of the first molar in congenital syphilis are irregular and the enamel of the occlusal third of the tooth appears to be arranged in an agglomerate mass of globules rather than in well-formed cusps.

H

Hyposensitization is the therapy involves the injection of increasing doses of allergen. Following treatment, there is an increase in serum levels of allergen specific IgG and suppressor T cell activity while specific IgE levels tend to fall. However, since allergic humans are clinically diagnosed after sensitization and this may explain the relative lack of success of desensitization in many subjects.

Hypothesis is a proposed explanation of an observed phenomenon or it is a conjectural statement of the relationship between variables.

Hypothyroidism is a condition where secretion of thyroid is diminished. It may be due to atrophy of thyroid gland or failure of thyrotropic function of pituitary gland. It may lead to three types: Cretinism-hormone failure occurs in infancy, juvenile myxedema—it occurs in childhood, myxedema—it occurs after puberty. *Clinical Features:* Cretinism and myxedema may be present at birth, constipation and hoarse cry may result, delayed fusion of epiphysis, hair become dry and sparse. Cretinism leads to mental defects, generalized edema and other changes. Base of skull is shortened. Face fails to develop in longitudinal direction. Mandible is underdeveloped. Tongue is enlarged by edema fluid. Development of teeth is delayed.

Hypoxia is low oxygen level.

Hysteric tremor tends to involve a limb or the whole body and is worsened by the examiner's attempt to control it.

Hypodontia *see* Partial anodontia.

Histologic pocket depth *see* Biologic pocket depth.

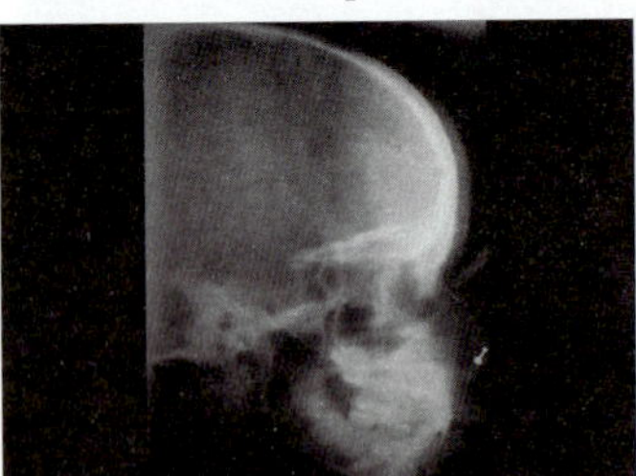

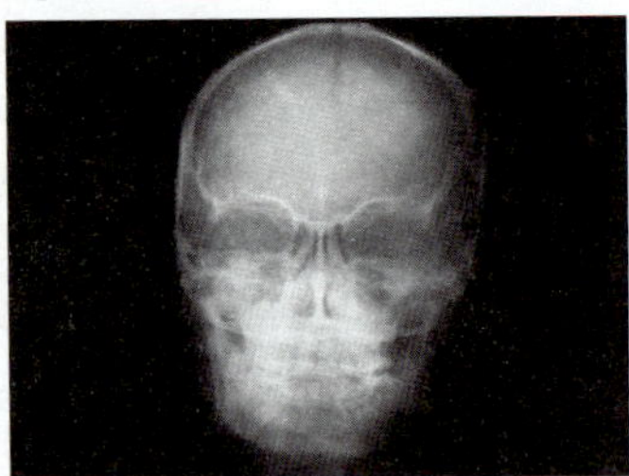

Fig.: *Open sutures seen in case of hypothyroidism*

I

Ice immersion is a procedure in which the part to be treated is immersed in an ice solution such as hand, feet and elbows. Solution is made up of 50% water and 50% ice. It has to be single less than 10 minutes immersion or shorter immersion making a cumulative time of 10 minutes.

Ice packs: Crushed or flanked ice may be placed inside a specially made terry towel bag. It may be done by folding towel into an appropriate shape. The wet ice pack is placed on the top of the part to be treated. It should not put pressure to obstruct the circulation. Reduced circulation may lead to ice burn.

Id was described by Sigmond Frued in 1905 in psychosexual theory. In Latin, it means 'it' Greek–primal urges, it is the basic structure of personality which serves as reservoir of instincts (or) their mental representative. Present at birth, impulse ridden and drives immediate pressure gratification.

Ideal occlusion is a complete harmonious relationship of the teeth and masticatory system.

Identification dot is a small raised dot that appears in one corner of intraoral film. It is used for film orientation.

Idiocy is the result of congenital defective mental faculty. The person may have negative existence and may be devoid of any will power, memory, emotion and initiative power. He is not able to protest himself. IQ is between 0 to 10.

Idiopathic dysguesia like atypical facial pain and idiopathic xerostomia is considered a manifestation of depression. Taste dysfunction is reported as a complaint by burning mouth syndrome.

Idiopathic thrombocytopenic purpura is an uncommon disease of remissions and exacerbations when platelet count is low; excessive bleeding may occur after dental extraction. Bleeding time is prolonged.

Iodophors are intermediate level hospital disinfectants with tuberculocidal action. These are effective within 5–10 minutes. These may discolor surface or metals.

Idoxuridine is used as anti-herpetic agent in treatment of mouth and eye infections due to Herpes simplex ions.

Illegitimate child is the one who is born out of wedlock or not within a competent line after the cessation of relationship of husband and wife or when procreation by the husband is not possible due to congenital defect or getting vasectomy done.

ILS (Inferior labial sulcus) is the point of greatest concavity in the midline of the lower lip between labrale inferior and soft-tissue pogonion.

Imbecility is the term used for children who have IQ between 20-40 but can speak in articulated language. They are intellectually poor and often dangerous to society.

Imipramine is used in treatment of mental depression and effect is produced in 4-10 days. It can be given once daily. It results in papillary dilatation, paralysis of accommodation, dryness of mouth, postural hypotension and urinary retention.

Immunity means resistance to disease certain white cells release antibodies and antitoxins into blood plasma. Many causative factors such as micro-organisms, bacteria and animal toxins can produce antibodies and antitoxins. All such factors are known as antigens.

Immunization is the deliberate artificial exposure to disease to produce acquired immunity.

Immunodeficiency is a type of immunopathological condition that involves deficiency in number, function or interrelationship of involved WBCs and their products. It may be congenital or acquired. When person's immune system is not functioning opportunistic infections invade the host.

Immunogenesis any substance that is capable of inducing an immune response is called an immunogen and is said to be immunogenic.

Immunology is the study of the ways in which the body defends itself from infectious agents and other foreign substances in its environment. It encompasses many layers of defense including physical barriers like skin, protective chemical substances in the blood and tissue fluids and the physiologic reaction of tissues to injury or infection.

Impacted tooth: Teeth cannot erupt due to physical obstruction.

Impaction-bony: Tooth that is blocked by both bone and tissue.

Implant is a titanium post that is implanted into bone. A crown,

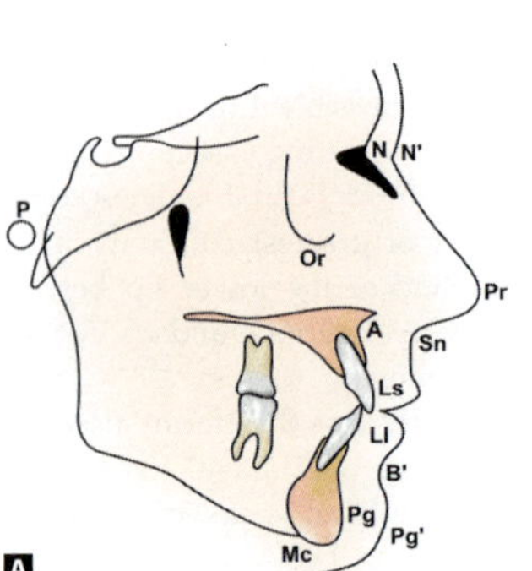

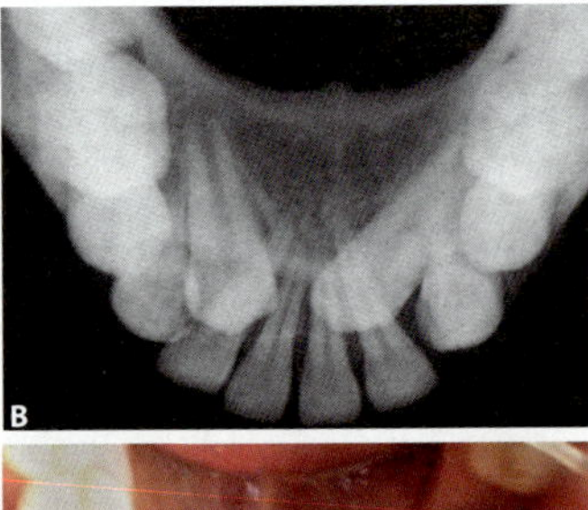

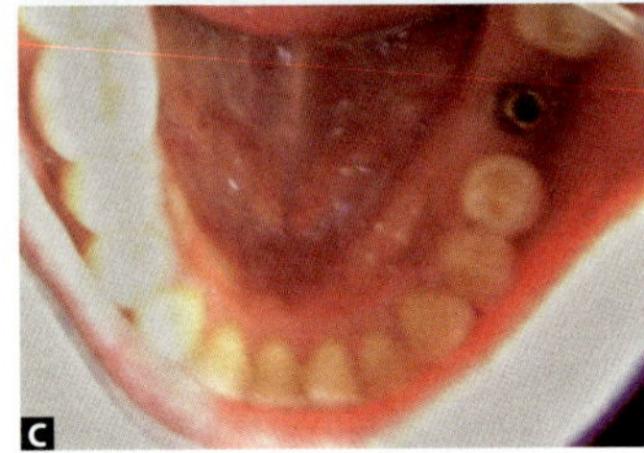

Figs A to C: *(A) Inferior labial sulcus; (B) Bilaterally impacted canines; (C) Implant placed in the alveolar bone*

bridge, or denture is then placed over the implant to restore function and esthetics.

Implantation: The placement within body tissue of a foreign substance.

Implied contract is established between patient and doctor. An expressed contract is informed consent given in writing or verbally. Gardian's consent is given when patient is minor or is not mentally competent to do so. Written consent is an expressed consent.

Impotence is the inability to have sexual intercourse. While sterility is the inability of male to get children as in female, it is the inability to conceive the child. A person can be sterile without being impotent.

Impression is the negative replica of an oral cavity.

Impression compound is a solid material which is softened by heat to a plastic consistency suitable for impression taking. In mouth, it hardens rapidly on cooling. Slab form is softened in hot water and sticks which are softened over a flame. It gives a full denture by means of a perfect peripheral seal. Disadvantage is that it cannot be withdrawn from undercut areas without distortion.

Impression material: These are used to make an accurate replica of oral tissues. Area involved varies from a single tooth to the whole dentition. Impression gives a negative reproduction of tissue and by filling it positive case is made. Die is used to prepare inlays or bridge.

Impression paste is used to make impression of dentures. It is supplied in 2 tubes. One containing white zinc oxide mixture and the other containing red eugenol mixture. Equal lengths of mixtures are mixed together with a spatula to give a uniform pink mix. Disadvantage of it is that not very useful for partial impressions.

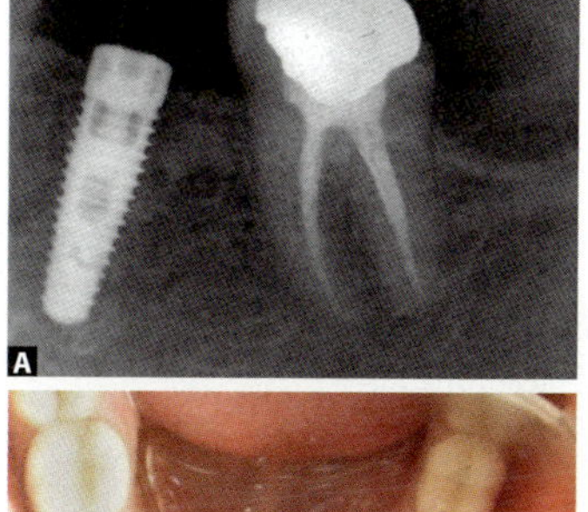

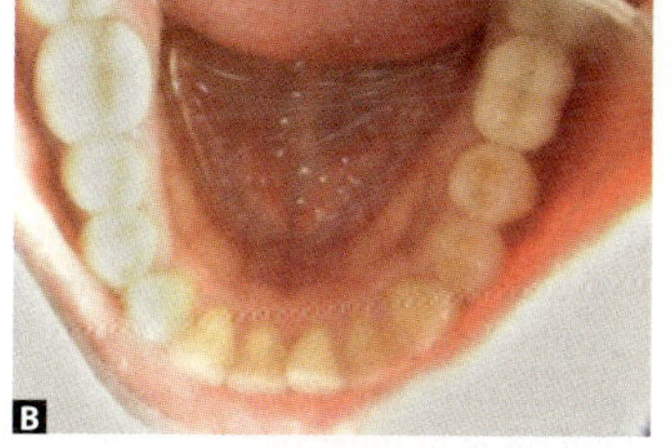

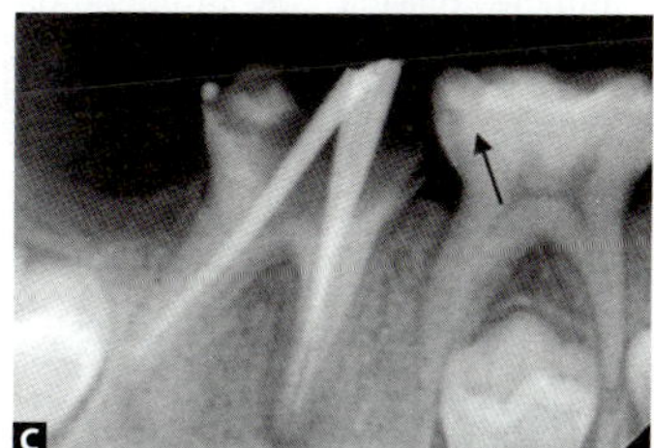

Figs A to C: *(A) Radiographic view of an implant; (B) Postoperative picture of implant along with the placement of crown; (C) Incipient proximal caries*

vesiculobullous lesions on trunk and extremities. The pigmentation begins to fade with-in a year. There may be associated local and generalized baldness, optic atrophy. There is delayed tooth eruption. No treatment is required.

Incus is the bone in the middle ear. It has a main part or body and two processes: long and short. The long process is directed downwards parallel to the handle of the malleus. The short process is directed backwards.

Independent 't' test: A parametric test of differences between two independent samples.

Independent variable is a term used for variable that the researcher has a control over the presumed cause of a measured effect. In experimental research, at least one independent variable is manipulated.

Index (Esther M Wilkins) is an expression of clinical observation in numerical values which is used to describe the status of the individual or group with respect to a condition being measured.

Index (Russel AL) has been defined as a numerical value describing the relative status of a population on a graduated scale with definite upper and lower limits, which is designed to permit and facilitate comparison with other populations classified by the same criteria and methods.

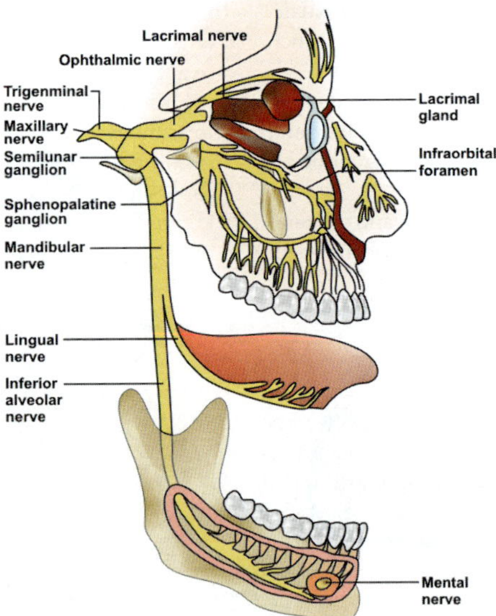

Fig.: *Incisive nerve*

Impression tray formed in the general shape of the mouth, used for taking impressions. These are of two types. Partial trays are used for impressions of partial dentures and edentulous trays are used for full dentures. These are semicircular in cross-section.

Impulse refers to dental radiography, a measure of exposure time. 60 impulses occur in one second.

Inrecoverable strain original length will come back after removal of the applied force or the material may remain deformed in such case, the strain is not recoverable.

Interleukin-1 is a pro-inflammatory, multifunctional cytokine, which among its many biological activities, enables ingress of inflammatory cells into sites of infection, promotes bone resorption, stimulates eicosanoid (specifically PGE2) release by monocytes and fibroblasts, stimulates release of matrix metalloproteinases, that degrade proteins of the extra-cellular matrix, and participates in many aspects of the immune response.

Interleukin-6 is a cytokine that stimulates plasma cell proliferation and, therefore, antibody production and is produced by lymphocytes, monocytes and fibroblasts. Levels of IL-6 have been shown to be elevated in inflamed tissues, higher in periodontitis than in gingivitis tissues and higher in GCF from refractory periodontitis (Yamazaki (1994). IL-6 has been shown to stimulate osteoclast formation. Thus, this cytokine may in large part, account for both the predominance of plasma cells in periodontitis lesions as well as bone resorption.

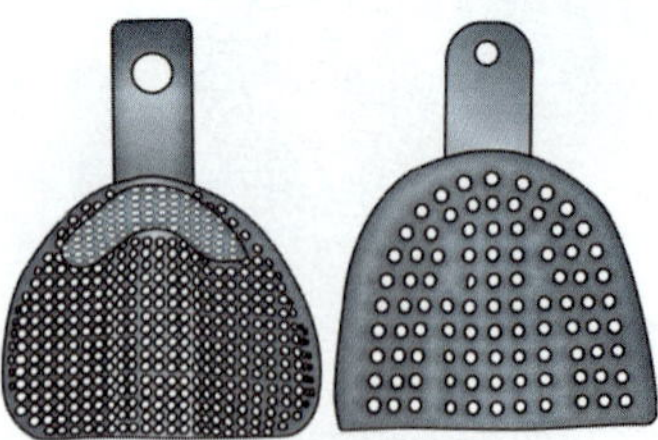

Fig.: *Impression tray*

Interleukin-8 is a chemo-attractant that is mainly produced by monocytes, is response to lipopolysaccharide, IL-1 or tumor necrosis factor alpha (TNF-α). It is present at high levels in periodontitis lesions, mainly associated with the junctional epithelium and macrophages. In addition to serving as a chemo-attractant for neutrophils, it appears to selectively stimulate matrix metalloproteinase activity from these cells, thus in part accounting for collagen destruction within periodontitis lesions.

In vitro: Outside living body/in a test tube.

In vivo: In the living body, plant or animal.

Inborn immunity: Immunity to disease that is inherited.

Incidence is defined as the number of new cases occurring in defined population during a specified period of time.

Incident is number of new cases of a disease in a defined population at a certain period of time.

Incipient interproximal lesion extends less than halfway through the thickness of enamel. The term incipient means beginning to exist or appear. An incipient lesion is seen in enamel only.

Incipient stroke *see* transient ischemic attack.

Incipient malocclusion may be defined as a condition, which shows a tendency to develop into a deviation from the normal dentofacial or occlusal relationship.

Incisal edge the cutting edge, ridge, or surface of anterior teeth.

Incisal edge: Biting edge of an anterior teeth.

Incisive foramen is an opening or hole in bone located at midline of the anterior portion of hard palate, posterior to maxillary central incisor. It appears radiolucent.

Incisive nerve refers to the nerve that originates at mental foramen and innervates those teeth anterior alveolar nerve.

Incisor the central and lateral incisors; the first and second teeth from the midline of the mouth.

Incisor liability: The succession of smaller primary incisor with larger permanent incisor has been called incisor liability. Numerically, it is the size difference between the four permanent maxillary incisors teeth and four primary incisor teeth. According to Baume. It is 7.6 mm in maxilla and 6.0 mm in mandible.

Inclination angle: The inclination angle gives an assessment of the maxillary base. It is the angle formed by the Pn line and palatal bone. A large angle expresses upward and forward inclination, whereas small angles indicate down and back tipping of the anterior end of the palatal plane and maxillary base. This angle does not correlate with growth pattern.

Inclination of the nasal base: The angle formed between true vertical (e.g. SnV) and the long axis of the nostril varies from about 90° in men to as much as 105° in women.

Incontinentia pigmenti also known as Bloch-Sulzberger syndrome and is rare X-linked dominant disorder of skin, hair, teeth and CNS. There develops erythematous and

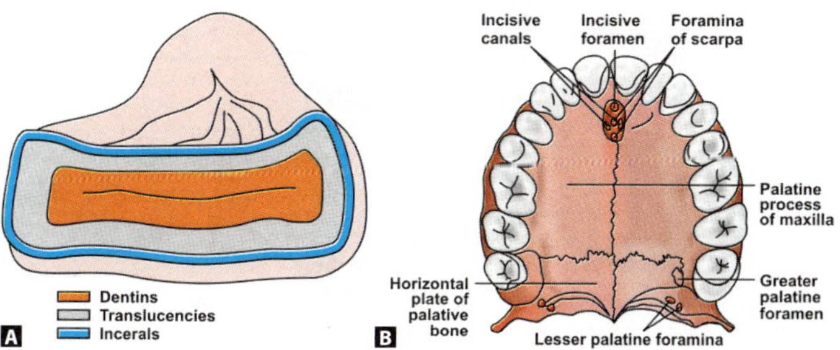

Figs A and B: *(A) Incisal edge; (B) Incisive foramen*

I

Indirect transmission of disease is said to have occur when the transmission of microorganism has taken place through dirty hands, soiled laundry, contaminated instruments touching during dental procedure.

Indomethacin is an anti-inflammatory agent with analgestic and anti pyretic effect and is absorbed well when given orally. Bone marrow depression has been reported. Side effects include GIT upsets, headache and dizziness with oral ulcerations. It is not given in dental disorder.

Inert: No inherent power of action, motion or resistance.

Infancy: Refers to the 1st year after birth and the first 4 weeks of which are designated as the newborn or neonatal period.

Infancy caries: A rapidly progressing type of dental caries that affects the primary teeth of children, usually during the first 2 years of life and as early as the first year. In children with infancy caries there is a unique distribution of dental decay. The 4 maxillary anterior incisors are affected first; these teeth are anatomically so positioned in the mouth as to be most frequently bathed by a feeding for, if unchecked, the decay may extend to the maxillary and mandibular molars. Initially, the lower anterior teeth may not be involved because of the protective environment of the mandibular salivary secretions and the cleansing action of the tongue muscles. Infancy caries is most often seen in children with an unusual dietary history such as the addition of syrup, honey or sucrose to the formula of the use of a pacifier dipped in honey or other. It has been reported that prolonged and unrestricted night time breast-feeding can result in increased caries rates.

Infantile beri beri: It results in infants between second and sixth month. Illness develops acutely and is rapidly fatal. Child becomes restless, often cries, passes less of urine and becomes puffy. Child may become cyanosed suddenly with tachycardia and dies within 24-48 hours. He may develop convulsions and coma.

Infantile swallow: Until the primary molars erupt, infant swallows with the jaws separated and the tongue toward using facial muscles (orbicularis oris and buccinators). This is a non-conditional congenital reflex. During the normal infantile swallowing the tongue lies in between the gumpads and the mandible is stabilized by an obvious contraction of the facial muscle. The buccinator muscle

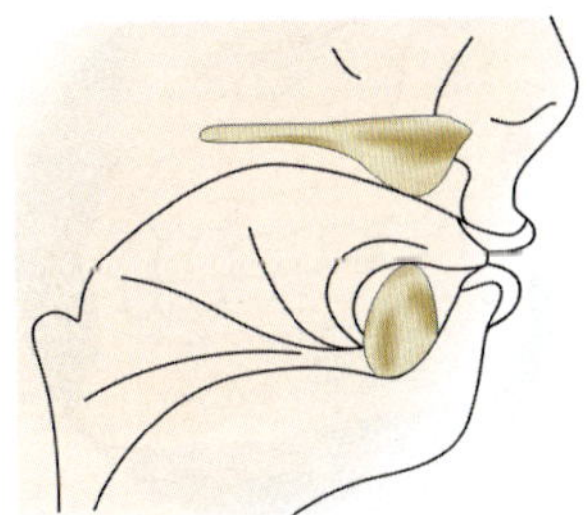

Fig.: *Infantile swallow*

is strong in infantile swallow as it is during nursing. The normal infantile swallow is such in the neonate and gradually disappears with the eruption of molars in the primary dentition.

Infectious mononucleosis: Its symptoms include, fever, sore-throat, malaise and glandular enlargement. Fauces may show exudates. Spleen is enlarged. Hepatitis may be seen. Liver may be enlarged. In severe cases myocarditis, neuritis and encephalitis may develop.

Infectious waste consists of blood, blood products, contaminated sharps or microbial waste.

Infective conjunctivitis: The patient presents with red eye with discomfort and a foreign bodysensation in the eye. There is sticking together of lid margins during sleep. Chemosis of conjunctiva is present. Mucopurulent discharge is seen at the inner canthus lower fornix or at the root of eyelashes.

Infective dose: The number of organisms required to cause an infection is termed as the infective dose.

Infective oral ulcer is due to tuberculosis usually dorsum of tongue. Shape is angular or stellate. Floor is pale in color with thick mucus like material in base of ulcer. Edge is irregular with undermined border. No extra specific treatment is required.

Inferior alveolar nerve block is a local anesthetic technique used for anesthetizing inferior alveolar nerve, lingual nerve and its terminal branches, i.e. mental and incisive.

Inferior alveolar nerve is a branch of the posterior division of the mandibular nerve. At its upper end, the nerve lies deep to the lateral pterygoid. Emerging at the lower border of this muscle, the nerve runs downwards and forwards deep to the ramus of the mandible. Reaching the mandibular foramen, it passes through it into the mandibular canal. It runs forwards in this canal just below the teeth, and ends at the mental foramen by dividing into incisive and mental branches.

Inferior alveolar neuritis is the information of inferior

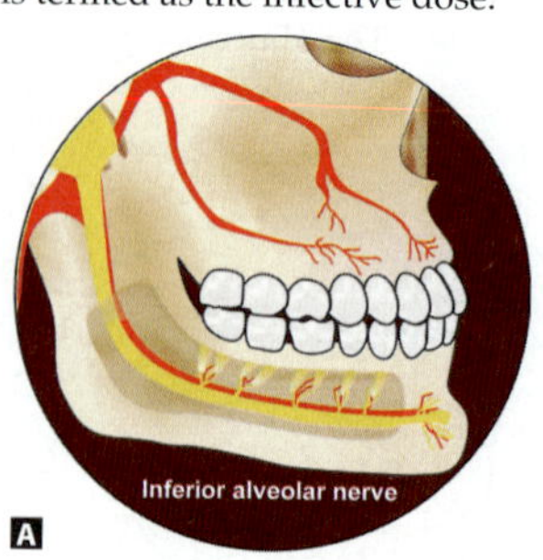

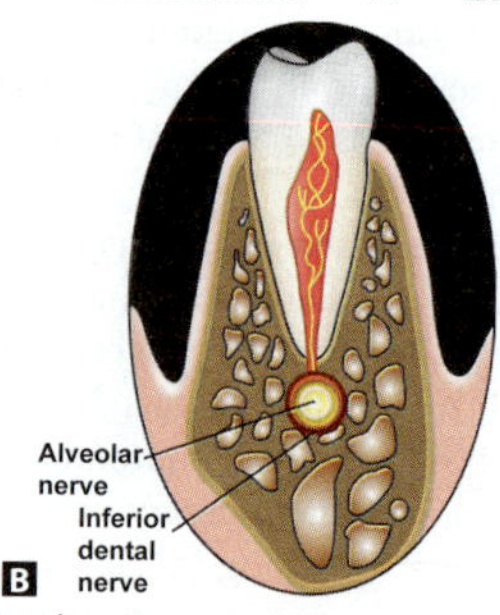

Figs A and B: *Inferior alveolar nerve*

alveolar nerve. It involves the mandibular dental nerve within the mandibular canal. It may result due to trauma, surgery or dental sepsis. Pain may be felt in all structures innervated by these nerve fibers. No autonomic or muscle symptoms are present.

Inferior sagittal sinus lies within the lower free margin of the falx cerebri as shown. It begins anteriorly and ends posteriorly by joining the straight sinus.

Inferior thyroid artery is a branch of the thyrocervical trunk. It runs upwards for some distance and then turns medially to reach the thyroid gland. The artery is distributed mainly to this gland through an ascending and a descending glandular branch.

Inferior vena cava is one of the two large veins carrying blood into right atrium.

Inflammation is a nonspecific response to injury and occurs as redness, heat, swelling pain and loss or normal tissue function. While systemic signs of inflammations are fever, leukocytosis and enlargement of lymph nodes. It is the reaction of the body to the

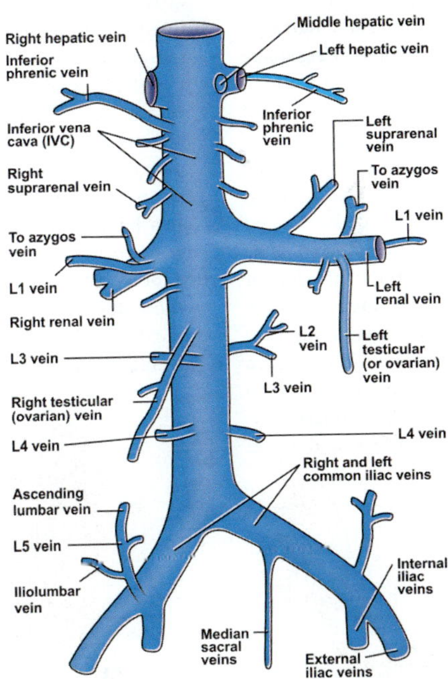

Fig.: *Inferior vena cava*

irritation. It is a defence reaction and not actually a disease. White cells are body's main defence mechanism hence there is always an increase of blood flow to the infected part. WBC's fight against invading bacteria. Cardinal signs of inflammation are swelling, redness, heat, pain and loss of function pain caused by increased pressure of blood on nerves. Affected part is unable to function properly.

Inflammatory gingival enlargement: Chronic inflammatory enlargement this is caused by prolonged exposure to dental plaque. It originates as a slight ballooning of the interdental papilla and/or marginal gingiva. In early stages, a line preserving shape bulge is seen around the teeth. It progresses slowly uniting the part of the crowns. Is it usually painless, unless complicated by acute infection or trauma. Occasionally, discrete, sessile or pedunculated mass may be present, which may be interproximal or on the marginal or attached gingiva. Painful ulceration may occur by the folds of the mass and adjacent gingiva. The gingiva may be deep red or bluish red in color, soft and friable in consistency, soft and shiny surface and bleed easily. Histologically, connective tissue shows preponderance of inflammatory cells. There is vascular engorgement with new capillary formation. Involved tissue is glossy, smooth and edematous and bleed readily. Fetid odor may occur. Drifting of teeth occurs in long-standing cases. In mouth breathers maxillary anterior gingiva is affected. Local treatment is of value.

Inflammatory pocket wall is said to be occurred where there is presence of inflammatory fluid and pocket wall appears red, soft, spongy and friable with the smooth and shiny surface.

Influenza commonly known as flu is a viral infection that starts suddenly with all signs of fever, cough and running nose like common cold. Fever is often associated with chills or rigor like malaria. Body ache is too much. Several strains of influenza have been discovered. There is no specific test to diagnose it.

Infrabony pocket is the term used where the base of the pocket is apical to the level of adjacent alveolar bone.

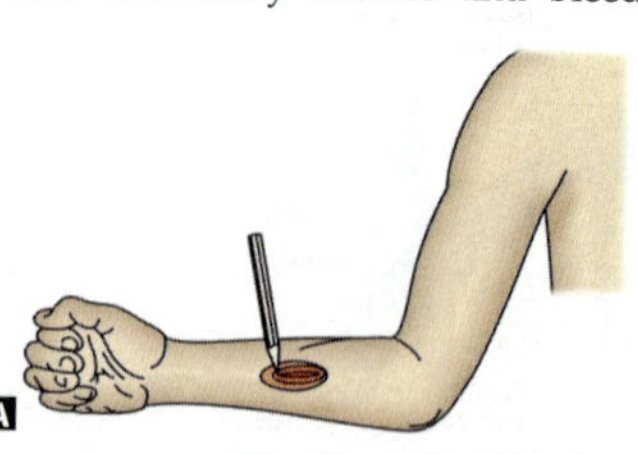

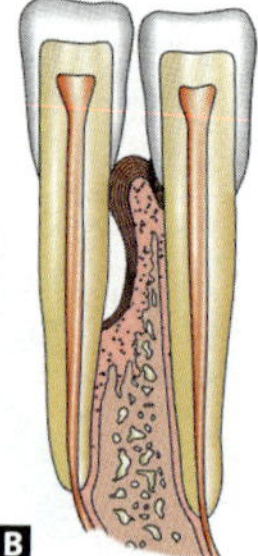

Figs A and B: *(A) Inflammation; (B) Infrabony pocket*

Infrared soldering is a technique used for soldering appliance through an infrared light source. Here focused light beam is used. The light supplies the sufficient heat to bring the parts to the soldering temperature and melt the solder.

Infratemporal fossa is a space that lies lateral to the pterygoid process, it has a greater wing of the sphenoid that forms the roof and communicates with the temporal fossa. The anterior wall of the infratemporal fossa is formed by the posterior surface of the maxilla. Just behind the basilar part the occipital bone has a large foramen magnum, through which the cranial cavity communicates with the vertebral canal.

Infundibulum is a stalk that passes through an aperture in the diaphragma to join the inferior wall of the third ventricle.

Ingot: Cast rod of alloy.

Inhalation is the flow of air in to the body also known as inspiration.

Inhalation anesthetic agents nitrous oxide is the gas which is constantly used with at least 20% oxygen. It requires a specific equipment to mix the gas in the specific proportion. Any drug or equipment necessary for resuscitation should be easily available in emergency.

Inhalation transmission: Inhalation of microorganism aerolised from a patient's blood or saliva when doctor is using high speed of ultrasonic equipment.

Inherited taste disorder: Familial dysautonomia is rare, found in Jews. Affected children are usually hypotonic, easily being disturbed, excessive sweat and mucus production. Such children are not having vallate and fungiform papillae. Tongue is devoid of taste receptors.

Initially the immune system generates diversity by combining high polymorphic gene segments to form receptor molecules. Tolerance like immune recognition is Ag specific.

Injury breach of biological tissue due to intentional or accidental attack. Injury to oral tissues results in tissue damage. Physical injury

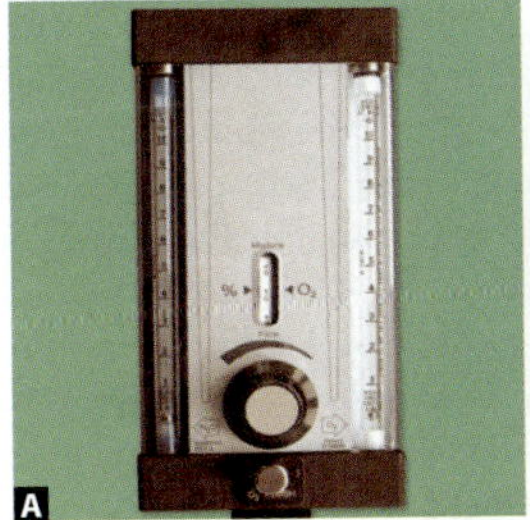

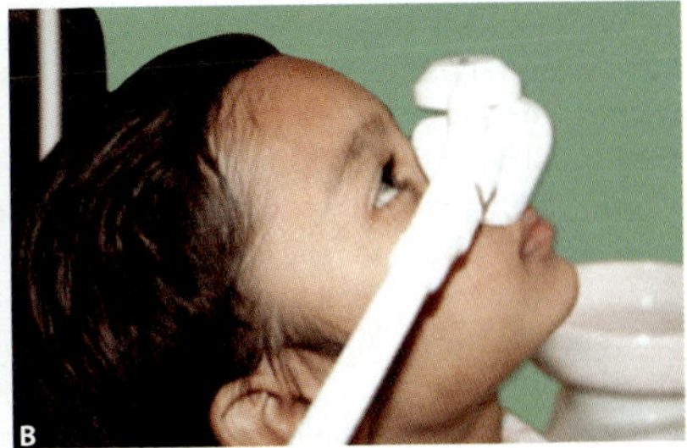

Figs A and B: *(A) Nitrous oxide equipment; (B) Patient receiving nitrous oxide*

can affect teeth, soft tissue and bone. Chemical injury occurs due to use of caustic materials. Microorganisms can cause injury by invading oral tissue.

Inlay a gold, porcelain, or composite custom-made filling cemented into the tooth. If it covers the tips of the teeth, it is called an onlay.

Innate refers to any inborn resistance that is present the first time the pathogen is encountered. It does not require previous exposure and is not modified significantly by repeated exposures to the pathogen over the life of an individual.

I

Inoculation refers to introduction of microorganism into living tissues and culture media.

Inositol also known as vitamin B_8. Its high concentrations are found in muscles of heart and brain. Therapeutically inositol is useful for depression, bipolar disorder, Alzheimer ADHD, PCOS, insulin resistance, weight gain and sterility.

Insertion is the point where muscle attaches to the bone.

Insidious refer to coming on gradually.

Inspiration center that is present in medulla oblongata sends signal to cause inspiration.

Intrabony defect can be described as three-wall bony defect.

Integrin mediated phase develops slowly but leads to stable long-lasting molecular contacts that prevent further movement of neutrophils and cause it to flatten out against the endothelium. Once attached, neutrophils actively move themselves between endothelial cells to migrate out of the venule. Emigration and chemotaxis are facilitated in part by binding of neutrophil surface integrins to fibronectin and other components of extracellular matrix.

Integrins are a group of heterodimer proteins with alpha and beta polypeptide chains. Integrins bind a variety of ECM cells as well as non-integrin adhesion molecules such as vascular cell adhesion molecule found on stoma cell surface. They allow progenitors to bind tightly to marrow stoma and are responsible for sequestering progenitor cells in appropriate microenvironment. Contact of integrin with its ligand also transmits a signal into the integrin expressing cell, which can stimulate its growth and other activities.

Intellectual disability is a disability characterized by significant limitations both in intellectual functioning and in adaptive behavior, which covers many everyday social and practical skills. This disability originates before the age of 18. Intellectual functioning—also called intelligence—refers to general mental capacity, such as learning, reasoning, problem solving, and so on (AAIDD 2002). According to the American Academy for Cerebral Palsy and Developmental Medicine, cerebral palsy is described as a group of disorders of the development of movement and posture, causing activity limitations that are attributed to nonprogressive disturbances that occurred in the developing fetal or infant brain. The motor disorders of cerebral palsy are often accompanied by disturbances of sensation, cognition, and communication perception or by a seizure disorder. The term cerebral pasly describes the group of disorders of movement and posture due to the lesion of immature brain (Bax in 1964).

Intelligence quotient refers to the relationship between intelligence and chronological age.

Intention tremor also known as cerebellar tremors and it is the manifestation of cerebellar disease, the superior cerebellar peduncle.

Intercostal muscles refer to respiratory muscles found in between ribs.

Interradicular refers to between the roots.

Inter-transitional period refers to mixed dentition period where the maxillary and mandibular arches consist of sets of deciduous and permanent teeth. Between the permanent incisors and first permanent molars are the deciduous molars and canines. This phase during the mixed dentition period is relatively stable and no change occurs.

Interceptive orthodontics can be defind as phase of science and art of orthodontics employed to recognize and eliminate potential irregularities and malpositions in the developing dentofacial complex. These procedures are employed to lessen or to eliminate the severity of developing malocclusion (either due to heredity or extremes or intrinsic factors, e.g. serial extraction).

Intercuspation: Interlocking a cusp-to-fossa relationship of the maxillary to mandibular teeth.

Intercuspal position (ICP) refers to that position of mandible when there is maximal intercuspation between the maxillary and the mandibular teeth.

Interdental eyelet wiring is a wiring technique where eyelets are constructed with a help of artery forceps, these eyelets are fitted between two teeth and push the wire on the lingual/palatal aspect

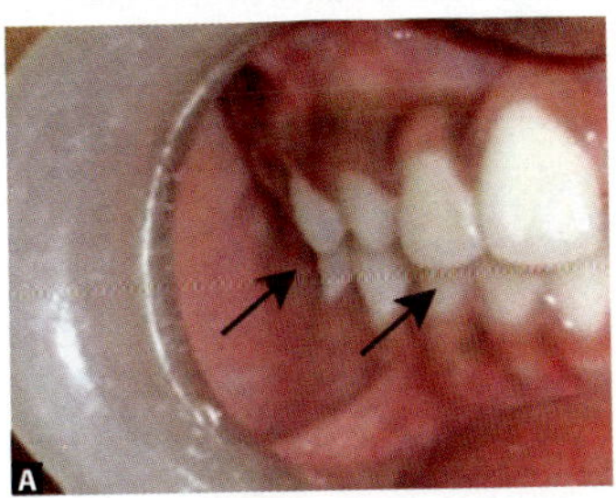

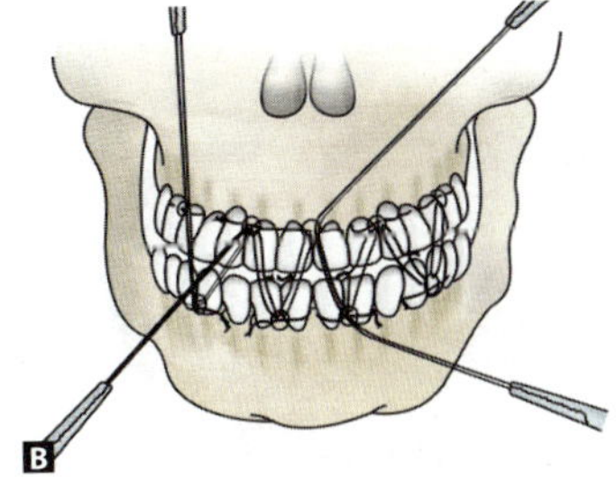

Figs A and B: *(A) Intercuspation; (B) Interdental eyelet wiring*

as eyelets tend to get displaced. The free ends are then passed from the adjacent proximal contact, the distally placed free-end wire is passed through the eyelet and then it is twisted along with the mesially placed free wire. To connect the upper and lower jaw, the wire is passed through the upper and lower eyelets and then plaited together at the lower border of the mandibular teeth.

Interdental gingiva also known as papillary gingiva occupies the gingival embrasure which is the interproximal space beneath the area of tooth contact, the shape of the papilla is in the shape of reverse triangle, i.e. the tip of the papilla is towards the contact point or have a "col" shape in the adult dentition, which is more susceptible to infection. In the primary dentition, interdental spacing is common. Hence saddle areas are present resulting in a well-keratinized interdental surface. This may be the reason for lower prevalence of periodontal lesions in children because these areas are less vulnerable to development and progression of the inflammatory spaces.

Interdental knives are knives used in the interdental area. These are spear-shaped knives that has cutting edge on both the sides of the blade that are available in double-ended or single-ended blades, e.g. Orban knife no 1-2 and Merrifield knife no 1-4.

Interference refers to any contact in ICP or other movements, that prevents the remaining occlusal surfaces to achieve stable occlusion.

Interlabial gap: The vertical distance between the upper and lower lip ranges between 0 and 3 mm.

Intermaxillary fixation (IMF) is a method where the immobilization is achieved by the help of intermaxillary wiring, a clinical union of bone can be expected within four weeks and without using general anesthesia.

Intermittent fever: When fever is present only for few hours during the day.

Internal bevel incision is the incision used in periodontal surgeries. It is the incision from which flap is reflected to expose the underlying bone and root. It starts from the designated area on the gingiva and is directed to the area at or near the crest of the bone.

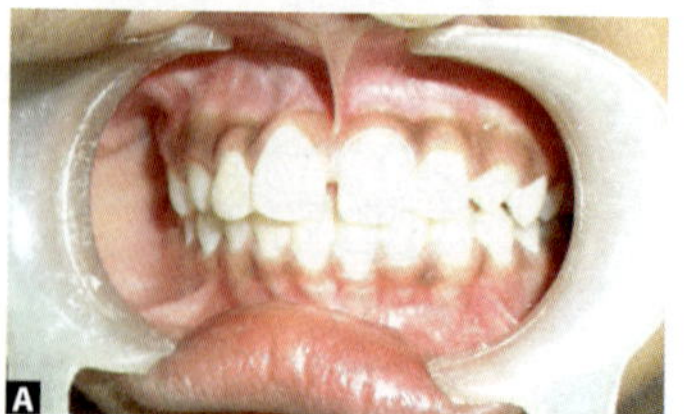

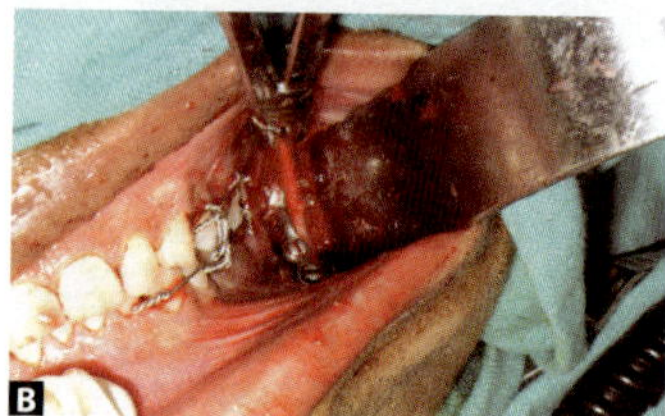

Figs A and B: *(A) Interdental gingiva; (B) Intermaxillary fixation*

Internal carotid artery is a terminal branch of common carotid artery that begins at the upper border of the thyroid cartilage and ascends to reach the base of the skull where it enters the carotid canal.

Internal ear is in the form of a cavity within the petrous temporal bone having a very complex shape. This bony cavity (or bony labyrinth) has a central part called the vestibule. Continuous with the front of the vestibule, there is a spiral-shaped cavity, the bony cochlea. Posteriorly, the vestibule is continuous with three semicircular canals.

Internal jugular veins are the chief veins of the head and neck. Present on either side, the upper end of the vein lies in the jugular foramen on the base of the skull. The lower end of the vein lies behind the sternal end of the clavicle where the internal jugular joins the subclavian vein to form the corresponding brachiocephalic vein.

Internal resorption is an insidious process when the afflicted pulp is completely symptom free. Symptoms of internal resorption depend primarily on whether the process had broken through the external tooth surface. The pulp that erodes through the root surface may give vague pain on mastication. Percussion may be of little value pulpectomy is the only treatment for internal resorption. The cause is unknown. No early symptoms are present. Generally only one tooth is affected. On X-ray, involved tooth shows a round or oval radiolucent area in central portion of tooth. If tooth is not treated, complete performation may take place.

I

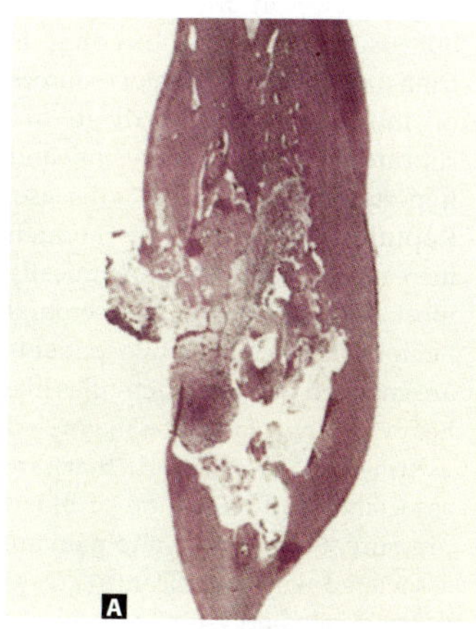

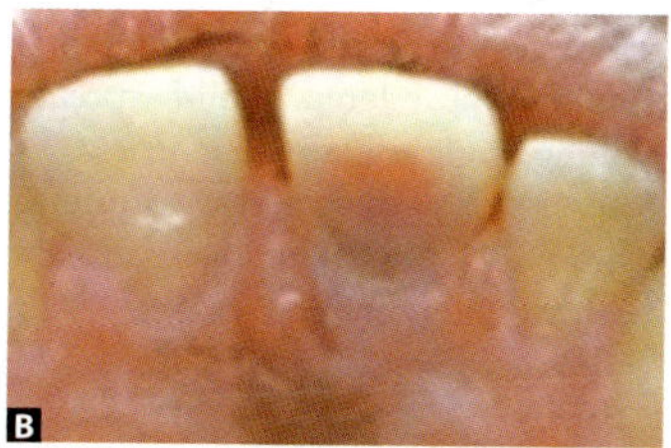

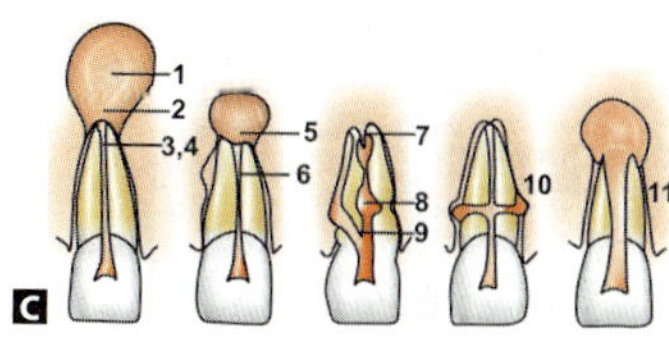

Figs A to C: *(A and B) Histological and clinical or view of internal resorption; (C) Patterns of internal resorption*

Interneuron refers to the nerves that conduct impulses from sensory neurons to motor neurons.

Interoceptors are the pain receptors which are located within the body cavities, they serve involuntary bodily function below conscious levels, e.g. Free nerve endings: perception of visceral pain and other sensation. Pacinian corpuscles – perception of pressure.

Interpret to offer an explanation.

Interproximal the space between two adjacent surfaces.

Inter-radicular fibers occur in a multirooted tooth as they fan out from the cementum of the tooth into the furcation area.

Interstitial brain edema: During acute hydrocephalus due to sudden or persistently high intraventricular CSF pressure, the ependyma gets damaged and CSF escapes to the periventricular white matter. Interstitial space known as interstitial edema. Fluid spreads along angles of lateral ventricle.

Intervertebral disk rupture produces gradual or sudden low backache with or without sciatica. Pain radiates to legs. Pain is increased by coughing, spasm and reflexes are decreased on affected side. Patient leans towards the affected side.

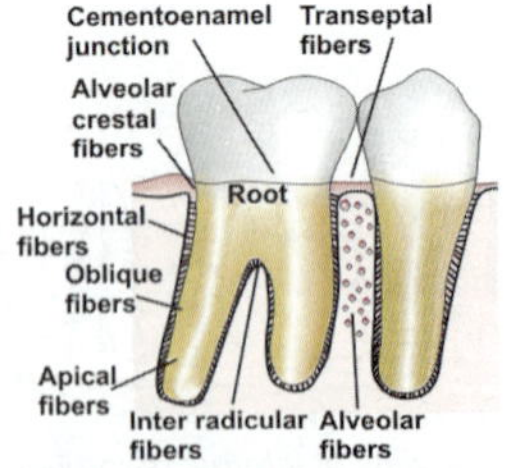

Fig.: *Inter-radicular fibers*

Intestinal tuberculosis cecum, mesenteric glands and peritoneum are generally involved. Miliary TB is the primary lesion. Common presenting symptoms are abdominal pain, malabsorption, diarrhea, low-grade fever and loss of appetite. Ulcers are circular and may cause obstruction. Mantoux test may be positive. Ascites is exudative in nature with raised protein and plenty of leukocytes. Treatment is with INH, rifampicin, pyrazinamide and streptomycin for 3 months and INH and rifampicin for another 9 months.

Intracerebral hemorrhage is also called apoplexy. Most commonly seen in individuals over 50 years of age. Intracerebral hemorrhage may develop in any blood vessel, but usual source of bleeding is from arteries. Two major sources of intracerebral hemorrhage are ruptured arterial aneurysms and hypertensive vascular disease. Rupture occurs with sudden increase in local pressure. Clinically most cases of intracerebral hemorrhage occurs while patients are engaged in normal activities like heavy lifting, factors categorized as physical stress and that are associated with elevation of blood pressure. Both anxiety and pain are associated with significant increase in heart rate and blood pressure of patient making development of an hemorrhagic CVA more likely.

Intractable pain: Pain unresponsive to usual methods of pain management.

Intradermal nevus is congenital development of tumor-like malformation of the skin/mucous membrane. Function of nevus cells is to produce melanin. *Clinical features:* These are commonly known as mole of dark brown color. It is slightly raised. Intraoral lesions are commonly seen over hard palate or gingival. These grow slowly. Under microscope, nevus reveals cluster of nevus cells confined within connective tissue. No mitotic activity is seen. These generally don't require any treatment.

Intraligamentary anesthesia is a technique of depositing local anesthesia within periodontal ligament. Some people find an inferior dental block unpleasant due to tongue and lip being made numb. So injection is given directly down the gingival crevices. It immediately anesthetize the tooth.

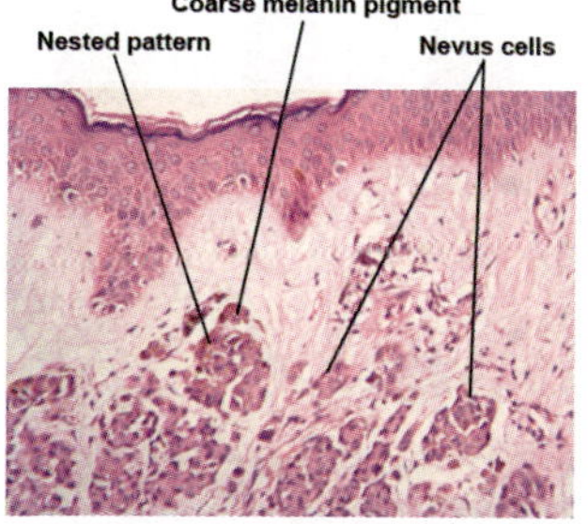

Fig.: *Intradermal nevus*

Intramembranous ossification is a physiological process of bone formation where bone is formed directly in membranous tissue.

Intraocular pressure means pressure within eye.

Intraoral is inside your mouth.

Intrapulpal injection is a local anesthetic technique used to deliver anesthesia directly into the pulp. It is useful for mandibular teeth anesthetization as local anesthesia technique rarely obtain profound anesthesia due to high bone. This injection controls pain, both by applying pressure and utilizing the pharmacologic action of local anesthetic agent.

Intrathecal baclofen is a drug that is administered directly into the cerebrospinal fluid (CSF). Intrathecal baclofen administration is useful for the severely involved spastic child, dystonic child, or child who has mixed disease to enable sitting in the wheelchair decrease spinal deformity, and increase the comfort level and ease of care.

Intravenous anesthetics is simpler and leads to rapid pleasant induction. Recovery is swift without nausea and vomiting and there is lack of pulmonary irritation. IV anesthesia can be used for induction of anesthesia as a sole agent for very short procedure. It should not be used for maintenance of anesthesia. Extra venous injection may produce local necrosis. Overdose and too rapid injections are its cautions.

Intravenous sedation refers to the sedative drug directly infected into a vein. It is given to reduce anxiety in an over-anxious patient. This may be insufficient for certain restorative and minor surgical procedure. Intravenous diazepam is commonly used. It is injected into a bigger vein to avoid thrombophlebitis. Diazepam produces muscle relaxation and also a dry mouth.

Intrusion is the term given to displacement of tooth in an apical direction.

Invagination is to enclose within.

Invasive refers to spreading to surrounding tissue of benign tumors that are generally confined to a fibrous capsule or well circumscribed. Capsule is formed by atrophy of cells at the periphery of expansile growth. Malignant tumors don't respect normal anatomical boundaries. In some malignant tumors invasion is seen only under microscope.

Investment material is a special gypsum product that is able to withstand extreme heat.

Iodine deficiency T_3 and T_4 production decreases because iodine is necessary for the synthesis of these thyroid hormones. Low plasma levels of T_3 and T_4 cause the secretion of TSH. A persistent secretion of TSH causes the thyroid gland to enlarge, producing a goiter.

Iodine: It forms thyroid hormone. Its deficiency results in goiter. One third iodine of whole body lies in thyroid. An ovary also contains more of iodine. Whole blood contains 3 to 30 microgram. It is constituent of thyroxine, an active principle of thyroid gland. It plays an important role in energy metabolism and in growth of body. Adult body contains 50 mg of iodine. Cabbage, cauliflower and radish are goitrogenic not allowing food iodine available to body.

Iodophors are complexes of iodine and surface active agents such as non-ionic detergents, quaternary compounds and macromolecules. The iodine is held in a loose combination and about 70-80% may be available when the solution is diluted. Iodophors are non-toxic, non-irritating, non-staining and miscible with water in all proportions. They do not produce sensitivity and are, therefore, used in prophylaxis.

Ion is an electrically charged particle at atom that gains or loses an electron.

Ionizing radiation: Radiation capable of producing ions including electromagnetic radiation.

Iontophor is the process of introducing a drug through the dental

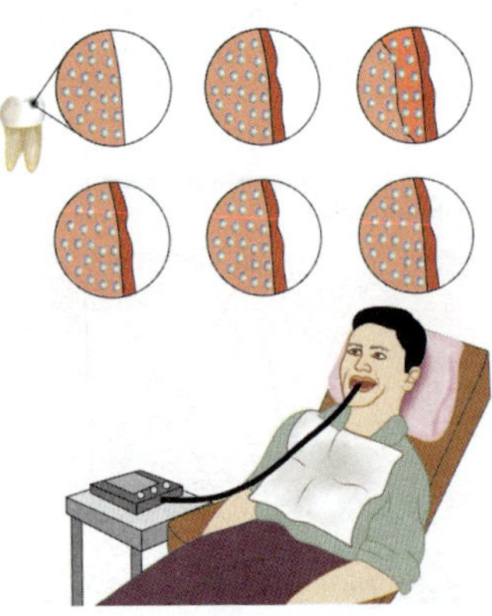

Fig.: *Iontophoresis*

enamel by use of an electrical current; often used in the treatment of dentin hypersensitivity.

Iris refers to the circular dark part seen in the center of the eye. The iris is seen through a transparent disc-like structure—the cornea which covers it. It forms a diaphragm placed immediately in front of the lens. At its periphery it is continuous with the ciliary body. In its center there is an aperture, the pupil. The iris is composed of a stroma of connective tissue containing numerous pigment cells, and in which are embedded blood vessels and smooth muscle (see below).

Iron deficiency anemia is a chronic microcytic hypochromic type of anemia and exists most commonly. It may cause pale skin and generalized weakness. Some may develop splitting and cracking of hair. Palpitation, dizziness and sensitivity to cold may develop. It occurs due to: Inadequate absorption of iron and excessive loss of iron. *Oral Manifestations:* Pallor of oral mucosa and gingiva. Atrophic mucositis, loss of tongue papillae, glossitis, Angular cheilitis is seen. Total RBC count is low. Stool should be examined for occult blood. Ferrous sulphate in sufficient quantity helps.

Iron in pregnancy: Total of 300 mg of iron is needed for the growth of fetus, 70 mg for placenta and 500 mg for the synthesis of hemoglobin with increased blood volume. Iron accumulates at the rate of 0.5 mg/daily in first trimester. It may increase 3 to 4 mg/day in second and third trimester. This extra iron need cannot be met through diet so it has to be supplied from outside.

Iron refers to a mineral that is required by our body for performing many functions. It is needed for formation of blood and is absorbed in the upper portion of duodenum. When hemoglobin level is short absorption is higher otherwise it is lower. Total iron in body is 3-4 gm and daily requirement is 20 mg. Idiopathic hemochromatosis results in excessive iron absorption. Deficiency of iron result is anemia.

Irreversible index refers to index that measures conditions that will not change. Irreversible index

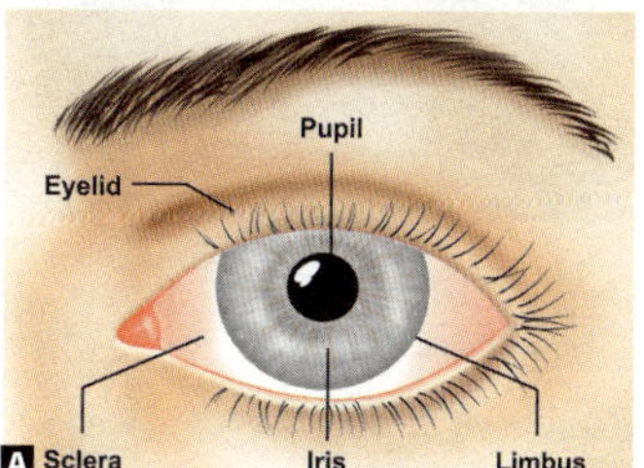

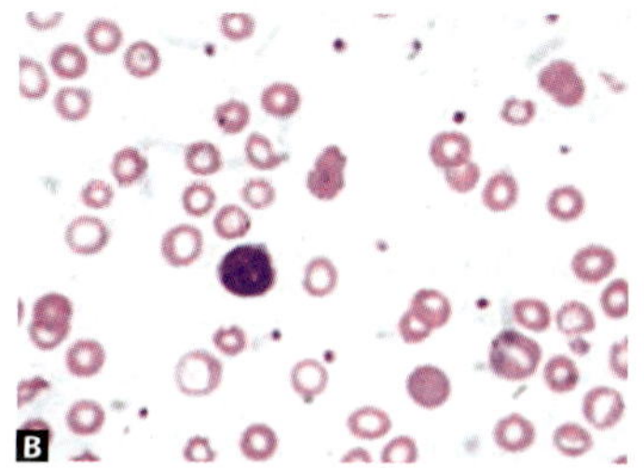

Figs A and B: *(A) Iris; (B) Iron deficiency anemia*

scores cannot decrease in value on subsequent examinations, e.g: An Index that measures dental caries.

Irreversible pulpitis is a persistent inflammatory condition of the pulp, symptomatic or asymptomatic, caused by a noxious stimulus". It has both acute and chronic stages in pulp.

Irrigation is the technique of using a solution to wash out your mouth.

Irritable bowel syndrome is principally a motility disorder of intestine due to response to cholecystokinin after food. First group has abdominal pain and constipation, second group has watery diarrhea without pain, and third group has both. Some to 3-4 times in morning to clear their bowel. In some, bloating heart burn and palpitation.

Irritation fibroma refers to fibroma.

Ischemic stroke refers to obstruction with the blood vessel 80% strokes are ischemic. In severe case, ischemic cell death may cause infarction. T1A results from brief occlusion of an artery with restoration before irreversible damage occurs. Symptoms include monocular loss of vision and contralateral weakness. Symptoms develop within a few seconds. Loss of consciousness is very rare and signs are focal causative factor may be atheroma and thrombosis.

Isograft is a graft harvested from an identical twin. There is no rejection of this graft.

Isokinetic is an exercise in which the muscle generates force against a variable resistance and the speed of movement is maintained by a present controlled device.

Isometric is an exercise in which the muscle generates force but there is no observable movement. It is like pushing a wall.

Isotonic is an exercise in which muscle generates force against constant resistance and movement results.

Isotonic solution is the one that has the same concentration as the solution to which it is compared.

Isotope: Any or two or more forms of a chemical element which have different mass numbers because their nuclei contain different numbers of neurons. Radioactive isotopes are widely used as tracers.

Isotropic is occuring equally in all directions.

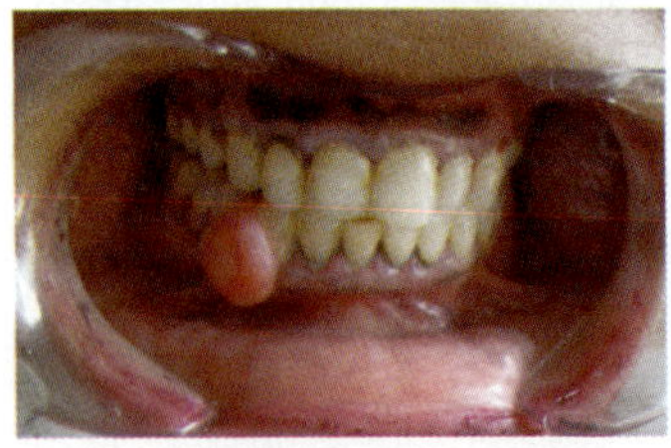

Fig.: *Fibroma*

Jacket crown is used for front teeth which are too mutilated to be restored by ordinary filling. Such cases have extensive caries, fractured crown and discoloration. Outer coating of natural crown is removed to leave a stump of dentin on which artificial crown fits like a jacket.

Jackscrew is a small device generally used for expansion of maxilla and mandible. It is used as a removable appliance to perform interceptive orthodontic procedure. The device can be placed in anterolateral position or in midline to achieve minor tooth movements.

Jacksonian epilepsy is a neurological disorder that includes the convulsions seen only in one area of the body.

Jadassohn: Lewand Owsky syndrome is recognized by congenital gross thickening of finger and toe nails. Along with it leukokeratosis is noted. Nail lesion is noted just after birth with a horny brownish material at nail bed. Oral leukokeratosis affects dorsum of tongue which becomes thickened and grayish white. Histologically these are similar to white sponge nevus. Frequent oral aphthous ulceration may develop.

Jaundice is a yellow pigmentation of skin and sclera of eye due to formation of excessive bilirubin. Bilirubin is formed from hemoglobin when the old RBCs are broken down by spleen. There are three types of jaundice, i.e. Hepatocellular jaundice, obstructive jaundice and hemolytic jaundice.

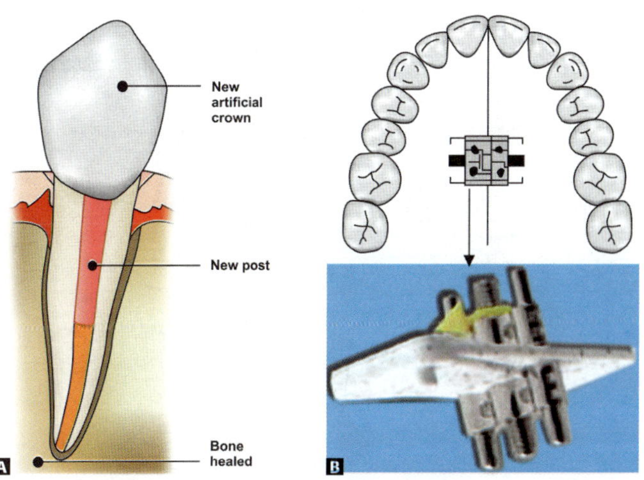

Figs A and B: *(A) Jacket crown; (B) Jack screw*

Jaw is a common name for the maxilla or mandible.

Jaw thrust is the maneuver used to obtain the airway.

Joint refers to that part of the body where the meeting of two bones occurs in order to establish movement.

Junctional epithelium is collar like band of stratified squamous non-keratinized epithelium which is formed by the merger of oral epithelium and reduced enamel epithelium (REE) during the tooth eruption Internally it is attached to the tooth by the means of epithelial attachment or internal basal lamina and externally it is attached to the gingival connective tissue by the means of external basal lamina.

Juvenile periodontitis was the term given by Chaput in 1967 and Butler in 1969 and can be defined as a disease of periodontium occurring in an otherwise healthy adolescent which is characterized by rapid loss of alveolar bone and by migration and loosening of the

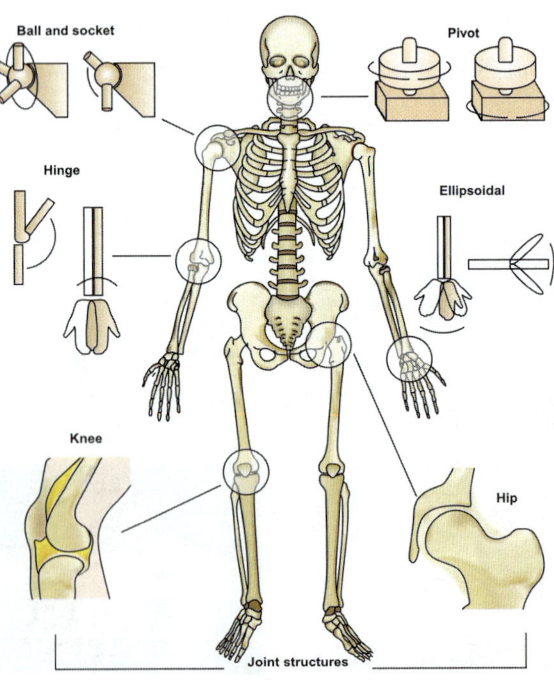

Fig.: *Various types of joint*

teeth in the presence or absence of either secondary epithelial proliferation and pocket formation or secondary gingival disease. Rapid periodontal destruction of selected teeth occurs at an early age. It involved severe periodontal destruction with an onset around puberty. The localized form (JP) occurs in otherwise healthy individuals with destruction classically localized and around the first permanent molars and incisors, and not involving more than two other teeth generalized juvenile periodontitis (GJP) also occurs in otherwise healthy individuals but involves more than 14 teeth that is being generalized to an area or the entire dentition.

Juvenile rheumatoid arthritis is a condition that involves joints, connective tissue and viscera. Peak incidence is 1-4 years. Child develops fever, lymphadenopathy, hepatosplenomegaly, abdominal pain and pleura pericarditis. Any form of arthritis in younger age for more than 3-4 months. Subcutaneous nodules, symmetric joint involvement, morning stiffness and osteoporosis without erosions are diagnostic. Aspirin is the drug of choice.

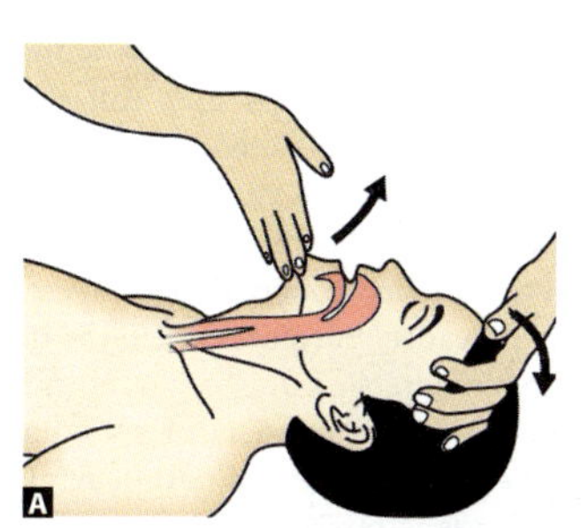

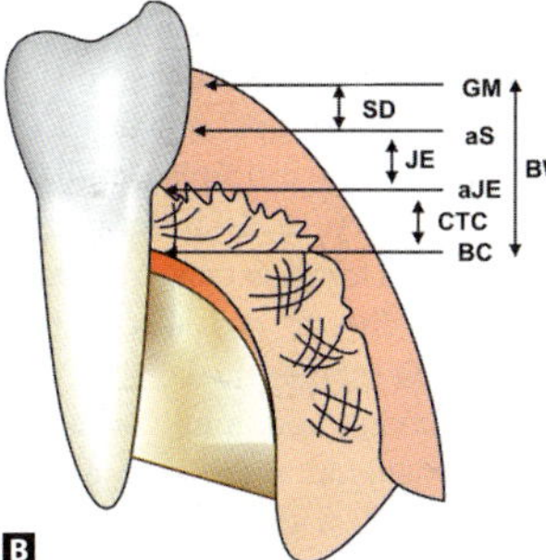

Figs A and B: *(A) Jaw thrust maneuver; (B) Junctional epithelium*

Kala azar is characterized by fever, hepatic and splenic enlargement. Fever is having double daily remission. There is dusky pigmentation which is noted on feet, hands and abdomen. There will be generalized enlargement of glands. Blood shows leukopenia and Leishman-Donovan bodies. Specific complement fixation test will become positive.

Kaolin is a fine powder used in pharmacy in ointments and coating pills.

Kaposi's sarcoma is a malignant neoplasm arising from endothelial cells of capillaries. *Clinical Features:* With AIDS, lesions are multicentric. It affects skin, lymph nodes, bone and viscera. It develops after age of 50. Tumor shows multiple capillaries. Inflammatory cell infiltration is common. Homosexuals are affected more easily. It has three stages: (1) Patch stage—It is the initial stage having red, pink or purple. These develop over oral mucosa; (2) Plaque stage—Patch converts into plaque. Lesion is large and raised; (3) Nodular stage—There develops multiple nodular lesions on the skin. Being multicentric surgery is not feasible. Radiotherapy and chemotherapy is given.

Keloid is a painless and progressive enlargement of scar. Itching is a prominent manifestation. Area in front of sternum face and neck are commonly involved. It is reddish and elevated from surface. It is firm and irregular with claw-like processes invading healthy skin.

Keratoacanthoma is a fast-growing neoplasm that resembles squamous carcinoma. Lesion is an elevated umbilicated lesion with a depressed central core. It measures 1.0 to 1.5 cm in diameter. It starts as a small, firm nodule and within 2 months develops to a full size. It may heal spontaneously. The size of the lesion will vary from 1 cm to several cm. There will be a central keratin filled crater. Many suspect a viral cause. Surgical excision is the treatment.

Keratomalacia consists of softening of entire thickness of part or whole process is rapid one and may lead

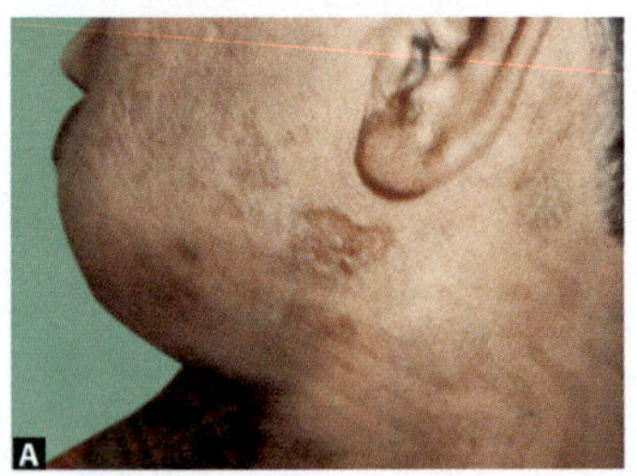

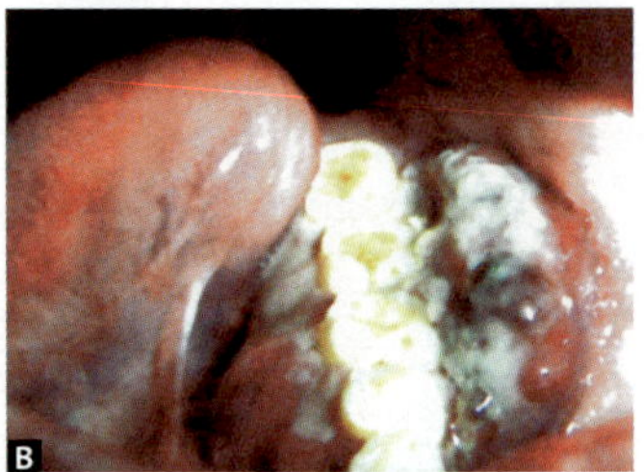

Figs A and B: *(A) Kaposi sarcoma (patch stage) affecting skin; (B) Kaposi sarcoma (nodular stage)*

process is rapid one and may lead to necrosis, ulceration and destruction of eye-ball.

Keratosis follicularis is a genodermatosis transmitted as autosomal dominant characteristic. It is manifested during childhood. Skin lesions appear as small, papules which are red. When macerated, they produce foul-smelling masses. Oral lesions develop as minute, whitish, papules most commonly found on gingiva and tongue. It is rare and inherited as an autosomal dominant condition. In less severely affected cases, intraoral lesions are keratotic. In severe case dermal inflammatory exudates and a ten-dency to cobblestone changes is seen.

Kerosene poisoning: Thinking it as water by mistake children can drink it. There will be burning pain in the throat and feeling of warmth. A smell of kerosene oil in the vomited matter is characteristic. Patient develops cough and becomes drowsy. Face may be pale or cyanosed. Pulse is feeble and respiration may be hurried convulsions may be seen in some children. Bronchopneumonia may be developed.

Ketamine is related to ary cyclo alkyl amines which produce dissociative anesthesia. Patient loses consciousness rapidly but with only slight depression of normal reflexes. Analgesia and amnesia are marked but there is poor muscular relaxation. Dreams and hallucinations are common. Recovery period is slow. Analgesic effect remains for hours.

Ketoacidosis is mostly found as a complication of diabetes mellitus. In it low blood pH is caused by the presence of an abnormally large number of ketone bodies produced when fats are converted to form of glucose to be used for cellular respiration.

K-flex file was introduced by Kerr manufacturing company in 1982. It was realized that square blank of file results in total decrease in the instrument flexibility. To maintain shape and flexibility of this file, K-flex file was introduced. K-flex file is rhombus in cross-section having two acute angles and two obtuse angles. Two acute angles increase sharpness

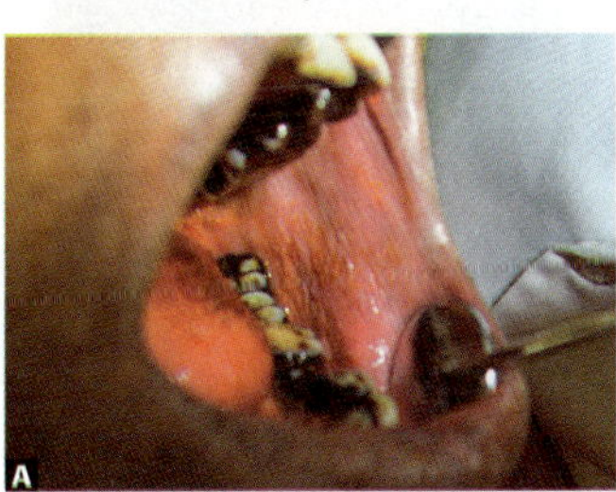

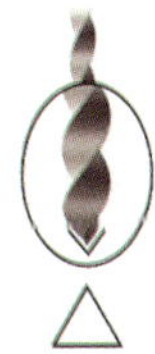

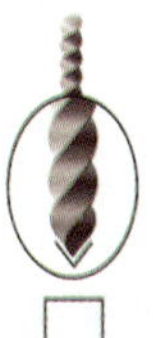

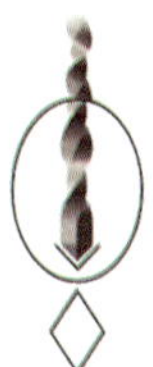

Figs A and B.: *(A) Keratosis follicularis; (B) K files*

and cutting efficiency of the instrument. Two obtuse angles provide more space for debris removal. Also the decrease in contact of instrument with canal walls provide more space for irrigation. It is used with filing and rasping motion.

Killian's dehiscence refers to a gap here between the thyropharyngeal and cricopharyngeal fibers.

Kinesics means body language

Kirkland curette refers to a heavy surgical curette often required during the surgical procedures for the removal of granulation tissue, fibrous interdental tissue and tenacious subgingival deposits.

Kirkland knives/periodontal knives/ Gingivectomy knive is a representative of knive commonly used as gingivectomy. They are available either as single-ended or double-ended instruments. The entire peri-phery of kidney-shaped knive is the cutting edge of the instrument.

Kramer curette refers to a heavy surgical curette often required during the surgical procedures for the removal of granulation tissue, fibrous interdental tissue and tenacious subgingival deposits. It is available in number 1, 2 and 3.

Krushkal Wallis test is the non-parametric version of one way analysis of variance.

Kyphosis refers to an excessive backward curvature of spine. It results in lump or a more gradually rounded back. It may be a result of osteoporosis, fracture of vertebra or tuberculosis.

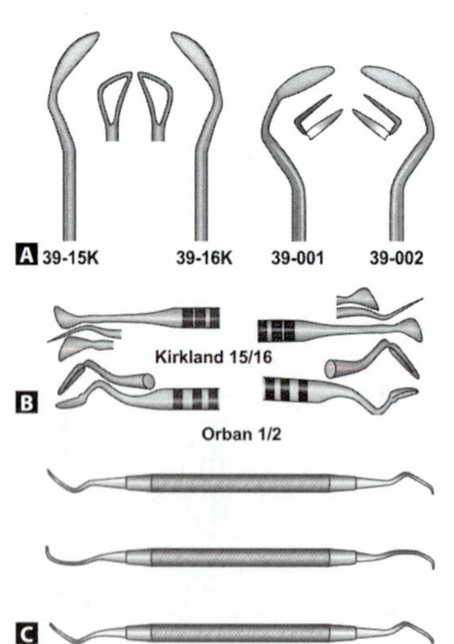

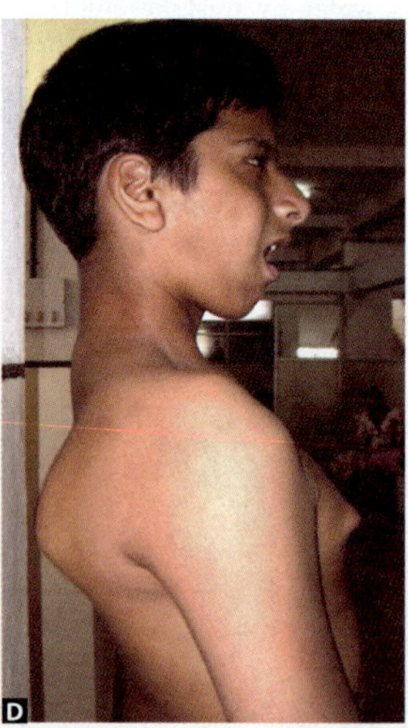

Figs A to D: *(A) Kirkland curette; (B) Kirkland knives; (C) Kramer curettes; (D) Kyphosis*

Labial is relating to the lip; another name for the facial surface of anterior teeth (next to the lip).

Labioversion refers to abnormal protrusion of maxillary incisors towards the lips.

Lacrimal apparatus is a system that consists of the organs concerned with the secretion and drainage of this fluid. Lacrimal fluid is secreted by the lacrimal gland and is poured into the conjunctival sac at the superior conjunctival fornix.

Lacrimal gland refers to the gland that produces tears, located in upper lateral portion of orbit.

Lacrimal papilla is a small conical elevation present just lateral to the lacrimal caruncle.

Lactational mastitis refers to infection of breast of nursing mother is caused by introduction of infection into breast through cracked nipple. Nursing mother develops pain in breast, chills and fever. Condition may be treated with antibiotics and wet dressings.

Lactobacilli are Gram positive, non-spore-forming rods that generally grow best under micro-aerophilic conditions. Isolation and enumeration of oral lactobacilli have been facilitated by use of selective agar medium which suppresses the growth of other oral organisms by its low pH (5.4).

Lactose intolerance is an intestinal condition that causes symptoms like cramping, abdominal distension and gas problem. There is an absence of body enzyme lactase which breaks down lactose into glucose and galactose. In this condition lactose descends directly to the large intestine where intestinal bacteria break it down into acid and gas causing discomfort.

Lag screws are used for rigid immobilization where the thread of the screw engages only in the inner plate of bone. The hole is drilled in the outer cortex and is slightly of a larger diameter than the threaded part. Once tightened, the head of the screw engages in the outer plate and the fracture is compressed.

Lamina propria is a layer of connective tissue that lies just under the epithelium of the mucous membrane.

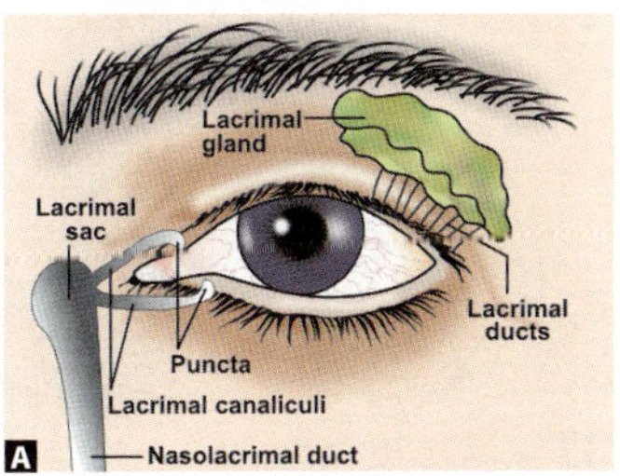

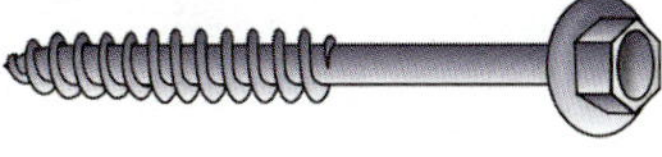

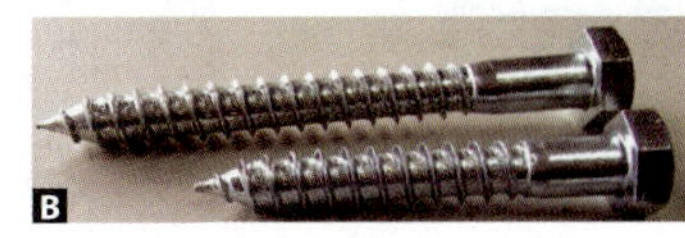

Figs A and B: *(A) Lacrimal system; (B) Lag screw*

Laminate veneer is porcelain, or composite covering which is bonded to restore discolored, or damaged teeth.

Land refers to the area between the flutes which projects axially from central core to the cutting edge.

Landau reflex can be elicited by suspending the neonate in the prone position by putting a hand under the abdomen. The normal response consists of extension of head, trunk and hips. When the head is flexed the trunk and hips also flex.

Langhan's giant cells are big and have large number of nuclei. Nuclei are vesicular. Nuclear arrangement is in the form of horse-shoe. Cytoplasm is in abundant. Mostly are seen in tuberculosis.

Language is a system of codes and patterns that have meaning. A language is a system of units with certain properties called the linguistic information stored in the memory store of both listener and speaker.

Laparoscopy is the visualization of pelvic and abdominal viscera can be done without major injury to abdominal wall. It can be done by using a fibreoptic, telescope illuminated by a light source.

Laryngitis refer to inflammation of larynx. This could be due to abnormal use of vocal cord or excessive smoke. Rest to the voice is helpful. Symptoms will clear in a few days. Carcinoma of larynx produces hoarseness of voice.

Laryngoscope is an instrument that is used to examine the interior of the larynx in a living person.

Laryngoscopy is the procedure carried out to examine interior of a larynx with the help of laryngoscope.

Laryngospasm refers to involuntary muscular spasm of adductor muscles of larynx. It can be identified by high pitched inspirations and dyspnea. It is caused by partial or complete spasm or the vocal cords. In complete spasm breath sounds maybe absent and abdominal heaving becomes prominent.

Larynx is a hollow tube with a flap of epiglottis protecting the airway from aspiration of food material. Highly mobile vocal cords function

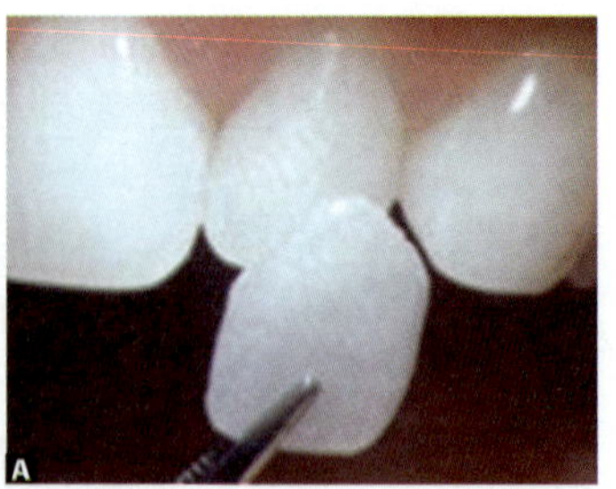

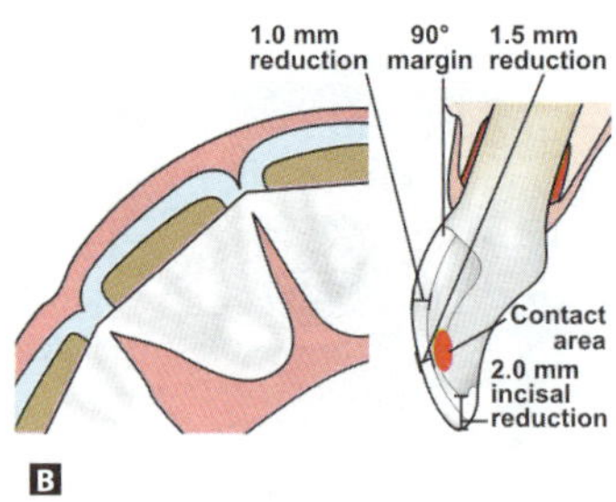

Figs A and B: *(A) Veneers; (B) Laminate preparation*

in phonation. Larynx is divided into supraglottis, glottis and subglottis. Only the true vocal cords are covered by nonkeratinized squamous epithelium.

Laser (Light Amplification by Stimulated Emission of Radiation).

Laser burns are the burns caused by lasers. There are basically thermal burns where laser energy is used for other purposes like hair removal or resurfacing or vascular or pigmented lesions and heat released is dissipated into the normal skin leading to skin burns. The damage to the skin will depend upon the energy released by the laser, therefore, these can be superficial burns which are more common or deep dermal when the energy used is very high which take a long time to heal. Therefore wet gauze should be kept in the surrounding skin thus isolating the treatment field as in resurfacing and treating pigmented or vascular lesions. In case of hair removal, cold air blast is need to be given along with the laser beam to nullify the effects of heat.

Laser Doppler flowmetry (LDF) was developed by Tenland in 1982 and later by Holloway in 1983. The technique depends on Doppler principle in which a low power light from a monochromatic laser beam of known wavelength along a fiberoptic cable is directed to the tooth surface, where the light passes along the direction of enamel prisms and dentinal tubules to the pulp.

Laser welding means where the heat for welding is supplied by focused beam of light generated by a laser. Laser light can be focused on small regions and can apply high energy in a very short period of time. There is very little heating of total appliance except at the point of application.

Late adolescence is a period of transition as the young person (adult) consolidates his identity and comes to grips with his future.

Late shift: Many children lack the primate spaces and thus the erupting permanent molars are unable to move forward to establish class I relationship. In these cases,

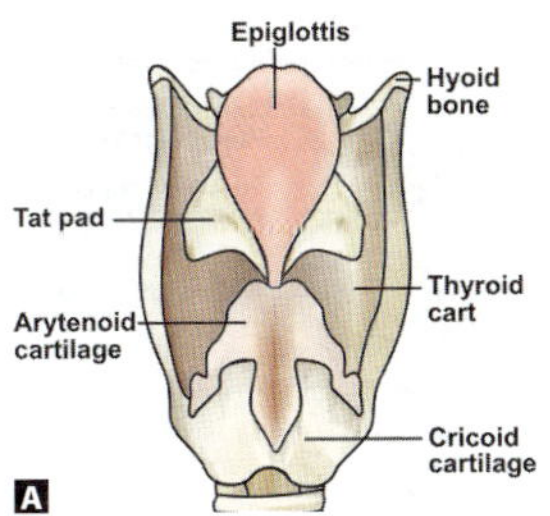

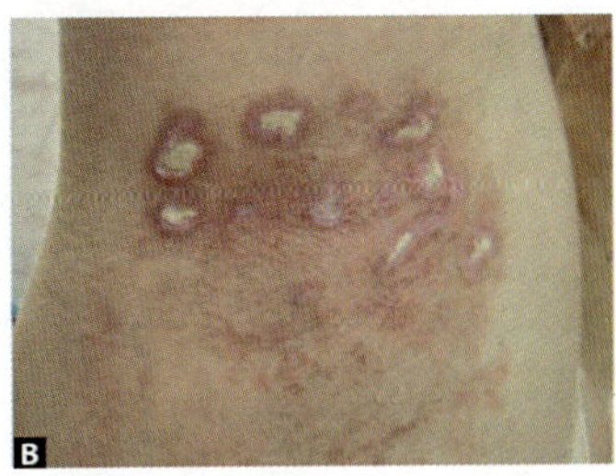

Figs A and B: *(A) Larynx (posterior view; (B) Laser burns*

when the deciduous second molars exfoliate, the permanent first molar drift medially utilizing the leeway space. This occurs in the late mixed dentition period and is thus called late shift.

Latent concealed not open.

Latent image the invisible image produced when film is exposed to X-rays. It remains invisible until film is exposed.

Latent syphilis refers to the term given to hidden syphilis. This generally happens when the secondary syphilis is not treated and the diseases enter the latent stage. It is characterized by positive serological tests for syphilis, absence of clinical manifestations and normal CSF.

Lateral fossa is a smooth depressed area of maxilla located between the canine and lateral incisor. It appears radiolucent.

Lateral periodontal abscess is a painful condition where the soft tissue around the tooth gets infected and inflamed. It generally develops in pre-existing periodontal pocket. Bacteria multiply in the depth of the pocket causing irritation. Cortical plate may be destroyed. Abscess resembles an abscess elsewhere and has to be drained out. Extraction of tooth is advised only in advanced cases.

Lateral periodontal cyst is a well-recognized type of developmental odontogenic cyst. It develops chiefly in adults. No particular sign and symptoms appear and lesion is discovered accidently. Surgical excision is to be done without removing the tooth.

Lateral pterygoid is a muscle of mastication. The muscle has two heads: upper and lower. Their fibers run more or less horizontally

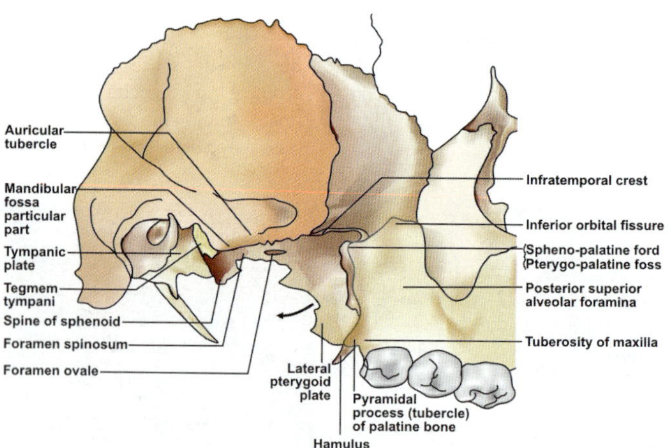

Fig.: *Lateral pterygoid*

and converge posteriorly to reach the neck of the mandible.

Lateral refers to the side or away from midline.

Lateral towards the outside.

Lateral pterygoid plate is a wing-shaped bony projection of sphenoid bone located distal to the maxillary tuberosity region.

Lateral sulci are the prominent grooves between the deciduous canine and the deciduous first molar segments.

Laterotrusion refers to movement of mandible laterally to the right or left from ICP.

Laterotrusive side refers to the side of either dental arch corresponding to the side of the mandible moving away from midline.

Lefort I refers to the horizontal fracture above the level of nasal floor. The fracture-line runs backward from the lateral margins of the anterior nasal aperture, it also passes along the lateral wall of the nose and lower third of nasal septum to coincide with lateral fracture behind the tuberosity.

Lefort II refers to those fractures which run from the middle area of the nasal bones on both the sides, crossing the frontal process and into the medial wall of each orbit.

Lefort III refers to those fractures which run from near the frontonasal suture transversely backwards, parallel with the base of the skull and involves considerable depth of ethmoidal bone including the cribriform plate, as it crosses the orbit, it involves optic foramen and inferior orbital fissure, from the base of inferior orbital fissure, the fracture extends into two directions; backwards across the pterygomaxillary fissure and laterally across the lateral wall of orbit.

Lead poisoning occurs as professional hazard. It may cause serious GIT disturbances. Peripheral neuritis also develops. Encephalitis may also occur. X-ray may show deposition of lead on bones.

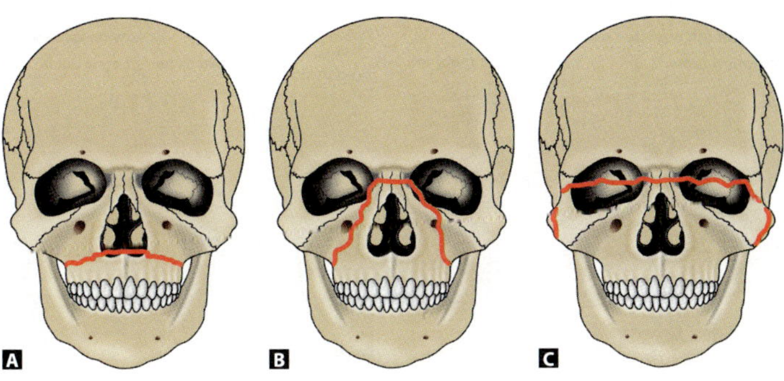

Figs A to C: *(A) Lefort I; (B) Lefort II; (C) Lefort III*

Lead line on tooth occurs. Gray/ bluish black line of sulfide pigmentation is seen over gingiva. It is more diffuse than bismuth. Excessive salivation and metallic taste develops.

Lean tissue mass includes muscle other body tissues, body fluids and bone usually calculated as total body mass minus fat mass.

Ledges are the plateau like bony margins caused by resorption of bony thick plates

Ledging is an iatrogenic ledge formation in the canal during the BMP which prevents positioning of an instrument to the apex in an otherwise patent canal.

Leiomyoma is a benign neoplasm of smooth muscle cells. Majority of these cases are found on posterior portion of tongue. Palate and buccal mucosa may also be involved. *Clinical Features:* These grow slowly and are painless pedunculated mass. Mass does not ulcerates and maintain the normal color. Submucosal nodules may be seen. These are firm and yellow in color. Lesion can be multi-nodular. These are composed of spindle-shaped smooth muscle cells. Surgical excision including surrounding normal tissue is practiced. After surgery, it does not recur nor transforms into malignancy.

Leiomyosarcoma is a malignant tumor of smooth muscle origin. It is rare in oral cavity. The check and floor of mouth are the common sites. It looks like leiomyoma except number of mitosis. Patient may hardly survive for 3-5 years.

Lentulospirals are used for applying sealer cement to the root canal walls before obturation. They can be used as hand or rotary instruments.

Lepromatous leprosy is a skin lesion of macules, nodules and papules. Lesions are multiple and bilaterally symmetrical. There is loss of outer eyebrows, thickened and corrugated skin of face and forehead. Skin biopsy, ear lobe clipping and nasal smear examination helps.

Leprosy is a chronic granulomatous infection caused by an acid fast bacillus. *Mycobacterium leprae* causes

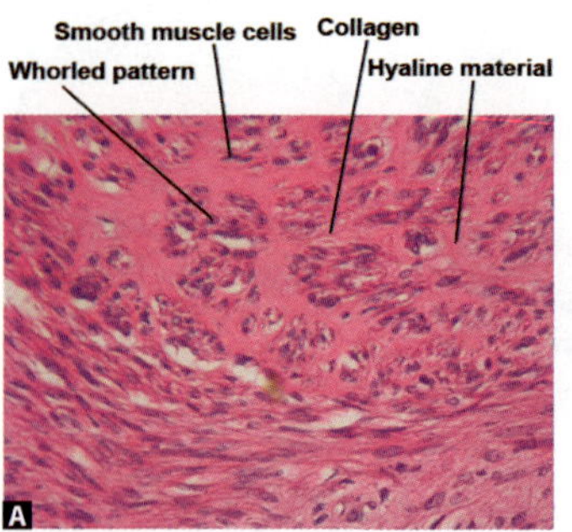

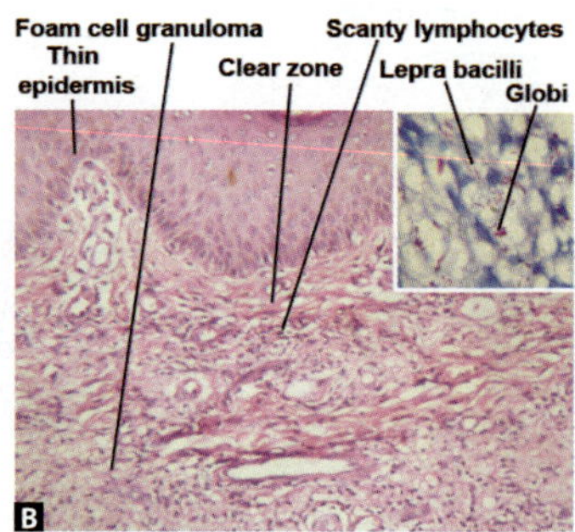

Figs A and B: *(A) Leiomyoma in hyaline changes; (B) Lepromatous leprosy*

granulomatous infection of skin and peripheral nerves. Incubation period is 3 to 5 years. Clinically, it can be classified into lepromatous leprosy and tuberculoid leprosy. Onset is insidious. To start a small area of impaired sensation or numbness is developed. There is lack of sweating and lack of hair in involved area surrounding cutaneous nerve is thickened. Oral lesions consist of tumor-like masses called lepromas developing on lip, tongue and hard palate. Gingiva may enlarge and teeth may become loose. Long-term chemotherapy is suggested.

Leptin is a body fat signaling hormone-like protein secreted in blood stream. It is transported to satiety center in the hypothalamus. There it blunts the appetite when calorie intake is sufficient to maintain ideal fat store.

Lesion refers to any wound or local degeneration.

Lesser occipital nerve arises from the descending branch of the ventral ramus of the second cervical nerve. The origin lies deep to the sternocleidomastoid muscle. The nerve forms a loop round the accessory nerve. It then runs upwards and backwards for some distance along the posterior border of the sternocleidomastoid. Higher up it lies superficial to the muscle between it and the deep fascia.

Lethargy means sleepiness.

Letterer-Siwe disease is an acute, often fulminating histiocytic disorder. Patient will have constant low-grade spiking fever with malaise and irritability. Oral lesions are ulcerative with gingival hyperplasia. Prognosis in Letterer Siwe disease is extremely poor.

Letters are symbols that represent sounds. Letters, in particular combinations, form words, with each word standing for something.

Leukemia is a malignant disease with increased proliferation of WBCs at the cost of other cells. It is more common in younger age groups. Some may be of immature form. Myeloid leukemia involves granulocyte series. Lymphoid

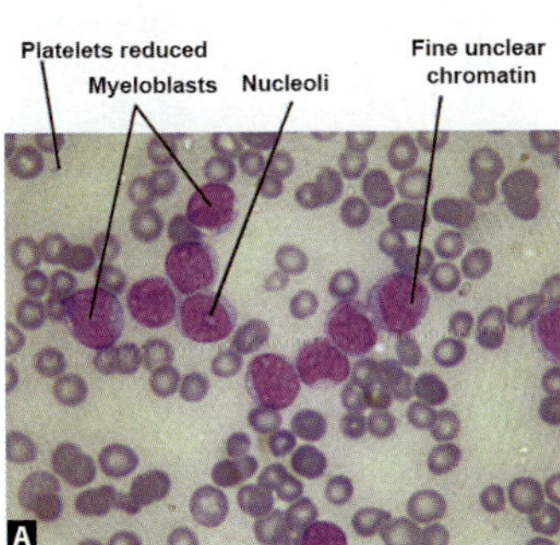

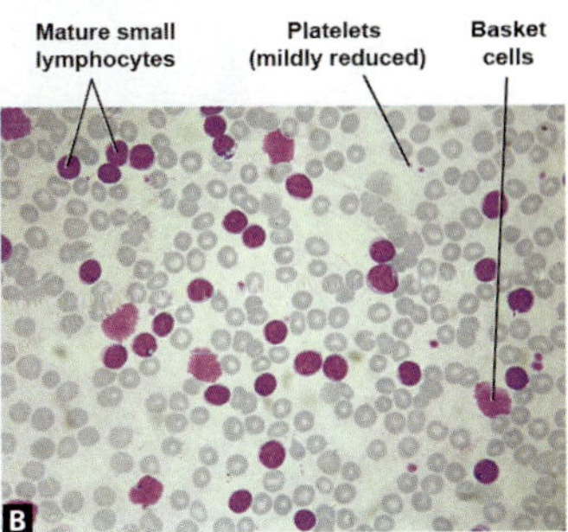

Figs A and B: *(A) Acute myeloblastic leukemia; (B) Chronic lymphocytic leukemia*

leukemia involves lymphocytic series and monocytic leukemia involves monocytic series. Each one of them may be acute, subacute or chronic. Exact cause is not known. But exposure of high doses of radiation therapy, phenyl butazone, chloramphenicol may lead to it. Some families have more incidences of leukemia. These have been classified into acute and chronic. *Clinical Features:* Generally either children or old people are affected. Persistent fever of unknown origin, spontaneous bleeding from gingiva, multiple large ulcers may develop on mucosa, candidiasis, histoplasmosis and HSV infections are common in leukemic patients. Teeth may start loosening, alveolar destruction may take place, Leukemic cell infiltration may cause atypical dental pain. There may be prolonged bleeding after extraction.

Leukoedema is a white lesion of oral cavity which clinically resembles early leukoplakia. It varies from film-like layer to greyish white cast with a coarsely wrinkled surface. It is more prominent in bicuspid to occlusal line; etiology is not known. Intraorally, the buccal mucosa retains its normal softness and flexibility. It exhibits a greyish white folded opalescent appearance. Leukoplakia is more common to develop. Since it is a variant of normal mucosa, it does not require any treatment.

Leukoplakia is a premalignant condition. It occurs as a white patch over mucous membrane of lip, hard and soft palate, floor of mouth and gingiva. Patches of leukoplakia may vary from non-

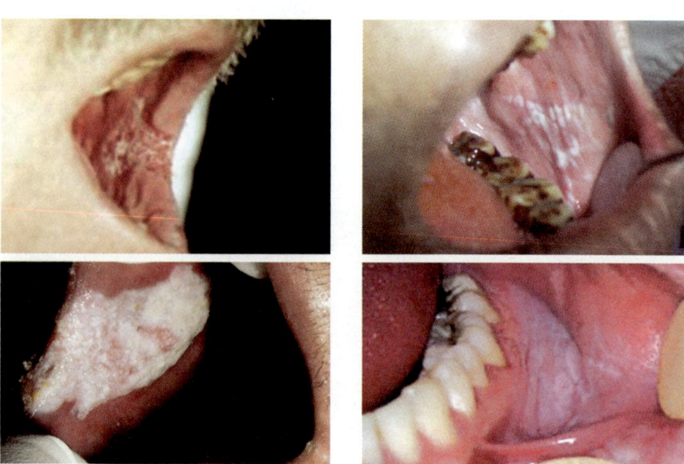

Fig.: *Leukoplakia involving buccal mucosa, angle of the mouth and buccal vestibule*

palpable to thick white translucent indurated lesion. These may be fissured or papillomatous. It may be localized or diffuse and is of 3 forms. Homogeneous leukoplakia is a localized lesion. If extensive, it is of consistent pattern. It may be wrinkled or papillomatous. Verrucous leukoplakia is an oral white lesion in which surface is broken up by multiple papillary projections. Nodular granular is hairy mixed white and red lesion. In it lesions are scattered over an atrophic patch of mucosa. Leukoplakia can be developed on any part of oral cavity but is more common on buccal mucosa and gingiva. 50% lesions affect cheeks. Tobacco, alcohol, mechanical irritants are causative factors. If floor of mouth is involved, then chances of transforming into malignancy are more. Microscopically one finds cellular dysplasia. Benign leukoplakia shows hyperkeratosis and chronic inflammatory cell infiltration. Cytological study is of little importance. Topically applied toluidine blue shows the areas which are more likely to show carcinomatous changes. Biopsy is to be done from that area. Surgical excision done with or without grafting remains the standard treatment for leukoplakia.

Leukostasis syndrome in this condition WBC count may go up to one lac per cu/mm. Person may develop headache and stroke-like symptoms. Many patients may be asymptomatic. Spleen may be enlarged hugely. Unexplained leukocytosis, basophilia and thrombocytosis may be present. Bone marrow is hypercellular with markedly increased granulocyte precursor specially metamyelocytes and myelocytes.

Levator anguli oris is a facial muscle that arises from canine fossa just below infraorbital foramen and is inserted over angle of mouth.

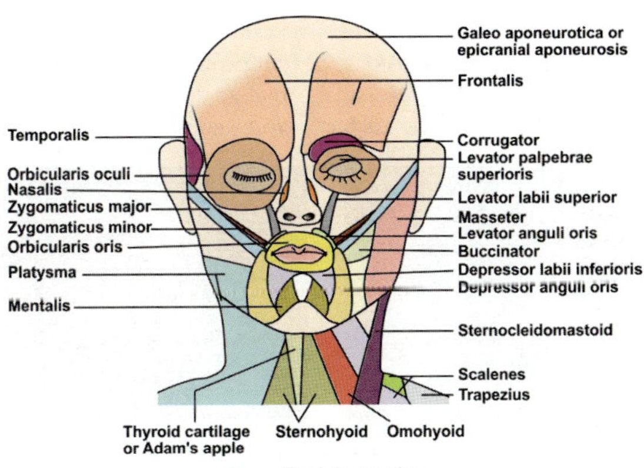

Fig.: *Facial muscles*

Its action is to raise angle of mouth and produces nasolabial furrow.

Levator labii superioris is a facial muscle. It arises from lateral surface of zygomatic bone and passes downward and medially into muscular substance of upper lip. It elevates the upper lip and produces nasolabial furrow.

LI (Labrale inferius) is the median point in the lower margin of the lower membranous lip.

Lichen planus is a common dermatosis developing on mucous membrane which appears as small, angular, flat topped papules only a few millimeters in diameter. Papules are sharply demarcated. Center of papule may be slightly umbilicated. Its surface is covered by greyish white line known as Wichame's striae. Face generally remains uninvolved. Early symptom is pruritis causing severe itching. Causative factor of lichen planus is immunologically induced degeneration of basal layer of epithelium. There are three basic types of erosions, keratosis, erosions and bulla formation. Psychogenic problems play an etiological role. During deep emotional problems, remissions and exacerbations are seen. It may be associated with diabetes. Generally it is a bullous form of disease and a painless lesion, the reticular form is slightly elevated, fine, whitish line. Lines are fine radiating of lacing nature. Cheeks and tongue are generally affected. In the popular form lesion is less than 1 mm in size. It is whitish elevated lesion. Bullous lichen planus is rare. It presents coexisting bullous pemphigoid. Atrophic lichen planus is inflamed area covered by red, thinned epithelium. Erosive lesion is a complicated atrophic process when thin epithelium is ulcerated. Main histological features of lichen planus are: Areas of hyperparakeratosis, liquefaction degeneration, dense epithelial band of lymphocyte damage of basal cell layer is the diagnostic point. The lesions of oral lichen planus appear, regress and reappear in unpredictable fashion. Lesions are too diffuse to remove surgically and may transform into malignancy. Antihistamine rinses and corticosteroids are useful.

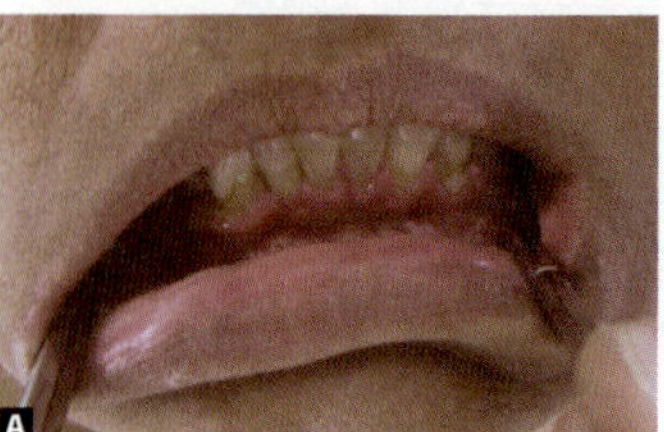

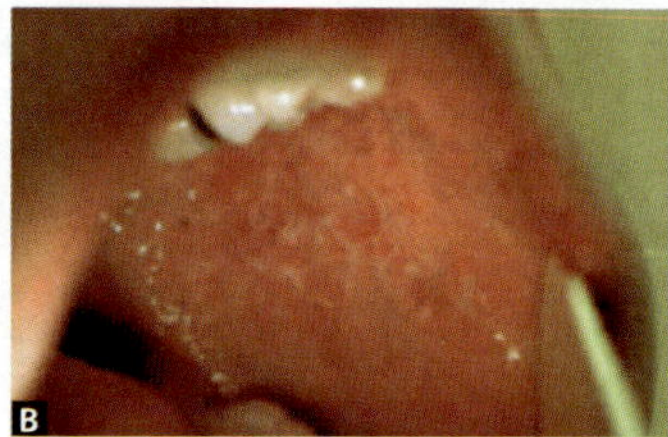

Figs A and B: *(A) Lichen planus of labial vestibule; (B) Lichen planus of buccal mucosa*

In resistant cases intralesional injections of trimcinolone acetonide are useful. Retinoids may be given in addition.

Lichenoid drug reactions these white patches are identical clinically to lichen planus and are caused by a mucosal reaction to certain drugs. Drugs include phenothiazines, dental amalgams and dental composites, nonsteroidal anti-inflammatory drugs and anti-hypertensive.

Life expectancy is the average number of years lived by an individual or group born in the same period.

Ligatures are fine wires or elastic bands used to tie or ligate the arch wire to the brackets.

Light activated denture base material is used to fabricate dentures with light activation. Advantage of it is reduced polymerization shrinkage, possible better fit than conventional base material and not much of equipment is required. But disadvantage is an increased elastic deformation during mastication.

Light cure system chemical cure composites cannot set until two are mixed together. Light cure materials such as durafill or pecafil need exposure to bright light for setting. A special lamp is used and it makes a material set in about a minute. No mixing is required. Just a thin layer of composite is needed to fill a shallow cavity and one application of curing light is needed.

Lightening injuries refer to injuries due to thunder and lightening have variable affects. It may not always be fatal but patient may fall unconscious and stop breathing. However these patients withstand prolong periods of apnea and respond very well to immediate CPR. Burn markings are characteristic for lightening injuries. There is a spidery pattern of skin burns which is caused by the current passage along pathway of skin dampness where the resistance is the lowest.

Lightning degradation of high molecular weight complex organic molecules that reflect specific wavelength of light responsible for the color of the stain into lower molecular weight and less complex

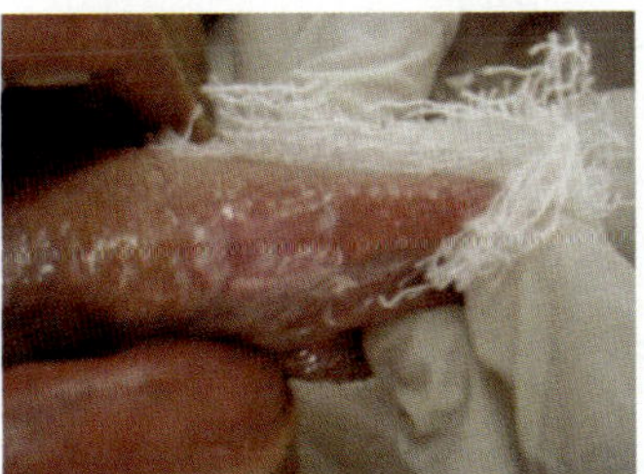

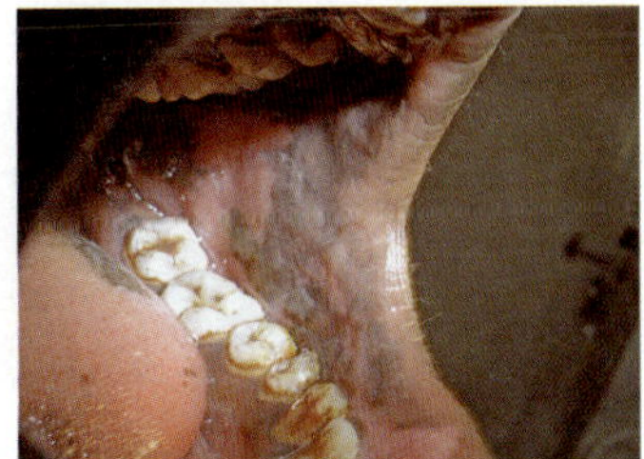

Fig.: *Lichenoid reaction on the lateral border of tongue and angle of the mouth*

molecules that reflect less light is called lightning.

Lignocaine is a local anesthetic agent and was introduced in 1948. It diffuses rapidly and onset is rapid. It produces anesthesia within 2-3 minutes. It is easily absorbed from mucous membrane. It is an effective surface anesthetic. It is doubly more potent than prilocaine. It is also available in spray form and also a cream in concentration of 5%. Saliva can washout its effects.

Limb placement reflex: When the front of the leg below the knee, or the arm below the elbow is brought into contact with the edge of the table, the child lifts the limbs over the edge.

Limbic system is also known as emotional brain. It is a collection of various small regions of brain that act together to produce emotions.

Lime is the cheapest of all disinfectants. It is used in the form of fresh quick lime or 10-20% aqueous suspension of milk of lime. Feces and urine can be disinfected by mixing 10-20% aqueous suspension.

Linea alba is a white line extending anteroposteriorly on buccal mucosa along occlusal plane. It can be found.

Linear epitopes: When all the amino acids or sugar residues that form an epitope are positioned in linear sequence. Not affected by heat and denaturation.

Lines of cleavage and surgery: In certain regions of the body, collagen fibers tend to orient more in one direction than another. Lines of cleavage (tension lines) in the skin indicate the predominant direction of underlying collagen fibers. The lines are especially evident on the palmer surfaces of the fingers, where they are arranged parallel to the long axis of the digits. An incision running parallel to the collagen fibers will heal with only a fine scar. An incision made across the rows of fibers disrupts

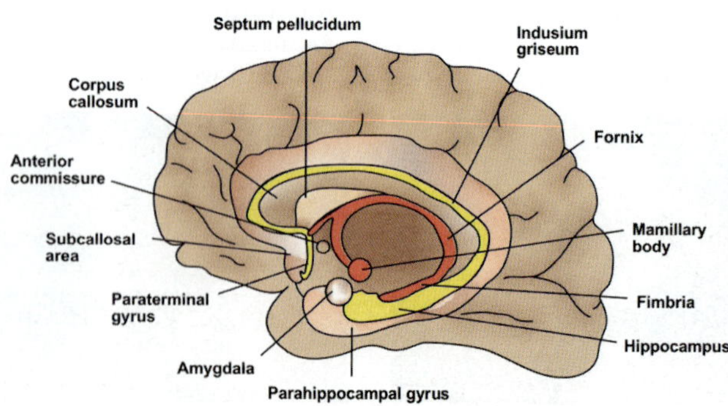

Fig.: *Limbic system*

the collagen, and the wound tends to gape open and heal in a broad, thick scar.

Lingual refers to the surface of a tooth nearest the tongue; relating to the tongue.

Lingual nerve arises from the posterior division of the mandibular nerve. Its upper part runs downward deep to the lateral pterygoid muscle. It is joined here by the chorda tympani nerve. Runs downwards and forwards between the medial pterygoid and the ramus of the mandible. It then enters the mouth. Within the mouth, the nerve lies deep to the mucous membrane just below the third molar tooth.

Lingual thyroid nodules in this condition, the remnants follicle of thyroid tissues are found in substance of tongue. It is a benign condition during puberty. It lies in mid of tongue. It appears deeply situated having a smooth surface. It has a color of mucosa. If size is 2 to 3 cms, it may result in dysphagia, dysphonia and hemorrhage with pain.

Lingual tonsils are accumulations of lymphoid tissue on the root of the tongue. They may extend as far back as epiglottis and laterally through palatine tonsil.

Lingual varicosities these are prominent purplish blue sports, these are usually observed on the ventral and lateral surfaces of tongue. Clinically red to purple dilated vessels or clusters are seen. It has no relation with jugular venous pressure or obstruction to portal venous system. These are generally seen in old age.

Lingual vein accompanies the lingual artery and joins the internal jugular vein near the greater cornu of the hyoid bone.

Lining mucosa is present in non-masticatory regions such as floor of mouth, enteral surface of tongue, soft palate, cheeks, lips and alveolar mucosa. It is not attached to bone.

Lip: Lysis is a metabolic break down of fats for energy.

Lip biting and lip sucking is an oral habit that, sometimes, appears after forced discontinuation of thumb or digit sucking. Lip biting most often involves the lower lip which is turned inwards and pressure is exerted on the lingual surfaces of the maxillary anteriors. Clinically it may appear as proclined upper anteriors and retroclined, hyper-

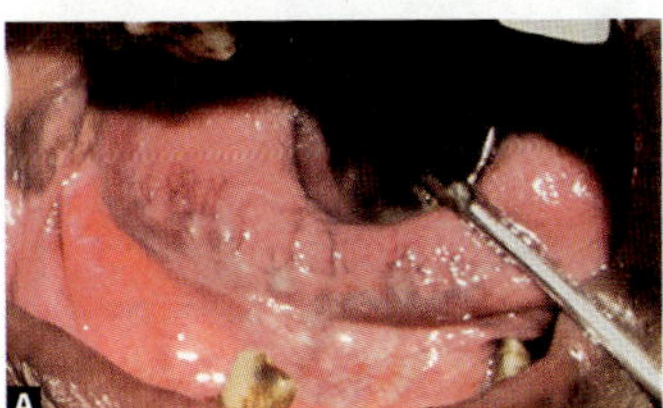

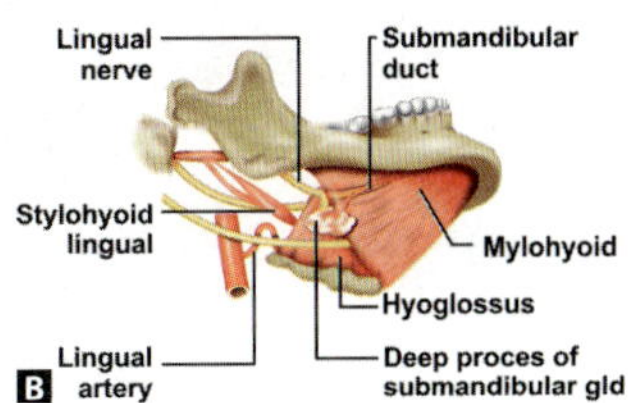

Figs A and B: *(A) Lingual varicosities; (B) Lingual nerve*

trophic and redundant lower lip or a cracked lip.

Lipemia is the presence of abnormally high concentrations of lipids in blood.

Lipoid proteinosis is a condition occurring due to disturbance in mucopolysaccharides metabolism. These produce yellowish hay nodules of size 0.5 cm. Such lesions may develop on eyelid. In oral mucosa yellowish papular plaques develop. Lips become thick. Painful parotitis may occur repeatedly. No specific treatment is available.

Lipoma is a slow-growing tumor of adipose tissue. It is composed of mature fat cells. Cheek, tongue, floor of mouth and salivary glands are frequently involved. *Clinical Features:* It is a single, lobulated painless lesion attached by peduncle. Epithelium is thin showing blood vessels. It is composed of mature fat cell with varying collagen strands. These are yellowish in color with smooth surface. There is no surrounding capsule. Simple surgical excision helps. Recurrence is uncommon.

Liposarcoma is not a common malignant mesenchymal neoplasm. It is a slow, silent growth, submucosal or deep in location. Lesion is firm, lobulated suggestive of cyst. It may be myxoid type, round cell type and plesmorphic type.

Lipostrophy is the breakdown of subcutaneous fat at the site of repeated insulin injection.

Lipping is the term given to the bulging of bone contour due to peripheral buttressing bone formation.

Lisinopril is an angiotensin converting enzyme (ACE) inhibitor that is used to treat hypertension.

Listerine is an essential oil or phenol mouthwashes have been used for more than a century. Phenol as an antiseptic made a breakthrough in 1867 under John Lister. Phenolic compounds used alone, or combined with mouth rinses and throat lozenges have proved to be safe. The action of phenols depends

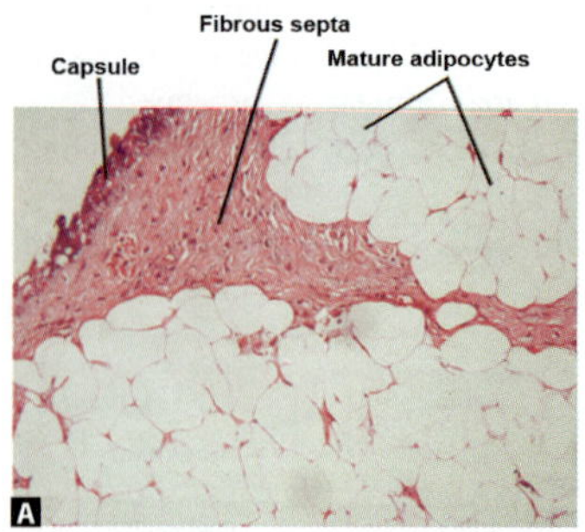

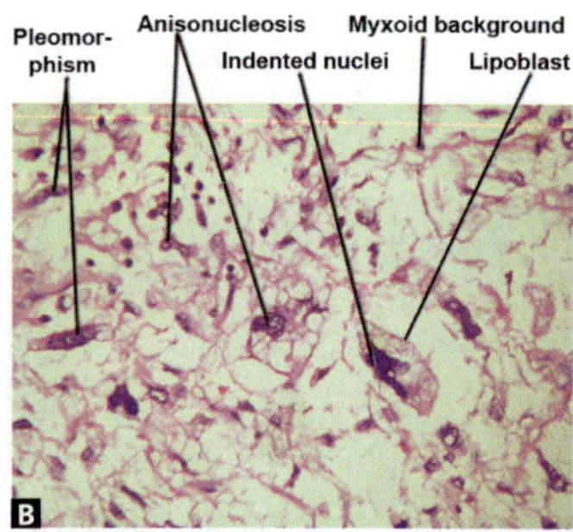

Figs A and B: *(A) Lipoma; (B) Liposarcoma*

upon the concentration and contact time. Composition: menthol 0.04%, thymol 0.06%, eucalyptol 0.09%, benzoic acid 0.015%, ethyl alcohol 6-26%. Listerine is contraindicated for those patients on metronidazole/ tinidazole as it contains alcohol.

Liver abscess is commonly caused by *E. coli.* It is slow-growing with fever. Pain may be a complaint. Jaundice, tenderness in right upper abdomen with leukocytosis is commonly noted. Cephalosporin and metronidazole help but abscess larger than 5 cm may require drainage.

Loading dose is the larger dose of a drug given initially to control the disease effectively.

Lobar pneumonia is a localized injection of terminal air spaces. The usual homogeneous lung opacification is limited by fissure and affected lobes retain normal volume and show air bronchograms. *Streptococcus penumoniae* causes typical lobar pneumonia. Consolidation may not spread uniformly in lobe.

Lobe refers to center of tooth formation.

Local anesthetic infiltration is a method of administrating local anesthesia that is given over apex of tooth to be anesthetized. Needle is inserted below the mucous membrane. Infiltration applies to nerve endings while nerve block is

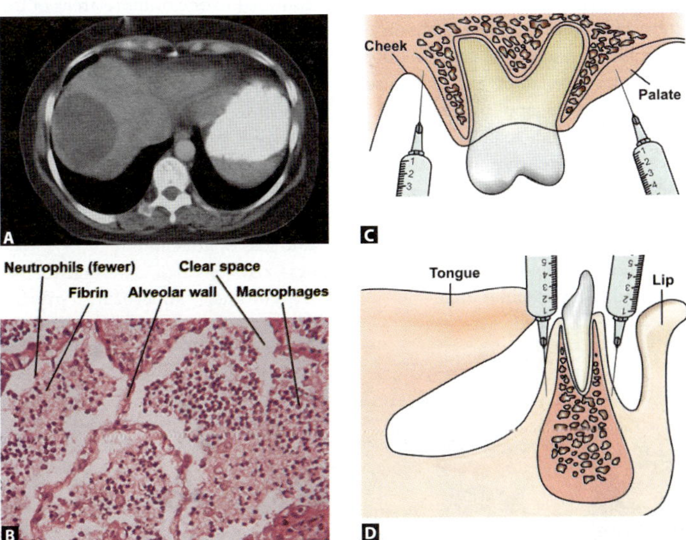

Figs A to D: *(A) Liver abscess; (B) Lobar pneumonia; (C) Local infiltration maxilla; (D) Local infiltration mandible*

done to trunk of nerve. It is effective for all upper teeth.

Local anesthesia refers to relieve the sensation of pain in a localized area.

Local dental anesthesia is widely used in dental practice. It is produced in a number of ways by paralyzing sensory nerve endings by producing tissue ischemia, application of cold or putting pressure on nerve trunks. Local anesthetics are thought to act by stabilizing the cell membrane. These prevent inward movement of sodium ions. Most local agents are tertiary amines. Lignocaine and procaine are good agents.

Local muscle soreness is a condition with a local cause. It has a low pain threshold due to strain, injury, infection of inflammation. Some pain is thought to result from accumulation of metabolites after excessive use. Both ischemia and hyperemia are believed to relate to pain genesis.

Localized aggressive periodontitis see Juvenile periodontitis.

Localized diffuse gingivitis is the one which extends from the margin to the mucobuccal fold but is limited to a particular area.

Localized enamel hypoplasia is a type of hypoplasia occasionally seen is unusual in that only a single tooth is involved, most commonly one of the permanent maxillary incisors or a maxillary or mandibular premolar. There may be any degree of hypoplasia, ranging from a mild, brownish discoloration of the enamel to a severe, pitting and irregularity of the tooth crown.

Localized gingivitis is said to occur where the inflammation is confined to a single tooth or a particular area.

Localized juvenile periodontitis (LJP) see Juvenile periodontitis.

Localized marginal gingivitis is confined to one or more areas of the marginal gingiva.

Localized papillary gingivitis is confined to one or more interdental spaces in a particular area.

Localized periodontitis is said to have occurred when less than thirty percent of the areas assessed in mouth demonstrate the bone loss and loss of attachment.

Localized scratch dermatitis is a chronic, superficial pruritis

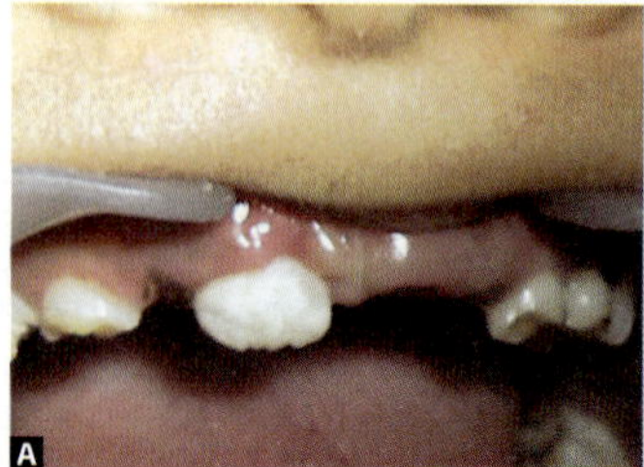

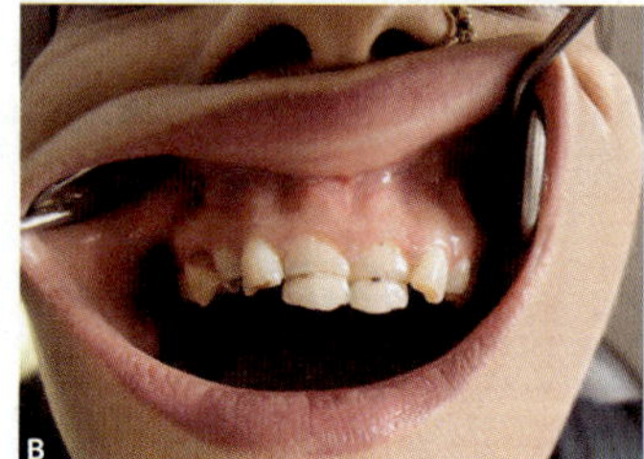

Figs A and B: *Local enamel hypoplasia*

inflammation of the skin with dry scaling. There will be pigmented lichenified plaques with oval and irregular shapes. There is a strong psychogenic component. Outer zone of patch may have brownish discrete papules and a central zone. The involved skin will be red, moist and hyperpigmented. Diagnosis is mostly clinical. Topical corticosteroids are most useful. Zinc oxide paste can be locally applied.

Logo therapy refers to spiritually, essentially oriented therapy that seeks to achieve healing and health through meaning.

Long buccal nerve block is a local anesthetic technique used for anesthetizing buccal mucosa of mandibular molar teeth.

Longitudinal study is measurement of same person or a group at regular intervals, over a period of time.

Loose tongue is also known as frenum insufficiency. Patient mostly has been operated for tongue tie. Tongue becomes loose and difficult to control. Dysarthria is present and signs of airway obstruction take place during sleep.

Loosely adherent subgingival plaque is an unattached bacterial plaque found adjacent to the gingival epithelium or pocket lumen.

Lorazepam is a drug belonging to a group of barbiturates and is 4 times more potent than diazepam. Half-life is 12 hours. Onset of action is 30-60 minutes. Psychomotor impairment is seen for 12 hours. 2 mg orally of it is equivalent of 10 mg oral diazepam. 5 mg dose of it may cause disorientation.

Loss of tooth is referred to if tooth is extracted and not replaced artificially opposing tooth becomes useless and it has nothing to bite. It loses its beneficial effect of cleaning and mastication. If several teeth are missing, mastication will be affected to produce malmutrition. Loss of one tooth can result in plaque accumulation and in caries in at least six other teeth.

Low blood pressure refers to inadequate intravascular pressure to maintain oxygen requirement of body's tissues. It may be drug-induced. Normal blood pressure varies typically a reading below

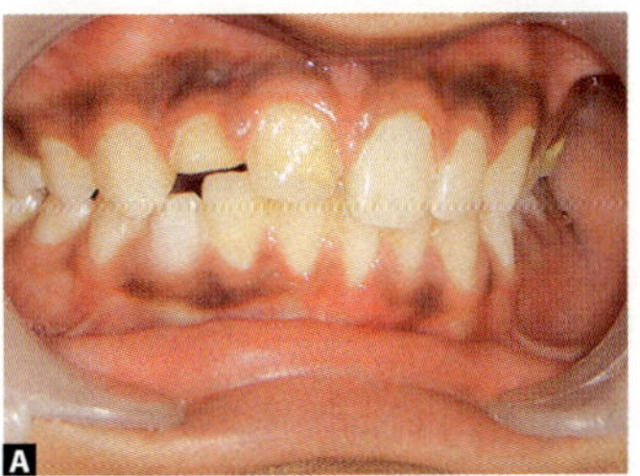

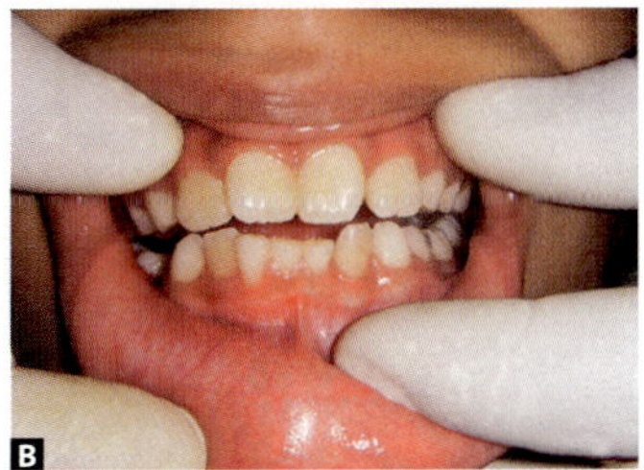

Figs A and B: *Loosely adherent subgingival plaque*

L

90/60 mm Hg or a drop of 30 mm Hg from baseline is considered low BP. Dehydration and hemorrhage may result in low BP.

Low-level fracture *see* Lefort I.

Low testosterone levels presents as disturbed sleep pattern, loss of sensitivity of erogenous zones, cold and shriveled penis. Patient starts gaining weight which is difficult to loose it. Seminal volume will be reduced with reduced facial hair growth.

Low-voltage electrical burns are the electrical burns that are caused by low voltage (240 ac) domestic appliances. Though more common than the high voltage burns, they may be deceptive in appearance as they may penetrate deeply. They are very commonly seen in infants crawling on the floor or in children who take the electrical wires into their mouth and chew them. They suffer severe damage to the lips, tongue and mouth and though the legion may be small the reactive edema may interfere with breathing and may require tracheostomy.

Lower lip prominence is the most prominent point of the lower lip (Li) should be 2 ± 1 mm anterior to Sn-pog line.

Ls (Labrale superius) is a point indicating the mucocutaneous border of the upper lip. The most anterior point of the upper lip (usually).

Ludwig's angina is a cellulitis of submaxillary submandibular space and floor of the mouth. In Ludwig's angina submandibular and submaxillary spaces are involved. Second and third molars are involved. There is difficulty in swallowing with varying degrees of trismus. There develops swelling of mouth. Structures in floor or mouth are swollen and tongue is pushed up and back. Laryngeal edema may be present. Swelling is firm, painful and diffuse. Person is not able to swallow or eat. Cavernous sinus thrombosis result's in subsequent meningitis. Antibiotics are useful.

Lumbar puncture is a procedure, where a hollow needle is inserted into subarachnoid space between l3–l4 to avoid spinal cord. A sample of CSF is withdrawn and examined

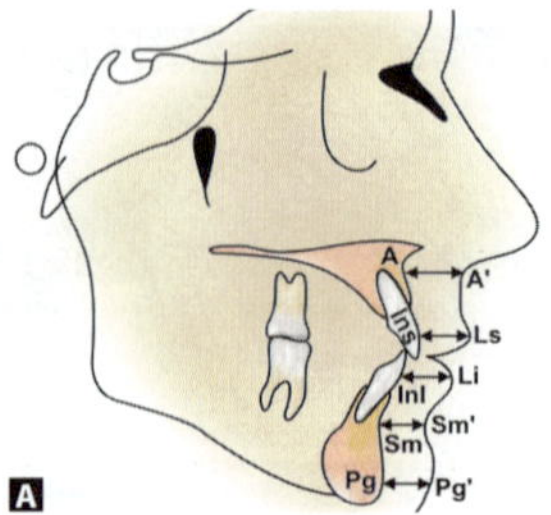

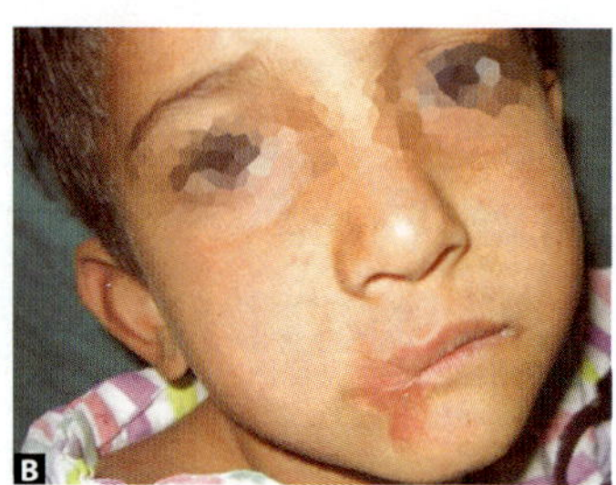

Figs A and B: *(A) Ls (Labrale superius; (B) Electrical burn*

under microscope to rule out pathologies.

Lumbar stenosis vertebral canal space inside the ring is greatest when all the rings line up on top of each other. These vertebrae line up best when you stoop forward. Space gets smaller when you stand up and smallest when you bend backwards. Arthritis or injury makes it further smaller. People with lumbar stenosis feel better when their spine is bent forward.

Lung abscess is a type of suppurative pneumonia characterized by destruction of lung parenchyma by the inflammatory process generally leading to micro-abscess formation. When a large collection of pus occurs within the lung parenchyma lined by chronic inflammatory tissue, the condition is known as lung abscess.

Lupus erythromatosus there may be a genetic predisposition. There occur many remissions and exacerbations. Superficial painful ulceration may occur with crusting or bleeding. Margins of lesions are not demarcated. Often white striae radiate out from margins. Central healing results in central scarring.

Lupus miliaris disseminates faciei – there develop dark red to brown acneiform papules. These are non tender brownish red papules. There is no tendency to form pustule. No foreign material or remnants of microbes can be detected.

Lute is cement-like material which fills and seals gap.

Luting is a mixing consistency of cement which is used for bonding or cementing two unlike substances together.

Lymph nodes are round and nodular shape organ that are distributed throughout our body and forms the important part of our immune system. They perform biological filtration of lymph on its way to circulatory system. These are the part of body network, which filters antigen from tissue fluid and lymph during its passage from the periphery to the thoracic duct. These are located at branches of lymphatic vessels. Human lymph nodes 1-25 mm in diameter and round or kidney-shaped. Indentation is present

L

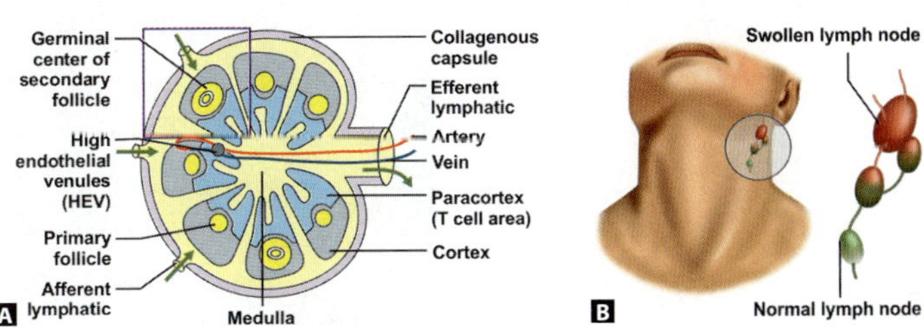

Figs A and B: *Lymph node*

on the concave surface, where efferent blood vessels leave the node. Lymphatic afferent vessels enter through the convex surface. They have a collagenous capsule, radial trabeculae, B-cell rich cortex, T-cell rich paracortex and a central medulla with T-cell, B-cell and plasma cells. Para cortex: rich in inter-digitating cells, APC, large quantity of MHC class II antigen. Medulla: cords separated by large sinuses where scavenger phagocyte cells along sinuses remove antigen from lymph. Cortex: primary and secondary follicles/stimulated with germinal centers contain dendritic APCs and some macrophages. Involved with development of B-cell response and B-cell memory.

Lymphadenopathy refers to enlargement of lymphs. Lymph node enlargement occurs due to increase in number and size of lymphoid follicles, proliferation of macrophages or infiltration by abnormal cells. Enlargement of lymph nodes more than 1 cm is always pathological. Supra-auricular, supra clavicular mesenteric glands and mediastinal nodes are always pathological. Lymphadenopathy may be localized or generalized.

Lymphangioma is a benign neoplasm due to proliferation of lymphatic vessels. It can be a simple lymphangioma, cavernous lymphangioma, cellular and systemic lymphangioma. Most of lesions are present at birth. They are similar to hemangioma except the fact that these vessels are filled with clear, protein-rich fluid containing a few cells. Lymphangioma may occur in the skin of mucous membrane of head and neck region. These may vary in size. Lesion is composed of numerous cytically dilated cavernous, lymphatic spaces, many of which contain lymph. In the neck, it is known as cystic hygroma. Mostly tongue is involved. These are not having clear-cut outline. Deeper lesions appear as diffuse nodules.

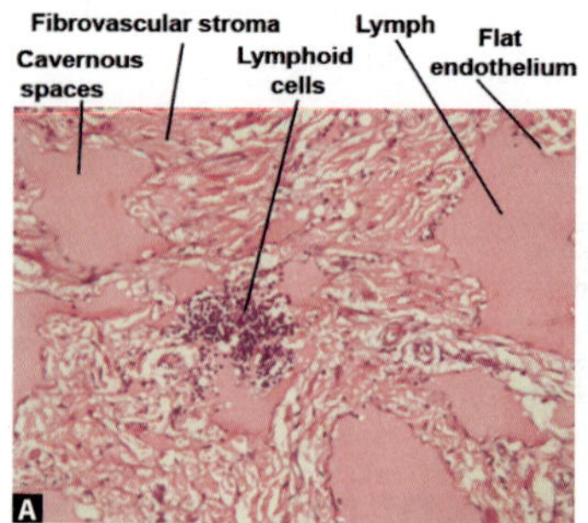

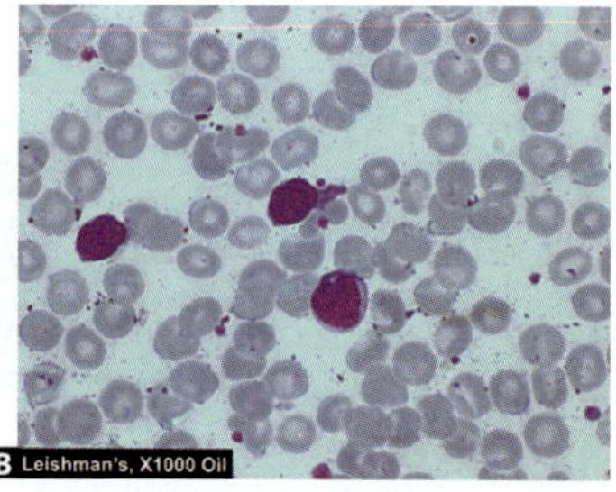

Figs A and B: *(A) Lymphangioma of tongue; (B) Lymphocytes*

Clinical Features: These are painless, nodules or vesicle-like lesions over oral mucosa. Color of lesion is lighter than surrounding mucosa. On palpation 'crepitation' sound is produced. Lymphangioma of tongue produces macroglossia. Surgical excision is the treatment of choice. It is radio resistant.

Lymphangitis is the inflammation of lymph vessels with pain in limb, pyrexia and toxaemia. Pain is throbbing or burning in nature. Pain is felt along with vessel. Superficial lymphatics of upper or lower limb are affected. Overlying skin may have edema. Regional lymph nodes are painful and enlarged. It is frequently accompanied by streptococcal or staphylococcal infection mostly in distal arm of leg. Malaise, sweating, chills and fever of 37.5 to 40oc is noted. Regional lymph nodes are enlarged and tender. Lymphangitis acute phase is seen in pyogenic infections mostly due to streptococci or other pyogenic microorganism. Skin becomes red and there is edema and tenderness over area. It may totally recover without any sequlae. In the process of healing the lymphatic may become fibrosed.

Lymphedema is anything that obstructs the lymphatic vessel draining a limb cause edema of upper or lower extremities. It involves dorsal surfaces of hands and fingers or the feet and toes. Erythema is pitting initially and becomes brawny and non pitting with time ulceration, stasis and pigmentation may develop. If it persists it stimulates an overgrowth of fibrous tissue and has a brawny consistency and does not pit on pressure.

Lymphocytes are the primary white blood cells involved in immune response are lymphocytes. These cells recognize and respond to an antigen. Lymphocytes are derived from stem cell which is located in bone marrow. These constitute 20 to 25% white cells. Two main types of lymphocytes are called B-lymphocytes and T-lymphocytes.

Lymphoepithelial cyst appears as a small, asymptomatic, well circular and elevated nodule on floor of mouth. It may be of a few m.m. in size. Lesion consists of a cavity lined by stratified squamous epithelium. Lumen of cyst contains lymphocytes and amorphous coagulum. Treatment includes local surgical excision. It seldom recurs.

Lymphokines are the products of lymphocytes. They have different functions. They can help monocytes to be changed in macrophages. They encourage macrophages to remain in area of injury to destroy foreign cells.

Lymphoproliferative disorders are characterized by monoclonal proliferation and accumulation of malignant lymphocytes. These include lymphoblastic leukemia, chronic lymphocytic leukemia, and Non Hodgkin's lymphoma.

Lysis is the destruction of cells resulting from damage to the plasma membrane.

Lysosomal storage syndrome development of childhood gingival enlargement, widened alveolar ridges and widely spaced teeth certain viscera are enlarged.

Lysosome is a membrane-bound organelle visible by electron microscopy that contains acid hydrolases capable of breaking down macromolecules. Lysosome has: diameters ranging from 50 nm to 1 m. A single membrane consisting of a phospholipid bilayer that undergoes selective fusion with other membranous organelles, an ATP driven h+ pump in the membrane, which acidifies the lysosomal matrix to pH 4.5–5.5, hydrolases in the inner matrix that are active at acid pH and breakdown carbohydrates, lipids, and proteins.

Macrodontia is a developmental anomaly; one or more teeth is/are physically larger than normal. This term should not be used when normal-sized teeth are crowded within a small jaw. In such cases, the term relative macrodontia is more appropriate. Regional/localized macrodontia is occasionally seen on the affected side of the mouth in patients with hemifacial hypertrophy. Macrodontia of single tooth is seen, but is rare. Rhizomegaly/radiculomegaly are an uncommon type of macrodontia in which the root/roots of a tooth are considerably longer than normal. This condition is observed commonly in mandibular canines. It is associated with pituitary gigantism. Macrodontia of single tooth is not very common.

Macroglobulinemia is a variant of multiple myeloma. It develops in old age. Person develops weakness, lymphadenopathy and enlargement of liver. Hemorrhage from nasal cavity and oral cavity develops. Oral ulcers on tongue, buccal mucosa and gingiva are seen. There is no specific treatment.

Macroglossia refers to enlarged tongue. Congenital macroglossia is due to over-development of tongue musculature. Secondary macroglossia may be due to diffuse lymphangioma or hemangioma. It is found in acromegaly too. There is no particular treatment of it.

Macrognathia refers to abnormally large jaw. It may be associated with acromegaly and Paget's disease. Some cases follow hereditary pattern. Prognathic patient forms long rami with less steep angle with body of mandible. There will be increased height of ramus, increased gonial angle, decreased maxillary length, prominent chin button and varying soft tissue contours. Surgical correction is possible.

Macrolides are broad-spectrum antibiotics to which resistance develops rapidly. They inhibit protein synthesis by binding to the ribosome and are bacteriostatic at usual doses but bactericidal in high doses.

Macrophages are the monocytes that have left the blood stream, entered

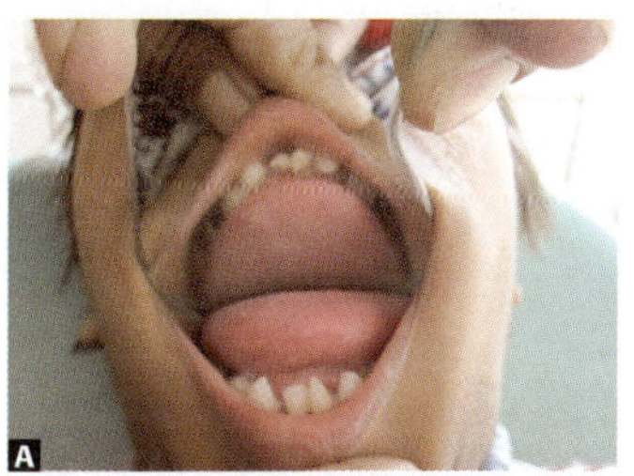

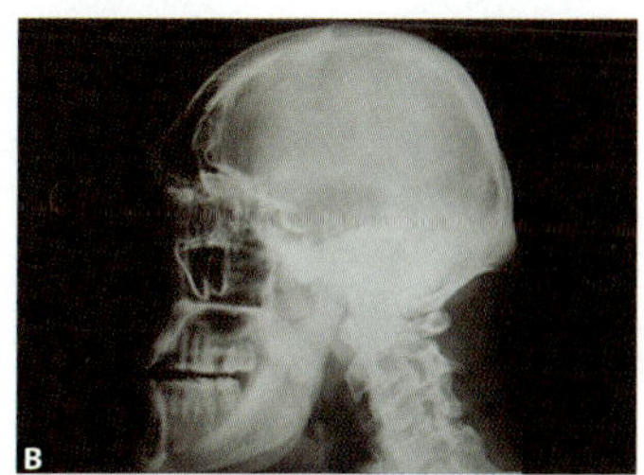

Figs A and B: *(A) Macroglossia; (B) Macrognathia*

the tissues, and differentiated into various subpopulations. Many are found in close proximity to blood vessels. They are active in endocytosis and phagocytosis. Because of their mobility and phagocytic activity, they are able to act as scavengers, removing extravasated red blood cells, dead cells and foreign bodies from the tissue.

Magill intubation forceps is used to grasp the objects which have fallen into back of the patient's throat.

Magnesia core material is compatible with the high expansion porcelains normally bounded to metals.

Magnesium is the essential trace element. Human body contains 2000 mEq of magnesium. Half of it is in bones and half is in soft tissues. Highest concentration is in liver and striated muscles. Daily intake is 36–48 mg. Nuts, peas, beans fruits and fish are rich sources. Plasma magnesium ranges from 1.5–2 mEq/L.

Magnetic resonance imaging (MRI) is an advanced diagnostic aid and has the great advantage over CT that the patient is not subject to X-radiation. Anatomical details are very well-shown. Very good pictures of spinal cord and lumbar roots are seen. Different pictures can be obtained by varying the repetition time and radiofrequency signal (TR) T1W1 images better anatomical details and T2W1 gives better pathological findings.

Mahler's theory (1933) categorizes the early childhood object relation to understand personality development. The period of childhood is classified into three stages: Normal autistic phase, Normal symbiotic phase, Separation individualization phase.

Maize is a stable diet of poor class Indians. It is rich in carbohydrate and fat but is poor in essential amino acid tryptophan. Due to constant use, it may lead to pellagra. Mixing of milk, egg or wheat flour will help. Yellow maize is rich in carotenoid pigment.

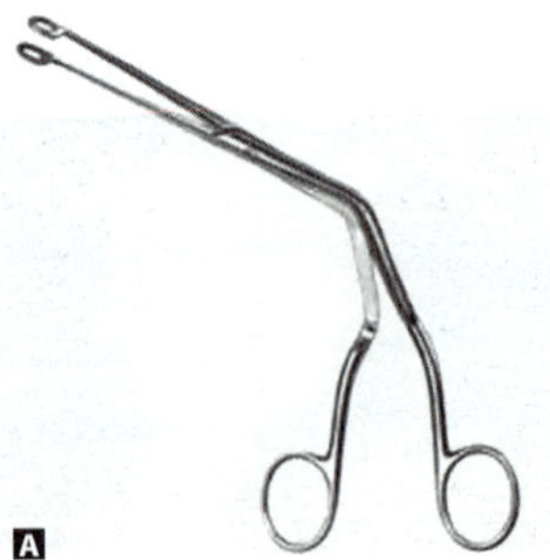

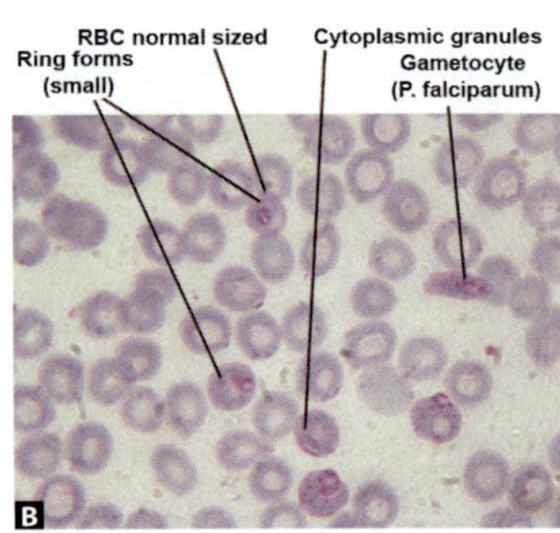

Figs A and B: *(A) Magill's intubation forceps; (B) Malaria parasite (P. falciparum)*

Malaise refers to any vague feeling of illness, uneasiness or discomfort.

Malaria is a parasitic infection caused by *Plasmodium vivax, P. falciparum, P. ovale,* and *P. malariae*. Globally around 1.5–3 million people die each year due to malaria, mostly due to *P. falciparum* infection. Currently malaria is appearing in the areas from where it had disappeared. Malaria is manifested as a type of fever occurring with rigors. It has 3 stages: Cold stage, hot stage, sweating stage. Cold stage lasts 15 minutes to 2 hours and is followed by hot stage in which fever may go very high. On an average, hot stage lasts for 4–8 hours. It is followed by sweating stage which lasts for 1–4 hours. Patient may have fever, vomiting and excessive thirst. Patient feels exhausted. In malignant malaria fever may be accompanied by severe headache, diarrhea and toxemia. There may be successive bouts of fever followed by severe cachexia. Splenic enlargement will be there.

Malformation is a primary structural defect that results from a localized error in morphogenesis, e.g. Peg-shaped lateral.

Malignant hypertension patient may be normotensive or hypertensive. Both kidneys show flea bitten

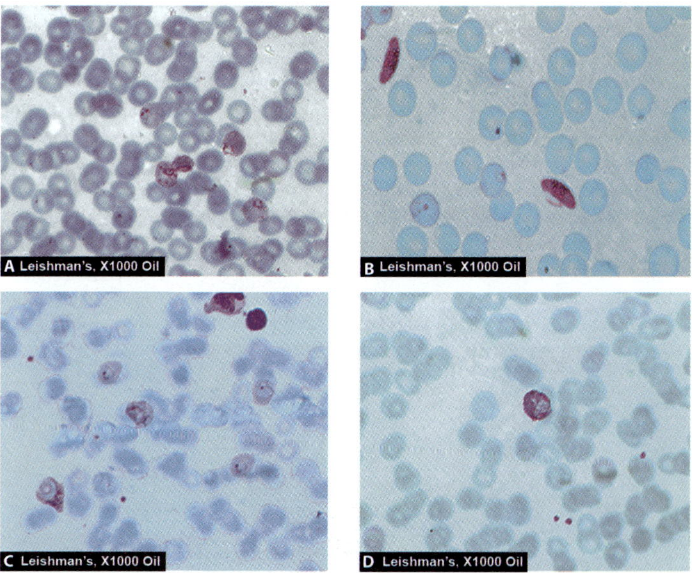

Figs A to D: *(A) Ring stage of P. falciparum (B) Gametocytes of P. falciparum; (C) Ring stage of P. vivax; (D) Amoeboid form of P. vivax*

appearance. In acute form kidney may be swollen and pin-point hemorrhages may be seen. Hypertension may result in episodes of unconsciousness or convulsions. Urine shows marked proteinuria and hematuria.

Malignant hyperthermia is a rapid onset of extremely high fever with muscle rigidity.

Malignant large intestine is a problem of rich society. Excessive fat and deficient fibers are the causative factor. Dietary fat enhances bile acid synthesis and level of sterol in intestine. Colonic bacteria convert this sterol into secondary acids which are thought to be carcinogens.

Malignant lymphoma is a neoplastic proliferative process lymphopoietic portion of RE system lymphomas and leukemias of lymphocytes and histiocytes are identical.

Malignant melanoma develops from melanocytes of skin or mucous membrane. Although the role of melanocytes is to protect the skin against development of skin cancer, but the cancer arising from the protective cell is most malignant tumor. Sunlight appears to play an important role in producing it. Commonest sites involved are hard palate and gingiva. *Clinical Features:* Most of the lesions are pigmented and are dark brown in color. It starts as macular pigmented focal lesions. Initially it grows very fast into large, painful diffuse mass. Surface ulceration is very common. Small satellite lesions may develop at periphery. There is widespread of tumor cells in lung, liver, bone and brain. Radical surgery and prophylactic neck dissection is advised. Still survival chances are bleak.

Malignant oral ulcer: Oral tumors may present as ulcers. Tobacco and alcohol consumption may cause squamous cell carcinoma. Oral epithelial dysplasia and lichen planus are the predisposing factors. These become painful when infected. Swollen nontender glands in neck may be seen. Loosening of teeth in carcinoma of gingiva is seen. Ulcer develops on tongue, floor of mouth and buccal mucosa. Shape may be round crescent or irregular. Edges are raised, rolled

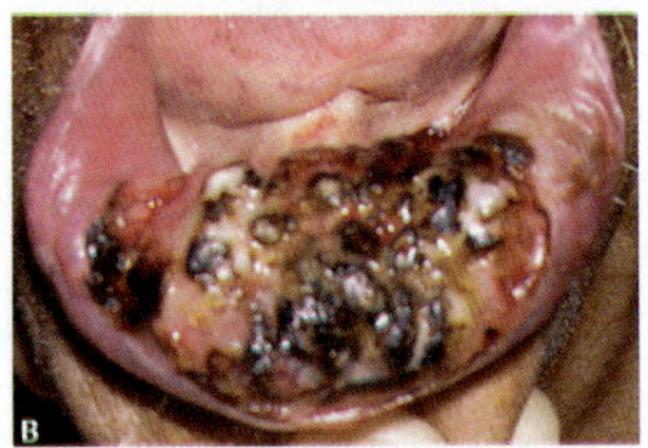

Figs A and B: *(A) Malignant melanoma of palate; (B) Malignant oral ulcer of labial sulcus*

and everted. Base is indurated and fixed. Floor is granular and ragged.

Malignant salivary gland tumor: Their incidence is much slow. Peripheral malignant salivary gland tumors can occur anywhere in lining of oral cavity but seldom in gingiva. Central variety is still rare. It generally develops between the age group 40-70 years of age. It grows slowly. When tumor infiltrates bone, it produces radiolucency.

Malignant schwannoma arises from nerve sheath cell. Some may develop from neurofibromatosis. Complaint may be of a mass, while some may develop pain. Radiographs will show diffuse radiolucency characteristic of malignant infiltrating neoplasm. It can be treated by surgery and by radiation.

Malingerer is the one who pretends to be sick or in pain for a motive.

Malleus is outermost and largest of three bones of middle ear. It is so called because it resembles a hammer (mallet = hammer). It has an upper rounded part called the head to which is attached a relatively long handle (or manubrium). At the junction of the head with the handle, there is a slight constriction called the neck. Just below the neck, the bone gives off two processes: anterior and lateral.

Malocclusion is any deviation from the ideal positioning of the teeth or jaws.

Mamelons are small elevations of enamel present on the incisors as they erupt.

Mammary duct ectasia is a dilatation of collecting ducts in subareolar region. It is a disease of at or about nenophase. Dilated ducts are bluish in color about 3-5 mm.

Mandible is the bone of the lower jaw and bears the lower teeth. It is a U-shaped bone anteriorly. Two rami—right and left that project upwards from the posterior part of the body. The bone has two surfaces internal and external surfaces. The body of the bone is known as alveolar process that bears the teeth, and a lower border that is called the base. The ramus has a posterior border, a sharp anterior border, and a lower border

M

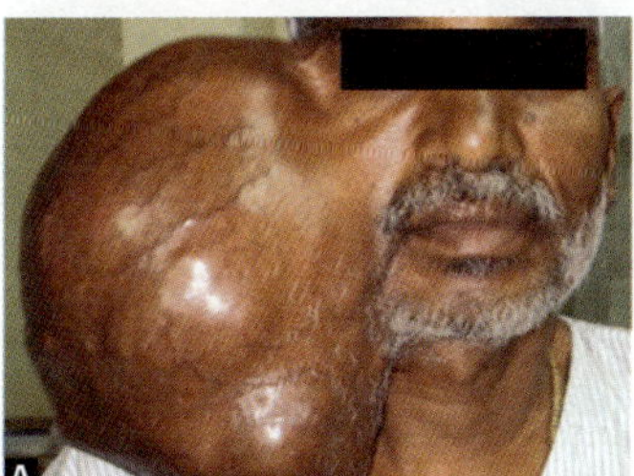

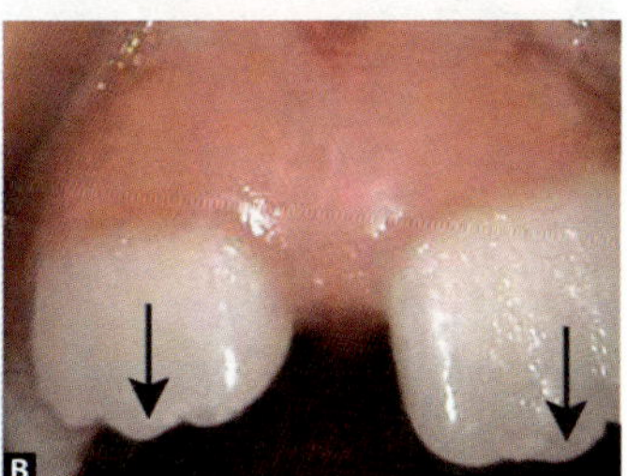

Figs A and B: *(A) Malignant tumor of parotid salivary gland; (B) Mamelons*

that merges with the base of the body. The medial margin of the foramen is formed by a projection called the lingual. The inner surface of the body of the mandible is marked by a ridge called the mylohyoid line that divides the inner surface of the body of the mandible into a sublingual fossa and a submandibular fossa.

Mandibular fracture commonly referred as fractures of jaw or breach in the mandibular bone. They amount to 20% of all fractures of face condyle and angles are two most commonly fracture sites. Multiple fractures do take place.

Mandibular nerve is the third branch of trigeminal nerve. The mandibular nerve is formed by union of two roots. The sensory root arises from the lateral part of the trigeminal ganglion, and leaves the skull through the foramen ovale. The motor root also passes through the foramen ovale and unites with the sensory root just below the foramen.

Mandibular nerve block is a local anesthetic technique used for complete anesthetizing the mandibular nerve.

Mandibular prognathism refers to a condition when the lower jaw is anterior to upper jaw. Radiologically, a line perpendicular to the constructed horizontal is dropped from glabella. The distance of soft-tissue pogonion from this vertical line is measured. Average distance of Pog′ is 0 ± 4 mm.

Mandibular subperiosteal implant is metal-frame implants that are surgically placed on top of the mandibular ridge.

Mandibulofacial dysostosis is the congenital condition where growth of this arch is defective so that the bones concerned remain under-developed, and the face is deformed.

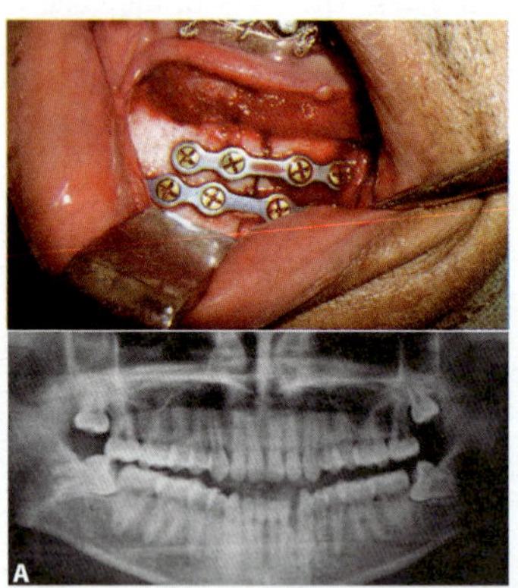

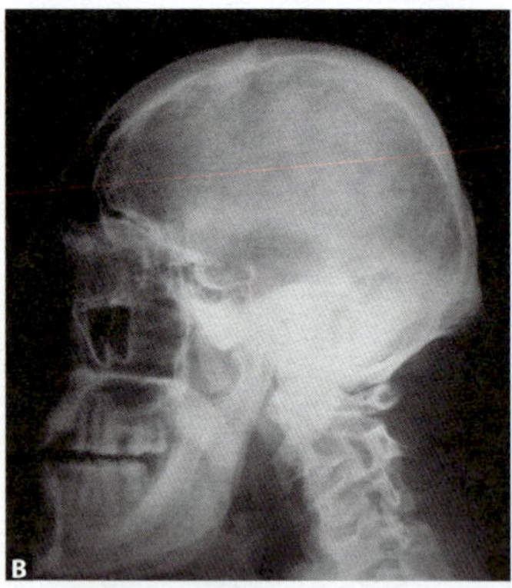

Figs A and B: *(A) Clinical and radiological view of mandibular fracture; (B) Mandibular prognathism*

Mania is an abnormal psychological state of mind with overexcitement and elevation of mood.

Mannitol is an osmotic agent that is freely filterable at the glomerular level. It is not reabsorbed by renal tubules. It has high diuretic potential so when given early in course of acute renal failure, it tends to flush out cellular debris and prevents tubular cast formation. Initial test dose is 12.5 to 25 gm over 3.5 minutes. Repeat after 1-2 hours. It is used in head injury. Mannitol is also an artificial sweetener occurring in seaweed, this alcohol is metabolized very slowly by oral microbes and, therefore, thought to have less cariogenic effect. It is used in toothpaste, mouth rinses and as a dusting agent in chewing gum.

Marasmus is a disease occurring due to protein energy malnutrition or due to general starvation. It arises from inadequate calorie intake. There is a failure to gain weight followed by loss of weight until emaciation results. Skin becomes wrinkled due to loose subcutaneous fat. Face becomes shrunken and wizened like a monkey. Abdomen may be distended. There may be associated vitamin deficiency.

Marginal gingiva also known as unattached gingiva is the terminal edge of gingiva which surrounds the teeth in a collar-like fashion. It also includes the gingival crevice or the sulcus and a free gingival margin. The free gingival margin is thicker and rounder around the primary teeth than

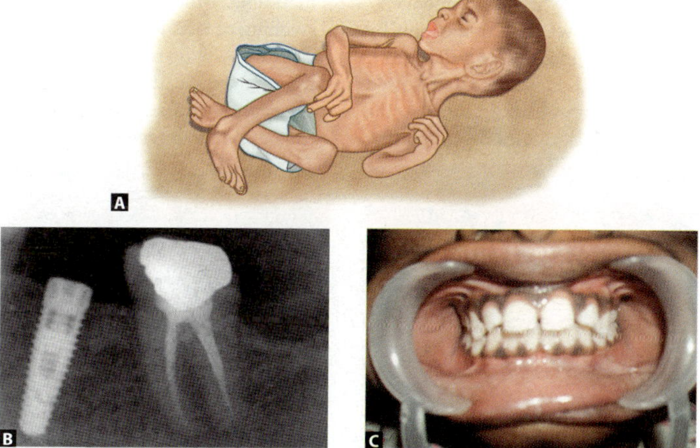

Figs A and B: *(A) Marasmus; (B) Mandibular subperiosteal implant; (C) Marginal gingiva*

in the permanent teeth, due to the morphological characteristics such as the cervical bulge and the underlying construction at the cementogingival junction, in contrast to the knife-edge margin seem in permanent dentition.

Marginal gingivitis is said to occur where the marginal gingiva is inflamed.

Margination is the process by which neutrophils adhere to vessel wall and is divided into three phases: Selectin mediated phase, activation phase/chemoattractant and Integrin-mediated phase.

Maryland bridge is permanent restoration that replaces missing teeth with minimal tooth preparation. These replace just one or two front teeth. The pontic has a porcelain bond in front with back side metal flanges resting against palatal surface of the abutments.

Maser (Microwave amplification by stimulated emission of radiation).

Masserann kit is a device that is used instrument retrieval within the canal. It has assorted end-cutting trepan burs which are large and rigid meant to be used only in coronal portion of straight canals.

Mastication is conditioned reflex, learned initially by irregular and poorly coordinated, chewing movements. The TMJ and periodontal ligament of the erupting dentition establishes a stabilized chewing pattern. It is also the first stage of digestion occurring in mouth. Food is broken up into pieces and mixed with saliva. Tongue helps to roll the mixture of food and saliva into a semi-liquid ball to be swallowed. Teeth help in chewing food and its chewing.

Masticator space refers to the space existing between the masseter muscle, pterygoid muscle, tendon of insertion of temporalis muscle, ramus of the mandible and the posterior part of the body of the mandible. Infection results in swelling of face, trismus and pain.

Masticatory pain refers to the pain upon chewing. It has the clinical characteristics of deep somatic rather than neurogenic pain. It may

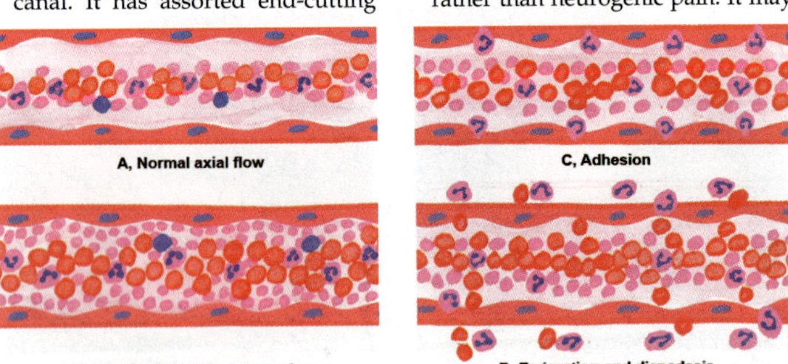

Fig.: *Sequence of leukocyte events in response to acute inflammation*

be induced by jaw movements. Pain may be severe but trigging by superficial touch and slight movement. Masticatory pain is not arrested by mandibular local anesthetic block.

Mastoid condyle is the marked prominence of bone located posterior and inferior to the temporomandibular joint.

Mat foil is a combination of mat gold and gold foil in which a layer of gold is sandwiched between layers of gold foil. Mat foil has rapid filling properties and is suited for the use as an internal filling material in a cavity.

Mat gold refers to the noncohesive form of gold material that has more mass than gold foiled and so can be used internally in a restoration and is often used to rapidly fill the preparation. It adapts well to the cavity wall and disadvantage is the bridging and surface pits are difficult to prevent. Mat gold is no softer than pure gold.

Materia alba is the soft accumulation of bacteria and tissue cells that lack organized structure of plaque which can be easily displaced.

Maternal deprivation syndrome is a form neglect that could be either intentional or of unintentional nature that results in failure to thrive.

Matrix band is a stainless-steel strip fabricated into a loop to fit around the prepared tooth and does not need a retainer.

Matrix metalloproteinases are a family of metal binding proteinases synthesized by connective tissue cells and also by hemopoietic cells including monocytes and macrophages, keratinocytes, endothelial cells, etc. They are usually secreted as a proenzyme form requiring extracellular activation. Metalloproteinase's can synergistically digest all the macromolecules of tissue matrices, although they are not necessarily produced together in

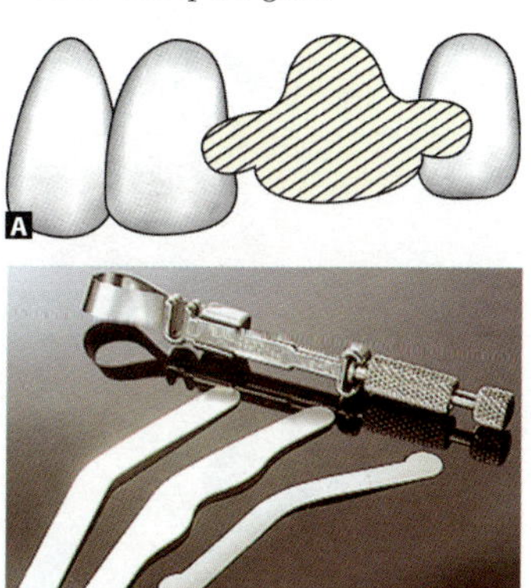

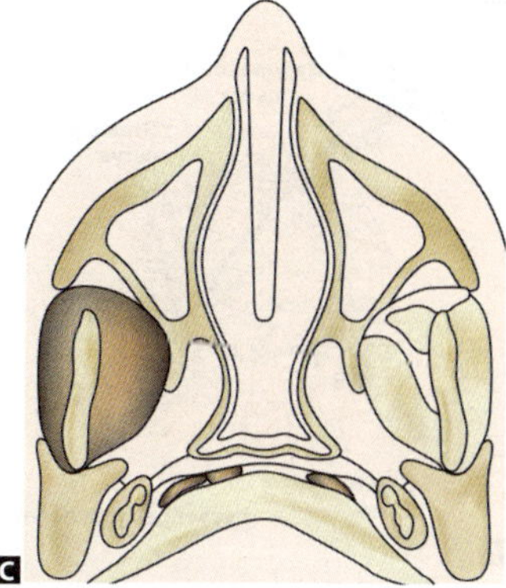

Figs A to C: *(A) Maryland bridge; (B) Matrix band; (C) Masticator space*

any specific situations. Major subgroups of MMPS are -> Interstitial collagenases (MMP 1, 8 and 13), Gelatinases (MMP 2 and 9), Stromelysins (MMP 3, 10, and 11), Membrane bound group (MMP 14, 15, 16 and 17), Matrilysin (MMP 7) and Metalloelastase (MMP 12).

Maturation is the qualitative change or aging.

Maxilla is the facial bone that forms the mid-face.

Maxillary antrolith refers to the calcified masses within the maxilla may occur at any age. Sometimes it is marked by pain, sinusitis and foul discharge. It is a complete or partial calcific encrustation of an antral foreign body. It has to be removed surgically.

Maxillary artery is one of the terminal branches of the external carotid artery. It begins behind the neck of the mandible, within the substance of the parotid gland. It is divided into three parts. The first part passes deep to the neck of the mandible to reach the infratemporal fossa. The second part of the artery runs superficial to the lower head of the lateral pterygoid muscle. The third part of the artery passes between the upper and lower heads of the lateral pterygoid muscle to pass through the pterygomaxillary fissure thus entering the pterygopalatine fossa.

Maxillary nerve is the second branch of trigeminal nerve leaves the middle cranial fossa through the foramen rotundum to reach the pterygopalatine fossa. The maxillary nerve is purely sensory. It arises from the middle of the distal edge of the trigeminal ganglion. Piercing the dura forming the distal edge of the trigeminal cave, it comes to lie in the lower part of the lateral wall of the cavernous sinus. It is entirely sensory in function supplies

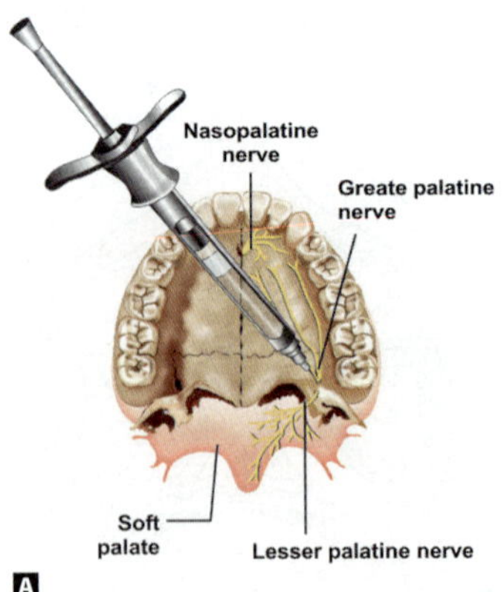

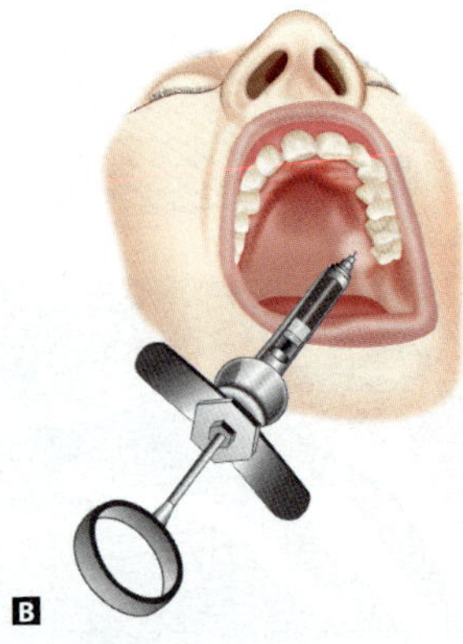

Figs A and B.: *Maxillary nerve block*

the skin of middle part of face, nasal cavity and side of nose, lower eyelid, upper lip and mucous membrane of nasopharynx, soft palate, tonsil, maxillary gingiva and teeth.

Maxillary nerve block is used for anesthetizing the maxillary nerve of trigeminal nerve.

Maxillary prognathism refers to when the maxillary jaw is present anterior to mandibular jaw radiographically can be described as a line perpendicular to the constructed horizontal is dropped from glabella. The distance of subnasale from this vertical line should be 6 ± 3 mm.

Maxillary sinuses are pyramid-shaped air-filled spaces that lie within the maxilla. On the medial aspect of this bone there is a large maxillary hiatus. The sinus usually opens into middle meatus of the nasal cavity by an opening in the lower part of the hiatus semilunaris.

Maxillary tuberosity is a rounded prominence of bone that extends posterior to the third molar region. It appears radiopaque on X-ray.

Mc′-Soft tissue menton: Lowest point on the contour of the soft-tissue chin.

Mean is the sum of observations divided by the number of observations.

Meaningful habits are habits that have a psychological bearing.

Measles (Rubeola) is an acute paramyxoviral infection. It is a cause of major morbidity and mortality in children worldwide. Measles is a highly infectious disease. It spreads through infected droplets. Patients in pre-eruptive and catarrhal phase are most infectious. The incubation period is about 7-14 days. Illness confers permanent immunity, child develops fever, cough, lacrimation and eruptive lesions of skin/mucosa. These appear as macule/papule which enlarge and coalesce. Oral lesions develop 2-3 days earlier of cutaneous rash. Intraoral lesions are known as Koplik's spot. These spots occur on buccal mucosa and are small, irregularly shaped appearing as bluish white specks surrounded by bright red margin.

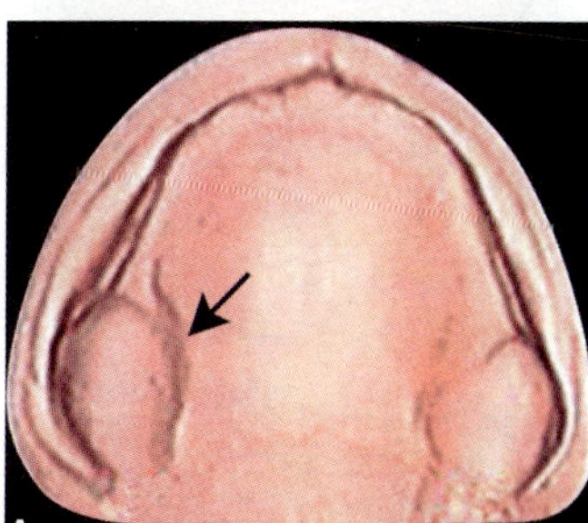

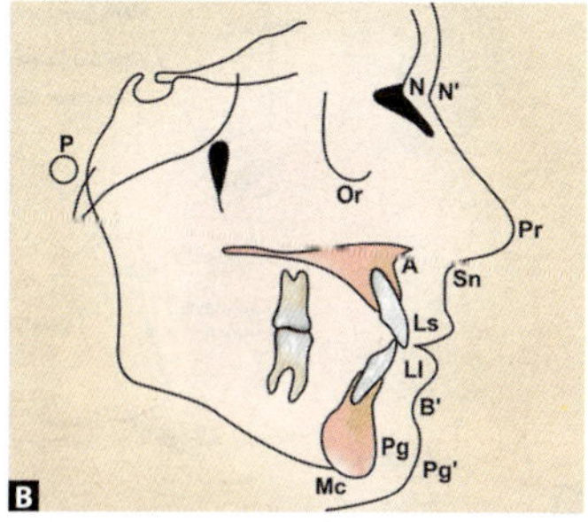

Figs A and B: *(A) Maxilla tuberosity; (B) Soft tissue menton Mc*

Mechanical antidotes refer to agents that counteract or neutralize the effect of poison and make them inactive by mechanical action, e.g. fine powdered charcoal in a dose of 4-8 gram acts mechanically by absorbing and retaining within its pores organic and to a less degree of mineral poison. One gram of charcoal absorbs about 500 mg of strychnine.

Meckel's syndrome is a rare, lethal genetic disorder characterized by renal dysplasia polydactyly hepatic developmental defects with pulmonary hyperplasia. Midline clefting of tongue is a feature of this syndrome. Tongue is also thrown into multiple nodular or papillomatous projections.

Medial means relating to the middle or medial plane.

Medial pterygoid muscle is a muscle of mastication. The fibers of this muscle run downwards and backwards. Anteriorly, some fibers of the muscle lie superficial to the lower head of the lateral pterygoid muscle. These fibers constitute the superficial head of the medial pterygoid muscle. The medial and lateral pterygoid muscles lie deep to the ramus of the mandible. The ramus separates the medial pterygoid muscle from the masseter.

Median is the middle score of a ranked distribution.

Median palatal cyst is a non-odontogenic fissural cyst of hard palate that arises from epithelium along the line of fusion of palatal process of maxilla. It lies in midline of hard palate. Treatment is by surgical removal and curettage.

Median rhomboid glossitis is a congenital abnormality due to failure of tuberculum impar to withdraw before fusion of 2 hours of tongue hence a structure devoid of papillae lies in between them. It is seen as an ovoid or rhomboid-shaped reddish patch on dorsum of tongue anterior to circum-vallate papillae. It is flat but slightly raised area.

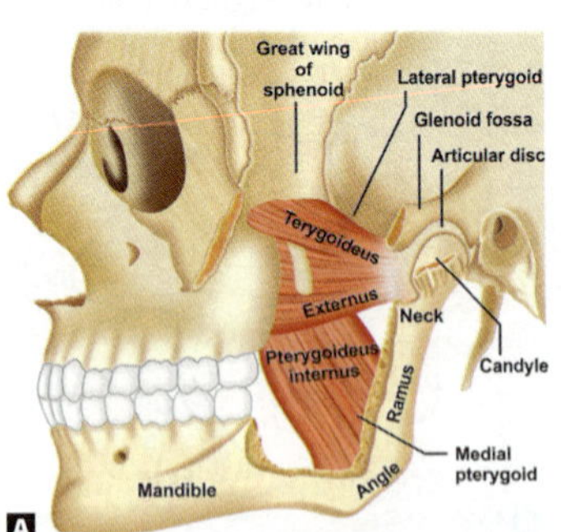

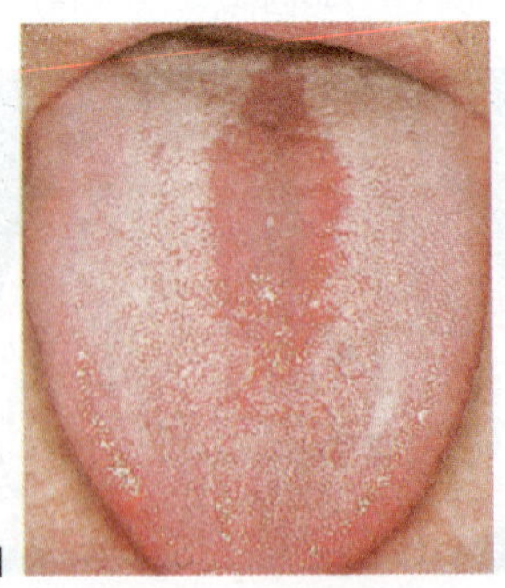

Figs A and B: *(A) Medial pterygoid muscle; (B) Median rhomboid glossitis*

Medical ethics are the special rules and regulations from the point of view of morality which a medical man should obey. Its violation is not an offence legally but is disgraceful and shameful from the point of view of profession.

Medical history refers to the history of any medical condition or any recent hospitalizations.

Medical neglect failure to provide the medical facilities to child is a form of medical neglect. Despite the known history of disease, failure to render treatment. Not maintaining proper immunization schedule and subjecting them to disease. Dental neglect, as defined by the American Academy of Pediatric Dentistry, is the "willful failure of parent or guardian to seek and follow through with treatment necessary to ensure a level of oral health essential for adequate function and freedom from pain and infection." The medical record is the chart that documents patient's experiences in the hospital from admissions to discharge. It contains relevant information regarding the patient's medical history and current conditions and details the plan for patient care from admission through discharge. The purpose of medical record purpose is to communicate cleanly and sufficiently. The medical record contains five major parts: (1) Admission notes, (2) Preoperative notes, (3) Operative and postoperative orders, (4) Progress notes, (5) Discharge notes.

Medication is the use of medicine.

Medication order: Name and directions for giving a drug.

Medicolegal autopsy is a legal procedure done to determine the identity of a person, to know the cause and time of death. It is also helpful in case of mutilated or skeletal remains to recognize the sex of it.

Mediotrusive side refers to the side of either dental arch corresponding to the side of the mandible moving towards the midline

Medulloblastoma is the commonest variety of primitive neuroectodermal tumor. It amounts 25% of child tumors usual location is inferior portion of cerebellar vermis.

Mega dose is an amount at least 10 times greater than RDA. In mega doses, vitamins act as drugs.

Megadontia refer macrodontia.

Megalodontia refer macrodontia.

Melanin is a nonhemoglobin derived brown pigment which is responsible for the normal pigmentation of skin, hair, gingiva and the rest of the oral mucous membrane. It is generally present in all individual and is very prominent in black individuals.

Melanocytes are the dendritic cells present in the basal and the spinous layer of gingival epithelium. They are mainly responsible for the production of a pigment called melanin which consequently attributes to the darker pigmented gingiva.

Melasma is a facial hypopigmentation seen commonly in pregnancy. There will be blotchy macules involving cheeks, temples and forehead. Sunlight increases the pigmentation while at the end of pregnancy, it dissolves out. During oral contraceptives also, it may develop.

Melatonin is an important hormone produced by pineal gland believed to regulate onset of puberty and menstrual cycle.

Memory b-lymphocytes refers to resting.

Memory cells are the cells that remain in reserve in lymph nodes until their ability to secrete antibodies is needed.

Menarche is the beginning of menstrual function or it is the first menstruation which marks the onset of puberty in the female. It usually occurs between the age of 11 to 16 years.

Meningeal carcinomatosis refers to the diffuse infiltration of meninges to the leptomeninges through the cerebrospinal fluid (CSF). Lesions such as lymphoma, melanoma and adenocarcinoma of breast are noted. Seizures and cranial nerve palsy are seen. Intrathecal injection and craniospinal irradiation are noted.

Meninges are a collective term given to the coverings around the brain and spinal cord, i.e. the dura mater, the arachnoid mater and the pia mater. Between the arachnoid mater and the pia mater, there is the subarachnoid space.

Meningioma is a tumor of arachoid cell of meninges. These are well-circumscribed extra-axial lesions that cause symptoms due to mass effect on underlying structures. These are completely resectable. Calcification in these is sufficient to make it radio-opaque. On CT, there are seen as well-defined hyperdense solid mass.

Meningitis means inflammatory changes in the meaninges and the subarachnoid space. Involvement of brain parenchyma along with meninges is known as meningoencephalitis. Meningitis is generally due to infective causes. These could be viruses, bacteria, or fungi. Meningitis can be classified into three main categories-Acute purulent

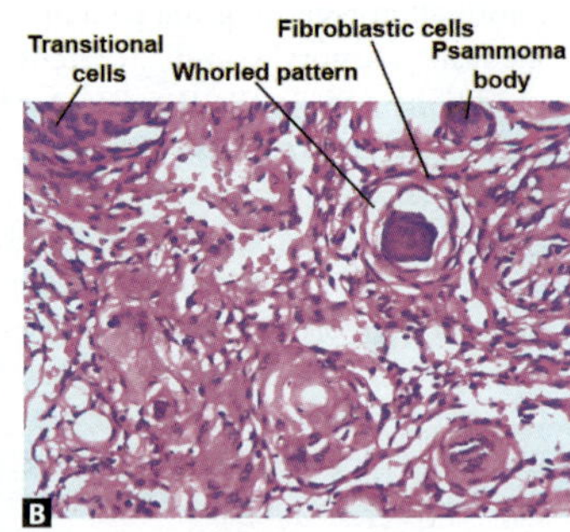

Figs A and B: *Meningioma (A) Macroscopic; (B) Microscopic*

(pyogenic, septic, bacterial), viral (aseptic), and chronic meningitis (tuberculous, fungal).

Menopause is the period during which menstruation ceases and female reproductive cycle comes to an end. Contrary to certain fears sexual desire and enjoyment are maintained.

Mental health is not mere absence of mental illness. Mental health is a state of balance between the individual and surrounding world, a state of harmony between oneself and others, coexistence between realties of self and that of other people and that of the environment.

Mental nerve is the branch of inferior alveolar nerve which exits in mandible through its foramen. It innervates chin and mucous membrane of lower lip.

Mental retardation (MR) is one of the most common developmental disabilities. It a condition, a syndrome, a symptom, a source of pain and bewilderment too many families. Mental retardation is also a condition or syndrome defined by a collection of symptoms, traits, or characteristics. It has been defined and renamed many times throughout history. This is not a disease, nor should it be confused with mental illness. Mental retardation (MR) is defined as an overall intelligence quotient lower than 70, associated with functional deficit in adaptive behavior, such as daily-living skills, social skills and communication.

Mentalis is a paired muscle located at the lower end of chin. Its shape is conical at the side of frenulum of lower lip. It raises and protrudes the lower lip and wrinkles the skin of chin.

Mentalis space refers to the space existing in the region of mental symphysis, where the mental muscle, depressor muscle of the lower lip and the angle of the mouth are attached. Infection to this area results in the large swelling of the chin.

Meprobamate is a common propanediol derivative used in treatment of anxiety and tension. It acts as muscle relaxant too, but is less potential than diazepines. It reduces muscle tone but can cause tolerance and physical dependence. It produces sleep, ataxia and hypotension.

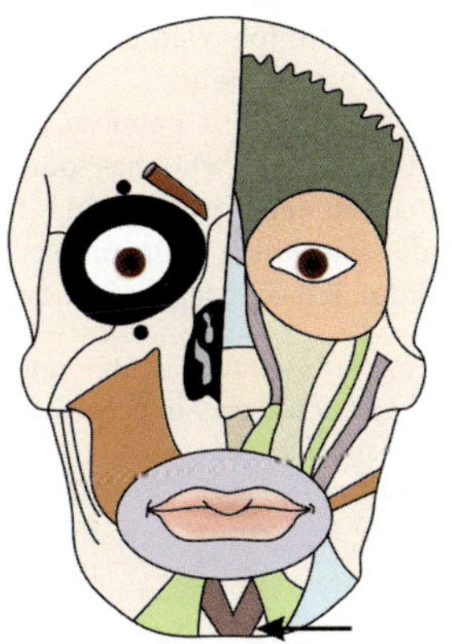

Fig.: *Muscles of facial expressions showing mentalis*

Mercury is a metal, component of amalgam fillings.

Mercury toxicity occurs due to excess dose of mercury. Fatal dose is 3-5 grams of mercuric chloride and fatal period is 3-5 days. Mercury toxicity may be acute or chronic. It develops gastric disturbances, excitability, headache and mental depression. Patient may develop fine tremor. Nephritis is common. There is an increased flow of saliva. Salivary glands may be swollen. Tongue may be swollen and painful. Loosening of teeth may occur. Treatment is supportive only. Symptoms include metallic taste in mouth with a feeling of constriction and choking in throat. It is followed by burning sensation. Mucous membrane becomes white and swollen. Vomits may contain slimily mucous with blood, stools become watery with mucous and blood. As treatment BAL 300 mgm 1 M at once followed by 150 mgm during next 12 hours.

Mercy killing is a painless killing of that person who has outlived his utility and is suffering from a disease which is incurable and painful. It has no legal sanction.

Merrifield's Z angle is an angle formed by the intersection of Frankfort horizontal (FH) and a line connecting the soft-tissue chin (Pog′) and the most protrusive lip point (may be upper or lower lip). Average value, 80 degree (± 9).

Mesh size is a numerical grading of particle size. larger numbers, e.g. 320 denote fine particles and smaller numbers denote coarse particles.

Mesial is the surface of the tooth nearest the midline of the dental arch.

Mesial step terminal plane refers to the occlusal relation in primary dentition where the distal surface of the lower second deciduous molar is more mesial than that of the upper. Thus the permanent molar erupts directly into 'Angles' Class I occlusion. This type of mesial step terminal plane must commonly occur due to the early forward growth of the mandible. If the differential growth of the mandible in a forward growth persists it can lead to Angles Class III molar relation and if the forward mandibular growth is minimal, it can establish a Class I molar relationship.

Mercury alloy ratio is the ratio of amongst of mercury to be mixed with an amalgam alloy.

Mercury	Hg	50%
Silver	Ag	35%
Tin	Sn	13%
Copper	Cu	0-3%
Zinc	Zn	0-1%

A

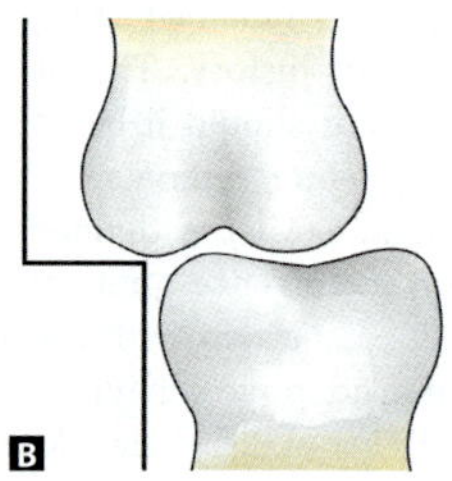

Figs A and B: *(A) Composition of amalgam; (B) Mesial step*

Mesiodens is the most common supernumerary tooth located between maxillary central incisors near the midline. Also refer to supernumerary teeth.

Meta-analysis refers to a statistical technique where the research results across several different studies are synthesized in a quantitive way. Advantages are that it has greater statistical power confirms data analysis and considers based resources.

Metabolic acidosis refers to a condition when the body produces too much acid or kidneys fail to remove acid from the body fluids. In mild case it may be asymptomatic while in severe case patient may develop hyperpnea. Cardinal clinical findings include hyperventilation. There will be increased depth and respiration frequency. Lips will become dry and parched tongue may be present especially in diabetic acidosis. Acidosis depresses cardiac response to catecholamines. It reduces red cells. Anorexia and fatigue are common. Confusion and stupor may occur. In acute renal failure organic acid retention causes fall in plasma bicarbonate by 1-2 mEq/L/day. Patient may have circulatory shock.

Metabolic alkalosis develops due to loss of acids from kidneys or stomach. It has raised plasma bicarbonate and pH. There is mild rise in $PaCO_2$. Urine pH below 7. Urine chloride less than 10 mEq/L. There may be tetany, apathy and confusion.

Metal ceramic crowns are the type of crowns where the dental porcelain can be bonded to variety of metal alloys. These alloys fall into three categories: precious metal alloys, semi-precious metal alloys and base metal alloys. The advantages of these crowns are strength, minimal palatal reduction, adaptability; wherein the disadvantages include esthetics, strength, loss of tooth substance and the cost.

Metal is a crystalline material that consists of positively charged ions in an ordered closely packed arrangement and bonded with a cloud of free electrons.

Metalizing is a coating of impression material with a powdered metal to make it electrically conductive.

Metallic stains due to drugs are generalized unlike other stains and may affect all the surfaces of

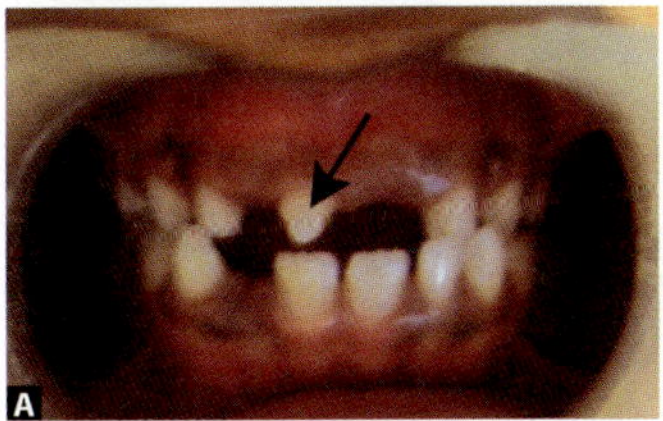

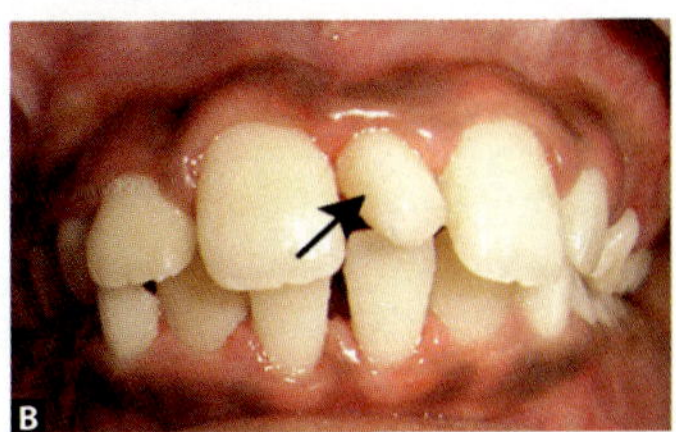

Figs A and B: *Mesiodens in primary and permanent dentition*

M

the tooth, these drugs enter the plaque substance and impart its color to plaque and calculus, e.g. consumption of iron will give rise to black or brown stains, manganese will give rise to black stains.

Metallic stains due to industries: Cervical third of the anterior teeth are primarily affected by the inhalation of metallic dust through mouth bringing them in contact with teeth, these metals along with bacterial plaque impart their color to the plaque present which occasionally may penetrate the tooth substance and give rise to endogenous stains. Copper will give bluish green stains, nickel will give green stain, and cadmium will give yellow or golden brown stains.

Metamerism is the change in color matching of two objects under light source is called Metamerism. Two objects that are marched under one light source but not under other light sources form a metameric pair.

Metaplasia is conversion of one type of differentiated tissue into another type of differentiated tissue. Metaplasia can be of epithelial or connective tissue type. Metaplasia of columnar to squamous epithelium occurs in respiratory mucosa.

Metastasis is a spread of tumor from one site of organ to another with no direct continuity with the main or primary tumor mass. Tumor thus formed is a secondary deposit. Metastatic spread can occur through lymphatic channels, blood vessels. Metastatic spread is the hallmark of malignant neoplasm. Benign tumors never metastasize.

Metastasis melanomatous nodes: Patient is a young person between 20 to 30 years. Lymph nodes are firm, massive but not tender. These are mobile in early stage but later become fixed.

Metastatic calcification is the deposition of calcium in normal viable tissue due to hypercalcemia. It is due to hyperparathyroidism, vitamin D intoxication and osteolytic bone secondaries. Gastric mucosa, lungs, blood vessels and kidneys are involved. Deposition is around the tubules in kidney.

Metastatic carcinomatous nodes are the solitary or multiple nodes are involved. It is hard but not tender. To start these are mobile and fixed.

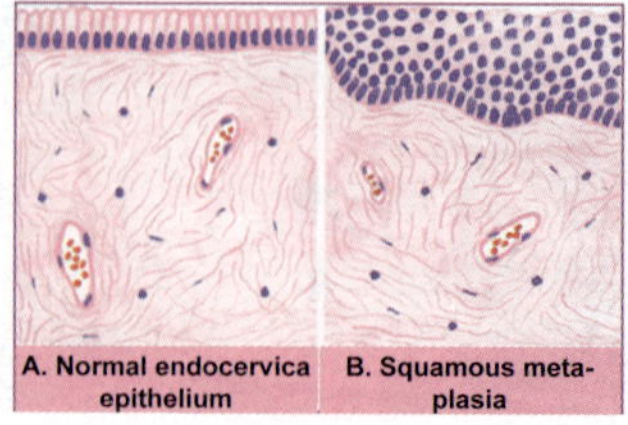

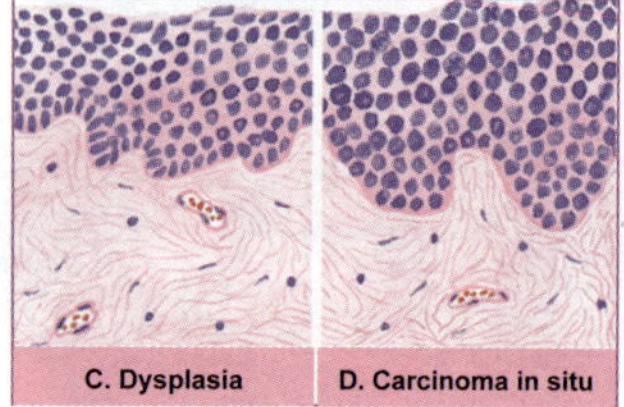

Fig.: *Various stages of metastatic cell differentiation*

It may macerate or fungate. Primary lesion may be known.

Metastatic liver neoplasm refers to the primary neoplasm of liver that has spread to the other sites of the body. Metastatic tumors are much more common. Cancer of breast, stomach, pancreas, kidney, and uterus are most to metastasize. Weight loss, anorexia and fatigue are the common complaints. CT scan is a better tool to diagnose it. Survival is 3 months to 3 years.

Metastatic tumors of jaw are formed by cells that have been transported from the primary tumor to site not connected to original tumor. These are not frequent and may be asymptomatic. If mandibular nerve is involved, there may be paresthesia of lip or chin. Teeth may become loose. Expansion of jaw is a constant finding. Mandible is affected more than maxilla. On X-ray these produce metastatic lesion. Diffuse destruction may lead to pathological fracture. Prognosis is not good.

Metastatic vertebral tumor is a secondary tumor that has spread from the primary tumor causes low back pain. Typically pain begins abruptly with cramping muscular pain. Pain is worst during night and is not relieved by rest.

Methadone was discovered in 1940 in Germany and produces mild analgesia. It is well-absorbed form

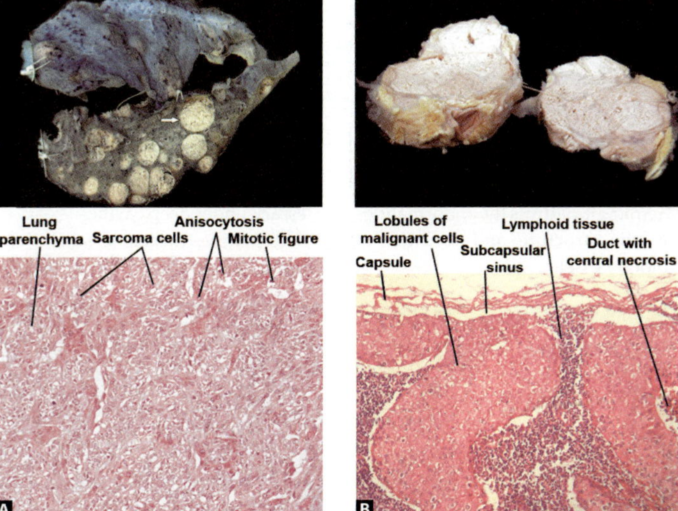

Figs A and B: *(A) Metastatic sarcoma of lung; (B) Metastatic carcinoma of lymph nodes*

GIT Its effective oral dose is 5-15 mg depending on severity of pain. Side effects are less common.

Methohexitone is a barbiturate derivative and used as IV anesthetic agent. It is two and half times more potent as thiopentone. It is prepared by mixing the powder in sterile distilled water. Average induction dose is 1.0 to 1.5 mg/kg body weight. It is the best anesthetic induction agent. It can be best used singly for extraction of tooth. If it is injected extravenously it may cause necrosis and ulcer formation.

Metronidazole is an antibiotic active against wide range of anaerobic micro-organism specially bacterial and parasitical origin. It is used in ulcerative gingivitis. It is well-tolerated when given orally except some GIT upsets.

Microabrasion is a drill-free technique using an instrument resembling a tiny sand blaster that delivers tiny aluminium oxide particles to the surface of teeth.

Microangiopathy is the abnormalities in the structure and function of blood vessel.

Microdontia is a developmental anomaly where the teeth are physically smaller than usual. Widely spaced normal sized teeth may appear small within the jaws that are larger than normal and is termed as relative microdontia. But this, in true sense, represents macrognathia, not microdontia. If all the teeth in both the normal sized arches are smaller than normal, it is referred to as generalized microdontia. True generalized microdontia is seen in pituitary dwarfism, Down's syndrome. Isolated microdontia/ microdontia involving one or two teeth are far more common than generalized types. Most commonly affected teeth are maxillary lateral incisor or maxillary third molars. Maxillary lateral incisors typically appear peg-shaped crown (conical).

Microfilled composite resins compositive resin of smaller size. Conventional resins are 500 times greater than that of particles in microfilled resin. Some pulpal protection is necessary under deep cavities.

Micrognathia means a small jaw. Either a maxilla or mandible may

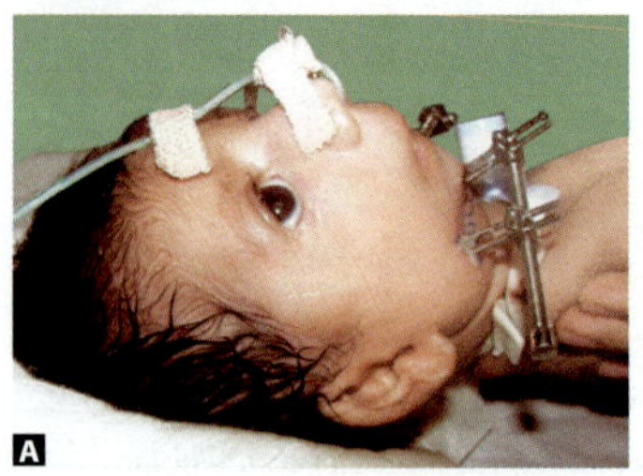

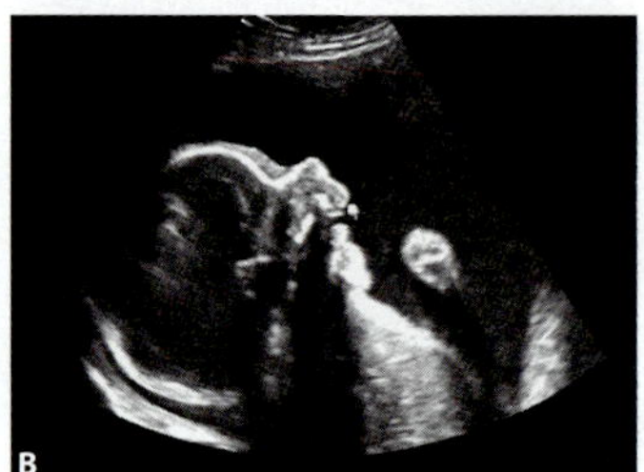

Figs A and B: *Micrognathia (A) Clinical; (B) Radiological*

be affected. True micrognathia may be congenital or acquired. In case of maxilla deformity is of middle third of face retracted. Congenital micrognathia is difficult to explain. Acquired type is due to disturbance of temporomandibular joint. There is severe retrusion of chin, steep mandibular angle and deficient chin button.

Micron: 0.001 mm or 0.00004 inch or 1/1000 millimeters.

Microphage *see* neutrophils.

Microshock: Low voltage but high amperage electricity.

Microstomia refers to a condition where patient presents with an abnormally small opening of mouth associated with functional disability. Shape of opening is circular and it appears as if patient is whistling. It may be congenital or may develop after burns.

Microwave diathermy is a deep heating modality and uses a form of electromagnetic radiation. Microwaves penetrate more deeply than do infrared rays but don't pass through the tissues in any appreciable density. Average depth of penetration is 3 cm. These are effectively absorbed by water so there is an appreciable heating of tissues having rich blood supply. It is very good in traumatic and inflammatory lesions. So it is useful in trauma and rheumatic condition. Skin must be dry because water is heated rapidly. Wet dressings should be avoided.

Mid-sagittal plane is also known as midline the vertical plane that divides the body into two equal left and right halves.

Middle adolescence refers to the children falling into the age group of 13-17 years. Participation in teenage subculture and peer group identity. It follows the onset of puberty.

Middle cerebral artery ischemia is the largest branch of internal carotid artery and supplies the lateral surfaces of frontal, parietal and temporal lobes. Complete occlusion results in contralateral

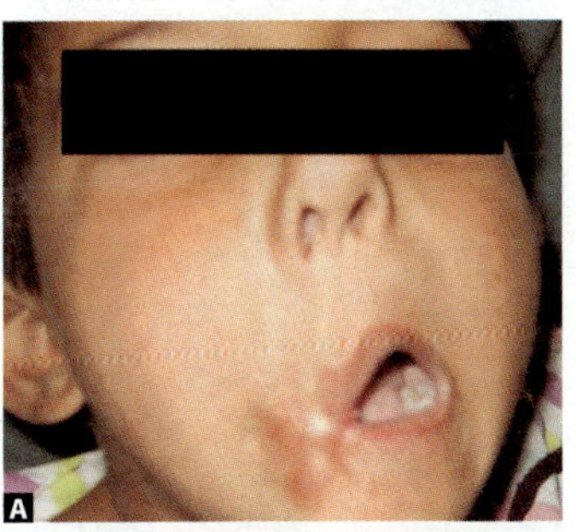

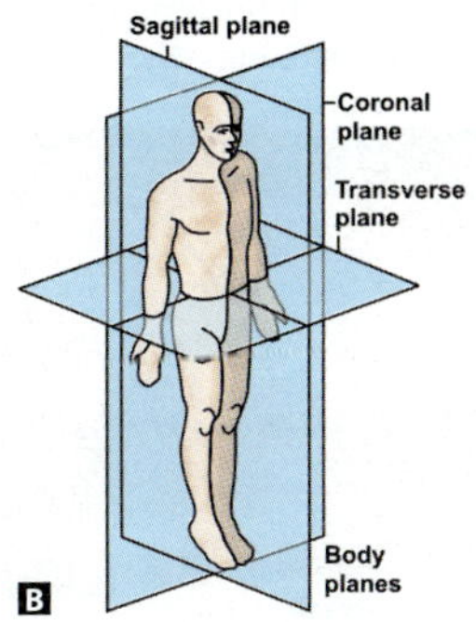

Figs A and B: *(A) Microstomia; (B) Various body planes, note mid-saggital plane*

M

sensory loss, motor weakness with positive Babinski sign of upper motor neuron lesion.

Middle cranial fossa is the centermost part of the base of the skull that has a raised median part formed by the body of the sphenoid bone, the lesser wings are attached to the sides of the body of the sphenoid, and the greater and lesser wings are parted by the superior orbital fissure that continues into the orbit.

Middle ear is also called the tympanic cavity or tympanum. It is a space lying in the petrous temporal bone. The middle ear is separated from the external acoustic meatus by the tympanic membrane.

Middle superior nerve is a branch of infraorbital nerve within the infraorbital canal, provides sensory innervations to maxillary premolars, periodontal tissue facial soft tissue and bone.

Middle superior alveolar nerve block is used for anesthetizing the middle-superior alveolar nerve and its terminal branches. It is given for anesthetizing the maxillary first and second premolars and mesiobuccal root of the first molar.

Midline is the imaginary line through the middle of an object which divides it into two equal parts.

Miescher's syndrome also known as cheilitis granutomatosa is characterized chronic swelling of lips. There develops diffuse swelling of lip, vermilion border scaling, fissuring, vesicle or pustule formation may take place also known as Melkersson rosenthal syndrome when associated with facial palsy and plicatd tongue.

Migraine is a familial disorder characterized by recurrent paroxysmal attacks of headache. It is one of the most disabling diseases. Often there is a strong family history. It is a paroxysmal unilateral headache, preceded by visual and sensory phenomena. It may be accompanied by nausea and vomiting. It is due to vasospasm in extra- and intra-cranial arteries. It starts just after waking up. Visual aura is common. It may be hemianopic field defect, transient blindness.

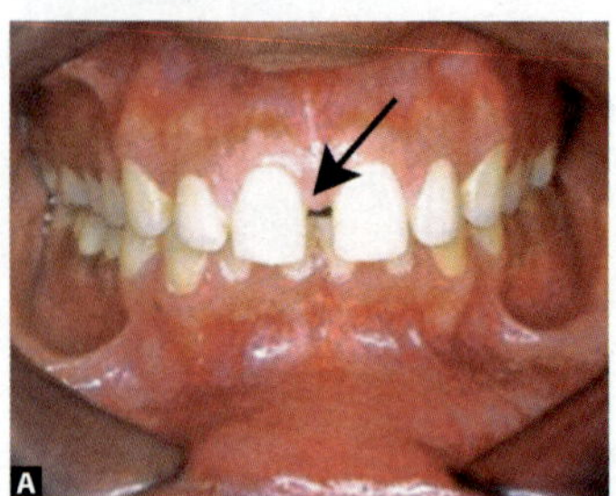

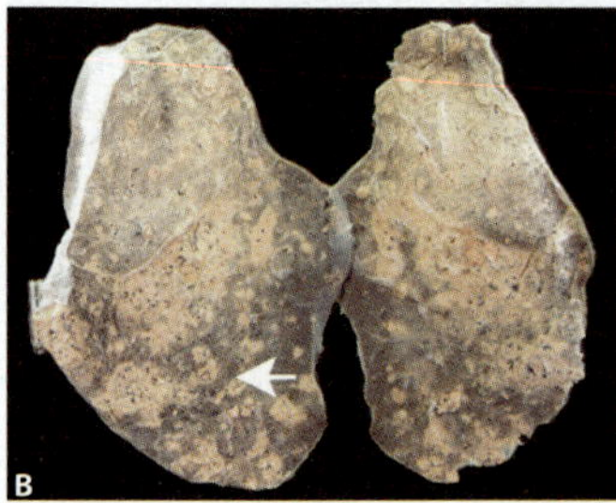

Figs A and B: *(A) Midline diastema; (B) Lung section showing miliary tuberculosis*

Sensory aura includes tingling, numbness and pins and needles in corner of mouth. In classical migraine, headache is characteristically associated with premonitory sensory, motor or visual symptoms (aura). Headache without aura (common migraine) is more frequent type of migraine. The headache typically starts with nonspecific prodromal symptoms like malaise and irritation followed by an aura of a focal neurological event. There is severe throbbing hemicranial headache with nausea, vomiting, photophobia and phonophobia.

Migraine without aura is of an abrupt onset without aura. Nausea and vomiting are common. It is strongly familial. Headache may awaken patient from sleep. Photophobia and homophobia are common. In status migrainous hospitalization may be needed.

Migrainous neuralgia *see* cluster headache.

Migratory glossitis refer geographic tongue.

Mikulicz's disease shows both inflammatory and neoplastic characteristics. There is enlargement of parotid or submaxillary gland. There may be fever, loose tooth and oral infection. Mass may increase or decrease in size.

Miliary tuberculosis lung is due to hematogenous spread of infection. X-ray may show small, discrete nodules 1-2 mm in diameter distributed throughout both lungs. These nodules may enlarge and coalesce.

Milk is a complete and ideal food and is a balanced diet. It contains 3.5% proteins. Carbohydrates are in form of milk sugar. Human milk contains more sugar than cow's milk. It is poor source of vitamin C and does not contain vitamin E. It is good source of calcium but is a poor source of iron. Fat is in the form of glycerides in emulsified form.

Mineral elements are the trace elements that are essential for normal functionary of the body. Body contains 24 minerals. About 4–6% of body weight is made up

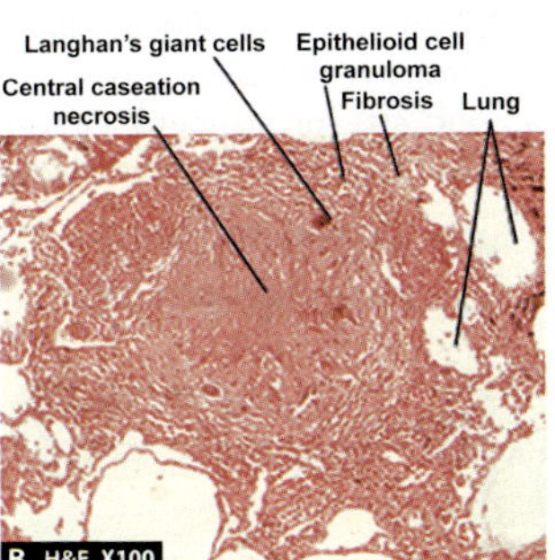

Figs A and B: *Histological section showing miliary tuberculosis of lung*

of mineral elements. Bones and teeth store these. These maintain acid-base balance, control of water balance, contraction of muscles and clotting of blood. This helps in formation of bone and teeth formation.

Mineral trioxide aggregate is a multipurpose material was developed by Dr Torabinejad in 1993. It contains tricalcium silicate, dicalcium silicate, tricalcium aluminate, bismuth oxide, calcium sulfate and tetracalcium aluminoferrite. pH of MTA is 12.5, thus having its biological and histological properties similar to calcium hydroxide. Setting time is 2 hours and 45 minutes. In contrast to $Ca(OH)_2$, it produces hard setting nonresorbable surface. Because of being hydrophilic in nature, it sets in a moist environment. It has low solubility and shows resistance to marginal leakage. It also exhibits excellent biocompatibility in relation with vital tissues.

Mini-bladed curettes are the modification of extended shank or after five curettes. They are half the size of standard Gracey curettes; they have shorter blades which allow easier insertion and adaptation into deep pockets, furcation areas, developmental grooves, etc.

Miniplates were introduced by Champy et al in 1978 customized for mandibular fractures; they were initially available in stainless steel which has now been replaced by titanium. These noncompression miniplates are confined to outer cortex allowing the fixation of plates both subapically and the lower border. Post-healing these plates can be left in permanently without causing any trouble.

Minor oral surgery instruments include scalpal, periosteal elevator, tissue retractor, Kilner cheek retractor and Austin retractor.

Minor salivary glands are found deep to the mucosa of the upper and lower lip, cheeks, undersurface of the tongue, soft palate, dorsal surface of the tongue and lateral parts of hard palate behind the first premolar. These small glands have short ducts which open directly onto the surface of the mucosa by multitude of openings.

Mitotic activity is a process of cell division. It determines the response of a cell to radiation.

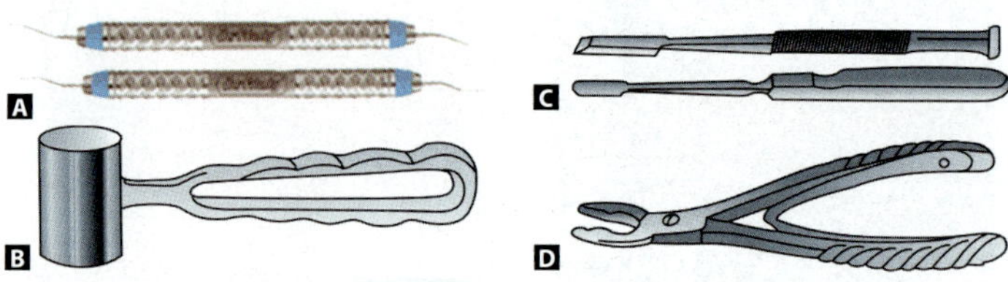

Figs A to D: *(A) Mini Gracey curettes; (B) Mallet (C) Bone chisel and file; (D) Bone forceps (bone instruments)*

Mitotic figures are seen in any proliferative tissue including benign tumors. A high mitotic index is not diagnostic of malignancy. Abnormal mitotic figures such as triploid and tetrapolar mitoses occur exclusively in malignant lesion.

Mitral regurgitation is a heart disorder where the mitral valve doesn't close tightly and allows the leakage of blood backwards. In acute regurgitation left atria pressure rises rapidly leading to pulmonary edema. When chronic, left atrium enlarges exertional dyspnea and fatigue progresses. Mitral regurgitation may predispose to infective endocarditis. There will be pan-systolic murmur maximal at apex radiating to axilla.

Mitral stenosis is a heart condition where the narrowing of mitral valve is seen. There will be dyspnea, orthopnea and paroxysmal nocturnal dyspnea. Prominent mitral first sound, opening snap and apical diastolic crescendo rumble ECG shows left atrial abnormality.

Mixed dentition: This type of dentition contains both the dentition as this is the transient phase where there is exchange of primary dentition to permanent dentition.

Mixing tip is used with an automix impression system.

Mm Hg: Millimeters of mercury a unit measuring pressure.

Mode is the most frequently occurring score within a distribution.

Moderate bone loss: Bone loss of 10 to 33% measured on a dental radiograph.

Moderate interproximal lesion extends greater than halfway through the thickness of enamel, but does not involve the DEJ. A moderate lesion is seen in enamel only.

Moderate periodontitis is said to have occurred when the periodontal destruction is generally considered moderate where 3 to 4 mm of clinical attachment loss has occurred.

Moderate pulpalgia may start spontaneously from such a simple act as that of lying down. Hot food or drink excites the pain. Warm water will not relieve the pain and cold water, sometimes, makes it worse. The pain is a true toothache. Pain is of nagging or of boring type. Pain to start is localized and later becomes diffuse or referred to another area. Pain does not resolve once the irritant is removed.

Modified DMFT index is an index used for assessing dental caries was

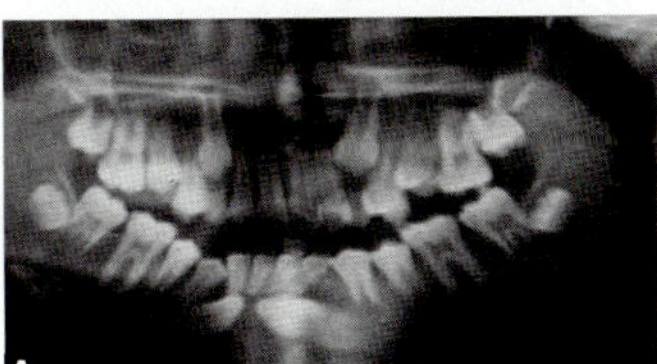

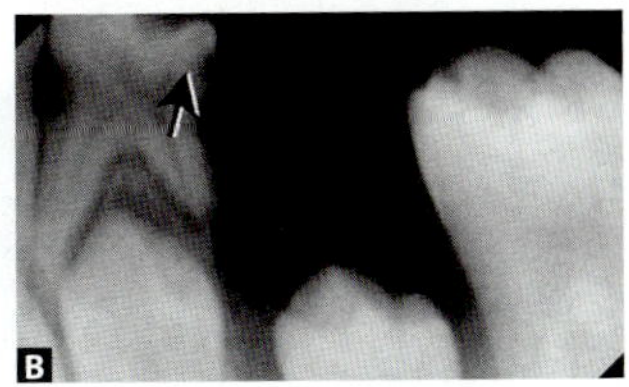

Figs A and B: *(A) Mixed dentition OPG; (B) Moderate proximal caries*

introduced by Joseph Z Anaise in 1983. The DMFT index by Klein and Palmer is one of the simplest and most commonly used indices in epidemiologic dental health status based on the number of decayed, missing and filled teeth. The index, however, does not provide an accurate description of previous dental care, nor does it provide information regarding the severity of the carious attack or the indicated treatment. Thus, a modification of the DMFT index was developed. The modification of DMFT index involved a division of the 'D' component into four separate categories. With the addition of these categories, the index remains simple, and yet provides description of one's previous dental experience. It further shows the extents of dental services needed by the population, which can be interpreted in terms of treatment hours and costs. Basically, this modified DMFT index involves the same operation procedures. Applied DMFT index involves the same operation procedures applied to the common DMFT index. The only difference is the scoring criteria for 'D' component of the index. In this modified DMF index, the 'D' component is divided into 4 separate categories.

M

Modified pen grasp ensures the greatest control in performing intraoral procedures. The thumb, index and the middle finger is used to hold the instrument as a pen is held. This grasp enhances control because it enables the clinician to roll the instrument in precise degrees, also it enhances tactile sensitivity.

Modulus of elasticity is a measure of material's stiffness. Stiffness is an important issue when selecting restorative materials because large deflections are undesirable. To withstand forces of mastication, material should have high modulus of elasticity.

Molars are the posterior-most teeth of the jaw. Their main function is chewing and grinding the food. Every quadrant has three molars that erupted by the 6, 14 and 18 years respectively. The third molar is also known as wisdom tooth.

Molar forceps are forces used for extraction of molar. These have pointed blades to fit the bifurcation of molar roots, upper molar forceps have one pointed blade to fit the

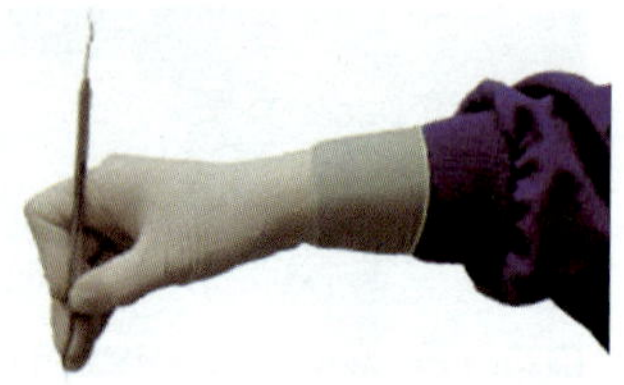

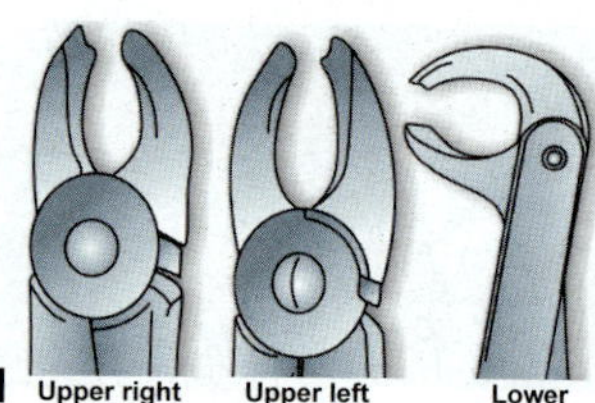

Figs A and B: *(A) Modified pen grasp; (B) Molar forceps*

bifurcation of buccal roots and a rounded blade to fit the single palatal root. Lower molar forceps have two identical blades. Left and right lower molars are extracted with it.

Molecular death means death of an individual cell of tissues of body. It takes sometime after the somatic death. The period between somatic death and cell death is rarely more than 3-4 hours. Signs of molecular death include loss of elasticity of skin, changes in eyes, cooling of body, flaccidity and lately rigor mortis.

Moller's index system was developed by Moller IJ and Poulsen S in 1964 is a standardized system for diagnosing, recording and analyzing dental caries data. The basis for the development of this system was to make available a system which could be used in many different situations. The advantages of the system seems to be its flexibility in meeting the varying needs of different types of clinical studies on dental caries.

Molluscum contagiosum is due to infection with a large DNA virus, a member of pox virus group. It causes small umbilicated 1-3 mm in diameter lesion which may express cheesy core on pressure. It is more common in children. Multiple, discrete elevated nodules occur on face and trunk. Disease appears to be spread by autoinoculation. Oral lesions occur on lips, tongue and buccal mucosa, surgical excision may be required.

Monellin is a protein derived sweetener. 3000 times sweeter than sucrose. It is extracted from an African berry.

Monocytes are the largest normal cell in blood. Nucleus may be round, kidney-shaped, oval or lobulated. Cytoplasm is slightly grey; chromatin is arranged in fine strands with sharply defined margins. It is also of same size as that of neutrophils, i.e. 10 um diameter but they are conventionally known as macrophages when they leave the blood as they begin to differentiate and grow larger in size up to 22 um diameter. They are best suited for communicating with lymphocytes and other surrounding cells.

Monomorphic adenoma is a benign encapsulated salivary gland. These are composed of uniform pattern of epithelial cells. These have no connective tissue like component. These are treated surgically.

Monoplegia refers to involvement of one side of the body and is believed to be a form of hemiplegia where one limb is significantly affected.

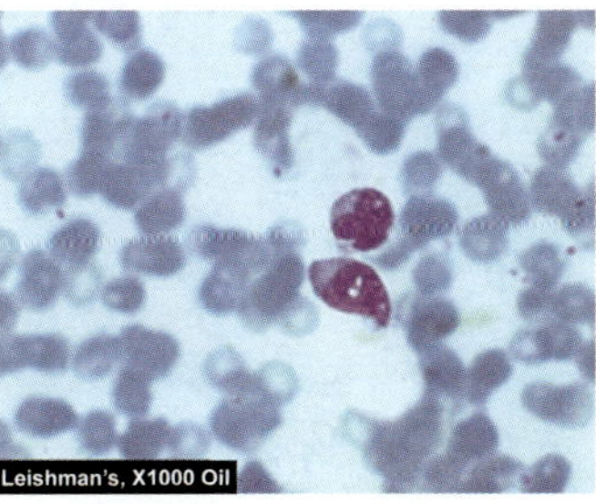

Fig.: *Monocytes*

Moral values are standards of conduct and thought influenced by family, religion, culture and society.

Morbidity is sickness/illness.

Morgue is the area where dead bodies are temporarily held or examined.

Morning sickness refers to nausea upon waking up in the morning. It develops in early pregnancy. Nausea and vomiting is seen. It may be due to hypoglycemia.

Moro reflex is a neonatal reflex. Any sudden movement of the neck initiated the reflex. This can be elicited by pulling the baby to a sitting position from the supine and suddenly let the head fall back to a short distance. This reflex consists of a rapid abduction and extension of the arm with the opening of hands. *Clinical Importance:* This gives an indication of muscle tone. The response may be asymmetrical if muscle tone is unequal on the two sides, or if there is a weakness of an arm or an injury to the clavicle. This reflex usually disappears in 2 to 3 months.

Morphine was first isolated in 1903 by Serturner. It is derived from Papaver somniferum. It chiefly affects CNS and bowels. 5-10 mg IV reduces pain within 20-30 minutes. There develops a feeling of drowsiness and euphoria. It is effective against all types of pain but not very effective in sharp intermittent pain. It depresses respiration. Cough reflex is also depresses and death is due to respiratory failure. Itching and urticaria may also develop. It develops tolerance and physical/psychical dependence. Heroin is more effective than morphine.

Morphology is the science that deals with form and structure without reference of function.

Mortal pulpotomy: Ideally, a non-vital tooth should be treated by pulpectomy and root canal filling. However, pulpectomy of a primary

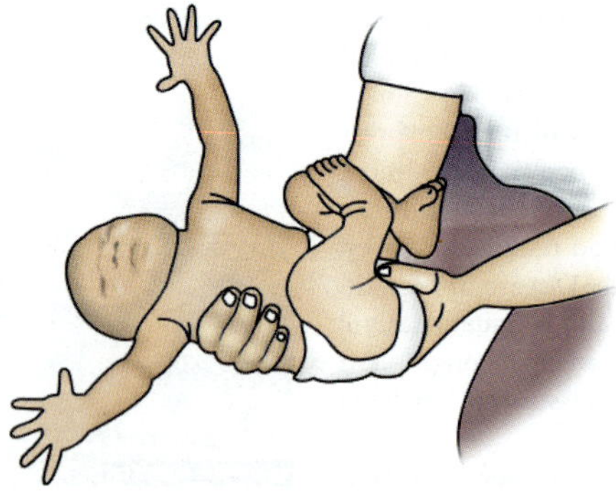

Fig.: *Moro reflex*

molar is often impracticable and a two-stage pulpotomy technique is, therefore, more commonly used. Necrotic coronal pulp is first removed and the infected radicular pulp is treated with a strong antiseptic solution, which is applied on a cotton pellet and sealed in the pulp chamber for 10–12 weeks. Beechwood creosote is usually used (Hobson 1970) but formocresol (Droter 1963) or camphorated monochlorophenol may also be used. Beechwood creosote is a mixture of cresol, glycol and other phenols, which is less irritant to the tissue than phenol itself.

Mortality means death.

Moss hypothesis: According to Moss the "bone" does not regulate its own growth. The genetic and epigenetic determines the growth of matrix, that is, muscle, nerve glands, teeth, neurocranial fossa, and nasal, orbital, oral, and pharyngeal cavities. This is primary while the growth of the skeletal unit is secondary. However, although the functional matrix principle describes what happens during growth, it does not account for how it happens. Functional matrices, which can be further divided into capsular and perosteal matrices, have the primary control for the growth of craniofacial structures. Bone responds to the matrices in a passive manner and doesn't have any primary growth potential.

Motions of instruments for cleaning and shaping. For effective use of reamers and files, following six different motions are given: (1) Follow motion is performed using files during initial cleaning and shaping. In this, file is precurved so as to follow canal curvatures; (2) Follow withdraw motion is performed with files when apical foramen is reached. In this, simple in and out motion is given to the instrument. It is done to create a path for foramen and no attempt is made to shape the canal; (3) Cart motion means transporting. In this, precurved reamer is passed through the canal with gentle force and random touch with dentinal wall up to the apical foramen. It is done to transport pulp remnants and dentinal debris; (4) Carve motion is performed with reamers to do shaping of the canals. In this a precurved reamer as touched with dentinal wall and canal is shaped on withdrawal; (5) Smooth motion is performed with files. In this, circumferential motion is given to smoothen the canal walls; (6) Patency motion is performed with files or reamers. Patency means that apical foramen has been cleared of any debris in its path; (7) Starting at the apex with fine instruments and working up to the orifice with progressively larger instruments, this is step-back technique; (8) Starting at the orifice with larger instrument and working up to apex with larger instruments, this is crown down technique. It is also called the reverse flaring technique by Weine, coronal two-third pre-enlargement by Cohen, and cervical flaring technique by Goerig.

Motor fibers are those fibers where impulses passing along such nerves cause the muscle to contract resulting in movement. They are also called efferent fibers (efferent = go away from).

Motor neuron transmits nerve impulses from brain and spinal cord to muscles and glandular epithelial tissue.

Motor nucleus of the trigeminal nerve lies in the upper part of the pons, in its dorsal part.

Mottled enamel was described first by F McKay in 1916. Ingestion of fluoride containing drinking water during the formation of tooth leads to it. Severity of it increases with increasing amount of fluoride. Above the level of 0.9 to 1.0 ppm fluoride may cause it. Mild changes manifest by white opaque areas. Moderate and severe change show pitting and brownish staining. Fracture enamel may be seen. Bleaching of affected teeth gives cosmetic relief.

Mould is a cavity into which molten metal is cast.

Mouth breathing is an oral habit where mouth has been attributed as a possible etiologic factor for malocclusion. The mode of respiration influences the positive of the jaw, the tongue and to a lesser extent the head. Mouth breathing can result in altered jaw and tongue posture, which could alter the oro-facial equilibrium thereby leading to malocclusion. It can be obstructive, habitual or anatomic in nature. Classified into a. Obstructive, b. Habitual, c. Anatomic.

Mouth should be applied only to the external opening which is also called the oral cavity.

Mouth guard is a removable appliance used to protect teeth from injury during sports.

Mouth rinse reduces the number of intraoral microbes by as much as 50 percent. There is an element of mechanical removal and reduction due to antiseptic too. Chlorhexidine is commonly used.

Mucin is a secretion of mucous cell a polysaccharide protein which when combined with water forms a lubricating solution.

Mucocele is a clinical term used to describe swelling caused

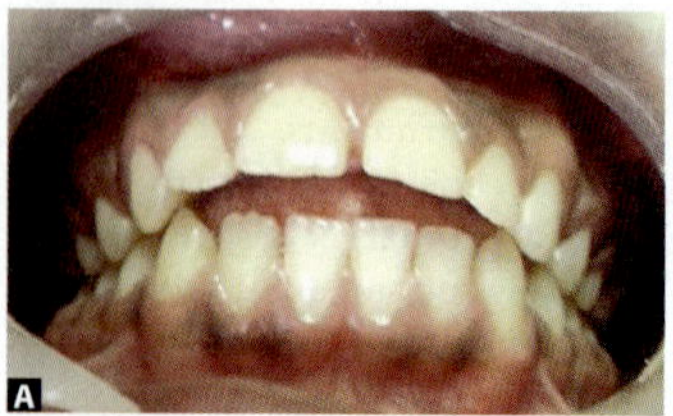

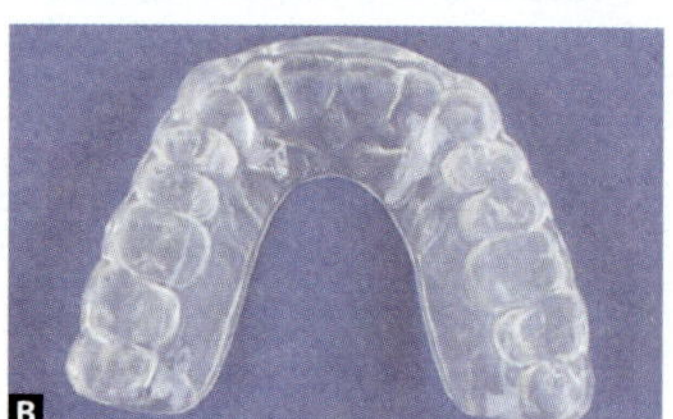

Figs A and B: *(A) Mouth breathing and tongue thrust; (B) Mouth guard*

by pooling of saliva at the site of damage or obstruction. It is generally of traumatic origin. It is of two types: (i) extravasation of mucocele or (ii) retention mucocele. It generally occurs on lower lip palate, cheek and tongue. Lesions may be fairly deep in tissue. Superficial lesion is a raised circumscribed vesicle Mucous extravasation type is common mucocele and is caused by laceration. Mucous retention type is due to obstruction resulting in cyst formation. Mucoceles show flattened epithelial lining. Treatment includes excision.

Mucocutaneous lymph node syndrome is a self-limiting febrile illness characterized by a systemic illness and has mucosal and cutaneous manifestation. Etiology is not known. *Clinical Features* include fever for 5-7 days, bilateral conjunctivitis, and peripheral edema. Sore-throat, headache, malaise and rash. Acute non-purulent swelling of cervical lymph nodes of 1.5 cms. Majority of cases are self-limit oral mucosal finding include dry fissured lips.

Mucoepidermoid tumor is an unusual type of malignant salivary gland neoplasm with varying degree of aggressiveness. Tumor generally involves parotid gland. *Clinical Features:* It is similar to pleomorphic adenoma, is a slow-growing, painless swelling, it has cystic feeling, X-ray will show unilocular or multilocular radiolucent areas in jaw, parotid tumor shows relatively, focal nodular swelling, swelling is mobile, facial nerve paralysis may develop, low-grade tumor shows fluctuation, but high-grade tumors are fixed to the adjacent areas, in a few cases tumor may be fast-growing with ulceration, hemorrhage and paresthesia.

Mucogingival surgery is the term given to describe the surgical procedures that were performed for the correction of relationship between the gingiva and oral mucous membrane with the reference to specific problems associated with attached gingiva, shallow vestibules and frenum involving marginal gingiva.

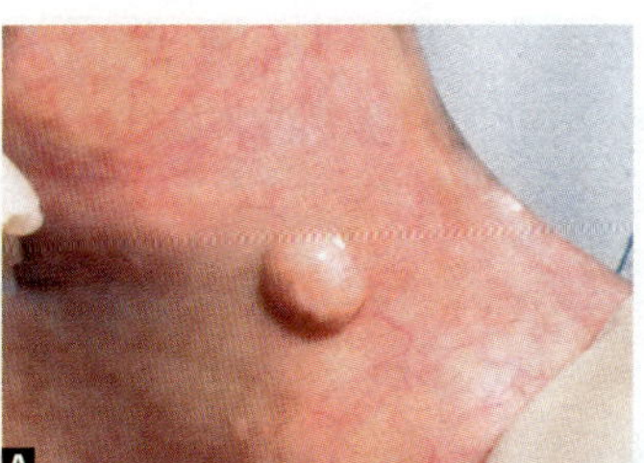

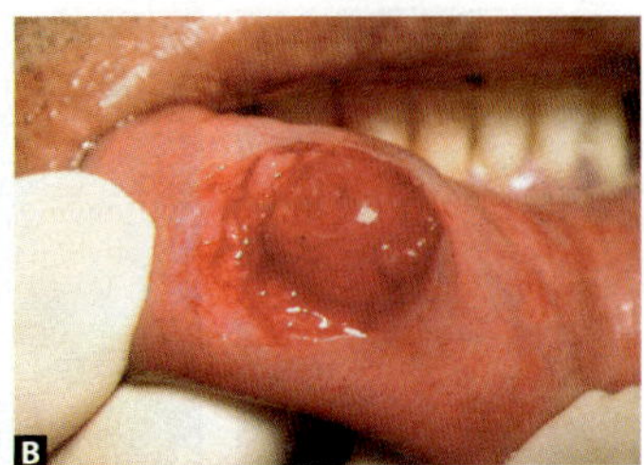

Figs A and B.: *Mucocele of buccal mucosa and labia mucosa*

Mucomycosis is caused by an infection with a saprophytic fungus. Fungus is generally non-pathogenic. It occurs normally in soil or as a mould on decaying food. There is development of ulcerative lesions. Denudation of underlying bones may develop. Negative cultures don't rule out the disease. Microscopically necrosis may be seen. Fungus invades arteries resulting in thrombosis and ischemia. Fungus may spread from oral and nasal area to brain causing death. In oral cavity, it results in ulceration of palate resulting necrosis. Ulcers may develop on gingiva, lip and alveolar ridge. Treatment includes surgical debridement of an infected area with Amphotericin-B for 3 months.

Mucoperiosteal flap *see* full thickness flap.

Mucoperiosteum is the soft oral tissue covering the bone that consists of mucosa and the periosteum.

Mucosa is the thin, outer pink or red membrane lining the inside of the oral cavity.

Mucositis is the direct cytotoxic action of chemotherapeutic agents on the oral mucosa resulting in atrophy or thinning of oral mucosa, erythema and ulceration.

Mucous membrane pemphigoid is an autoimmune disease affecting eye, skin and oral mucosa. Symptoms include painful, blood filled blisters which rupture to form ulcer. Rupture bullae is having well-defined margins. Floor is having an inflamed base.

Mulberry molars are suggestive of congenital syphilis. Buccal and lingual surfaces are normal but occlusal surfaces look like mulberry.

Müller burs are long shaft, round carbide tipped burs which are used in low speed handpiece. Their long shaft increases visibility of cutting tip. They are used for locating calcified canals because their long shaft is useful for working deep in the radicular portion. But since they are made up of carbide, they do not tolerate sterilization cycles and become dull quickly.

Multilocular cyst is the most frequently encountered entity in jaws.

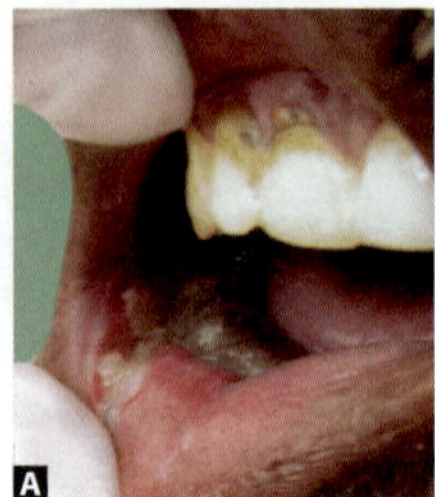

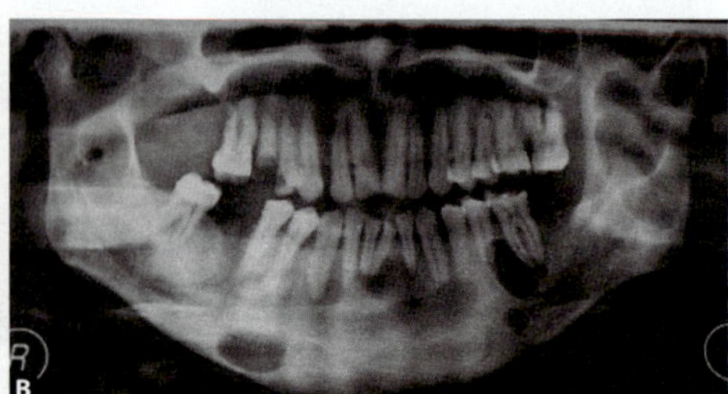

Figs A and B: *(A) Mucositis; (B) Multiple odontogenic keratocysts*

It is always of soap bubble type. It is a true cyst of jaws. Small cyst is usually asymptomatic; it increases slowly and may cause displacement of teeth. Root can be resorbed. If the overlying bone becomes thin, it may produce crackling sound. Later covering plate may be destroyed. It may contain thin, straw-colored fluid.

Multilocular lesion is the one which extends beyond the confines of one distinct area and is defined as many lobes. Odontogenic keratocyst is an example of multiocular lesion.

Multilocular radiolucencies are produced by multiple adjacent frequently coalescing and overlapping compartments in bone. Mostly these occur in maxilla. The term soap bubble, honeycombs and tennis racket are frequently used.

Multiple endocrine neoplasias are also known as MEN syndrome. It is inherited as an autosomal dominant. The lesion involves certain endocrine glands. They produce bumpy lips. Anterior 1/3rd of tongue is involved. These appear as tortuous masses of nerve fibers.

Multiple fractures refer to the fractures occurring at various sites resulting from single injury. The most common one is caused by the fall on the midpoint of chin resulting in fractures of symphysis and both the condyles.

Multiple myeloma is a malignant condition. There is an uncontrolled proliferation and disordered function of cells called plasma cells in bone marrow. Abnormal plasma cell expansion causes pain and destruction in bone. It may cause numbness and paresis when spine is involved. Multiple myeloma develops from bone marrow resembling to plasma cell. IL-6 is the major myeloma growth and C-reactive protein is a peripheral marker of IL-6. It develops in

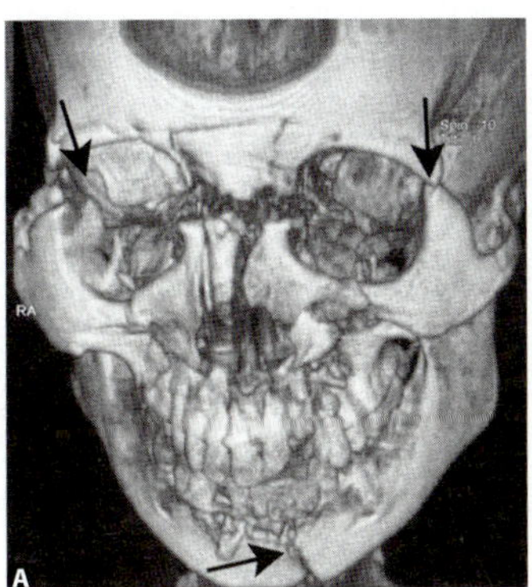

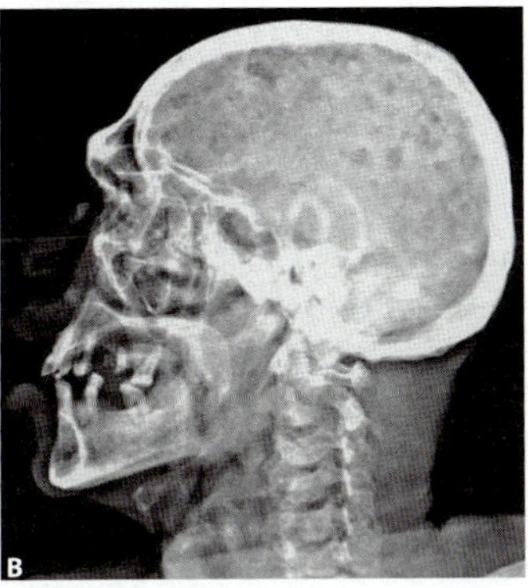

Figs A and B: *(A) Multiple fracture (panfacial); (B) Multiple myeloma of skull showing multiple punched out areas*

elderly age group. Pain is the early feature. Back pain, anemia and bone pain are common. Any movement increases pain. Pain is due to osteoclastic lesion. Pain increases with movement. Numbness of chin and lips may develop. Jaw swelling and pain may be confused with toothache. Jaw swelling crackling or pathological fracture may develop. Extraction of teeth results in severe hemorrhage. Collapse of vertebra or of a long bone is due to lytic lesion. Pathological fracture is common. Bence Jones proteinuria develops along with unexplained weakness, fatigue, osteoporosis ramus angle and molar region of mandible are the commonest sites involved. X-ray will show multiple sharply punched out areas. Size may vary from a few mm to 1 cm. There is no peripheral bone reaction. Chemotherapy is the treatment of choice.

Multiple organ failure is the condition in which two or more organ system gradually ceases to function.

Mumps is an acute contagious viral infection. There is unilateral or bilateral swelling of parotid glands. Submaxillary and sublingual glands may be involved. Incubation period is 2-3 weeks. Disease is preceded by chill, fever, pain below ear. Later on swelling becomes firm and rubbery salivary glands, complications include, orchitis, pancreatitis and otitis. Orchitis is unilateral; serum amylase level is increased.

Mumps-vaccine is highly effective live attenuated vaccine is available for prevention of mumps. Single dose 0.5 mL IM produces detectable antibodies in 95% vaccines. It should not be given to pregnant women or in severely-ill patient.

Munchausen syndrome by proxy is a form of child abuse in which a parent induces real or apparent symptoms of a disease in a child to meet his or her own emotional needs through the treatment process of the child. The disease is most commonly seen in mother to get desired attention in the society. It is also known as fabricated illness syndrome, pediatric symptom falsification, illness induction syndrome or factitious disorder by proxy. Munchausen syndrome is clearly a serious and life-threatening condition. Even though fathers have also been identified but majority of the abusers belong to the mother's category. Many consider it to be a psychiatric disorder by DSM-V, provisional criteria places it under factitious disorders by proxy, while some have described it as medical abuse.

Muscle relaxants are neuromuscular blocking agents producing their effect by interfering with the excitatory action of acetylcholine at the motor-end plate. These provide paralysis of voluntary muscles during clinical anesthesia. These are of two types: (i) non depolarizing neuromuscular blocking agents;

and (ii) Depolarizing neuromuscular blocking agents.

Muscle relaxation-Infra-red: Muscles relax when these are warm. Further relief of pain also relaxes muscles. After irradiation joint movement range also increases. Thus it helps in arthritis.

Muscle splinting pain is defined as rigidity of muscles occurring as a means of avoiding pain caused by movement of a part. Muscle splinting is involuntary contraction that tends to immobilize the part. At rest a splinted muscle relaxes. Splinting of masticatory muscles occurs as a protective mechanism to limit excessive functioning of TM joint.

Muscle strain causes mild to severe pain with movement. The reduction of movement may cause muscle weakness and atrophy.

Muscular contact position (MCP) refers to that position of mandible where the mandible is lifted into contact from resting position.

Musculoskeletal pain is non-inflammatory in origin. It results from muscle spasm, it is reactive, and it is protective, e.g. muscles splinting in a temporary protective mechanism resulting in muscle pain and weakness. Such splinting serves to rest the muscle until the symptoms have disappeared.

Mutism is a total inability to speak. It may be seen without any organic disease of CNS. It may be psychogenic in origin.

Mycobacterium leprae: Humans are the only hosts which reside in skin and nerves. Prolonged contact is required for transmission. It is aerobic, acid fast bacilli. These are not alcohol fast and no known toxins. Leprosy bacillus causes slow progressive chronic disease affecting skin and nerves.

Mycobacterium tuberculosis is responsible for TB and is found in infected humans mainly in lungs. Spread is by droplet. It is acid and alcohol fast, slender, beaded bacilli. Ziehl Neelsen stain is required to see them.

Myeloblast is round and large, about 14 to 18 mm in diameter. Nucleus is very fine of the cell. Nuclear chromatin is very fine and two to five nucleoli are present. Cytoplasm is basophilic.

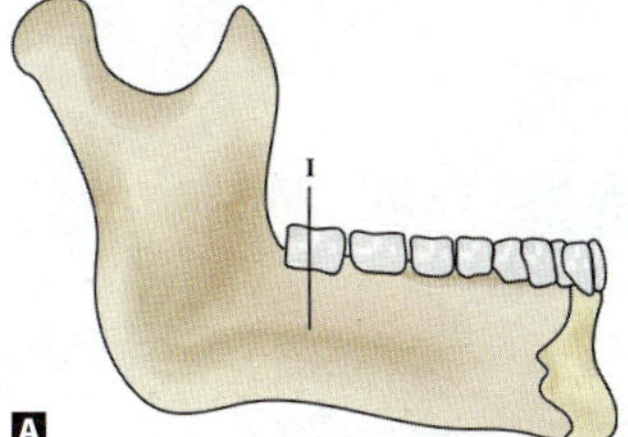

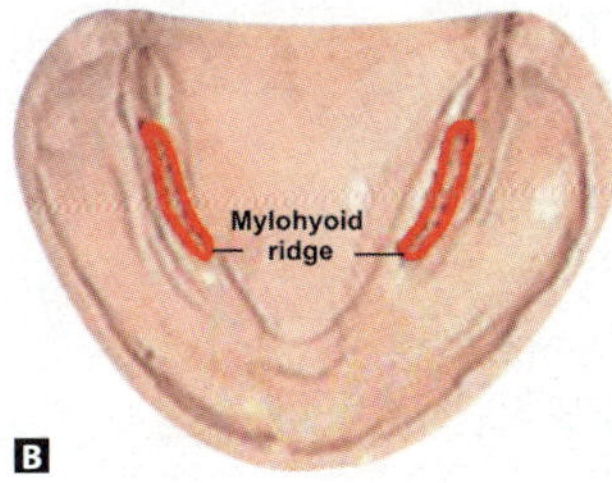

Figs A and B: *Mylohyoid ridge*

Myeloid is pertaining to bone marrow.

Mylohyoid ridge is a linear prominence of bone located on internal surface of mandible appears radiopaque.

Myocardial infarction is an area of ischemic necrosis of myocardium caused by insufficient blood supply due to coronary artery occlusion.

Myoclonic seizures are sudden brief bilaterally synchronous muscle contraction of face and trunk without loss of unconsciousness. They are shock-like muscle contractions that usually involved both sides of the body at the same time. They can occur in some healthy people as they fall asleep at night. This is called benign nocturnal myoclonus or sleep jerks. This form of a seizure is considered a nonepileptic type of seizure in spite of the fact similar movements occur in myoclonic seizures. Epileptic myoclonic seizures have a short duration and typically have no postictal phase. They can occur in both primary and secondary generalized epilepsies.

Myoclonus is a brief, involuntary random muscle contraction occurring either with rest in response to sensory stimuli. It may involve as single motor unit or group of units. Sudden brief lapses of contractions known as negative myoclonus. Myoclonic jerks may be focal, segmental or generalized. Etiologically myoclonus can be classified as physiologic myoclonus, essential myoclonus, epileptic myoclonus and symptomatic myoclonus.

Myoepithelioma is an uncommon salivary gland tumor. Parotid gland is mostly involved and palate is the common intraoral site to be involving tumor has to be removed surgically.

Myofacial pain comes from muscles and surrounding soft tissues. Injury or overuse results in painful muscle spasm may last long after an injury or muscle overuse. Muscles become short and tender. Pressing trigger points caused increased pain. Physical therapy and stretching exercises help.

Myofunctional appliance is defined as loose-fitting or passive appliance, which harneses natural forces of

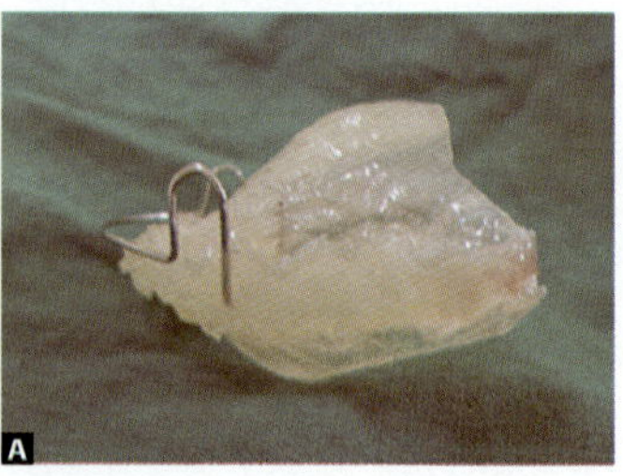
A

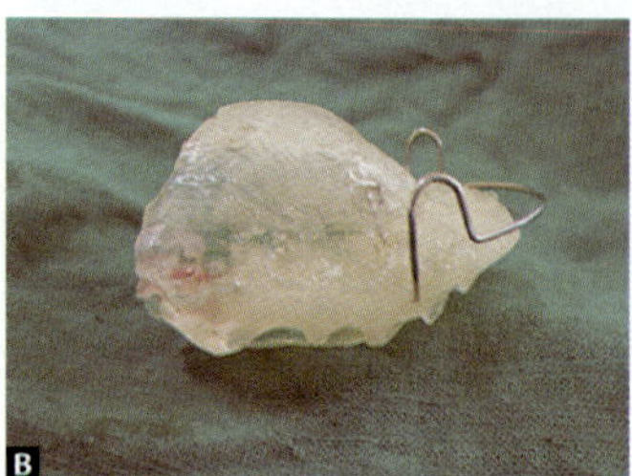
B

Figs A and B.: *Myofunctional appliance*

the oro-facial musculature that are transmitted to the teeth and alveolar medium through the medium of the appliance.

Myopathy is any disease or abnormal condition of muscle tissue.

Myosin is an actin accessory protein that functions as a molecular motor. There are several isoforms of myosin, and muscle and non-muscle forms have slightly divergent amino acid sequences. It is composed of two heavy chains and four light chains.

Myositis ossificans is the formation of bone within a muscle which is contused.

Myotonic appliances are functional appliances that depend on the muscle mass for their action.

Myxoma resembles primitive mesenchyme and is true neoplasm. Oral submucosal area, salivary gland and jaw bones are commonly affected. *Clinical features:* It is a slow growing invasive tumor that sometime reaches large dimensions. Jaw is distended. X-ray well shows a soap bubble appearance. Being locally aggressive radical surgery is advised.

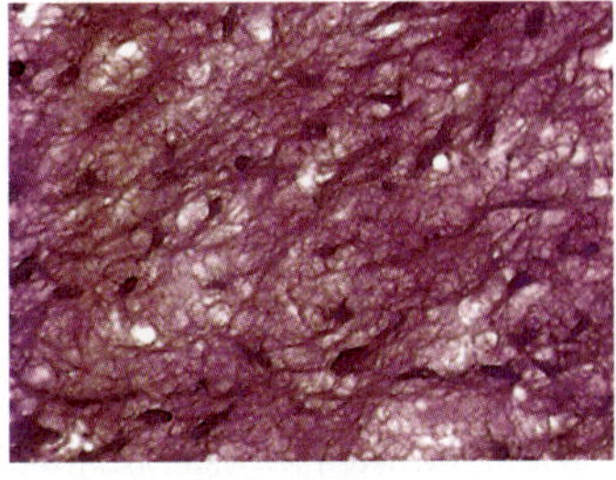

Fig.: *Myxoma*

M

N is the Nasion, the most anterior point of the nasofrontal suture in the median plane.

N′-soft tissue nasion is the point of greatest concavity in the midline between the forehead and the nose.

Nails are thin plates of stratified squamous epithelial cells. It contains a very hard form of keratin. These are found on the distal ends of fingers and toes. It has free edge, nail body and nail root. Extent of nail growth is represented by half-moon shaped lunula.

Nalgonda technique (named after the village in India where the method is pioneered) is a defluoridation technique based on chemical reaction where raw water is mixed with adequate lime and alum. The amount of lime depends upon the alkanity of the raw water if the raw water has adequate alkalinity the lime addition is not required. Alum solution is added after the addition of lime stirred gently for 10 minutes and the flocs formed are allowed to settle. This process of floc formation and setting requires one hour.

Nance method is one of the methods of performing serial extraction. This is similar to the tweeds technique and involves the extraction of the deciduous first molar followed by the extraction of the first premolars and the deciduous canine.

Narcolepsy sleep refers to a sleeping disorder. It may occur in inappropriate situations during conversation or meals. There develops a rapid sleep of poor quality. One develops hallucinations and sleep paralysis. Such potients have difficulty in sleeping at night.

Nasal cavity is the air filled space that consists of right and left halves separated by a nasal septum. The cavity opens, anteriorly, on the front of the skull through the anterior nasal aperture; and, posteriorly, on the base of the skull just above the posterior edge of the bony palate.

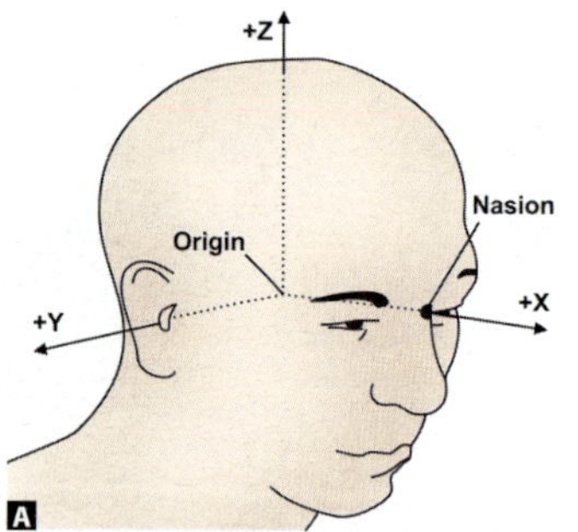

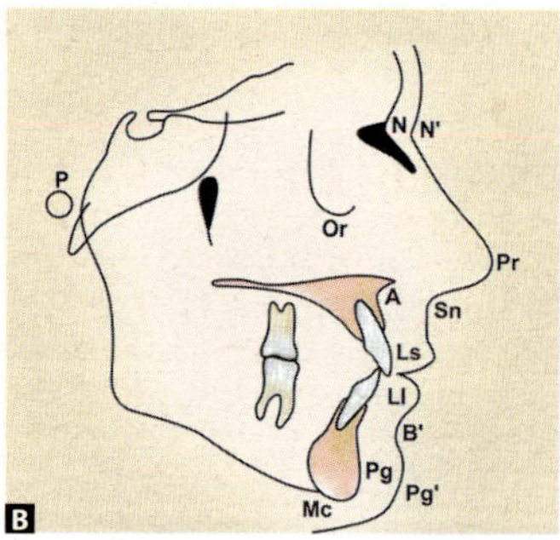

Figs A and B: *Nasion (A) Soft tissue (B) Hard tissue*

Nasal glioma is a tumor-like lesion in nose of children. It presents as a rounded projection in the nose. Microscopically, it is made up mature of glial tissue.

Nasal polyps are the proliferative masses from the mucous membrane of the nose. These may be unilateral or bilateral and can be divided into nonallergic and allergic. Nonallergic polyps consist of an edematous fibrous stroma. Variable infiltrate of lymphocytes, plasma cells and neutrophils are seen.

Nasal reflex is the stimulation of the face or nasal cavity with water or local irritants, produces apnea (stops breathing) in neonates—this leads to bradycardia and lowering of the cardiac output.

Nasofacial angle is formed by the intersection of a line drawn from glabella to soft-tissue pogonion with a line drawn along the axis of the radix of the nose. Average values are 30 to 35°.

Nasolabial angle is the angle formed by the intersection of a columella tangent and an upper lip tangent. Normal ranges from 90–110°.

Nasolacrimal duct is a tube about 18 mm long and is considered as a downward continuation of the lacrimal sac. It is in close approximation to the lateral wall of the nasal cavity. The wall of the nasolacrimal duct is made up of bone lined by mucous membrane.

Nasomental angle is constructed by a line drawn along the axis of the radix and a line drawn from the tip of the nose to soft tissue pogonion (e-line). Normal=120–132.

Nasopalatine nerve block is used for anesthetizing anterior portion of the hard palate (soft and hard tissues), extending from one side premolar to other side of first premolar.

Nasopalatine nerve is a branch of maxillary nerve that leaves the pterygopalatine ganglion and passes forward and downward entering the oral cavity through incisive foramen. It provides sensory innervations to the bone and lingual soft tissues in the premaxilla.

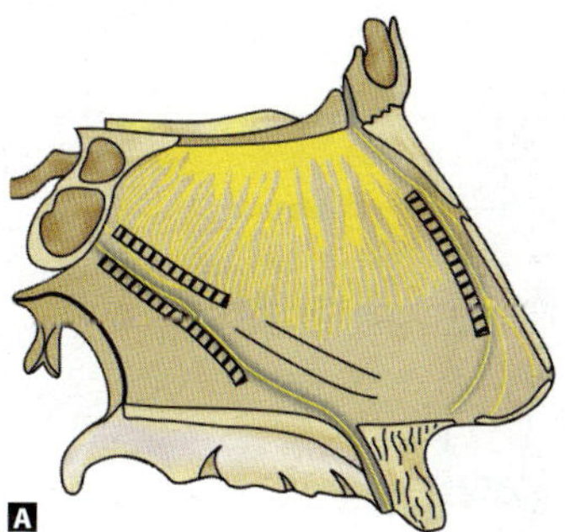

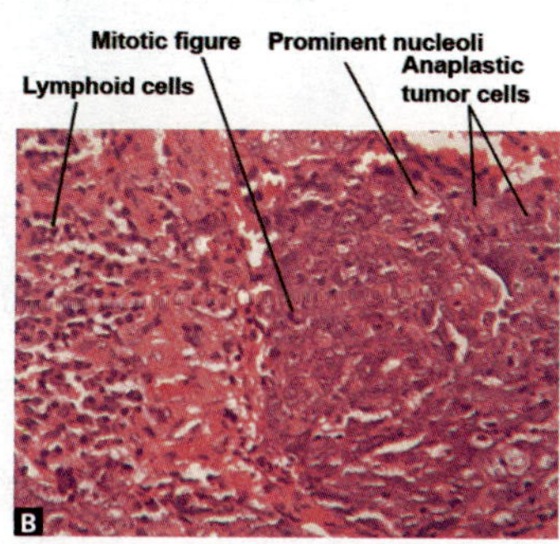

Figs A and B: *(A) Nasopalatine nerve; (B) Nasopharyngeal carcinoma*

Nasopharyngeal carcinoma refers to the tumor originating from nasopharynx. Symptoms include pain, restricted movements of jaw, ear complaints. There may be nasal stiffness, nosebleed and neck mass. Treatment requires radiation + chemotherapy.

Nasopharynx is the area lies behind the nasal cavities and in the widest part of pharynx. During swallowing the nasopharynx is closed below by the soft palate and at other times it is of free communication with oropharynx. Ostia of auditory tubes are in lateral walls.

Natural immunity *see* Innate.

Natural markers are the one that are left behind as a persistence of certain developmental features of bone, which are used as natural markers. Trabeculae, nutrient canals and line of arrested growth can be used for reference to study deposition, resorption and remodeling.

ND: YAG lasers as a solid active medium, a crystal of yttrium-aluminium-garnet doped with neodymium. Fiberoptically delivered in a free running pulsed mode. Most often in contact with the tissue. First laser designed exclusively for dentistry. Emission wavelength is 1064 nm. Highly absorbed by pigmented tissue and is about 10,000 times more absorbed by water than an argon laser. Common clinical applications are for cutting and coagulation of dental soft tissues with good hemostatic capability.

Neck tongue syndrome is characterized by unilateral upper nuchal or occipital pain with or without numbness in these areas. There is simultaneous numbness of tongue on the same side.

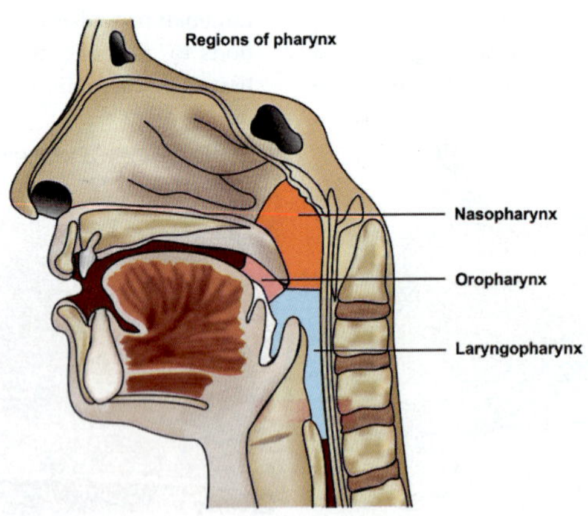

Fig.: *Nasopharynx*

Necrosis means the tissue death within the living.

Necrotic pulp refers to death of pulpal tissue. There are no true symptoms of complete pulp necrosis for the simple reason that pulp is destroyed along with its sensory nerves. Many cases of pulp necrosis are discovered because of discoloration of crown. This applies primarily to anterior teeth. The radiography may be helpful if a periapical lesion exists for its presence and usually indicates associated pulp death. On radiograph necrotic pulp may exhibit only slight periapical change. The tooth with a necrotic pulp may also be slightly painful to percussion.

Necrotic tissue is a nonliving tissue.

Necrotizing sialometaplasia is a benign inflammatory reaction of salivary gland tissue with unknown etiology. Acinar necrosis is fairly typical of coagulation. It develops due to infarction of tissues. It develops after 4th decade of life. Lesion generally presents as an ulcer. Most cases occur in palate. It is a painful lesion; mucus-secreting gland produces ulceration with rolled borders. Ulcer measures 2-3 cm in diameter. At the base, a few grey granular lobules are present. Some patients may complain of numbness or a burning type pain in that area. Biopsy will not show any sign of malignancy. So debridement will serve the purpose and the lesions will heal automatically within 1-2 months. There are no chances of recurrence.

Necrotizing ulcerative gingivitis (NUG) is an inflammatory destructive disease of the gingiva. NUG mostly occurs as an acute condition but mostly undergoes a diminution in severity, leading to a subacute stage. It is generally of sudden onset, clinically it appears as punched out lesions, with a crater-like depressions involving the papillary gingiva which subsequently involves the marginal gingiva as well, and spontaneous bleeding on slightest provocation is also noted. The lesion is extremely sensitive and patient may complain of pain which gets intensified on eating spicy food. Patient also complains of metallic foul taste and oral malodor.

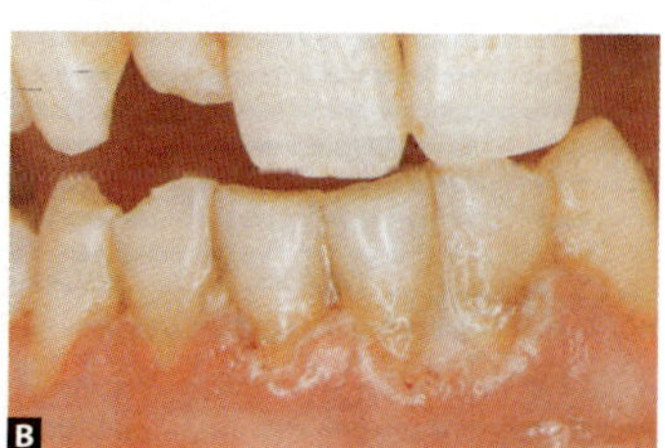

Figs A and B: *(A) Necrotizing sialometaplasia; (B) Necrotizing ulcerative gingivitis*

Necrotizing ulcerative periodontitis (NUP) is considered to be an extension of necrotizing ulcerative gingivitis into the periodontal structures leading to attachment and bone loss. The clinical pictures of NUP includes necrosis and ulceration of interdental papilla, gingiva appears erythematous, presence of oral malodor in addition to fever, malaise and lymphadenopathy. Stress, smoking and poor dietary nutrition are considered to be the main causative factors.

Needle holders are instruments which are beneficial during the suturing the flap or the tissue at the desired position.

Negative reinforcement involves removal of unpleasant stimulus following a response, e.g., if the parent gives in to the temper-tantrums thrown by the child, he reinforces this behavior.

Neglect is a failure of the parent or caretaker to provide the child's basic needs such as food, clothing, shelter and medical attention to the extent that the child's health and development is likely to be significantly harmed.

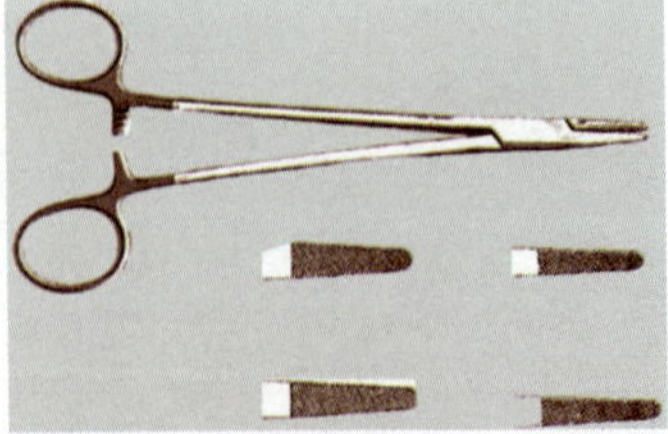

Fig.: *Needle holder*

Neonatal palatal cyst appears as small, white, raised nodules. Size may go up to 2 to 3 mm in diameter. These are true cysts lined by stratified squamous epithelium. They heal automatically and don't require treatment.

Neonatal seizures are seizures that occur in a body less than first 4 months of life due to abnormal electrical discharge. These may be focal or multifocal, clonic or focal tonic or generalized myoclonic.

Neoplasia is an abnormal mass of tissue, the growth of which exceeds and is uncoordinated with that of normal tissues. Neoplasia means the process of new growth. Neoplasms which progress and result in death of organisms are termed cancerous. Not all neoplasms are malignant. Those with a favorable clinical course and complete recovery are termed benign neoplasm.

Neoplasm is a proliferation of cells interfering with surrounding tissues; refers to cancer. The new growth comprised of abnormal collection of cells, the growth of which exceeds and is irregular. A malignant tumor arising from epithelial tissue is known as carcinoma, from gland is known as adenoma, from cartilaginous tumor, it is called as 'chondroma'.

Nephritic syndrome is a disorder of glomeruli and arises due to acute glomerular inflammation (glomerulonephritis, GN) and is characterized by sudden onset (days to weeks) of oliguria, edema, hypertension, hematuria, subnephrotic proteinuria (<3 g/day) and worsening renal function.

Nephroblastoma is an embryonic tumor derived from primitive renal epithelial and mesenchymal components. Abdominal mass is the commonest complaint with hematuria and hypertension. Tumor is single, large circumscribed mass firm usually solid. Tumor may become huge, i.e. 500-2500 grams.

Nerve block is a procedure done to block the nerve conduction by administration of local anesthetic agent. It is a one where several teeth in one quadrant or where local infiltration is not workable/useful. Nerve block is done in soft tissue before it enters the jaw to reach the teeth. Pain sensations from every part supplied by nerve are blocked. Inferior dental block is commonly done.

Nerve impulse is a signal that carries information along the nerves.

Nerve neuron is a single nerve cell while nerve contains many fibers of many neurons. Nerve contains many fibers bundled together with blood vessels and wrapped in connective tissue. Nerves are located outside the CNS.

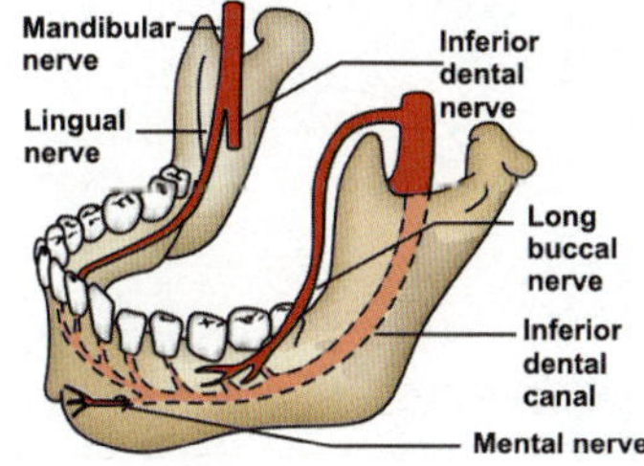

Fig.: *Nerves supply of mandibular teeth*

Nerve root compression also known as trapped nerve is that nerves which transmit pain impulses are compressed in spinal cord/roots. One feels unpleasant, burning pain often accompanied by painful sensations. Some features are due to direct nerve irritation; others are due to ischemia. Pain due to compression of peripheral nerve is referred to skin from which it receives sensory fibers. Root pain radiates throughout the dermatome of root concerned.

Nerve supply of lower teeth: Branches of mandibular nerve supply lower teeth.

Neuralgia trigeminal is a condition where it means pain associated with trigeminal nerve. Pain generally affects one side of face around eye, over cheek or into jaw and teeth. Pain is excruciating and is triggered by touching a specific area of the face, talk or chew the food. The pain is usually of short duration and lasts for few seconds. It is also known as 'Tic Douloureux' which has literal meaning of painful jerking. Usually characterized by paroxysmal, unilateral, sharp, lancinating pain typically confined to one or more branches of 5th cranial nerve. Even slight stimulation of "Trigger points' may elicit sharp, shooting pain.

Neurilemomma is benign, encapsulated tumor of nerve sheet. Schwann cells are the site of origin. It is a slowly growing lesion of long duration.

N

The lesion is painless. In mandible it is located as central lesion. There may be destruction of bone and extension of cortex. It requires surgical excision.

Neuritis literally means inflammation of nerve. It is usually observed as heterotopic pain in the peripheral distribution of the affected nerve. It may be caused by traumatic, bacterial and viral infection. In neuritis, the inflammatory process elevates the threshold for pricking pain but lowers it for burning pain. The characteristics of pain in neuritis are pain has a characteristic burning quality along with easily localization of the site. It may be associated with other sensory effects such as hyperesthesia, hypoesthesia, paresthesia, dysesthesia and anesthesia. Pain is nonpulsatile in nature. Pain may vary in intensity.

Neurofibroma arises from perineural fibroblasts. It is a dominant hereditary condition with overgrowth of nerve sheath. *Clinical Features:* These present as small and asymptomatic. These are submucosal with multilobulated surface. These are painless. On skin these are soft and firm freely mobile nodules. Nodular lesions vary in size and number varies widely. Radiographically is well-demarcated; unilocular or multi-locular radiolucent areas are seen.

Neurofibromatosis is a genetic disorder of the nervous system that disturbs the cell growth causing tumors. It has a hereditary impact and occurs in 2 forms, i.e. in one form numerous sessile or pedunculated, elevated nodules of variable size are scattered whereas in second, form deeper, more diffuse lesions of greater proportions are developed known as 'elephantiasis neuromatosa'. Transformation into malignancy is known. On buccal mucosa discrete, non-nucleated nodules of mucus colour are noted. Tongue may be enlarged. There is no satisfactory treatment.

Neurofilaments are those filaments that are found in neuron axons

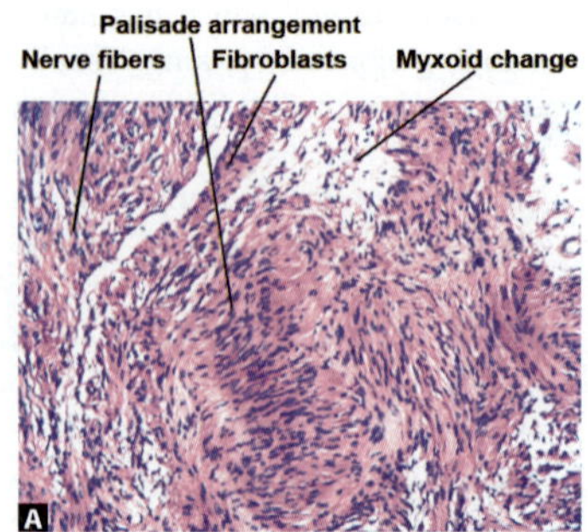

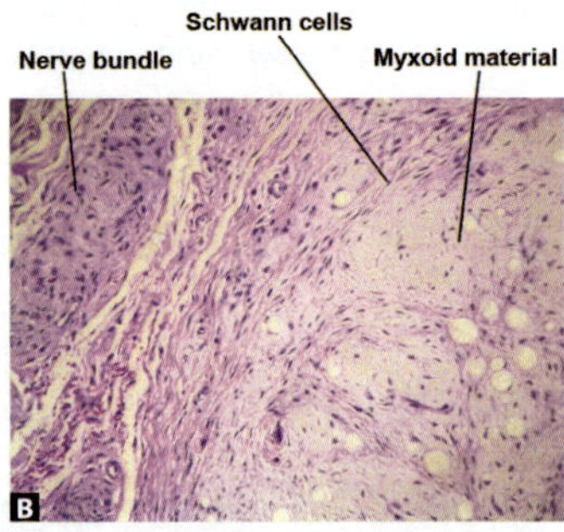

Figs A and B: *(A) Neurilemomma; (B) Myxoid changes in neurofibroma*

that account for the strength and rigidity of the axon.

Neurogenic pain may indicate a disease process affecting a particular nerve fibre.

Neurogenic sarcoma is a malignant tumor of Schwann cells. It has a poor prognosis. *Clinical Features:* These are rapidly growing and painful. It is an exophytic mass. Lips may be anesthetized. Expansion of mandible occurs. Lesions don't move and are fixed to underlying tissue. Nuclei are often pleomorphic and hyperchromatic. Neoplastic cells spread along the affected nerve.

Neuron is a nerve cell.

Neuropathic ulcer refers to ulcers due to underlying neuropathy, e.g. diabetic foot ulcer is classical ulcer. Ulcer may be single or multiple. It is generally on pressure point. Edge is punched out, pale and hard. There is purulent offensive discharge. Base is nontender.

Neuropathy is any abnormal condition characterization by inflammation and degeneration and peripheral nerves.

Neurotoxin: Tetanus, diphtheria and botulinium toxins are all neurotoxins and act via neuronal pathways.

Neurotransmitters are chemicals by which neurons communicate.

Neutral atom is an atom that has an equal number of protons and electrons.

Neutral crest cells are the one which arise from ectoderm along the lateral margins of neural plate and migrate extensively to form dental papilla.

Neutrophils are the predominant leukocyte in the blood accounting for about two-third of all the blood leukocytes. As neutrophils do not need to differentiate, they are best suited for rapid responses. Neutrophils have a size of 10 um diameter.

Nevoid basal cell carcinoma syndrome also known as Goltz syndrome and basal cell nerves syndrome is a hereditary condition characterized by jaw cysts, facies, calcification, bifid ribs and skin lesions. Multiple pink to brown papules appear on face. In 50% cases pitting of soles and palms is seen.

New attachment is the process of embedding the new periodontal ligament fibers into newly formed cementum and attachment of

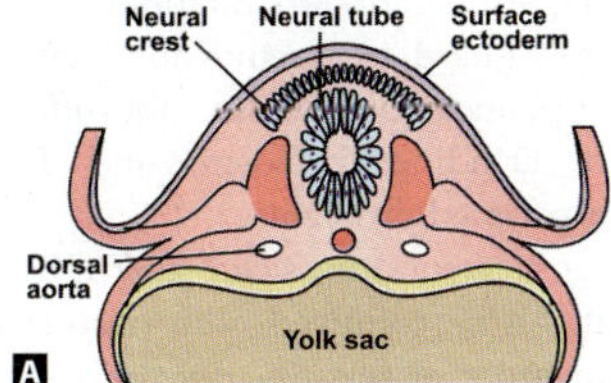

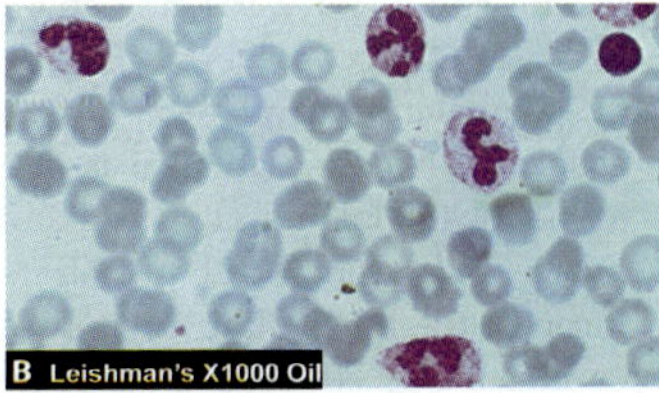

Figs A and B: *(A) Neural crest cells; (B) Neutrophils*

gingival epithelium to the tooth surface which was denuded by the disease.

Newton is a force required to give a mass of one kilogram in acceleration of one meter per second.

Niacin also known as nicotinic acid or vit B_3 can be formed from essential amino acid tryptophan. In human 1 mg niacin is formed from 60 mg dietary tryptophan. In body, it is converted into nicotinamide which is a component of coenzyme needed for carbohydrate metabolism. Liver, ground nut, pulses and fish are good source of it. Milling may remove most of it. Recommended daily allowance is 6.6 mg/1000 calories.

Nickel-titanium wires are the orthodontic wires that has weight percentage of 55% nickel and 45% titanium. Nickel titanium alloys with shape memory behavior activated at body temperature have been introduced. It has excellent spring back in bending particularly for super elastic and shape memory alloys. Super elastic alloys can be heat treated by clinician.

Nicotine poisoning is easily absorbed from the mucous membrane of the mouth when smoke is held in oral cavity for 2 seconds about 70% of it is absorbed. During deep inhalation about 90% of it is absorbed. Nicotine as such is one of the most fatal and rapidly acting poisons. It can even penetrate through the intact skin. Fatal dose of nicotine is 60 mg for an adult but even 4 mg may cause alarming symptoms in nonhabitual person. At the rate of one packet a day of 20 cigarette smoker inhales 100 mg of nicotine a week which, in a single dose, will kill the person as quickly as bullet.

NIDR monograph: The national caries program of the national institute of dental research has published a monograph, preventing tooth decay, to assist dentists, dental hygienists, public health administrators, school officials, and teachers implementing self-applied fluoride programs in schools. The monograph was prepared by the staff at the national caries program of the NIDR and describes in detail the methodology, strategy, and estimated cost of materials, addresses of suppliers, sample order forms, and checklists to ensure the success of such a program. It is highly recommended for public health officials and school personnel.

Nidus refers to the point of origin.

Night blindness refers to inability o see at night or in poor light. It has also known as nyctalopia. Retinol is essential component of pigment rhodopsin (visual purple) on which vision in dim light depends. Hence lack of retinol may result in impairment of dark adaptation.

Night guard is a removable acrylic appliance to minimize the effects of grinding (bruxism) and TMJ associated problems.

Night terrors is sleep disruption. It can be confused with nocturnal disorder of seizures due to frontal lobe epilepsy. Night terrors are likely to cause the child to sit up and scream. Involuntary motor components are unusual.

Ni-Ti alloys: (1) Shape memory, (2) Superelasticity, (3) Low modulus of elasticity, (4) Good resiliency, (5) Corrosion resistance, (6) Softer than stainless steel.

Ni-Ti rotary instruments was developed by Buchler 50 years ago. NiTi is also known as the NiTinol (NiTi Navol Ordinance Laboratory in US). In endodontics commonly used NiTi alloys are called 55 NiTinol (55% weight Ni and 45% Ti) and 60 NiTinol (60% weight of Ni, 40% Ti). First use of NiTi in endodontics was reported in 1988, by Walia et al when a 15 no NiTi file was made from orthodontic wire and it showed superior flexibility and resistance to torsional fracture. This suggested the use of NiTi files in curved canals. Disadvantages of NiTi files: Poor cutting efficiency. NiTi files do not show signs of fatigue before they fracture. Poor resistance to fracture as compared to stainless steel.

Nitrogen balance refers to a balance between the input and output of nitrogen. Negative protein balance exists when output is greater than input as in fever, starvation, etc. During growth pregnancy, protein need increases so is defined as a positive protein balance.

Nitrous oxide is a colorless, slightly sweetish gas with no odor. It is heavier than air. It has low solubility in blood and does not combine with hemoglobin. It has low anesthetic potency which limits its use as a sole anesthetic agents. Current limit recommended for all brief anesthetic procedures is 65% N_2O/35% O_2 at sea level. Its side effect includes mild depression of myocardial contractility. Recovery from nitrous oxide is quick. It does not produce muscle relaxation and it readily crosses the placenta.

Noble metals that are resistant to oxidation include gold, platinum, and palladium.

Nocturia is night time urination.

Nodular goiter is nodular on palpation. If it is present in more than 10% in an area, it indicates that condition is endemic. Iodine deficiency is the main cause.

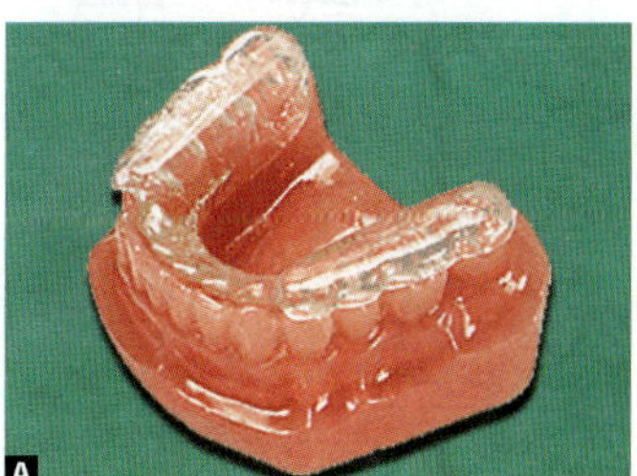

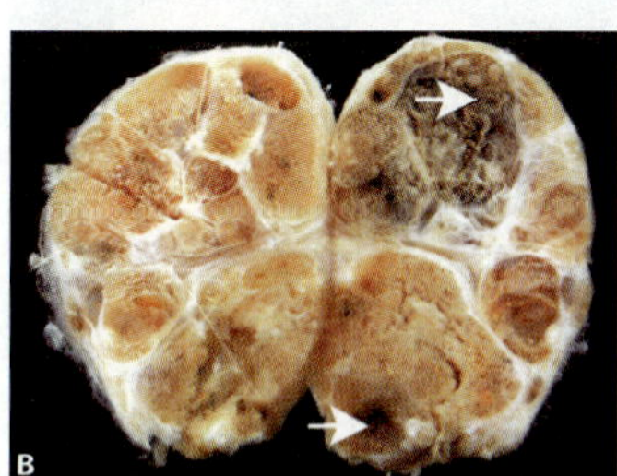

Figs A and B: *(A) Night guard; (B) Nodular goiter*

N

Nodular hyperplasia prostate is an overgrowth of prostatic glandular and fibromuscular elements. Enlarged prostate weighs more than 40 grams. Nodules show slit-like spaces containing milky fluid. Nodular hyperplasia causes elongation, compression and tortuosity of posterior uretra. It may lead to retention of urine and cystitis.

Nogenol is a material that was developed to overcome the irritating quality of eugenol. Base is ZnO with barium sulfate as radiopacifier along with vegetable oil. Set is accelerated by hydrogenated rosin, chlorothymol and salicylic acid.

Noise is an unwanted sound. Noise has been described as wrong sound, in the wrong place at the wrong time. Noise pollution is the cacophony of sounds leading to health hazard.

Noise-induced hearing loss (NIHL) refers to impaired hearing due to damage done by noise typically is centered at 3000, 4000, or 6000 Hz. As noise damage progresses, it starts affecting lower and higher frequencies.

Noma is rapidly spreading gangrene of oral and facial tissue in physically weak person localized to orofacial region. Tissue necrosis progresses after infection with anaerobic bacteria. It starts as a small ulcer of gingival mucosa. It may spread to jaws and cheeks. It starts around fixed bridge or crown. Commencement of gangrene is seen as blackening of skin. Smell is very foul. Mortality rate is higher. Broad spectrum antibiotics help.

Noncompression small plates are the small conventional orthopedic plates which were previously used for fixing mandibular fractures. These appear larger than the recently designed miniplates and offer no other advantage except compression to the fracture due to larger dimensions as when compared to miniplates.

Noncritical instruments are those that don't come into contact with body fluids and have low risk of transmitting infection. These can be put in low level disinfectant detergents

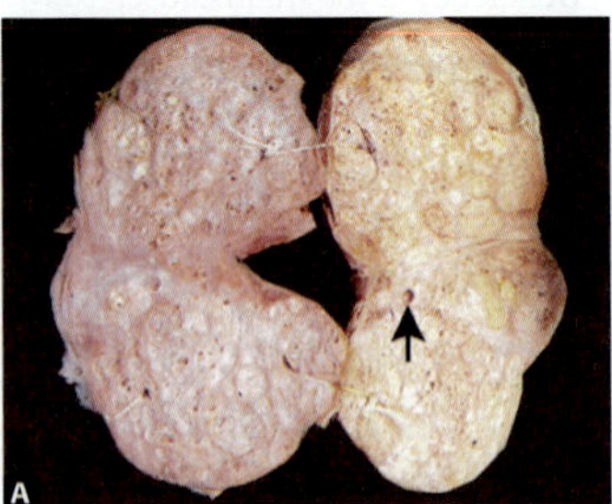

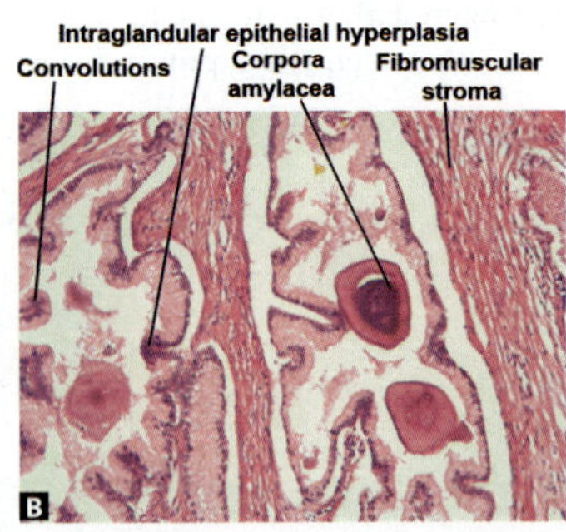

Figs A and B.: *Nodular hyperplasia prostate (A) Macroscopic; (B) Microscopic*

or simple washing will serve. These include jars, cavity liners, etc.

Nondisplaced flaps are the ones, when the flap is returned and sutured in its original position.

Non-experimental research in which there is no manipulation of an independent variable.

Non-Hodgkin's lymphoma is a heterogeneous group of neoplasm that arises from a monoclonal cell of lymphoid origin. These involve lymph nodes and lymphoid organs, extranodal organs and tissues. Patient of any age can be affected. Abdominal and mediastinal lymphadenopathy, fever, night sweats and loss of weight is seen. The cell type may be well-differentiated lymphocyte, poorly differentiated lymphocyte, mixed lymphocyte histiocytic, diffuse Histiocytes or lymphoblastic. Malignant cells may replace the node in a diffuse pattern. Mediastinal node involvement is common and enlargement of liver may develop. Multiple lymph nodes are firm and rubbery. Non-Hodgkin's lymphoma is also noted in AIDS patients. Oral lesion is fast-growing, painful and firm. There may be ulceration and bleeding. Swelling of gingiva and palate are common. In nodular pattern neoplastic cells aggregate so that cluster of cells are seen, while diffuse pattern is seen as monotonous distribution of cells. *Radiological Findings:* Floating teeth in radiolucent area may be seen. There will be diffuse, large, irregular areas of radiolucency with expansion and destruction. Biopsy of lymph glands gives an accurate diagnosis. Aggressive chemotherapy followed by radiotherapy helps.

Non-parametric tests are the statistical tests that don't rest on assumption related to the distribution of populations from which samples are taken.

Non-productive cough is a noisy cough, forceful expulsion of air from the lungs that does not yield sputum or blood coughing is ncessary protective mechanism of clearing airway.

Non-screen film is extra-oral film which does not require the use of screen for exposure.

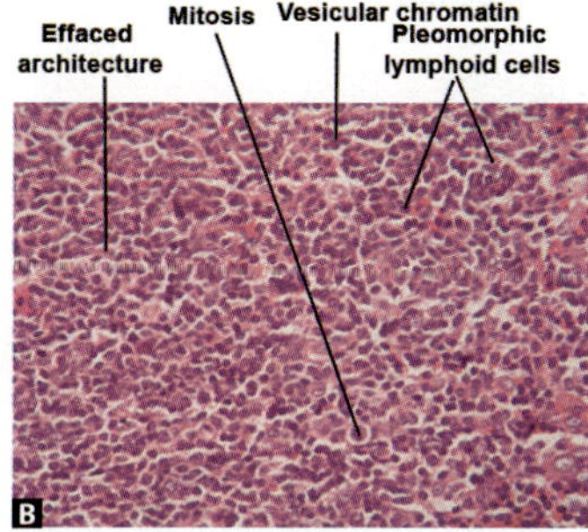

Figs A and B: *Non-Hodgkin's lymphoma of the palate (A) Clinical; (B) Histological*

Non-spastic cerebral palsy characterized by involuntary movement, that can be slow or fast often repetitive planned movement can intensify this effect.

Non-union refers to the fracture that is only not united but will not also unite by itself. Nonunion also includes the condition of fibrous union. It may occur due to infection, inadequate immobilization or unsatisfactory apposition of bone.

Non-vital pulpotomy refers mortal pulpotomy.

Non-compulsive habits they are habits that are easily learned and dropped as the child matures.

Non-pressure habits are ones which do not apply a direct force on the teeth or its supporting structures are termed non-pressure habits, e.g. Mouth breathing.

Non-spastic myofacial pain refers to no muscle spasm and pain is the only complaint. There is no muscular dysfunction. Palpable trigger may elicit acute pain at the trigger site when manipulated and may overshadow the referred pain momentarily.

Non-specific plaque hypothesis (Walter Loesche – 1976) states that periodontal disease results from the elaboration of noxious products by the entire plaque flora. When only small amount of plaque is present, the noxious products are neutralized by the host. Similarly when the large amounts of noxious products are produced, which would essentially overcome the host's defense. Periodontal disease was believed to result from an accumulation of plaque over time in conjunction with a decrease host response and increase host susceptibility of age. All plaque was thought to be alike and equally capable of causing disease.

Normal aging is a biological, sociological or psychological which are inevitable and occur as the result of maturation/passage of time.

Nuclei poisoning is the inactivation of nuclei of crystallization by the deposition of foreign material on their surface.

Nucleus ambiguous is situated in the medulla. It forms an elongated column that extends through

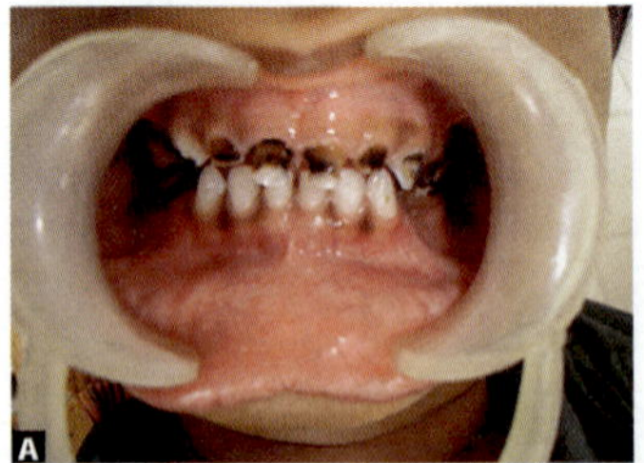

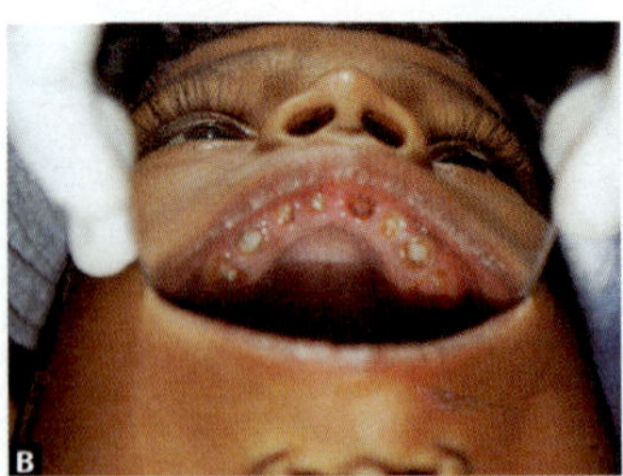

Figs A and B: *Multiple extensive caries due to nursing bottle syndrome*

both the open and closed parts of the medulla. It is a composite nucleus and contributes fibers to the glossopharyngeal, vagus and accessory nerves.

Nucosal flap refers to Partial thickness flap.

Nummular dermatitis is a chronic dermatitis with inflamed, coin shaped vesicular, crusted scaling and pruritic lesions. The discoid lesions start as pruritic patches of vesicles and papules that later ooze serum and form crusts. Lesions are widespread. No satisfactory treatment is available. Oral antibiotics are given empirically oral corticosteroids with ultraviolet – a may be required.

Nursing bottle *see* Infancy caries.

Nursing bottle syndrome: This occurs in babies on bottle feeding containing more of sugar. It results in multiple numbers of caries in many teeth mostly the lower one.

Nutritional neglect refes to children who are categorized as non-organic failure to thrive and acutely malnourished. Failure to supply essential nutrients necessary for the normal growth and development. The high mortality in developing nation is due to nutritional negligence. Obesity a manifestation of over nutrition is also a form of neglect due to failure of parents to realize the nutritive needs of growing child. This is generally a finding in a family of busy parents.

Nystatin is an antifungal medication acts by causing loss of potassium ion from pathogenic fungi. It is used in Candida infections of mouth and has to be applied locally.

O

Obligate aerobes ate the organisms which require oxygen for their growth, e.g. tubercle bacilli.

Obligate anaerobes bacteria can grow only in absence of oxygen, e.g. *Bacteroides, Fusobacterium.*

Oblique fibers refer to periodontal fibers that make the largest group in periodontal ligament. They extend from cementum to bone obliquely. They bear the occlusal forces and transmit them to alveolar bone.

Oblique ridge is a bony landmark in mandible that appears as a linear elevation that transverses a surface.

Obstructive mouth breathing is a habit usually a result of nasal obstruction such as nasal polyps, nasal tumors, chronic nasal inflammatory conditions, obstructive adenoids, and deviated nasal septum.

Obstructive sleep apnea is a sleep disorder related to upper airway collapse, leading to frequent apneas with sleep fragmentation. Obesity, alcohol and other sedative may cause it.

Obstructive voiding symptoms refer hesitancy; a delay in the initiation of micturation. Decreased force of stream results from the high resistance the bladder faces and is often associated with decrease in caliber of stream. Post-void dribbling may be due to benign prostatic hyperplasia.

Obunding material refers to the material is that reduces irritation or has a soothing effect on tissue.

Occipital lobe tumor causes contralateral hemianopia with sparing of macular vision. Dominant hemispheric lesions produce visual agnosias. Agnosia is loss of recognition of object. Visual ataxia is seen with extensive bilateral occipital lesion.

Occipital neuralgia is pain in the distribution of sensory branches of cervical plexus in neck. Trauma, neoplasm or infection is the most important cause.

Occipital sinuses are the air-filled spaces lie in the midline in relation to the floor of the posterior cranial fossa. Here the dura is raised into a fold called the falx cerebelli; and the sinus lies within this fold.

Occlude is to bring together.

Occlusal guard *see* night guard.

Occlusal plane is the imaginary surface on which upper and lower teeth meet.

Occlusal equilibration is the removal of all occlusal interfaces on the teeth.

Occlusal projection is a radiographic technique, a type of occlusal projection used to examine the anterior teeth of mandible. Occlusal projection maxillary topographic

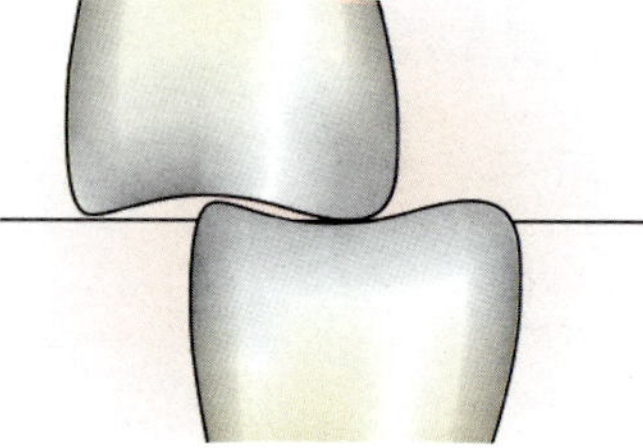

Fig.: *Occlusal plane*

is an occlusal projection used to examine the palate and anterior teeth of maxilla.

Occlusal refers to the chewing surface of teeth.

Occlusal rims are the wax spaces used during fabrication of removal prosthesis to determine the jaw relationship for missing teeth.

Occlusal sealants are defined as the application and mechanical bonding of a resin material to an acid-etched enamel surface thereby sealing existing pits and fissures from the oral environment.

Occlusal splints also known as biteguards or nightguards are removable dental applicances that is used for the treatment of MPDS, bruxism. The purpose of this appliance is to establish neuromuscular harmony in the masticatory system.

Occlusal surfaces are the chewing surfaces of posterior teeth.

Occlusal trauma refers to trauma of the occlusal table due to excessive force placed on a normal dentition, i.e. grinding and clenching of teeth. If left uncontrolled, occlusal trauma may result in rapid attachment loss and bone destruction.

Occlusion is the relationship of the teeth in a closed position in both the maxillary and mandibular arch.

Onlay is a laboratory processed restoration made of metal, porcelain or acrylic that replaces one or more of cusps of a tooth.

Oculo-dento-osseous dysplasia is characterized by micro-ophthalmus, iridal anomalies, bony anomalies of the digits and syndactyly, with enamel hypoplasia. The teeth show large multifocal hypoplastic defects and pitting-yielding a moth-eaten pattern radiographically.

Oculomotor nerve is a cranial nerve number three. It is a motor nerve and lifts upper eyelid, turns eyeball upward downward and medially. It constricts pupil and accommodates eye. This nerve emerges from the anterior aspect of mid-brain medial to cerebral peduncle. It enters the orbit through the superior orbital fissure.

Occupational exposure refers to the contact with blood or other infectious materials involving skin, eye or mucous membrane. Those results due to normal procedures done by dental professional.

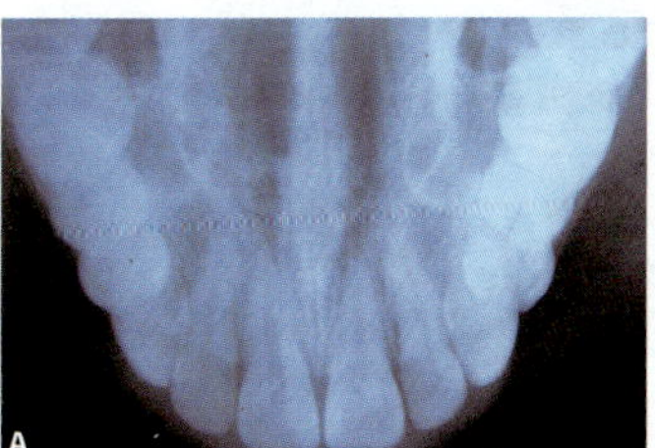

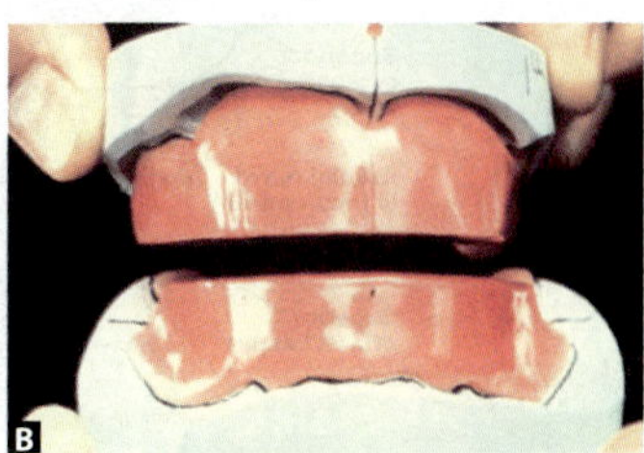

Figs A and B: *(A) Occlusal projection; (B) Occlusal rims*

Ochronosis refers to alkaptonuria.

Oculomotor nucleus arises from midbrain. The nuclei of the two sides form a single complex that lies in the central grey matter, ventral to the aqueduct.

Odontoblast layer of pulpitis is present immediately subjacent to the predentin, mainly composed of the cell bodies of the dentin forming odontoblasts. Actually it is composed of the cell bodies of odontoblasts along with capillaries, nerve fibers and dendritic cells. In the coronal portion of a young pulp the odontoblasts assume a tall columnar form. The tight packing together of these tall, slender cells produces the appearance of a palisade. The odontoblasts vary in height; consequently their nuclei are not at the same level.

Odontoblasts are the bone-forming/deposit cells. They are first type of cells encountered when pulp is approached from dentin. In the crown of the fully developed tooth, the cell bodies of odontoblasts are columnar and measure approximately 500 µm in height, whereas in the midportion of the pulp, they are more cuboidal and in apical part, more flattened. Ultrastructure of the odontoblast shows large nucleus which may contain up to four nucleoli.

Odontoclasia is a circular hypoplastic zone or line of primary enamel, which is susceptible to dental caries. The condition was first described in 1927 as a certain type of rampant caries among Hawaiian children.

Odontogenic cysts are defined as pathological epithelium lined cavity containing fluid or semi-solid material.

Odontogenic fibrosarcoma is malignant counterpart of fibroma. It occurs more frequently in children

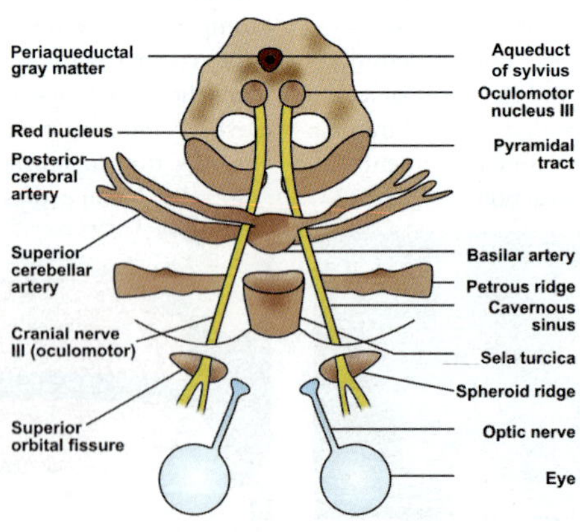

Fig.: *Oculomotor nerve*

and young adults. On X-ray, it produces expansile multilocular radiolucency. Treatment is surgical excision.

Odontogenic keratocysts are development odontogenic cyst of epithelial origin. They may develop at any age. Peak incident lies in 2nd and 3rd decade of life. Mandible is affected more. There is no characteristic clinical manifestation of keratocysts. Pain, soft tissue swelling and expansion of bone may be seen. Lesion may displace tooth. They are now reclassified as keratocystic odontogenic tumor.

Odontogenic myxoma is a benign tumor of bone developing only in jaws. It contains myxomatous tissue. It develops from mesenchymal portion of tooth germ. It is a central lesion of jaws. It is made up of loosely arranged spindle shaped and stellate cells. Intracellular substance is mucoid X-ray may show unilocular cyst like radiolucency, pericoronal radiolucency and a mixed radiolucent radiopaque image. Tennis racket appearance is very common. Very few tumors cross the midline. It generally develops between the age group of 25-35 years. Tumor develops slowly as painless expansion of jaw. Rarely there may be numbness of lips. Tumor may cause facial asymmetry. Sometimes it may perforate the cortices. Skin over tumor looks normal.

Odontoma is a benign tumor odontogenic origin. Etiology is unknown. It may be inherited or may be due to mutant gene.

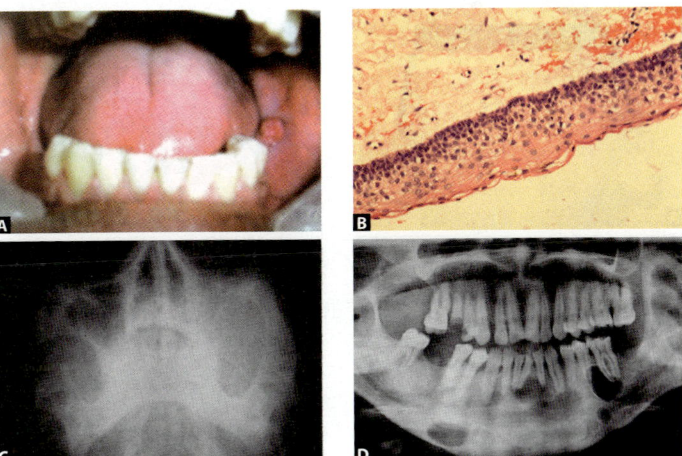

Figs A to D: *Odontogenic keratocyst (A) Clinical picture; (B) Histological picture; (C and D) Radiological picture showing multiple cysts*

It can be discovered at any age. Mostly it affects anterior maxilla. It is clinically asymptomatic. These are situated between the roots of teeth. It appears as calcified mass surrounded by a narrow radiolucent periphery. Ghost cells are present. Surgical removal helps and there is no recurrence.

Oedema is the swelling of tissue due to excessive fluid accumulation out side the cells.

Oedipus complex is said to have occured when young boys have a natural tendency to be attached to the mother and they consider their father as enemy. Hence they strive to imitate their father to gain the affection of the mother. Freud also described oedipal complex as a desire to have sexual relation with the mother. Name oedipal complex is derived from Greek mythology. Oedipus was king of thebes, unwittingly slew his father and married his mother. The little boy adopts his father's manners attitude, thinking that by becoming like his father, he can win his mother's sexual love.

Oesophagus is a tubular structure which starts at the lower end of the oropharynx. It descends through the lower part of the neck, and enters the thorax through its inlet.

Oil plants contain an abundance of natural oils which are having healing properties. Low levels of important fatty acids in diet may cause dry, flaky complex, weak nails and dull hair. Oils are good source of vitamin A, B, E and K.

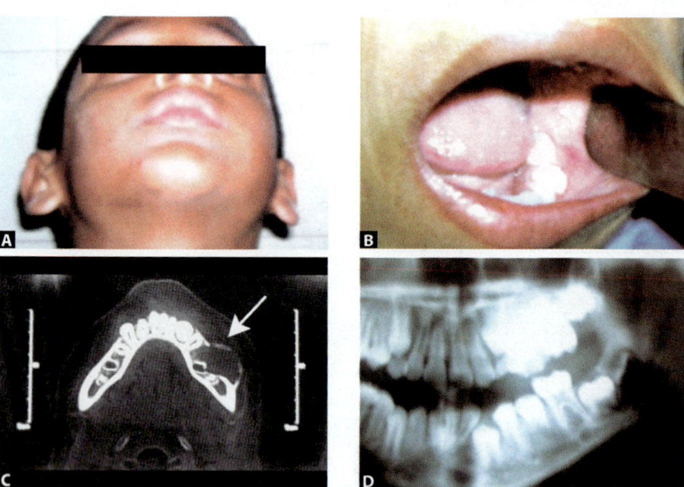

Figs A to D: *Odontogenic myxoma (A) Extraoral view; (B) Intraoral view; (C) Jaw expansion; (D) OPG*

Many natural oils also contain lecithin which has water retention properties. It delays aging by slowing down wrinkles.

Olfactory nerve is a nerve of small and cranial nerve number one. It originates as the central process of olfactory receptor nerve cells in mucous membrane of nose. It is a sensory nerve.

Oligodontia is a congenitally missing six or more teeth.

Oligomer is a polymer made up of two, three or four monomer units.

Omega-3 is a polyunsaturated fatty acid (PUFA) that reduces the chances of blood cells and platelets to form blood clots. It reduces LDL and increases HDL. It decreases production of triglycerides.

Omission refers to removal of the pleasant response after a particular response, e.g., if the child misbehaves during dental procedure. This favorite toy is taken away for short time resulting in the omission of the undesirable behavior.

Oncology is the science of neoplastic growth.

Open bite is a dental disorder that is said to have occurred when jaws are closed but the mandibular anterior teeth don't contact the lingual surfaces of the maxillary anterior tooth. It then refers to increased distance between the two arches.

Open chain exercise is the exercise in which the distal segment of the extremity does not bear weight.

Operant conditioning is significant extension of classical conditioning was arises from the studies of Skinner. Individual response is changed as a result of reinforcement (or) extinction of previous responses. Hence satisfactory outcome will be repeated while unsatisfactory outcomes will diminish infrequency. According to this theory, the consequence of behavior itself acts as a stimulus and affects future behavior. Since the behavior acts upon the environment called operant. Skinner described four basic types of operant, conditioning distinguished by the type of consequence.

Operational research is the application of scientific methods of investigations to the study of human organizations and services. Its aim is to develop new knowledge. It is a team work and involves several workers.

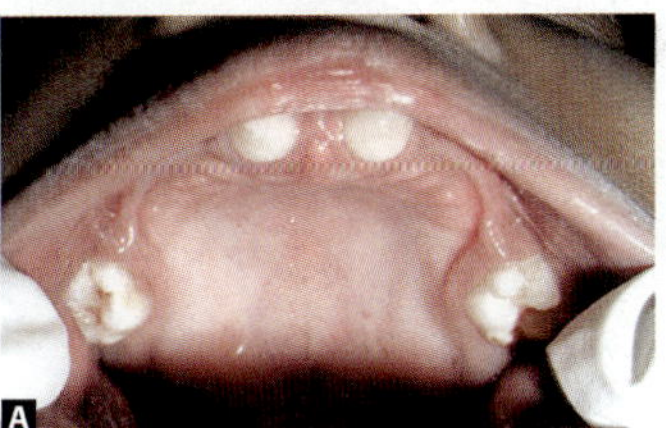

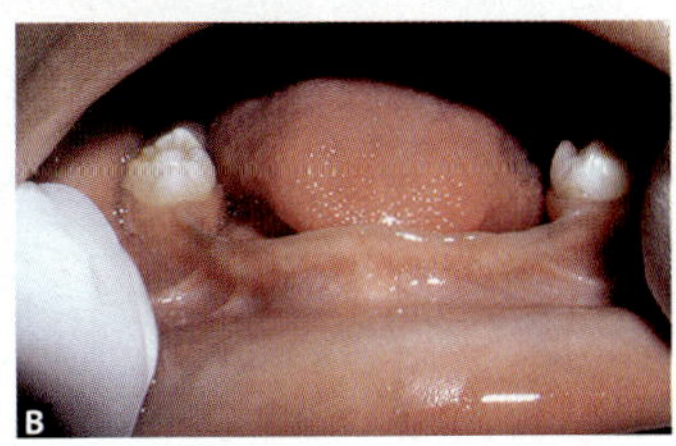

Figs A and B: *Oligodontia*

Ophthalmic nerve is the first branch of trigeminal nerve that arises from the trigeminal ganglion is the first branch of trigeminal nerve, pierces the dura of the trigeminal cave and comes to lie in the lateral wall of the cavernous sinus, below the trochlear nerve. The fibers of the ophthalmic nerve are purely sensory.

Ophthalmodynamometry is a technique measuring pressure in the retinal artery by applying a simple instrument to the globe of eye. It helps in diagnosing occlusion of the internal carotid artery. Pressure in retinal artery is reduced.

Opium poisoning refers to the excess level of opium in the circulating blood causing ill effects on the body. In case of morphine, these appear within a few minutes. In liquid form, it is quicker to act.

Opposing teeth are the teeth that are located in the opposite arch of the crown or bridge restoration onto the tooth preparation.

Opposite arch finger rest is a type of rest which can be established tooth surfaces of the opposite arch.

Optic disc is the area in the retina where the optic nerve fibers exit and there are no rods and cones.

Optic nerve is a cranial nerve of sight that is about 1.6 inches long. It leaves orbital cavity passing through optic canal. It is a sensory nerve. The nerve on both sides now joins one another to form optic chiasma. Here the nerve fibers that arise from medial side of retina cross the midline and enter the optic tract of the opposite side while the fibers from the temporal side reach the optic tract of the same side.

Optical caries monitor is an instrument, which quantifies incipient smooth surface lesions. It has been seen that *in vitro* lesions reflect much more light than sound enamel.

Optical pyrometer is a device to measure temperature by matching the color of an electrically heated

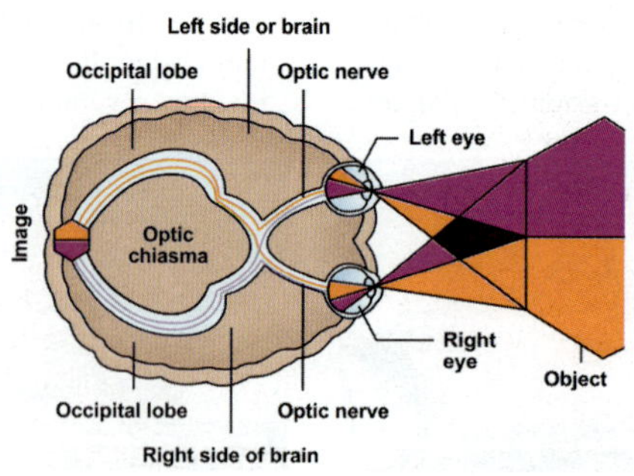

Fig.: *Optic nerve*

O

wire to the color of the surface being tested; current required is calibrated against temperature.

Oral cavity refers to the mouth.

Opacifiers are the white oxides added to decrease the transparency of the porcelain, usually tin oxide or titanium dioxide.

Oral drive theory postulated by Sears and Wise (1982) suggested that the strength of the oral drive is in part a function of how long a child continues to feed by sucking. Thus, sucking is the result of prolongation of nursing and not the frustration of weaning.

Oral habits are learned patterns of muscular contraction.

Oral health promoter is a person who explains disease, causes, homecare techniques.

Oral health status index (OHSI) is an index developed by Marcus M, Koch AL and Gershen JA in 1980. This index measure included the three components of the dmft (decayed, missing and filled teeth) and 15 other variables such as temporomandibular dysfunction, degree of periodontal disease and tumors. To calculate this measure for a population, a prior planning is needed to develop an examination protocol that includes all appropriate measurements. In a modified oral health index, "Marcus, Koch and Gershen" (1983, 1985 used weights for bone loss, missing free ends and decayed/ fractured and replaced teeth. This modified index is easier to use in epidemiological setting but its various components still need to be part of the planned protocol.

Oral herpangina is characterized by sore-throat, dysphagia, and stiff neck with loss of appetite. There develops small papulovesicular lesions about 1-2 mm in diameter with a grayish surface surrounded by red areolae in palate. Disease lasts for 4–5 days.

Oral hygiene is a routine measure that consists of keeping the teeth clean and free of food debris. It prevents accumulation and persistence of plaque which leads to dental disease. Tooth brush is an effective tool. Eating raw, firm and fibrous food/fruits as apples, pears and carrots also help to clean the teeth.

Oral hygiene index given by John C Greene and Jack R Vermillian while they were developing a plan to study variations in gingival inflammation in relation to the degree of mental retardation in children, as it became apparent that it would be necessary to separate out the effects of variations in oral cleanliness. In 1960, the "oral hygiene index" (OHI) was introduced—a "sensitive, simple method for assessing group or individual oral hygiene quantitatively". The oral hygiene index requires the user to make more decisions and to spend more time in arriving at the result. Therefore, an effort was made to develop another equally sensitive index which would reduce both the number of decisions and time required. This index was named the "simplified oral hygiene index" (OHI-S). The OHI and OHI-S were developed primarily to serve as systematic approaches to quantitating the oral cleanliness variable in population studies.

Oral is pertaining to mouth.

Oral indices (George P Barnes et al) are essentially sets of values, usually numerical with maximum and minimum limits, used to describe variables of specific conditions on a graduated scale, which use the same criteria and method to compare a specific variable in individuals, samples or populations with that same variable as is found in other individuals, samples or populations.

Oral irrigation is a procedure to direct a stream of water or therapeutic agent over the teeth, gingival tissues or into a periodontal pocket in order to remove the debris and reduce pathogens.

Oral malodor is a generic descriptor for foul smells emanating from the mouth which encompasses ozostomia, stomatodysodia, halitosis (either pathological and physiological, fetor oris or fetor ex ore). The latter term denotes local or systemic production of malodor.

Oral manifestation is a signs of disease in oral cavity.

Oral mucosa the lining of the oral cavity of mucous membrane composed of connective tissue covered with stratified squamous epithelium. It serves to protect these organs and to receive and transmit stimuli from the environment.

Oral pathology is concerned with the nature of diseases affecting oral structure. Doctor is known as oral pathologist.

Oral polio vaccine is a vaccine against poliomyelitis that is given orally by droplet method. It was discovered by Sabin in 1957. It contains an attenuated virus (type 1, 2 and 3) grown in primary monkey kidney or human. Diploid cell culture. Three doses are given at the interval of one month. It induces both humoral and intestinal immunity. It is cheaper and effective. It should not be given in acute infection.

Oral screen is a functional appliance that produces effect by redirecting the pressure of the muscular and soft tissue curtain of the cheeks and lips. It is also used to counteract deficiencies in lip posture and function and to prevent oral respiration when anterior and posterior oral seals are inadequate. It prevents child from placing the thumb or finger into the oral cavity during sleeping hours. It is also used to control tongue thrusting.

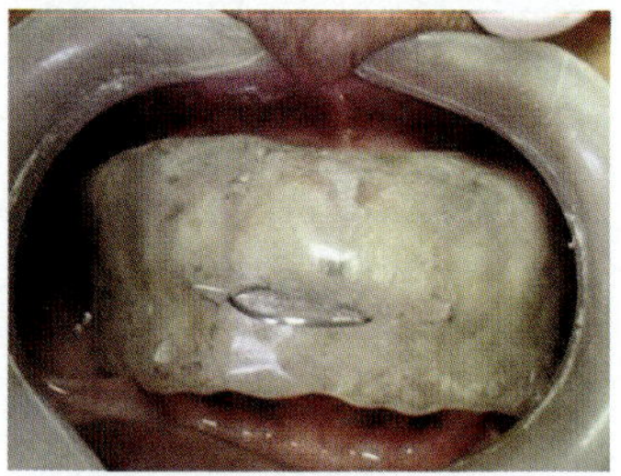

Fig.: *Oral vestibular screen*

O

Oral submucous fibrosis is a pre-cancerous condition and is a slow-growing disease in which fibrous bands are formed. Etiology is not known. There is a burning sensation of mouth when one consumes spicy food. Vesicles and later ulceration may develop. Salivation increases. Oral epithelium is atrophic. Systemic corticosteroids and local tropical hydrocortisone help.

Orange and red stains dental extrinsic stains that appear at cervical third, occur more frequently on anteriors than compared to posterior covering both facial and lingual surfaces of anterior teeth. These stains are generally caused by chromogenic bacteria. Stain a light thin material of brick-red orange color is seen on teeth. Its cause is not known. This stain is due to pigment producing microorganism. Stain is easily removed.

Orbicularis oculi are muscles present around the orbital aperture or orbicularis oris is a muscle surrounding the opening of the mouth in a circular fashion.

Order of use is the sequence in which dentist uses series of instruments.

Organogenesis is the formation of organs from the primary germ layer of an embryo.

Origin is the point where muscle attaches to bone. It usually refers to the proximal attachment of the muscle.

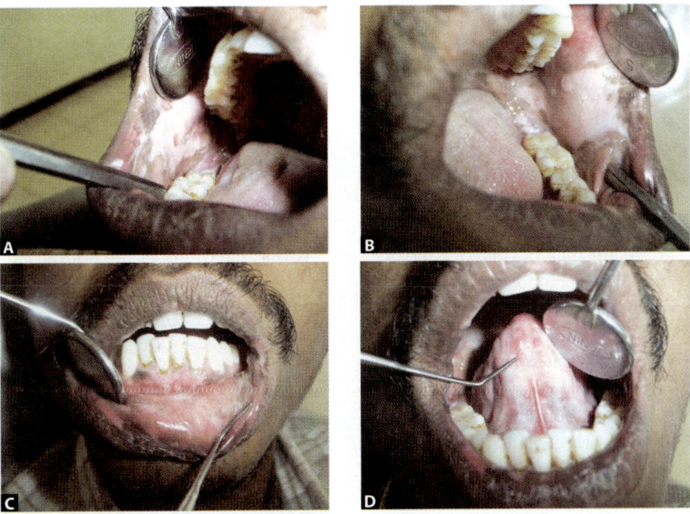

Figs A to D: *Oral submucous fibrosis (OSMF) (A and B) Buccal mucosa; (C) Labial mucosa; (D) Involving ventral surface of the tongue*

Orofacial dyskinesia is an extrapyramidal disorder or a complication of phenothiazines therapy. It generally develops after the age of 60. There develops involuntary, dystonic movements of facial, oral and cervical musculature. There may be lip smacking, lip licking or protrusion of lip.

Orofacial pain is the pain associated with structures of oral cavity.

Orthodontics is defined as the study of growth and development of the jaws and face particularly and the body generally, as influencing the position of the teeth; the study and action and reaction of internal and external influences on the development; and the prevention and correction of arrested and perverted development.

Orthopnea is the ability to breathe easily only in upright position.

Orthoses is any device which when in contact with the body improves the function of that part.

Orthostatic hypotension is a common cause of vasomotor syncope especially in elderly, diabetics or autonomic neuropathy. A greater than normal decline of 20 mm Hg in blood pressure is seen immediately upon arising from supine to standing position.

Orthostatic syncope also known as postural hypotension occurs within seconds or minutes of assuming upright posture. Patients are vulnerable on rising and after meals. It differs from vasovagal syncope in that the skin may be warm, pulse rate unchanged and sweating absent.

Osseointegration is a direct structural and functional connection between ordered, living bone and the surface of a load carrying implant or it can also be described as relationship between endosseous implants and bone where the bone is in intimate contact with implant but no ultrastructural contact is seen between the two.

Osseous craters are the concavities in the crest of the interdental bone confined within the facial and the lingual walls.

Osseous pain refers to pain originating from bone from this part are generally due to infection or injury. Such pains are more stable than myogenous pain. Acute septic osteitic usually is designated osteomyelitis. Pain is of throbbing quality. It induces necrosis by pressure against the unyielding walls. When cortex is penetrated, pain intensity decreases. When confinement is released by rupture or surgical drainage, pain intensity drops fast.

Ossicles of the ear are the term given collectively to the three small bones within the cavity of the middle ear.

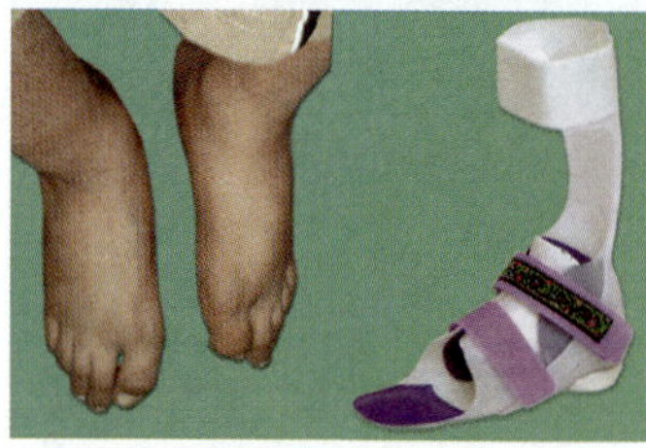

Fig.: *Orthosis for ankle and foot*

The ossicles are called the malleus (= like a hammer), the incus (= like an anvil, used by blacksmiths), the stapes (= like a stirrup in which the foot of a horse-rider fits). The three ossicles form a chain that is attached on one side to the tympanic membrane and internal ear.

Ossifying fibroma is a rare benign non-neoplastic condition composed of fibroblastic connective tissue. The color ranges from pink to red and can be frequently ulcerated are frequently found in paranasal sinuses especially antrum. These produce large densely calcified masses.

Osteolgenic sarcoma is a primary malignant tumor of bone. Patient is young between the age of 10–20 years. Pains and swelling are presenting features. Long bones are targets. Alkaline phosphatase enzyme will be raised. Metastasis to lung is through hematogenous route. Periosteal new bone formation occurs and is highly irregular. Sun ray appearance is characteristic. Osteogenic sarcoma of mandible is also noted.

Osteoarthritis is an old age degenerative joint disease without systemic manifestation. Disease may be primary in interphalangeal joints. Secondary may be post-traumatic. Bones X-ray may show subchondral sclerosis, cortical buttressing, trabecular hypertrophy, osteophyte, cysts and collapse. Erosive osteoarthritis occurs in menopausal women. Pain is worse on activity and is relieved on rest.

Osteoblasts are bone-forming cells located on bone surfaces and help in the growth and development of teeth and bones.

Osteochondroma is a bony exostosis projecting from external surface of bone having a hyaline lined cartilaginous cap. These are found in childhood and are asymptomatic. There develops hard, painless mass

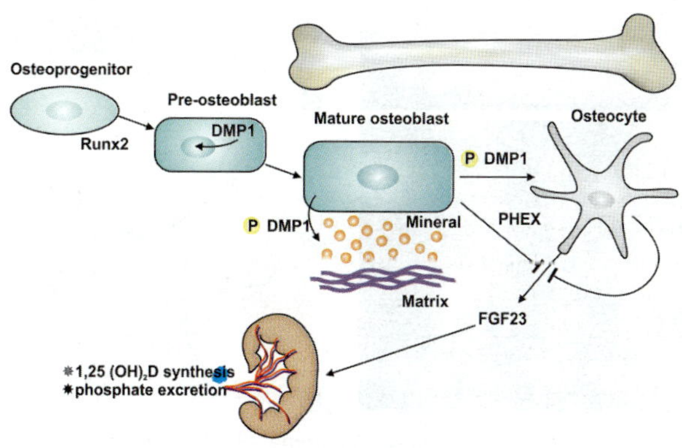

Fig.: *Osteoblasts*

near a joint of a long tubular bone. Cartilaginous cap shows irregularity and spotty calcifications. These project away from joint. When cap becomes more than 2 cm malignant, transformation may take place.

Osteoclastomas are brown tumors visible as distinct geographic radiolucencies. These are central, slightly expansile and septated looking like a destructive neoplasm. Mandible is mostly involved. These are marker of primary hyperparathyroidism. MRI may show fluid-fluid level.

Osteoclasts are bone-removing multi-nucleated cells which help to remodel bone.

Osteoconduction is the process by which formation of bone is seen. Osteoblasts occur from the margins of the defect on bone graft material that facilitate bone formation by bridging the gap between the existing bone and a distant location which is otherwise not possible.

Osteocyte is a mature bone cell responsible for maintaining bone tissue.

Osteogenesis imperfecta is a serious disease of unknown etiology. Disease is visual at birth. Bones are fragile and porous. Fractures occur while child learns walking. It develops due to defective matrix formation and lack of mineralization. Fetal collagen is not able to transform into mature collagen. There are 4 types. Two are autosomal recessive and rest two are autosomal dominant type. Moderate and deforming type—these are associated with

O

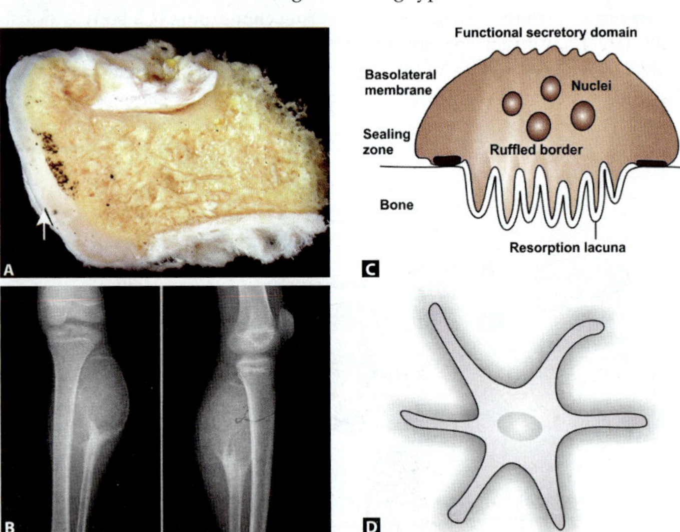

Figs A to D: *(A) Osteochondroma; (B) Osteoclastoma; (C) Osteoclast; (D) Osteocyte*

deciduous teeth and blue sclera. Child may have abnormal shape of skull, joint dislocations and defective heart valve. Mild not deforming type—patient, otherwise, is clinically normal. Person has blue sclera and dentinogenesis imperfecta. Neonatal lethal type—it is a serious form of disease. There are multiple fractures of bone. Severenon lethal type—patient develops fracture with slight trauma. Fractures heel early but deformity remains.

Osteogenic sarcoma is a primary malignant tumor of bone. Patient is young between the age of 10–20 years. Pain and swelling are presenting features. Long bones are targets. Alkaline phosphatase enzyme will be raised. Metastasis to lung is through hematogenous route. Periosteal new bone formation occurs and is highly irregular. Sun ray appearance is characteristic. Osteogenic sarcoma of mandible is also noted.

Osteoid osteoma is a benign tumor of bone. It rarely develops after the age of 30. Pain is severe. Radiographs will show small round radiolucent area surrounded

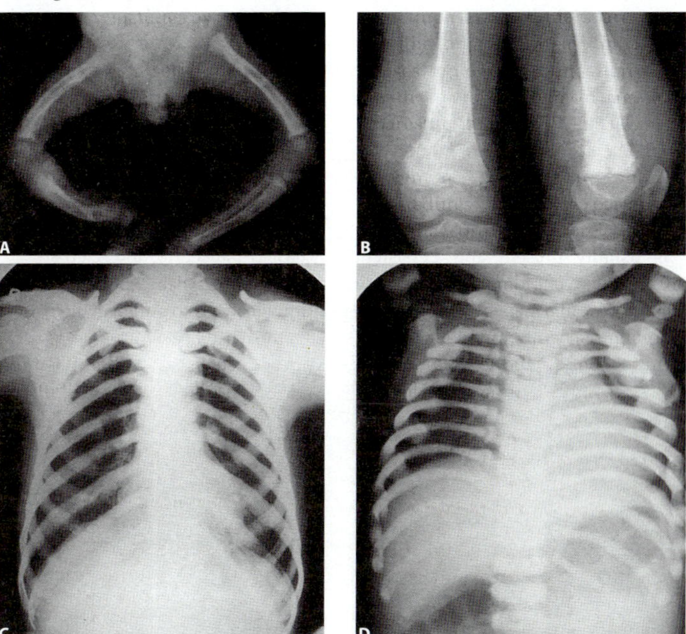

Figs A to D: *(A) Osteogenesis imperfecta with multiple, healing fractures; (B) Osteosarcoma; (C and D) Osteopetrosis ribs*

O

by a rim of sclerotic bone. Lesion is seldom larger than 1 cm. It consists of central nidus of compact osteoid tissue with calcification. Surgical excision is the treatment of choice.

Osteoinduction is a process where new bone formation occurs through the stimulation of osteoprogenitor from the defect that differentiates into osteoblasts.

Osteoinductive material is a material which causes the conversion of mesenchymal cells preferentially to bone progenitor cells.

Osteoma is a benign neoplasm. There is proliferation of cancellous bone in an endosteal or periosteum. It is not a common oral lesion. It shows a circumscribed swelling on jaw. It is not painful. Lesion is not capsulated and has to be removed surgically.

O

Osteomalacia is the counterpart of rickets in adults, commonly seen in women with pardah and menopausal females. Skeletal pain is usually present and persistent and ranges from backache to severe pain. Bone tenderness and muscular weakness are often present. Patient may find it difficult to climb stairs or getting out of chair. A waddling gait is not unusual. Osteoporosis which is atrophy of bone occurs and is due to defective formation of bone matrix. Bones become soft. X-ray shows severe asymmetric deformities of all stress bearing bones. Histological findings are nonspecific. Cortical bone becomes thin. Bone tenderness and muscular weakness are often present.

Osteopetrosis is a rare hereditary bone disease. There is lack of resorption of normal primitive osteochondrous tissue. Patient dies early. There may be severe anemia, liver and spleen are enlarged with palpable lymph glands. Leukemia and sarcoma are common sequelae. All bones are of homogeneous increased density. There may be bones within a bone. Ilium shows dense curved lines paralleling to iliac crest. Skull changes include calvarial and basilar thickening and sclerosis.

Osteopoikilosis is characterized by small, round or ovoid radio-opacities in juxta-articular region.

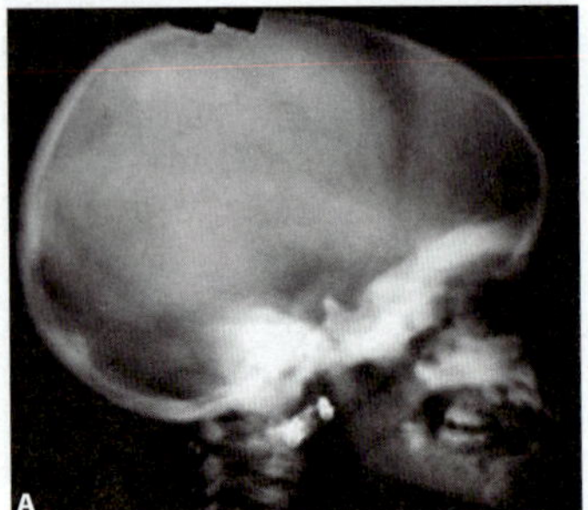

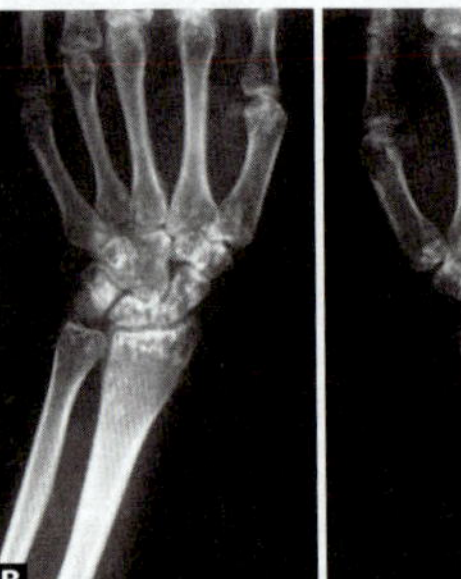

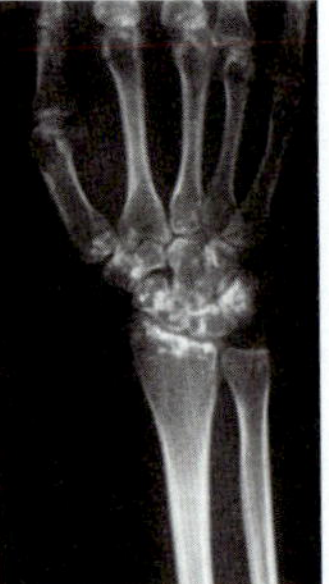

Figs A and B: *(A) Osteopetrosis skull; (B) Osteopoikilosis*

More of males are asymptomatic. Lesions are foci of bone which have failed to become cancellous. On X-ray lesions are symmetric of 1 to 8 mm in size. These are uniformly dense.

Osteoporotic compression fracture is a type of spinal fracture causal due to osteoporosis and is called compression fracture. On X-ray, anterior wedge is most commonly seen in thoracic vertebra and biconcave end-plate fracture in lumbar arc. Pain is so severe that person has to be admitted. Bracing is important to ambulate such patients.

Osteosarcoma is a very common neoplasm arising from bone. According to the site tumor has been divided into periosteal sarcoma, medullary osteosarcoma, parosteal osteosarcoma, soft tissue osteosarcoma. Maxilla is affected more than mandible. *Clinical Features* include: It s a fast growing, it develops a painful swelling of jaw, expansion and distortion of cortical plates may take place. Severe deformity of face leads to the displacement of teeth. Overlying skin becomes red and inflamed. Ulceration, hemorrhage and pathological fracture take place. *Radiological Findings:* In osteolytic type, it presents irregular, radiolucent areas giving rise to a moth-eaten appearance. Expansion, destruction and perforation of cortical plates are noted. Teeth are displaced in position.

Osteosclerosis refers to increased density of bone which can be detected radiographically due to increased density.

Otic ganglion is a small, flat oval shaped parasympathetic ganglion that is situated just below the foramen ovale medial to the trunk of the mandibular nerve. It is connected to the nerve to the medial pterygoid muscle. The middle meningeal artery and the roots of the auriculotemporal nerve lie close to it.

Outcomes research is an analysis of clinical practice as it actually occurs for the purpose of determining effectiveness of clinical methods by the researcher.

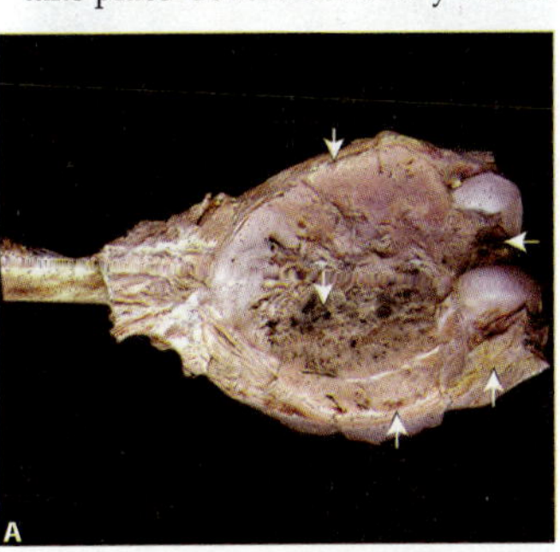

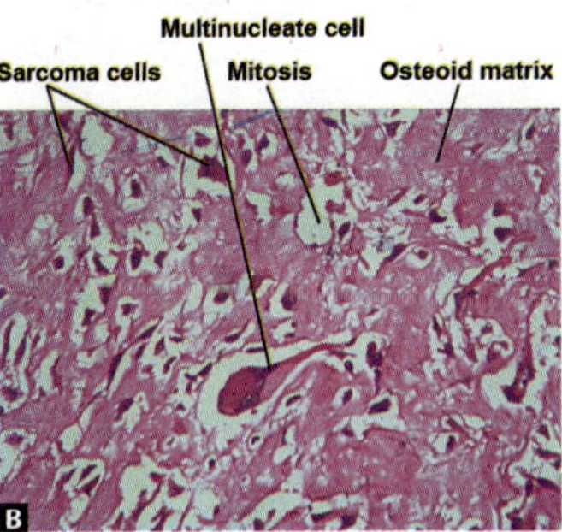

FigsA amd B: *Osteosarcoma (A) Macroscopic; (B) Microscopic*

Overbite is the amount of vertical overlap between the maxillary and mandibular incisors. The relationship can be described either in millimeters or more often as a percentage of how many the upper central incisors overlap the crowns of the lower incisors. The overbite in the primary dentition normally varies between 10% and 40%. When the incisor edges of the incisors are at the same level the condition is described as edge to edge or zero overbite.

Overdentures is a fabricated removable prosthetic appliance attached to the abutment cylinders. It is the one which is fitted on top of standing teeth or retained roots. Advantage of it is the presence of natural roots remaining in alveolar bone. As long as any roots remain there becomes hardly any loss of alveolar bone. Where there are no remaining roots implants can be used to support an overdenture.

Over infusion is over transfusion—may be of blood or saline. Respiration becomes shallow and rapid. Patient feels uncomfortable in lying supine. Neck veins are congested. There may be slight pitting edema. Crepts may be present on independent parts of the body. Patient may develop dieresis.

Overjet is the horizontal relationship or the distance between the most protruded maxillary central incisor and the opposing mandibular central incisor. The relationship is expressed in millimeters. If the maxillary incisors are lingual to the mandibular incisors the relationship is described as an under-jet. The normal range of overjet in primary dentition varies between 0 and 4 mm. In the same study by Foster the overjet was ideal in 28% of the cases and excessive in 72% of the children. Again the presence of excessive

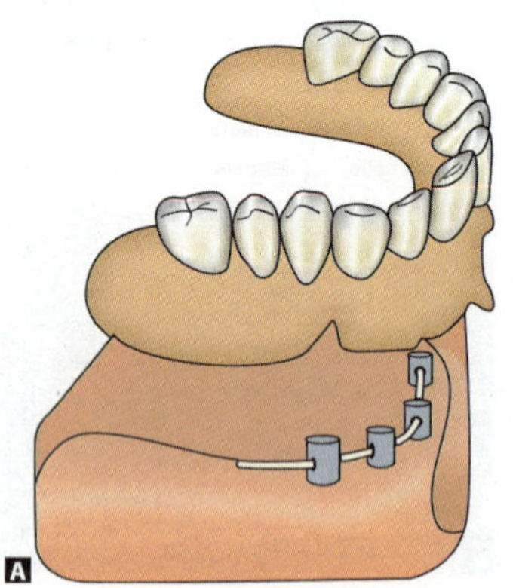

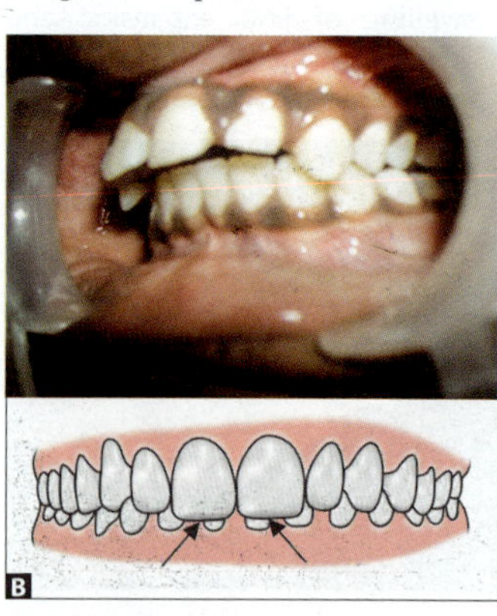

Figs A and B: *(A) Overdentures; (B) Overjet*

overjet was attributed to the effects of the oral habits.

Overuse is the chronic injury by repetitive stress.

Overextension is the extension of the boundary of appliance beyond physiological barriers that may produce discomfort and dislodgement of an appliance.

Overfilling is the total obturation of root canal system with excess material extruding beyond apical foramen.

Overgrowth *see* gingival hyperplasia.

Oviducts refer to fallopian tubes.

Oxidation is a chemical reaction that occurs when processing solutions are exposed to air. It is a chemical breakdown causing decreased concentration of solution strength.

Oxidized cellulose is gauze treated with nitrogen dioxide. On moistening the gauze adheres to the bleeding tissue and readily produces a clot.

Oxygen is a molecule composed of two oxygen items. Air we breathe contains about 21% oxygen. It is essential for life. O_2 we breathe is used by cells to extract or liberate the energy from food we eat.

Oxygen therapy is an administration of oxygen gas to individuals suffering from hypoxia.

Oxyphil adenoma is a benign tumor occurring in parotid gland in elderly age group. It is composed of polygonal cells with mitochondria in eosinophilic granular cytoplasm. Centrally placed nuclei are uniform, small and round. Salivary enlargement is a result of benign epithelial metaplasia.

Oxytalan fibers are made up of two immature forms of elastin: oxytalan and elaunin. These fibers run parallel to the root surface in a vertical direction, bend and attach themselves to the cementum in the apical one-third of the tooth.

Ozonated water irrigation is newer irrigant solution which is shown to be powerful antimicrobial agent against bacteria, fungi, protozoa and viruses. It is suggested that ozonated water may prove to be useful in controlling oral infectious microorganisms.

P

PA posteroanterior view of radiograph.

Palate *see* roof of the mouth.

Pachyonychia congenital is rare and inherited as autosomal dominant characteristic. It also refers to oral leukokeratosis as well as striking nail changes and develops shortly after birth. There is congenital gross thickening of finger and toenails as they become thick and hardened with brownish material at nail bed. Corneal dystrophy, thickening of tympanic membrane and mental retardation are reported. Dorsum of tongue becomes thickened and greyish white. Checks may also be involved on occasion. Hyperkeratotic calluses of palms and soles may develop. Oral lesions include focal or generalized white, opaque thickening of mucosa. Angular cheilosis also develops. Frequent oral aphthous ulceration may be seen. There is no treatment available.

Packed RBCs refer to concentrated forms of RBCs but are devoided of plasma by centrifugation. transfusion of these helps in raising hematocrit. Each unit of 300 mL consists of 200 mL of RBCs. One unit of packed RBCs will raise the hematocrit by 4%.

Paget's disease is a disease of middle age. Most of the patients are asymptomatic. There will be pain with multiple fractures. Milkman's syndrome involves local areas of demineralization within the bone. Pseudo-fractures may also be seen. Spinal cord and nerve root compressions may be seen.

Pain is a symptom in the completely subjective sense. It is a complex experience that includes a sensory discriminatory component.Pain is accompanied by the most widespread reactions and can sometimes be said truly to involve the whole being. The experience of pain is a subjective, private sensation, which can be described only imperfectly to others.

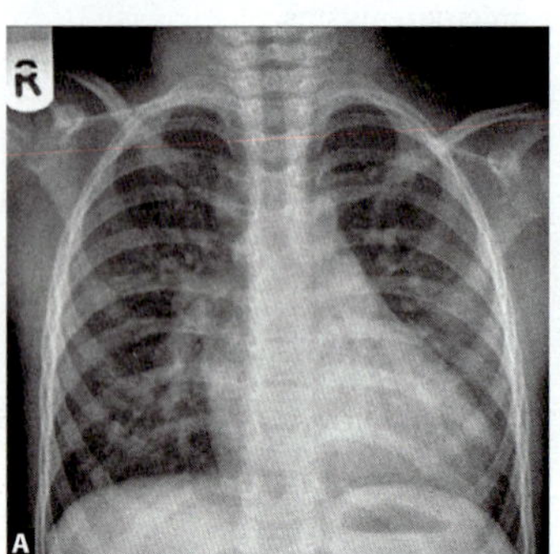

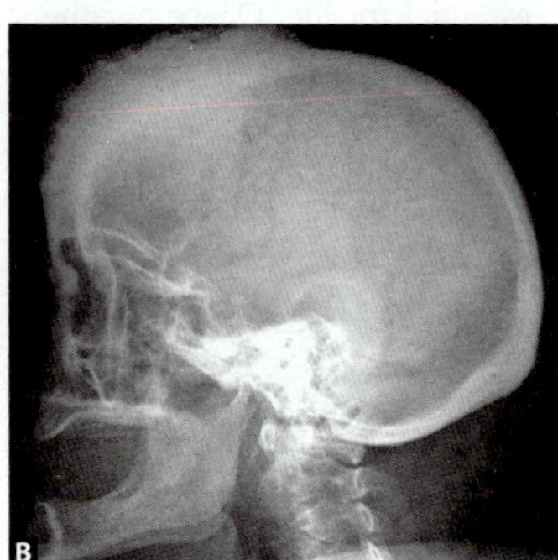

Figs A and B: *(A) Posteroanterior view; (B) Paget's disease*

Whereas it is possible to share other sensations by, for example, listening, testing or touching with reasonable certainty of the same experience as another person but this is not possible with pain. Pain also includes the reactions elicited by the stimulus. For instance, some of the reactions to a noxious stimulus include pain. Startle response, muscle reflex, vocalization, sweating, and increase in heart rate, in addition to blood pressure and behavioral changes. Therefore pain is a neuroscience characterized by; (1) The more sensory nerves that supply a region of body, the more acute the sensibility in the area; (2) The higher the ratio of motor nerves to muscles, the greater the possible control finesse.

Pain threshold is that point at which sufficient pain transmitting neurochemical reaches the brain to cause discomfort also. Pain threshold is the amount of stimulus which produces a sensation of pain.

Palatal papillomatosis is an unusual condition involving mucosa of the palate. It develops in edentulous patient with denture. Lesion presents with numerous red, edematous papillary projections. It may involve whole of hard palate. Each papilla is 1 to 2 mm in diameter. No specific therapy is available.

Palatal surface is the surface of the maxillary teeth nearest the palate.

Palate separates the oral cavity from the nasal cavity. It is divisible into an anterior, larger part—the hard palate; and a posterior part, the soft palate.

Palate soft is the posterior most portion of roof of mouth separating the mouth and pharynx.

Palatine tonsils are paired masses of lymphoid tissue lying in lateral wall of pharynx and form part of Waldeyer's ring. Each palatine tonsil (right or left) lies in the tonsilar sinus on the lateral wall of the oropharynx. Reactive lymphoid hyperplasia can result in their enlargement. It then produces difficulty in breathing.

Palatoglossal fold is a mucosal fold that connects the palate to the lateral margin of the posterior part of the tongue and is called the

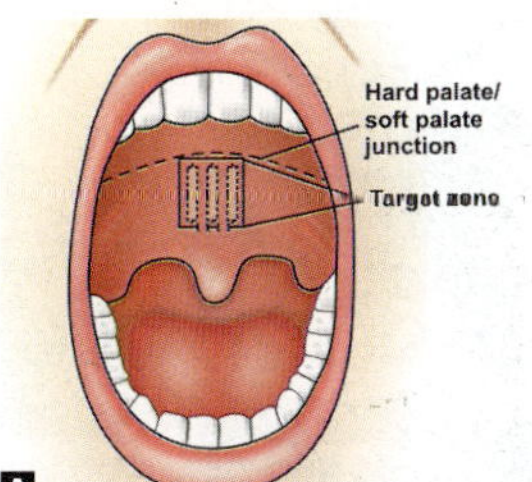

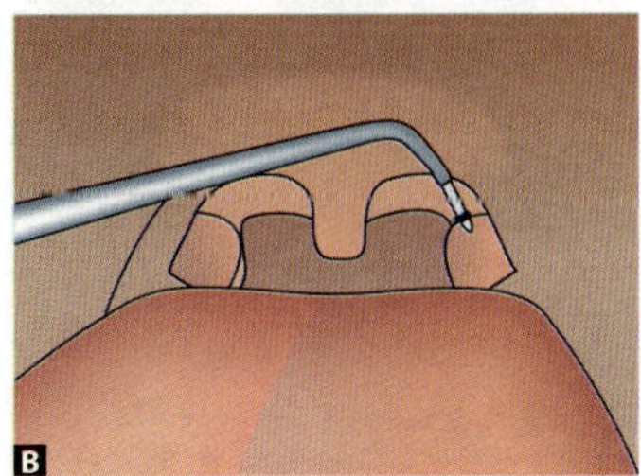

Figs A and B: *(A) Palate; (B) Tonsils*

posterior fold. Connects the palate to the wall of the pharynx and is called the palatopharyngeal fold.

Palladium-cobalt is an alloy that contains 88% palladium and 4 to 5% cobalt by weight. It has a higher coefficient of thermal expansion which is useful with certain porcelains. Disadvantage is of formation of dark oxide at margins.

Palladium-copper alloys were introduced in 1982. It contains 70 to 80% palladium, a little gold, 15% copper and 9% gallium. There is no change of color problem. It generally doesn't melt easily so casting becomes difficult.

Palladium-silver alloy usually includes 50 to 60% palladium with most of the balance being silver. It has good corrosion resistance. The disadvantage is that color changes to green.

Palliative refers to relief of pain but not a cure.

Pallor dullness of mucus membrane that usually indicates anemia but may be a sign of low cardiac output.

Palm down rest is the type of extraoral rest which can be established by resting the front surfaces of the middle and fourth finger on the skin overlying the lateral aspect of the mandible on the left side of the face.

Palm up rest is the type of extraoral rest which can be established by resting the back of the middle and fourth finger on the skin overlying the lateral aspect of the mandible on the right side of the face.

Palmer's notation is an identification system for teeth; widely used to designate individual teeth amongst orthodontists. Each of the four quadrants is given its own tooth bracket made up of a vertical line and a horizontal line. This system is a shorthand diagram of the teeth as if the patient's teeth were being viewed from the outside. The teeth in the right quadrant would have the vertical midline bracket to the right of the tooth numbers or letters, just as when looking at the patient—the midline is to the right of the teeth in the right quadrant.

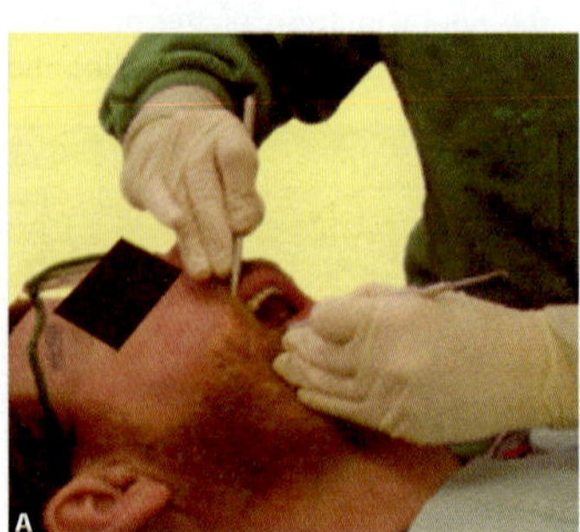

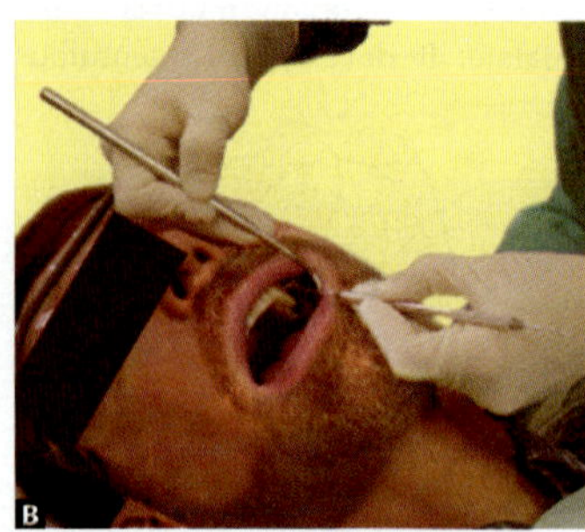

Figs A and B: *(A) Palm down; (B) Palm up rest*

Palpate is to examine and explore by touching.

Palpation is done using digital pressure to check any tenderness in soft tissue overlying suspected tooth.

Palpitation is an unpleasant awareness of the beating of the heart. Generally it may occur due to abnormalities in the rate, rhythm or force of contraction of the heart. Important causes of palpitation are atrial, junctional and ventricular tachyarrhythmias.

Panic disorder is an axiety disorder. Many patients with panic disorder have existing symptoms of depression with suicidal tendency. Person will develop chest pain, dyspnea, and palpitation. Sweating and trembling develops. Person develops fear of dying.

Panophthalmitis is a condition where there is development of intense pain, fever, malaise and complete loss of vision. Lids are edematous. There is chemosis of conjunctiva. Person develops proptosis and limitation of eye movements. Anterior chamber is full of pus.

Panoramic radiographs are X-ray films to obtain the wide view of upper and lower jaw and their associated structures. These are useful for viewing larger areas of maxilla or mandible on single film. These don't give minor details such as to detect interproximal bone loss or other fine changes.

Panorex refers panoramic radiographs.

Pantothenic acid was discovered in the year 1940. This vitamin is widely distributed in animals and vegetable foods. No specific deficiency. This vitamin loses 15-50% in canning, heat drying and cooking. Milling of wheat causes 50% loss of it.

Papillary gingivitis involves the inflammation of papillary gingiva and often extends into the adjacent portion of the gingival margin.

Papilloma is a common benign neoplasm arising from epithelial tissue. There develops an exophytic papillary growth of stratified squamous epithelium. They appear as a small finger-like projections giving a cauliflower-like shape of surface squamous epithelium; may be caused by human papilloma virus (HPV-6, HPV-11). *Clinical Features:* Slow-growing, small,

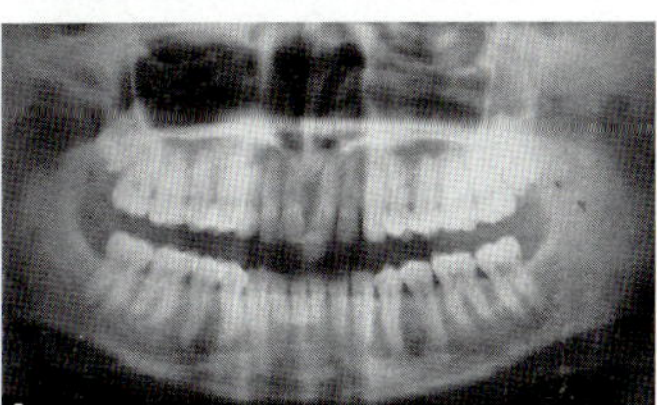

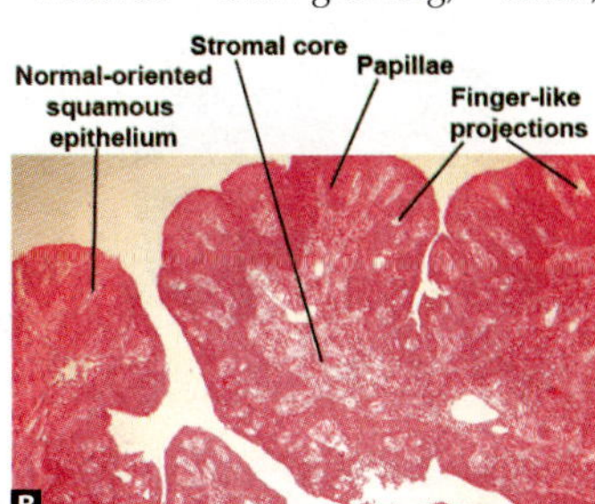

Figs A and B: *(A) Panoramic radiographs; (B) Papilloma*

painless cauliflower-like growth with many finger-like projections. Size varies from a few mm. to 1 cm. It is pedunculated, ovoid swelling white in color. Multiple papilloma of oral cavity is known as papillomatosis. It is not a premalignant condition. Surgical excision along with base is advised. Recurrence is very rarely seen.

Papilloma of tongue is an exophytic growth where patient present with a warty swelling of tongue of long duration. Mostly it is present on dorsum of tongue. It is pedunculated, mobile and soft in touch.

Papilloma of ureters may be single or multiple, small, papillary and branching pattern. Mitosis is absent and basal polarity is retained.

Papillon-Lefevre syndrome is characterized by hyperkeratotic skin lesion, severe periodontal destruction and calcification of the dura, the cutaneous and the dural changes generally occur before the age of 4 years. Premature loss of primary and permanent dentitions and ectopic calcifications, the syndrome is inherited and appears to follow an autosomal recessive pattern. Parents are not affected and may occur in siblings; males and females are equally affected. The syndrome is an autosomal recessive trait with a prevalence of about 1-4 per million of the population. Rapid and progressive periodontal destruction affects the primary dentition with an onset of about 2 years. Exfoliation of all primary teeth is usually before the permanent successors erupt and patients may be in mid to late teens.

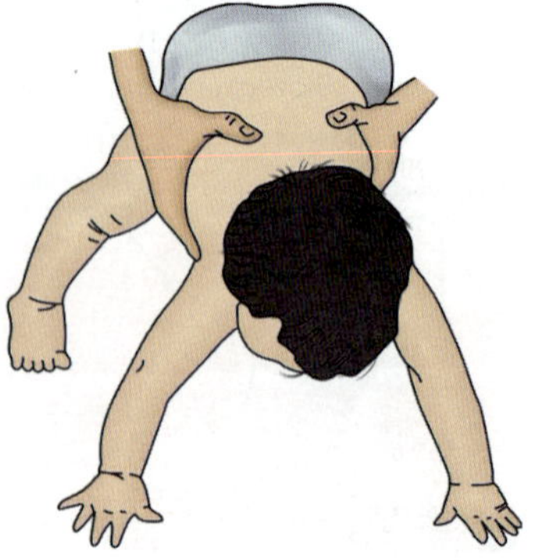

Fig.: *Parachute reflex*

Para-aminosalicylic acid is an antimetabolite of the tuberculosis bacteria. It has a weak effect.

Paracetamol is an NSAID and is more widely used as anti-pyretic and anti analgesic drug. Phenacetin has a disadvantage of creating papillary necrosis and methhemoglobinemia. Paracetamol also may produce fatal hepatic necrosis. It has very minimal anti inflammatory effect. One gram daily is a safer dose.

Parachute reflex is a neonatal reflex that appears about 6-9 months. This reflex is elicited by lowering the newborn in ventral suspension from for a short distance. Normal reflex includes extension of arms, limbs and fingers. In children with cerebral palsy, the reflex may be absent or abnormal.

Paraffin wax: Wax bath is available in many sizes. The melted wax needs to be maintained at temperature 40 to 44°C. It is the most convenient way of applying conducted heat to the extremities. Wax gives off heat slowly due to its low thermal conductivity. It has a sedative effect on the sensory nerve endings.

Parahemophilia is rare and hemorrhagic disorder. It is inherited as an autosomal recessive trait. Excessive epistaxis and menorrhagia is common. Intraocular hemorrhage or hemorrhage into CNS has been reported. Spontaneous gingival bleeding occurs with no specific treatment available.

Paramyxoviruses are large pleomorphic enveloped RNA viruses. These are responsible for measles, mumps parainfluenza and respiratory pneumonitis and bronchiolitis.

Paranasal sinuses are spaces present in the substance of bones related to the nasal cavities. Each sinus opens into the nasal cavity, and is lined by mucus membrane continuous with that of the latter. Because of this communication each sinus is normally filled with air.

Paraplegia refers to paralytic. Involvement of lower half of the body including both the legs is affected.

Parasitic or septic theory was described in 1843 by Erdl described filamentous parasites in the "surface membrane" of teeth. Shortly thereafter Ficinus, a Dresden physician observed filamentous microorganisms, which he called denticulate in material taken from carious activities. He implied that these bacteria caused decomposition of the enamel and then the dentin. Neither Erdl nor Ficinus explained how these organisms destroyed tooth structure.

Parathyroid glands are so called because they lie in close relationship to the thyroid gland. Normally, there are two glands, one superior and one inferior, on either side, there being four glands in all. However, the number can be more or less. Each gland is roughly

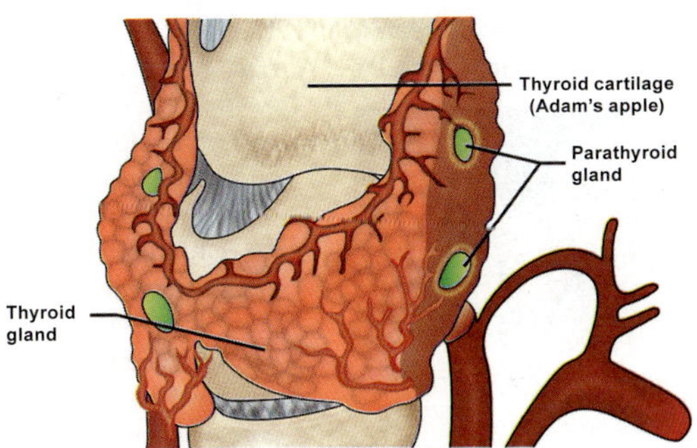

Fig.: *Thyroid and parathyroid glands*

P

oval and weighs about 50 mg. On each side, the superior parathyroid gland lies near the middle of the posterior border of the thyroid gland. It is relatively constant in position.

Paraviruses are icosahedral viruses with single stranded DNA.

Parching is a process of puffing, wheat, rice and maize are done like it. Material is suddenly heated. Water escapes by puffing out the grain. Murmure and popcorn are well-known parched products. This way starch becomes more digestible.

Parkinsonism is a clinical syndrome of bradykinesia, rigidity, tremor at rest and loss of postural reflexes. Bradykinesia is the diagnostic feature. There is difficulty in initiating voluntary movement. Expression is staring with drooling of saliva, hypophonia, micrographia. Gait is short and shuffling with lack of arm swing. Patient is unable to perform rapid and repetitive movement. It is difficult for him to change posture in bed or rise from a chair. Tendon reflexes are normal.

Parotid gland is one of the paired salivary glands that lie on the lateral side of the face in a depression below the external acoustic meatus, behind the mandible, and in front of the sternocleidomastoid muscle. It is roughly triangular on cross-section. It has a lateral or superficial surface, anteromedial surface, a posteromedial surface. At its upper end, it has a small superior surface. Its lower end is rounded and is called the apex. It is the largest of the three paired salivary glands. It is a bilobular serous gland overlying the masseter muscle. It extends upward to the level of the auditory canal and downward to the lower border of the mandible. Posteriorly it overlaps the sternomastoid muscles and anteriorly extends into the buccal pad of fat where it gives off its excretory duct. The salivary secretions are serous in nature and discharged into the oral cavity via the Stensen's duct. This duct emerges part from the anterior aspect of the gland crosses the masseter, pierces the buccinator muscle and opens in the vestibule of mouth opposite to the first molar tooth. The duct is about 5 cm long and 3 mm internal diameter.

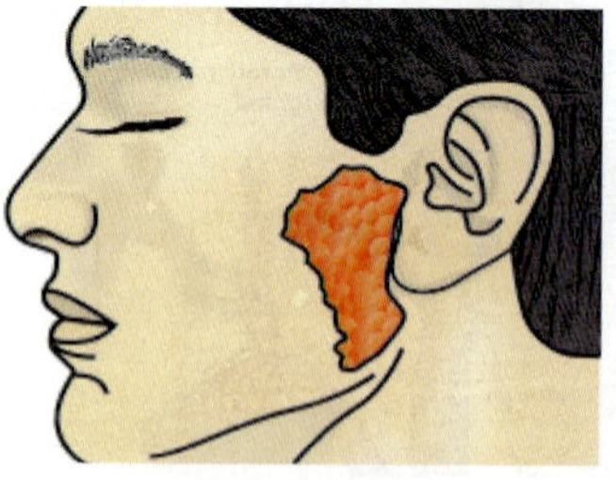

Fig.: *Parotid gland*

Pars posterior forms the posterior part of hypophysis cerebri contains numerous nerve fibers. It is directly continuous with the central core of the infundibulum, which is made up of nervous tissue. These two parts are together referred to as the neurohypophysis.

Pars tuberolis is an extension of the pars anterior surrounds the central nervous core of the infundibulum.

The pars tuberalis is part of the adenohypophysis.

Partial anodontia is the congenital absence of one or more teeth. Many cases of hypodontia appear to be genetically controlled. Environment also influences the final outcome or in some cases may be responsible completely for the lack of tooth formation. For example, trauma, infection, radiation, chemotherapy, endocrine disturbances and severe intrauterine disturbances have been associated with missing teeth.

Partial seizures are simple seizure; is a contraction of muscles in one part of body without loss of consciousness. Each contraction is caused by discharge of neurons in contralateral motor cortex when neuronal discharge is from sensory cortex, paresthesias hallucinations and psychic symptoms appear. Partial seizures involve a specific region of the brain. Focal seizures remain localized, in which paroxysmal neuronal activity is limited to one part of cerebrum. The individual's consciousness and awareness usually is somewhat disturbed and variable degree of amnesia may be evident. Partial seizures have highest incidence of a detectable cortical lesion. Focal seizure can turn into a generalized seizure in which case individual loses consciousness. Generalized seizures are clinically more dangerous in the dental office due to their greater potential for injury and post-seizure complication.

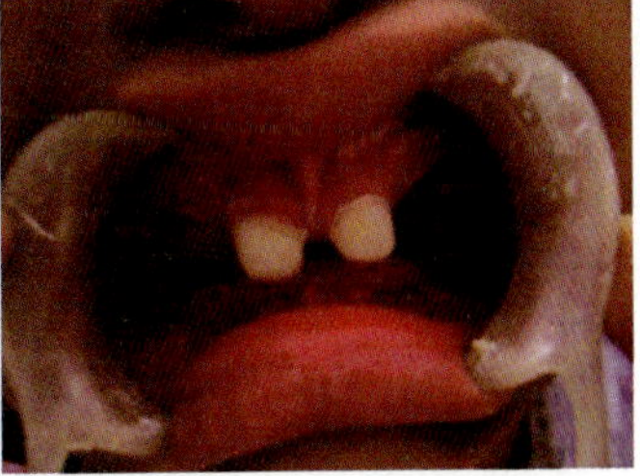

Fig.: *Partial anodontia*

Partial thickness flap refers to the flap that includes only the layer of epithelium and a layer of underlying connective tissue. The bone remains covered by the layer of connective tissue including the periosteum.

Partial thromboplastin time (PTT) is a test that measures the effectiveness of clot formation. This test is performed measuring the time it takes for a clot to form after the addition of a kaolin, a surface activating factor and a cephalin a substitute platelet factor to plasma. Normal PTT is 25-40 seconds. Greater than 50 seconds may cause severe bleeding. It is used to monitor heparin therapy.

Pascal is a metric unit of pressure. 1 MPa (megapascal) is = 1 MN/m^2.

Passive eruption describes the process by which teeth continue to erupt into the mouth as tooth structure is lost to attrition and wear.

Passive immunity is the one where the antibodies produced. Another person is used to protect against infectious disease. It can be natural or acquired. Natural passive immunity develops when antibodies from a mother pass through the placenta to the developing fetus. These antibodies protect a child till his immune system matures. While passive immunity can be acquired through an injection of antibodies against a microorganism to which person has not developed antibodies. This type of immunity is short-lived but acts immediately.

Passive modalities are therapeutic techniques that don't require the patient's active participation.

Paste is a vehicle that contains a drug.

Patent ductus arteriosus (PDA) is a congenital heart disease. There are no symptoms unless left ventricular failure or pulmonary hypertension develops. Heart may be slightly enlarged. Pulse pressure is wide and diastolic pressure is low. Continuous rough machinery murmur accentuated in late systole at the time of S2 is heard at left first and second interspace. Thrills are common.

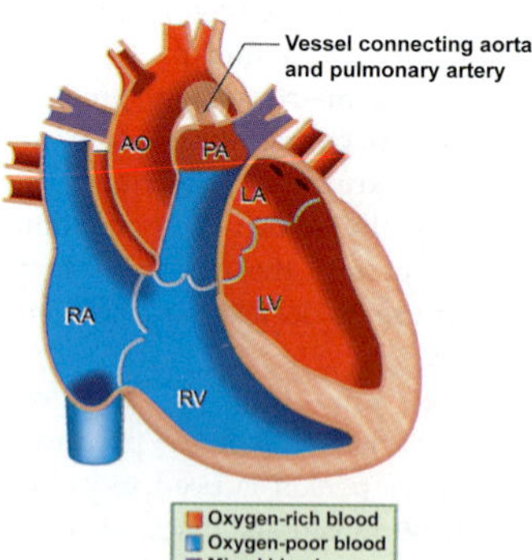

Fig.: *Patent ductus arteriosus*

Pathogen refers to a microorganism capable of causing disease.

Pathologic grief is the condition in which a person cannot tolerate a grief and resulting in illness.

Pathological fractures are the fractures resulting due to underlying pathology and not due to any type of trauma, e.g. fracture occurring due to osteomyelitis.

Pathological tooth migration refers to the tooth displacement that occurs due to imbalance among the factors that maintain physiologic tooth position is disturbed by the periodontal disease.

Pathology is the study of abnormal (diseased) tissue conditions.

Pathosis refers to disease entity.

Pattern is a set of constraints operating to preserve the integration of parts under varying conditions or through time. The interaction throughout the life between hereditary and environment determines the expression of patterns. The two aspects of normal growth pattern are: Cephalocaudal gradient of growth, Scammon's growth curve.

Pattern theory replaced the summation theory whereby the patterns of neural impulses set up by the noxious stimuli were considered important.

Peak aerobic power is the maximum power output or peak oxygen intake that a person can attain safely when performing a large muscle activity as on treadmill.

Peak expiratory flow rate (PEFR) can be measured by a portable meter and is helpful in the diagnosis and management of patients with asthma.

Pediatric dentistry (AAPD-1999) is an age defined specialty that provides both primary and comprehensive preventive and therapeutic oral health care for infants and children through adolescence, including those with special healthcare needs.

Pediatric dentistry is concerned with the preventive and therapeutic oral healthcare of children from birth to adolescence.

Pediatrics is related to child.

Pedicle graft is the graft that remains attached to its donor site.

Peeso Reamers are rotary instruments used mainly for post-space preparations. They have safe ended noncutting tip. Their tip diameter varies from 0.7 to 1.7 mm. They should be used in brushing motion.

Pellagra is a nutritional disease occurring due to the deficiency of niacin. Endemic among poor peasants fed on maize. Greater part of niacin in maize is not available. Moreover, principal protein of maize, zein is deficient in essential amino acid tryptophan, the alternative source of niacin. It may develop 6–8 weeks of deficiency of niacin. Pellagra has been called the disease of three D's dermatitis, diarrhea and dementia.

Pellicle is a thin deposit which may form shortly after eruption on the exposed surface of teeth, i.e. it is the first step in plaque formation; a clear, thin covering containing proteins and lipids (fats) found in saliva. It is fully formed in 30 minutes and reaches its mature thickness of 0.1 to 0.6 microns within a day. It is free of bacteria. Brown pigment is due to presence of tannins in the pellicle. Acquired pellicles are composed of mucoproteins containing lipid material.

Pemphigoid is the term that generally refers to the number of cutaneous, immune-mediated, subepithelial bullous diseases that are characterized by the separation of basement membrane.

Pemphigus is a serious chronic skin disease with vesicle and bullae of different sizes. Etiology is still unknown. It is of many types such as pemphigus vulgaris, pemphigus vegetans, pemphigus foliaceus and pemphigus erythematosus.

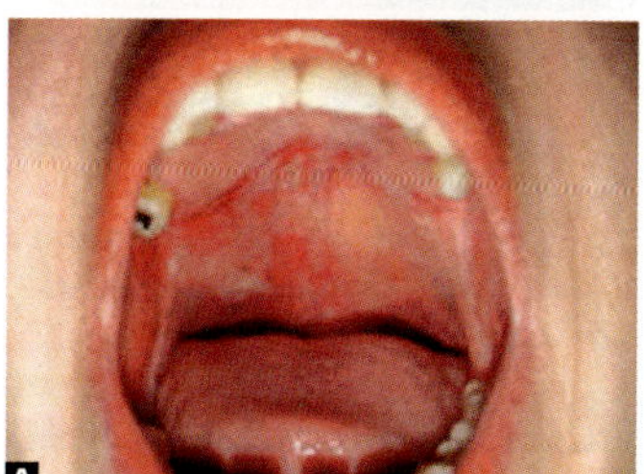

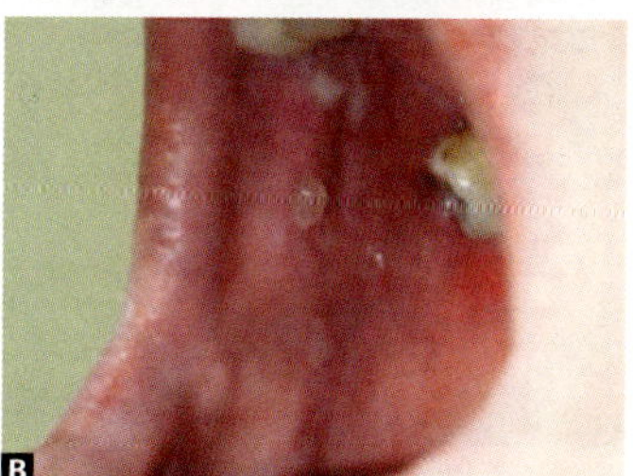

Figs A and B: *Pemphigoid*

Pemphigus erythematosus is a condition where there is occurrence of bullae and vesicles concomittant with the appearance of crusted patches. There may be fever and malaise. Even death may occur.

Pemphigus foliaceus is early bullous lesion rapidly ruptures and leaves masses of flakes or scales.

Pemphigus vegetans is a benign variant of pemphigus vulgaris. The fungoid masses are covered by purulent exudates. It shows inflamed border. It is of two types. Neumann type is more common. Early lesions present as large with denuded areas, while Hallopeau type is less aggressive and appear as pustules in the initial stage. These are followed by verrucous, hyperkeratotic vegetations. Gingival lesions appear as lace-like ulcers. Base is of granular/ cobblestone appearance.

Pemphigus vulgaris is an autoimmune disease. It is characterized by rapid appearance of vesicles and bullae. These lesions contain a thin watery fluid. Classically lesion may appear as a thin-walled bulla arising from mucosa. Bulla breaks rapidly and continues to extend peripherally. Pressure to an apparently normal surface will result in formation of a new lesion. On breaking of bullae, ulcers may appear shallow. A thin layer of epithelium peels away in an irregular manner leaving the denuded base. Edges of lesions continue to extend.

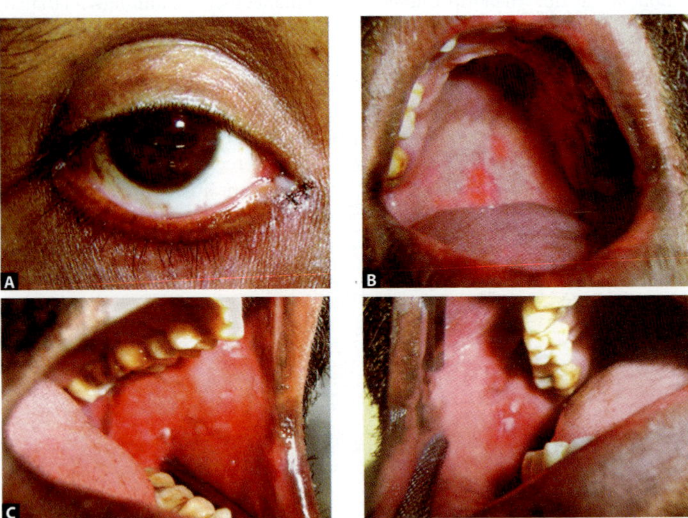

Figs A to C: *Phemphigus involving (A) Medial canthus of the eye; (B) Palatal mucosa; (C) Buccal mucosa*

Penetration coefficient is the combination of properties of viscosity, surface tension and contact angle which promotes rapid capillary penetration.

Penicillin contains a beta-lactam ring and inhibits the formation of peptidoglycan cross-links in bacterial cell walls (especially in Gram-positive organisms). This weakens the cell wall and water enters the cell by osmosis, causing cells to burst. Penicillin is bactericidal but can act only on dividing cells and is not toxic to animal cells, which have no cell wall.

PENS stands for percutaneous electric nerve stimulation is a pain management technique involving a combination of acupuncture needles and transcutaneous nerve stimulation.

Pentazocine produces analgesic drug with no potential abuse. It produces CNS analgesia, sedation and respiratory depression. Euphoria is not much. Some may feel nightmares and hallucinations. 30 mg IV of it is effective as 10 mg of morphine. It is more potent than morphine. It causes addiction.

Pentane is halogenated ether and was synthesized liquid. It is kept in opaque bottles to retard decomposition. It has a fruity odor. It is neither explosive nor flammable. It is the most potent of inhalation anesthetic drug. It is used with nitrous oxide/oxygen to produce any desired depth of anesthesia.

Pepsinogen is a component of gastric juice that is converted into pepsin by HCL.

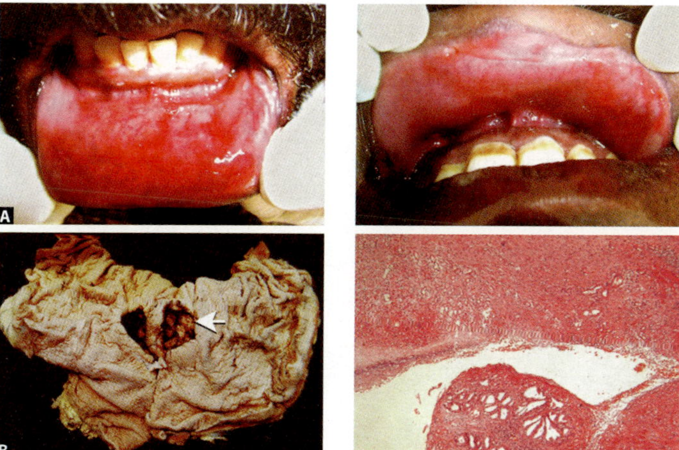

Figs. A and B: *(A) Phemphigus involving labial mucosa; (B) Macroscopic and microscopic presentation of peptic ulcer stomach*

Peptic ulcer applies to mucosal ulceration near the acid bearing regions of gastrointestinal tract. Most ulcers develop in the stomach or proximal duodenum. It may run in families. Smokers and anxiety-prone personalities are more prone to it. Emotional stress, disprins and other pain killers may cause it.

Perforated ulcer may be caused by nonsteroidal anti-inflammatory drug. Spillage of gastric content may cause severe peritonitis. There may be abdominal pain of sudden onset, nausea and vomiting. There will be hypovolemia, hypotension and fever with tachycardia.

Perforation refers to an opening between tooth and other oral structure. Perforations can occur at any stage while performing endodontic therapy that is during access cavity preparation or during instrumentation procedures leading to canal perforations at cervical, midroot or apical levels. (According to AAE) the perforation is defined as "the mechanical or pathological communication between the root canal system and the external tooth surface".

Periapical means around the apex of teeth.

Periapical abscess is an infection of the pulp of the tooth and tissues surrounding the base of the tooth. It is a suppurative process of dental periapical region. It may also develop due to traumatic injury. Tooth is extruded and becomes painful. Regional lymph glands are enlarged and fever develops. On X-ray, slight thickening of membrane is seen. Radiolucent area at apex is noted. Drainage if fails extraction of tooth is the remedy.

Periapical cemental dysplasia is a condition of unknown etiology. The lesion develops near the periodontal ligament around the apex of tooth and usually in a mandibular incisor area. It is discovered accidently during routine X-ray.

Periapical film is an intraoral film used to examine the entire tooth and supporting bone.

Periapical granuloma is usually described as a mass of chronically inflamed granulation tissue found at the apex of nonvital tooth. It is the most common sequelae of pulpitis.

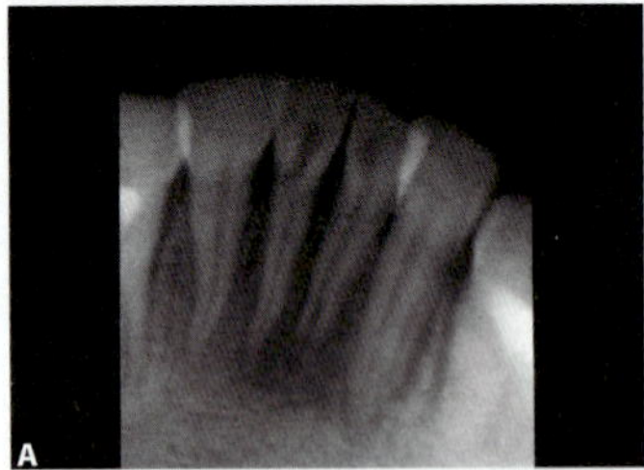

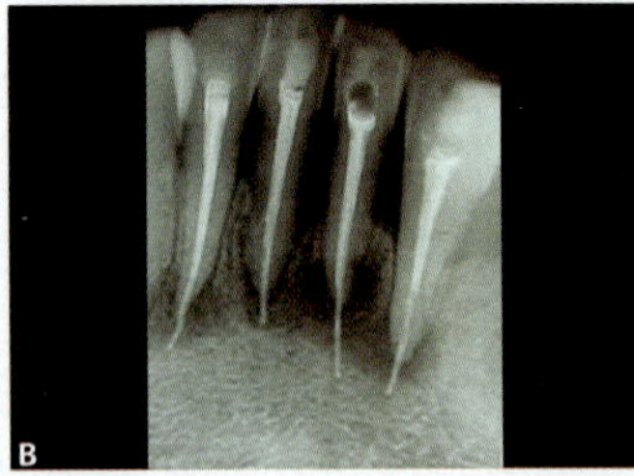

Figs A and B: *IOPA indicating (A) Periapical radiolucency; (B) Periapical abscess*

Due to infection a localized mass of granulation tissue is formed. There will be sensitivity to percussion and a mild pain on biting or chewing. Many cases may be asymptomatic. On X-ray, one can note thickening of periodontal ligament. Periapical granuloma appears as radiolucent area. It is slow-growing lesion.

Periapical radiograph is an intraoral film that shows the entire tooth and surrounding anatomy.

Pericarditis is a condition where acute rheumatic carditis serofibrinous pericarditis is often seen. Both layers of pericardium are thickened covered with thin fibrin giving bread and butter appearance. Chest pain is the most common presenting symptom. Pain increases in supine posture and is reduced in sitting posture. Person will develop dyspnea, fever, fatigue, abdominal pain and syncope. Pericardial rub is best heard over the left sterna border and is increased by sitting up and leaning forward. Healing produces fibrosis and adhesion between two layers.

Pericoronitis generally refers to inflammation of the gingiva in relation to the crown of an unerupted tooth, it generally occurs in a partially erupted or impacted third molar. The space present between the overlying flap and the erupting tooth provides an excellent environment for the accumulation food debris and nurturing of oral microorganisms which leads to infection and ultiately inflammation. The patient may have erythematous, edematous and suppurative type of lesion that is quite sensitive to pain along with radiating pain to nearby areas. There might be some amount of swelling at the angle of the mouth along with local lymphadenopathy of the affected side.

Perilymph is a watery fluid that fills the bony labyrinth of the ear.

Perio 2000 system: Diamond probe is a recently developed instrument, which combines the features of a periodontal probe with the silver sulfide sensor for detection of volatile sulfur compounds.

PER-IO-TOR are the instrument tips for scaling and root planing causing minimal removal of tooth structures.

Perio-aid is a toothpick holder, which is one of the most effective aids available for cleaning exposed furcation after periodontal therapy.

Perioalert: Immunoassay to detect serum antibodies to specific bacterial pathogens, monocytes response to LPS and peripheral neutrophil function. Site of sample is peripheral blood.

Periocare is a zinc oxide noneugenol periodontal dressing available in the form of paste-gel and setting occurs by chemical reaction. Paste consists of zinc oxide, calcium hydroxide, magnesium oxide and vegetable oils; Gel consists of resins, fatty acid, ethyl cellulose, lanolin and calcium hydroxide.

Periocheck is rapid chair side test kit developed to detect neutral proteases in GCF.

Periochip is a small, pale orange chip of baby's thumb nail 4 mm x 5 mm x 350 urn size, weighing 7.4 mg. The prescription chip contains 2.5 mg of chlorhexidine gluconate, of a biodegradable hydrolyzed gelatin matrix, cross-linked with glutaraldehyde and also containing glycerin and water.

Periocline is subgingival delivery system of 2% minocycline hydrochloride in syringable gel suspension formulation.

Period prevalence less commonly used method of prevalence. It measures frequency of all current cases existing during a definite period of time. It includes caries arising before, extending into the year as well as those cases arising during the year.

Periodex: 0.12% Chlorhexidine gluconate.

P

Periodontal means around tooth.

Periodontal abscess is a localized purulent infection within the tissue adjacent to the periodontal pocket that may lead to destruction of PDL and alveolus bone. It appears as an avid lunation of the gingiva along the lateral aspect of root. Gingiva appears red and edematous. Pus can be expressed from gingival sulfurs by digital pressure.

Periodontal flap refers to the section of gingiva or mucosa that is surgically separated from the underlying tissue to access the bone and root surfaces.

Periodontal ligament is a unique structure as it forms a link between alveolar bone and cementum. It is continuous with connective tissue of the gingiva and communicates with the marrow spaces through vascular channels in the bone. Periodontal ligament houses the fibers, cells and other structural elements like blood vessels and nerves.

Periodontal plastic surgery is defined as a surgical procedure performed to correct or eliminate anatomic, developmental or traumatic deformities of the gingiva or alveolar mucosa.

Periodontal pocket can be defined as pathologically deepened gingival sulcus exceeds 3 mm. Which occurs due to the destruction of supporting periodontal tissue.

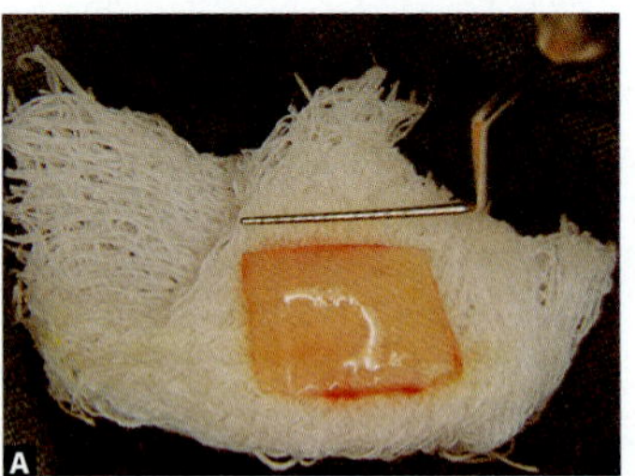

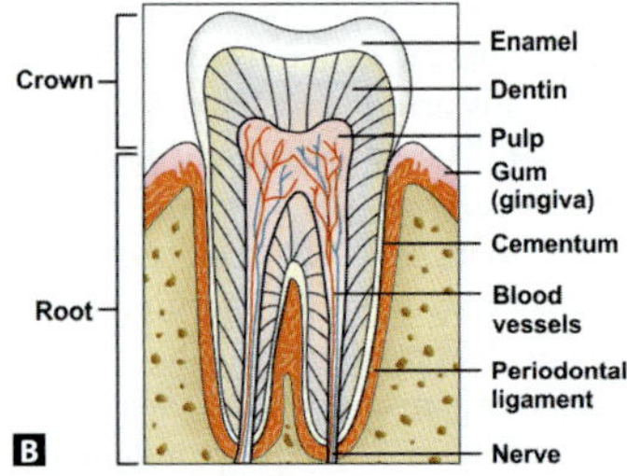

Figs A and B: *(A) Periodontal flap; (C) Peridontium*

Periodontal probe is the instrument that is used to locate and measure the pockets as well as to determine their course on individual tooth surface. The probe is a tapered rod like instrument, calibrated in mm with a round and a blunt tip. These probes are thin and the handle allows easy insertion into the pocket. Nabers probe is the best for evaluating the furcation areas.

Periodontal screening and recording (PSR) system is a device which is specially designed for faster screening and recording of the periodontal status of the patient. It uses a specially designed probe which has a ball tip of 0.5 mm and is color coded from 3.5 – 5.5 mm.

Periodontics is a branch of dentistry that is concerned with the diagnosis and treatment of disease of the supporting and surrounding tissues of tooth. Specialist is known as periodontist.

Periodontitis means inflammation of periodontium. Initially it starts as a simple marginal gingivitis as a reaction to calculus or plaque. There will be tiny ulceration of crevicular epithelium. Gingiva becomes more inflamed and swollen. Calculus may be present. Gingiva bleeds easily. Foul halitosis may be present. Teeth become mobile and dull on percussion. X-ray will show blunting of alveolar crest. If there is no excessive bone loss, the tooth can be saved.

Periodontium attaches the tooth to its bony housing. These are tissues that invest and support the teeth such as gingiva and alveolar bone. It provides resistance to forces of mastication, speech and deglutition. It defends against external noxious stimuli. It is the structures that surround and support the teeth.

Periodontoblastic space is a fluid-filled space located between the dentinal tubule and the cell-wall of the cytoplasmic part of the odontoblastic process. This interstitial fluid continues beyond the cytoplasmic part of the process and extends the full length of the tubule, surrounding remnants of the odontoblastic processes found in peripheral circumpulpal dentin. It plays an important role when tissue changes occur within the primary dentin.

Periodontology: The science that deals with the structures and

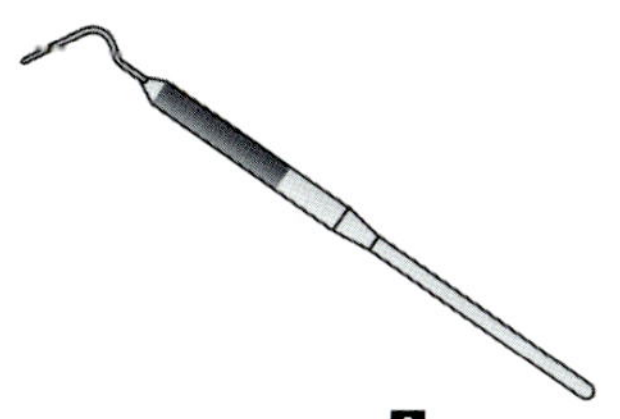

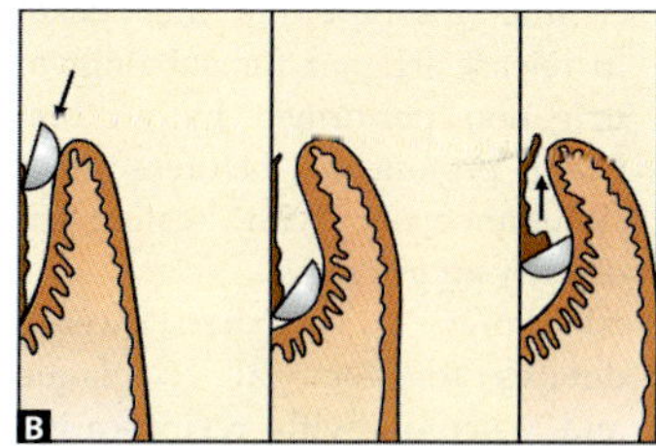

Figs A and B: *(A) Periodontal probes; (B) Periodontal scaling and root planning*

behavior of the periodontium in health and disease.

Periodontometer: Instrument used for detecting tooth mobility.

Periogard: Rapid chair side test kit for aspartate aminotransferase (AST). GCF collected is placed in tromethamine hydrochloride buffer is allowed to react with mixture of L-aspartic and a-Keto-glutaric acids for 10 minutes. If AST is present, the aspartate and α-glutarate are catalyzed to oxalacetate and glutamate.

Perioglass: Bioactive glass alloplast consisting of sodium and calcium salts, phosphates, silicon dioxide of irregular particles of 90–170 urn.

Periograft: Nonporous hydroxyapatite alloplast.

Periopac is premixed zinc oxide non-eugenol dressings. It contains calcium phosphate, zinc oxide, acrylate, organic solvents, flavoring and coloring agents, when this material is exposed to air or moisture, it sets by the loss of organic solvents.

Periopaper is blotter on which GCF is collected.

Periopik: Tip used for subgingival irrigation. It is a rigid metal cannula inserted into the pocket to release irrigant for subgingival irrigation performed by an oral health professional before scaling, simultaneously with scaling or directly after scaling.

Perioplaner/Periopolisher: Powered devices for removal of plaque and calculus with reciprocating motion.

Perio-probe: Electronic probe with a tip diameter of 0.5 mm and uses standardized probing force of 0.3–4 N.

Perioral dermatitis is an inflammatory disorder of facial skin of unknown cause in which papules and pustules are seen around mouth. There may be a clear zone around lip. There is no persistent erythema.

Perioscan is a chair-side diagnostic kit using BANA reaction to identify *Tannerella forsythia, P. gingivalis, Treponema denticola* and *Capnocytophaga species.*

Perioscopy consists of 0.99 mm diameter reusable fiberoptic endoscope over which is fitted a disposable sterile sheath. The new fiberoptic endoscope instrument fits into specially designed periodontal explorers with 24–46 power magnification and fiber-optic illumination, this device allows clear visualization into deep subgingival pockets and in furcations.

Periostat: It is subantimicrobial dose of doxycycline hyclate capsule of

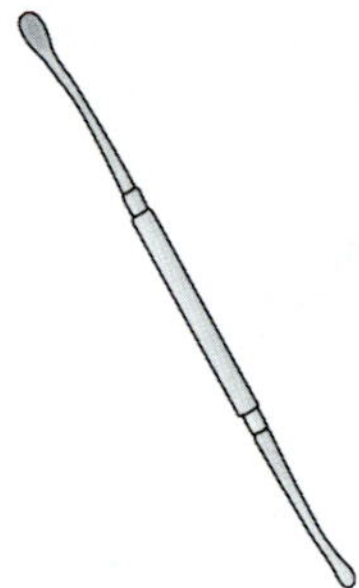

Fig.: *Periosteal elevators*

20 mg prescribed for patients with chronic periodontitis twice daily.

Periosteal elevator is a surgical instrument which is essentially used to reflect and move away the periosteum, once the incision is given, in order to expose the bone.

Periosteal suture is used to hold the apically displaced partial thickness flap.

Periosteum can be described as tissue covering the outer surface of the bone. Periosteum consists of inner layer which has osteoblasts surrounded by osteoprogenitor cells which has the potential to develop into osteoblasts and an outer layer which is rich in blood vessels and nerves.

Periotemp probe refers to the type of diagnostic probe that helps in detecting early inflammatory changes in the gingiva by detecting temperature rise. The probe detects pocket temperature difference of 0.1 degrees from the reference subgingival temperature. It consists of copper-nickel thermocouple connected to a digital thermometer attached to metal probe.

Periotest is device for determining tooth mobility by measuring the reaction of the periodontium to a defined percussion force which is applied to the tooth and delivered by a tapping instrument. Periotest scale ranges from – 8 to + 50:

– 8 to 9—Clinically firm teeth

10 to 19—First distinguishable sign of movement

20 to 29—Crown deviates within 1 mm of its normal position

30 to 50—Mobility is readily observed.

Periotriever: Highly magnetized instruments designed for retrieval of broken instrument tips from the periodontal pocket.

Periotron is the electronic machine used for measuring the amount of fluid or GCF collected on filter paper.

Periowave is a photodynamic disinfection system developed by Ondine Biopharma Corporation that utilizes low intensity lasers and wavelength-specific, light-activated compounds to specifically target and destroy microbial pathogens and reduce the symptoms of disease. The photosensitive compounds are topically applied in the gingival sulcus and the laser is used to activate the compounds and complete the disinfection.

Peripheral buttressing bone formation is the process of compensatory bone formation occurring on the external surface in an attempt to buttress bony trabeculae which is weakened by bone resorption.

Peripheral giant cell granuloma arises interdentally or from the gingival margin usually on labial surface. The growth may be sessile or pedunculated. It may vary in appearance from smooth regularly outshined mass to an irregularly shaped, multi-liberated mass with protuberates and surface indentations. It is usually painless unless painful ulceration occurs. It may be pain or spongy in consistency and color varies from pink to deep red or purplish red. Size ranges from 0.5 to 1.5 cm in diameter. It is seen as fusiform swelling. Ulceration is less common. It contains non-capsulated mass. Capillaries are numerous. Radiograph may show superficial destruction of alveolar margin. Surgical excision is needed.

Peripheral nervous system is where the nerves connecting the brain and spinal cord to other parts of body.

Peripheral neuritis is an inflammatory process occurring along the course of nerve trunk secondary to traumatic, bacterial, thermal or toxic causes. Neuritis of superior dental plexus has been reported when inflammation of sinus is present. The dental nerves frequently lie just below the lining mucosa or are separated by very thin osseous structure. These nerves are easily involved due to direct extension. Symptoms usually seen along with antral disease are pain, paresthesia and anesthesia of a tooth, gingiva or area supplied.

Peripheral neuropathy is a complication mostly occurring in diabetes. Neuron is the term for nerve. Nerves that go to your arms, legs, hands, feet are called peripheral nerves. Pathos means suffering. Many diseases diabetes, thyroid, rheumatoid and kidney disease can cause damage to peripheral nerves. Damage causes tingling, numbness, burning and pain. There are no medicines to improve the nerve function in peripheral neuropathy. Aerobic exercises can reduce the unpleasant feeling.

Peripheral odontogenic fibroma is a rare lesion. These are slow-growing often present for number of years. These are solid, firmly-attached gingival mass. Some lesions may contain a calcified stalk. Mature fibrous connective tissue stroma is present.

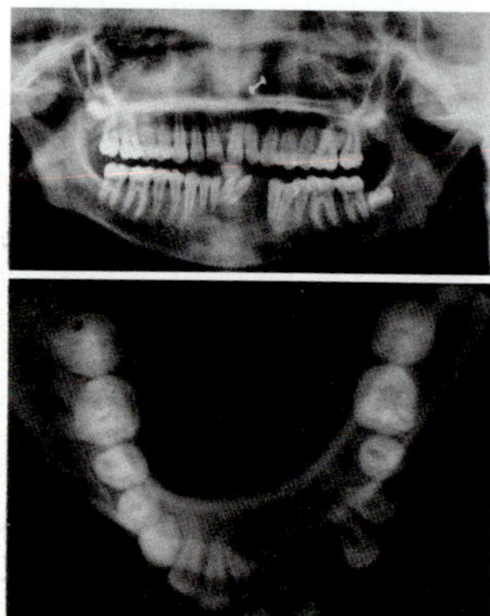

Fig.: *Peripheral giant cell granuloma*

Peripheral ossifying fibroma is a benign gingival overgrowth that is located in anterior maxilla and predominantly affecting women more common in younger age group. It is a well-demarcated mass on gingiva. It has sessile or pedunculated base. It is slightly reddened. Surface may be ulcerated. Several forms of calcification develop. Lesion may be surgically excised.

Peripheral vertigo also known as otologic or vestibular vertigo caused due to problem with vestibular system/nerve. It is generally asymptomatic with prominent nausea and recent upper respiratory tract infection, ototoxic drugs or Meniere's disease. Neurological examination may be normal. Nystagmus is horizontal or rotary.

Periradicular is around the root of a tooth.

Peristalsis is a wavelike, rhythmic contraction of the stomach and intestine that move food material along the GI tract.

Peritonsillar abscesses are infections; may come from tonsillar crypt or supratonsillar fossa. There may be pain, difficulties in swallowing, sore throat and fever cervical glands will be enlarged and possible trismus may develop. Tongue is coated with marked halitosis. Oropharynx may be narrowed.

Perleche also known as angular cheilitis presence of multiple ulcers at angles of mouth with burning sensation. Person is in habit of licking angles of mouth with burning sensations. In old age there may be mild leakage of saliva, ulcers are superficial.

Permanent alopecia is a full thickness burn, completely destroy the dermis and epidermis leaving translucent alopecia. Scarring or keloid formation leads to permanent alopecia.

Permanent dentition is the second dentition which replaces the complete set of primary dentition. This dentition consists of 32 teeth, i.e. 8 incisors, 4 canines, 8 premolars, 12 molars.

Permanent dentitions see permanent teeth.

Permanent teeth are the teeth that replace the deciduous or primary teeth.

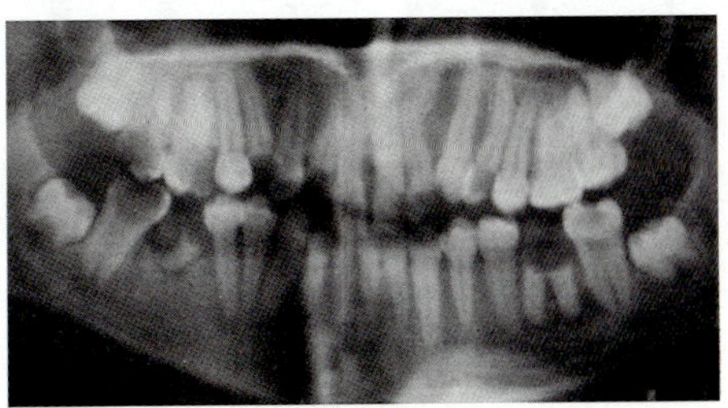

Fig.: *Permanent dentition OPG*

Pernicious anemia is due to impaired RBC maturation due to lack of B_{12}, it is a chronic, progressive, megaloblastic anemia of adults. *Clinical features:* It shows large RBCs. Hypochlorhydria, generalized weakness, anorexia, weight loss, dyspnoea, skin becomes smooth, dry and yellow. *Neurological symptoms* include tingling sensation in hand and feet, depression and irritability is seen in a few people. *Oral Manifestations:* Beefy red tongue, areas of patchy ulceration may be noted. Tongue may be fissured or lobulated. In some cases, it may become bald. A few patients may develop macular lesions in entire mucosa and may develop burning sensation. There may be hyperpigmentation of oral mucosa.

Persistent apical periodontitis is post-treatment apical periodontitis in an endodontically treated tooth. *Enterococcus faecalis* is found as most consistently reported organism in persistent apical periodontitis.

P

Pertussis is a disease of infants and preschool children below the age of 5 years. Infants below 6 months have the highest prevalence. Occurs in nasopharyngeal and bronchial secretions. It has three stages: Catarrhal stage lasts 10 days, paroxysmal stage lasts 2–4 weeks and convalescent stage lasts for 6–8 weeks. Complications include bronchitis, bronchopneumonia and bronchiectasis.

Pesso file is a long shank bur used in endodontic treatment.

Petechiae are capillary hemorrhage will appear red initially turning brown in a few days. Petechiae secondary to platelet deficiency or aggression disorders are usually not limited to oral mucosa.

Pethidine is a synthetic derivative of piperidine. It was discovered in 1939. Its actions are similar to morphine. Its primary action is on CNS and smooth muscle. Somatic and visceral pain is relieved together. It has anticholinergic properties also hence it is used

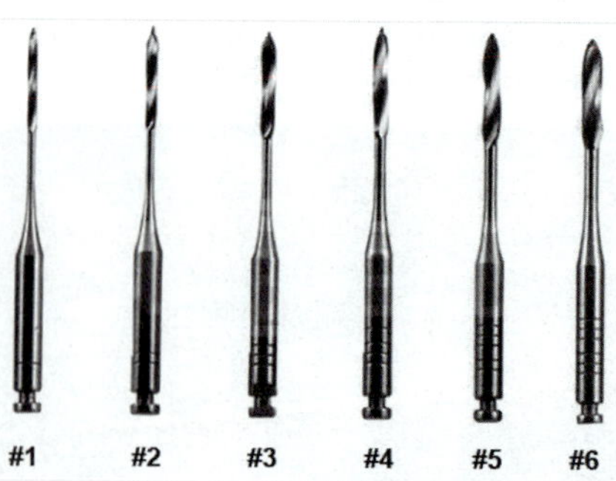

Fig.: *Pesso file*

for visceral pain also. Analgesia is achieved in 15 minutes after intake and lasts for 5 hours. 100 mg of pethidine analgesia is equivalent to 10 mg of morphine. It may produce drug abuse and dependence as there is a euphoric effect. It depresses respiration and does not slow rate of respiration. It is not very effective spasmogenic. It does not alter the size of pupil.

Petit mal seizures can be described as sudden cessation of conscious activity or loss of postural control. Individual looks blank for a few seconds. Person quickly regains his consciousness. Incidence decreases with age and seldom seen beyond 30 years of age. These seizures tend to occur shortly after awakening or during periods of inactivity. Clinically, consists of a brief lapse of consciousness, normally lasting from 5-10 seconds and only rarely beyond 30 seconds. Individuals exhibit no movement during the episode. EEG shows symmetrical 3 HZ spike and wave discharge throughout the brain during attack.

Petrovic's hypothesis (Servo system) explains the primary cartilage in which growth occurs by differentiation of chondroblasts can be modified with factors which affect the direction only and not the amount of growth. Secondary cartilage has a direct cell multiplication effect but more importantly indirect effects also play an important role, e.g. it explains the mode of action of the functional appliances directed at the condyle and the upper arch acts as a mould into which the lower arch adjusts itself such that optimal occlusion is established.

Peutz-Jegher's syndrome is an autosomal dominant characterized by hematomas of GI children often develop an oral pigmentation, multiple, focal, melanotic brown macules concentrated on lips. Macules may go up to 3-5 cms in size. Anterior tongue may be involved. Histologically these show basilar melanogenesis without melanocytic proliferation.

Phantom limb pain occurs after amputation of a limb, sensation may be felt for several months as that part is still intact. Pain is unpleasant and of intolerable nature.

Phantom pains occur in orofacial area. These pains are felt in missing structures as if still present. Edentulous areas are frequent sites of such pain. Some form of memory pattern remains present.

Pharmacokinetics deals with the study of drug in the body.

Pharmacology: Study of drugs.

Pharyngeal (branchial) arches, consisting of bars of mesenchymal tissue and separating from each other by pharyngeal pouches and clefts, initially give the head and neck their typical appearance, post-natal, the appearance of teeth and paranasal sinuses provide the face with its own personal characteristics. Each arch contains its own artery, nerve, muscles element and cartilage bar, or skeletal element. Endoderm of pharyngeal pouches gives rise to a number of endocrine glands and part of the middle ear.

Pharyngeal isthmus is the communication between the nasopharynx and the oropharynx. This isthmus can be closed (e.g., during swallowing) by elevation of the soft palate.

Pharynx is a median passage that is common to the alimentary and respiratory systems. It is divisible (from above downwards) into a nasal part (or nasopharynx) into which the nasal cavities open. An oral part (or oropharynx) which is continuous with the posterior end of the oral cavity. A laryngeal part (or laryngopharynx) which is continuous in front with the larynx, and below with esophagus.

Phenol compounds are disinfectants. Lipophilic viruses are susceptible but spores are resistant. If applied locally. It has a depolarized local anesthetic action. It may be used in alkaline phenol mouthwash containing 3% liquefied phenol.

Phenotype is the viable expression of the hereditary constitution of an organism.

Phenyl butazone is an anti-analgesic, anti-inflammatory drug used for the treatment of rheumatoid arthritis. It can produce bone marrow depression and gastrointestinal effects. These can produce oral ulcer hence should be avoided in dental diseases.

Phenytoin is a drug that is widely used in all epilepsies except petit mal epilepsy. It does not produce CNS depression. It limits the convulsions activity. Their side effect includes behavioral changes and megaloblastic anemia. Ataxia and diplopia are commonly seen. It may develop gingivitis.

Phenytoin gingival enlargement is an abnormal enlargement of gingiva due to use of phenytoin drug. Phenytoin (5–diphenylephentain) has been used to control seizures. Phenytoin selectively deposits int the cerebral cortex and stabilizes manual excitation by blocking or interfacing with Ca^{+2} influx across cell membrane. The clinical onset of gingival overgrowth is reported after 1 month of use of the drug. This reaches its maximum by 12 to 18 months.

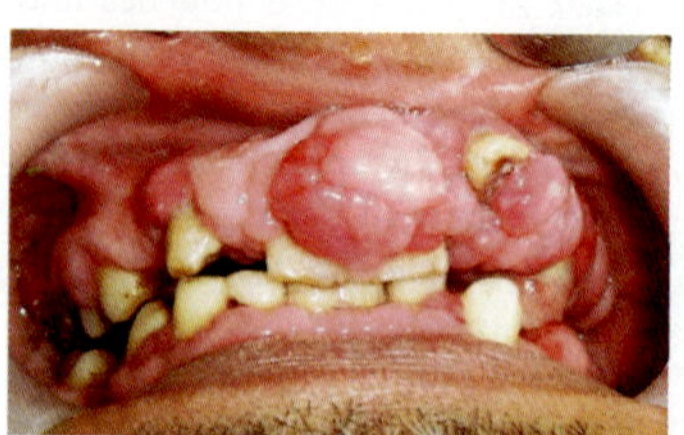

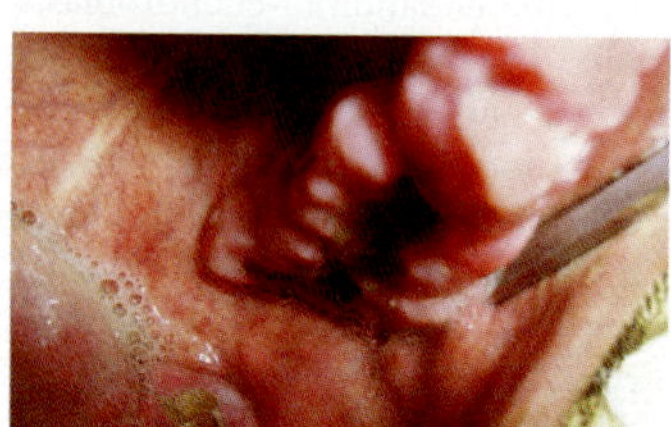

Figs A and B: *Phenytoin-induced hyperplasia*

Phenytoin gingivitis overgrowth involves interdental papillae which become bulbous and overlap the teeth. Typically gingiva is firm and becomes orange in color.

Pheumothorax is an accumulation of air in the pleural space causing collapse of the lung.

Phoenix abscess is defined as an acute inflammatory reaction superimposed on an existing chronic lesion, such as a cyst or granuloma. In other words, phoenix abscess is an acute exacerbation of a chronic lesion.

Phosphorescent re-emission or tissue fluorescence is a photochemical interaction which may be used as a diagnostic method to detect light reactive substances in tissue.

Phosphorus is a chemical element that is essential for most metabolic processes. Phosphorus depletion can occur from prolonged and excessive intake of aluminium hydroxide, antacid which binds dietary phosphate in the gut. Factures include anorexia, malaise and weakness.

Photoablation is a photothermal interaction which refers to the removal of tissue by vaporization and superheating of tissue fluids, coagulation and hemostasis.

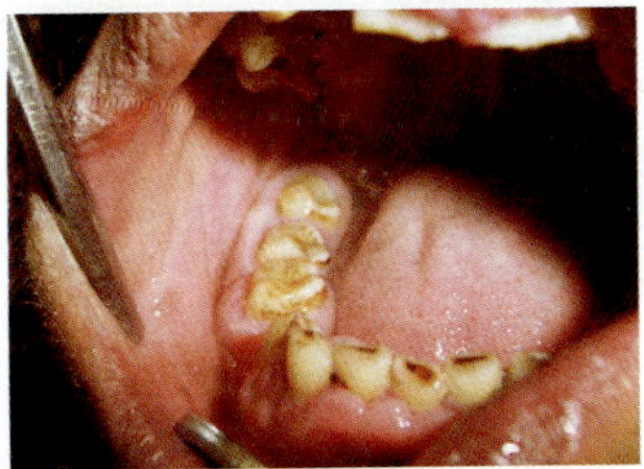

Fig.: *Phenytoin-induced hyperplasia*

Photo plasmolysis describes how tissue is removed through the formation of electrically charged ions and particles that exist in a semi-gaseous, high-energy state.

Photosensitization is sometimes an enhanced response of skin to UV irradiation. The agent responsible is usually a chemical present in skin which absorbs UV and transfers the energy to adjacent tissue molecules in a photochemical reaction.

Photo-acoustic interactions, which involve the removal of tissue with shock wave generation.

Photoactivated disinfection (PAD) is a breakthrough in the fight against pathogenic bacteria. It is a fast, effective and minimally invasive disinfection system which is considered to kill more than 99.99% of bacteria in the endodontic biofilm.

Photo-disassociation is the breaking apart of structures by laser light.

Photo-disruption see photo-disassociation.

Photodynamic therapy is a photochemical interaction which is the therapeutic use of lasers to induce reactions in tissues for the treatment of pathologic conditions.

Photopyrolysis is a photo-thermal interaction which means burning away of tissues.

Phrenic nerve is one of the most important nerves in the body as it is the only motor supply to the diaphragm. This nerve arises from the (ventral rami of) spinal nerves C_3, C_4 and C_5 the contribution from C_4 being the greatest. The nerve descends vertically through the lower part of the neck, and then through the thorax to reach the diaphragm. Some terminal branches enter the abdomen.

Phrynoderma means toad skin. A nutritional deficiency which develops due to Vit A, E, B and essential fatty acids. Phrynoderma is attributed to essential fatty acid. The disease characterized by horny papular eruption on the posterior and lateral aspect of limbs, back and buttocks also known as follicular hyperkeratosis.

Phycomycosis is of two types superficial and visceral. The only clinical manifestation of the disease is the appearance of a reddish black nasal turbinate. Infection of head organisms is characterized by classical syndrome of uncontrolled diabetes, cellulitis and meningoencephalitis. Diagnosis made at autopsy.

Physical abuse according to WHO is that which results in potential harm from an interaction and lack of interaction which is reasonable within the control of parent or person in a position of responsibility, power and trust.

Physical activity is an activity of any type which induces an increase over resting expenditure. It may be planned sport or unplanned domestic work.

Physician (According to WHO) is a person who, has been regularly admitted to a medical school duly recognized in the country and has successfully completed the prescribed courses of studies in medicine and has acquired the requisite qualification to be legally licensed to practice medicine using independent judgment to promote community and individual health.

Physiologic tongue thrust comprises the normal tongue thrust swallow of infancy.

Physiologic occlusion is said to be present where there are no signs of disease and is not indicative of any type of treatment.

Physiological saline solution is 0.9% sodium chloride solution which exerts an osmotic pressure equal to

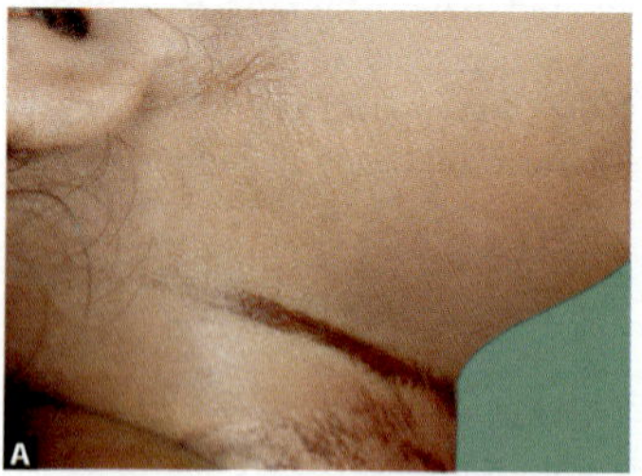

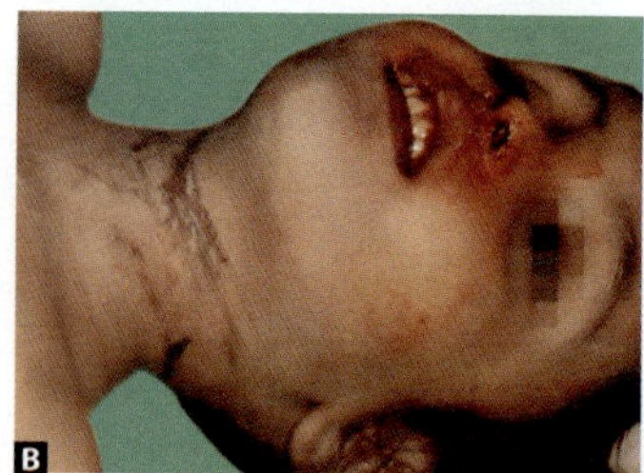

Figs A and B: *Physical abuse*

that of blood. It is compatible with blood.

Pigmented mole is a congenital developmental tumor-like malfor-mation of skin and mucus membrane. It is a superficial lesion of nevus cells. These may be congenital or acquired. Acquired have been classified as compound nevus, junctional nevus, spindle cell nevus and blue nevus. Treatment is not possible mole being multiple in number.

Pindborg tumor is an odontogenic tumor also known as calcifying epithelial odontogenic tumor (CEOT) was first discribed by Pindborg in 1958 develops in middle age; mandible is more affected than maxilla. This tumor is very similar to ameloblastoma. Radiographically it appears as either a diffuse or a well-circumscribed unilocular radiolucent area. Bony trabeculae may be irregular. Calcified flecks are distributed throughout the lesion, enucleation has to be done.

Pineal tumors are the tumors of pineal gland that seated very deep in brain are most common during childhood and produce precocious puberty in males. Tumor may compress aqueduct of sylvius to produce hydrocephalus and headache.

Pinealocytes are the small cells that form the pineal body.

Pit is a pinpoint depression in the occlusal surface of a tooth. It is defined as a small pinpoint depression located at the junction of developmental grooves or at terminals of those grooves. The central pit describes a landmark in the central fossae of the molars where developmental grooves join (Ash, 1993).

Pit and fissure caries are those originating in the pits and fissures found on the lingual surface of maxillary anterior teeth and on the buccal, lingual and occlusal surfaces of the posterior teeth.

Pit and fissure sealant is a material that is mainly composed of fluid resins that are applied to posterior occlusal surfaces of caries-prone teeth to seal pits and fissures from bacterial action. Principal monomer

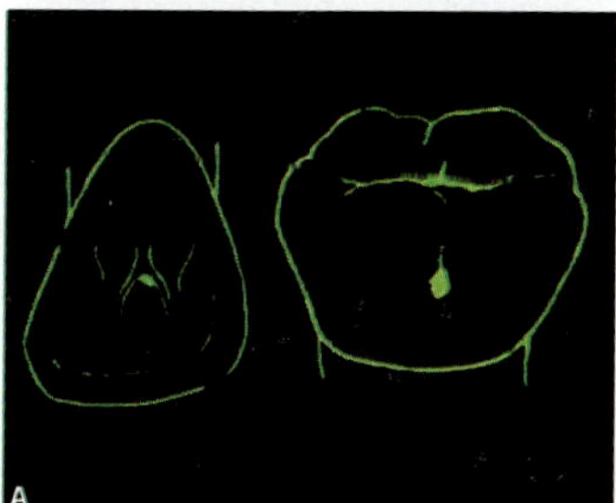

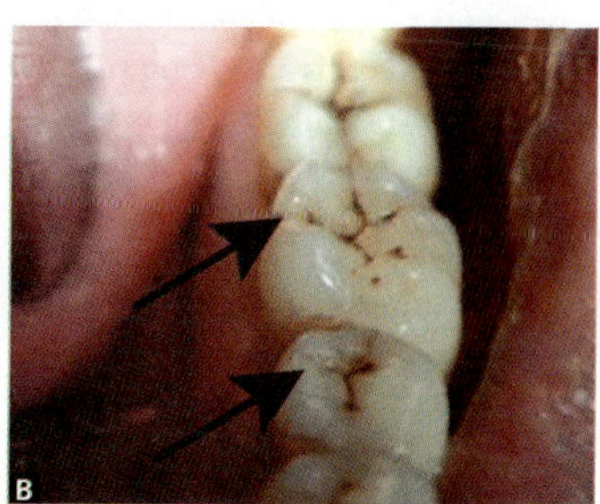

Figs A and B: *(A) Buccal pit; (B) Pit and fissure caries*

used in Bis GMA. It may be lightly filled with ceramic filler particles to improve wear resistance.

Pitch is the distance between two cutting edges. A file with short pitch has more flutes when compared to file with longer pitch. U-shaped grooves with radial lands of profile.

Pituitary tumors compress optic chiasma producing bitemporal hemianopia, optic atrophy and diabetes insipidus secretory tumors have Cushing's disease, gigantism or acromegaly.

Pityriasis Rosea is an unknown skin eruption of unknown etiology. There are superficial light red macules or papules. Lesions may accompany headache, low-grade fever and enlargement of lymph glands. Disease occurs seasonally. Lesions occur only on buccal mucosa. These are asymptomatic and require no treatment.

Placebo effect: Positive response from nonmedicine part.

Planing refers to smoothening of root to remove infective and necrotic tooth substance.

Plantar fasciitis: Planta is the Latin word for bottom of your foot. It is a tough band of tissue giving support to the arch of foot. Prolonged standing, excess activity may cause band tight causing pain. This pain is worst in the early morning and improves with continued walking. It is treated with anti-inflammatory medication.

Plaque is a highly variable entity resulting from the colonization and growth of microorganisms on the surfaces of the teeth and oral soft tissues and consisting of a number of microbial species embedded in an extracellular matrix. It sticks to tooth surface and has to be removed with food it provides nourishment for bacteria. Plaque grows thicker and results in caries and periodontal disease.

Plasma cell gingivitis is considered to be allergic response or hypersensitivity reaction to some component of chewing gum, dentifrice or diet. It is also known as atypical gingivitis plasma cell gingivostomatitis or plasma cell granuloma (localized form). *Clinical Features:* More common is young females. There is intense hyperemia and edema of free and attached gingival. Sharply demarcated from alveolar mucosa that appears red soft and friable with fissuring of commissures (chalets and glorifies common). Patient complains of burning recreations and is sensitive to dentifrices and legibly seasoned foods.

Plasma cells refer to effector cells.

Plasma dental probe is effective for tooth disinfection. Plasma emission spectroscopy identifies atomic oxygen as one of the likely active agents for the bactericidal effect.

Plasmacytoma is a solitary bone tumor and biopsy shows plasma cell histology. There is an absence of myeloma cells. Anemia is not present; clinical features are similar to multiple myeloma, i.e. pain, swelling and pathological fracture. Surgical excision followed by radiotherapy suits the patients.

Plaster of paris is a gypsum product, used to make models of teeth. It is a dry form and is commonly used for immobilization of fractures. The plaster sets in a given shape. Conversion is irreversible. It can be used as a slab or a cast. Plaster slab covers only a part of the circumference of limb. It is used for soft tissue injuries and for reinforcing plaster casts. Plaster cast covers whole of a circumference of a limb.

Plastic instruments are blunt double-end instruments having round or flat ends and are used for inserting fillings. One can manipulate linings with it.

Plasticizer is a small molecule that when added to a polymer lowers its glass transition temperature and increases the rate at which solvents penetrate the polymer.

Plate culture refers to the culture which is grown on a medium, usually agar or gelatin, on a Petri dish.

Platinized gold foil is prepared as gold foil except that a layer of platinum is sandwiched between two layers of gold and hammered. Platinum makes 15% of the alloy. It increases the hardness of the alloy. Disadvantage is that it makes finishing more time consuming.

Platysma is the most superficial muscle of the neck. Like the muscles of the face it lies in the superficial fascia. It is a remnant of an extensive sheet of subcutaneous muscle (called the panniulus carnosus) to be seen in some animals.

Plax is a prebrushing mouth rinse containing sodium benzoate and other nontoxic surfactants. It contains 7.5% alcohol. It reduces bacterial plaque.

Pleomorphic adenoma is a benign mixed tumor of gland. It can occur at any age. It accounts for more than 50% neoplasm of parotid gland. It is a slow-growing, well-delineated, exophytic growth. Neoplasm is solitary but in some cases

P

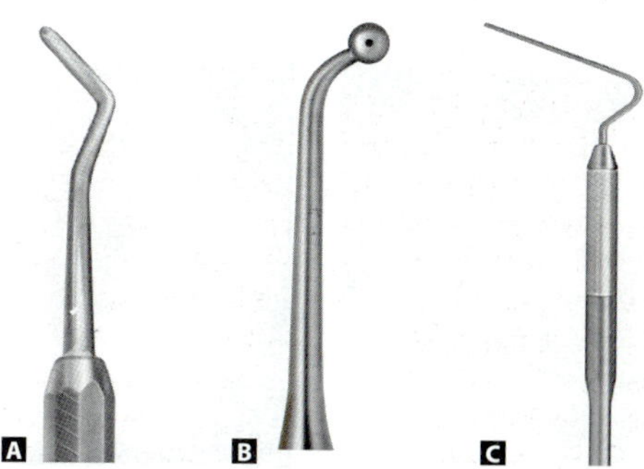

Figs A to C: *Plastic instruments; (A) Flat plastic; (B) Ball ended burnisher; (C) Pluggers*

there may be multiple recurrent lesions. Neoplasm is rubbery and painless. Overlying mucosa may remain intact. In lip, pleomorphic adenoma presents small, painless, well-defined, movable nodular lesion. *Clinical Features:* Well-circumscribed, lobulated, globular mass surrounded by capsule, cut surface is not smooth and shows cystic and hemorrhagic areas. There may be intermittent growth. It is not fixed to deeper structures. Size may or may not reach beyond 2 cms. Surgical excision is the line of treatment.

Plethysmography is a method for assessing the changes in volume and has been applied to the investigation of arterial disease because the volume of the limb or organ exhibits transient changes over the cardiac cycle. Plethysmography in limb or digit can be performed using air-filled cuffs or mercury in rubber strain gauges. As the pressure pulse passes through the limb segment, a wave form is recorded which relates closely to that obtained by intra-arterial cannulation. The same principle can be used to assess tooth vitality. Presence or absence of a waveform can indicate the status of the tooth.

Pleural effusion is defined as excessive accumulation of fluid in the pleural space. The collection of grossly purulent fluid is known as empyema. Presence of blood and lymphatic fluid in pleural space is called hemothorax and chylothorax respectively. Important causes of pleural effusion are pneumonia, tuberculosis, cardiac failure, cirrhosis and malignancy.

Plummer: Vinson syndrome is iron deficiency anemia develops due to chronic loss, inadequate dietary iron intake, faulty iron absorption or increased requirement for iron. It may develop at any age. One can notice cracks and fissures at corners of mouth, smooth red painful tongue with atrophy of filliform papillae. Koilonychia develops and nails become brittle.

P

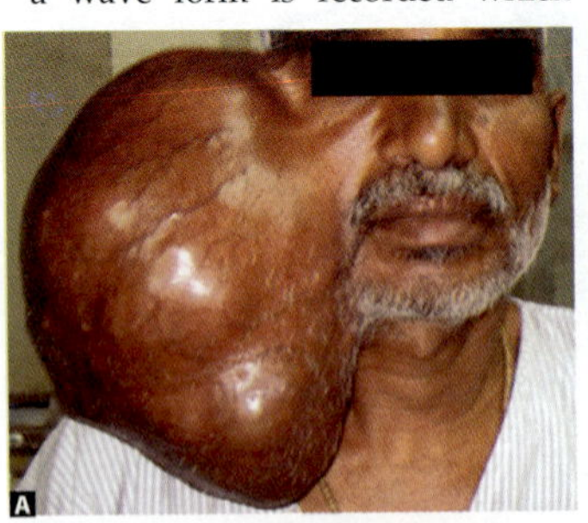

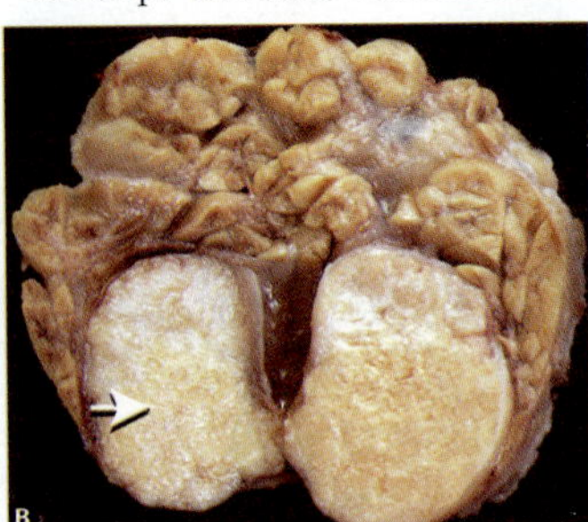

Figs A and B: *(A) Pleomorphic adenoma; (B) Pleomorphic adenoma salivary gland*

Anemia responds well to iron therapy and a high protein diet.

Plunging ranula is a slow-growing swelling in the floor of mouth as well as in one of the submandibular region below the angle of mandible. Cross fluctuation is present between oral and cervical swelling.

Pneumoconiosis may lead to mild chronic obstructive disease. Rare cases go into 'Progressive Massive Fibrosis'. In it large rubbery nodules of black fibrosis and dust are formed. Lesion develops as a radiating lesion around the bronchioles.

Pneumonia is defined as the infection of the lung parenchyma (alveoli and distal airways) and interstitium of the lung.

Pneumonitis is an inflammation of lung tissue caused by infective agent. Majority are caused by virus but bacteria and fungus may also cause it. Viral pneumonia causes mild cough, sometimes productive, mild fever and dyspnea. Symptoms of bacterial pneumonia are more marked. Patient looks ill, fever and chest pain develops. X-ray chest helps in diagnosis. Antibiotics such as erythromycin are helpful.

Pog soft-tissue pogonion is the most prominent or anterior point on the chin in the midsagittal plane.

Point angle is an angle in cavity formation formed by junction of 3 walls.

Point prevalence is a number of all current cases (old and new) of a disease at one point in time relation to a defined population. Point prevalent can be made specific for age, sex and other relevant factors.

Poison is any substance which, when induced by any route in particular quality, produces ill-health, disease or death.

Poisson's ratio is the ratio of transverse contraction per unit dimension to elongation per unit length.

Poliomyelitis is the disease where the causative agent is poliovirus which has three serotypes 1.2 and 3. Most outbreaks are due to type I virus. In a cold environment, virus can survive for 4 months, feces for 6 months. Cases are most infectious 7 to 10 days before and after onset of symptoms. Incubation period is 7-14 days. In paralytic polio of 1% cases virus invades CNS and causes varying degrees of asymmetrical flaccid paralysis. Fever with paralysis is highly suggestive of polio. There may be signs of neck and back muscles.

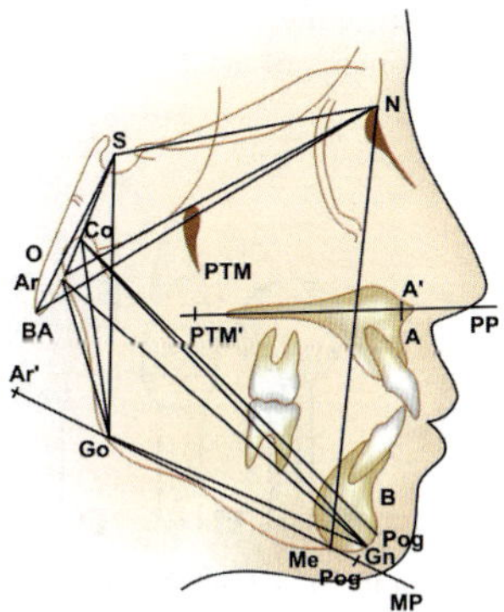

Fig.: *Ref. points and planes*

Paralysis is descending starting from hip to come down to knees. Paralysis reaches its maximum within 4 days. There is no specific treatment. Proper vaccination helps in prevention.

Polishing is a prophylactic procedure and is indicated when there are surface irregularities serving as plaque trap due to roughness of surface. It removes stain, plaque and acquired pellicle by using an abrasive polishing paste in a rubber cup attached to a slow-speed handpiece.

Polishing instruments are those instruments that are designed to perform the polishing and finishing action once the whole procedure is completed; it is mostly used with handpiece. Finishing burs and stones are used for smoothing cavity margins.

Polyacid-modified composite resins (or compomers) contain calcium aluminium fluorosilicate glass filler and polyacid components. They contain either or both essential components of a GIC, but are not water-based and therefore no acid–base reaction can occur. As such, they cannot strictly be described as GICs. They set by resin photo polymerization. The acid-base reaction occurs in the intraoral moisture and allows fluoride release from the material.

Polyarteritis nodosa is a noninfective necrotizing vasculitis involving the small and medium-sized muscular arteries of any organ. Nodular indurations and focal dilatations may be seen in course of affected arteries.

Polychromatic X-ray beam is a beam containing many different wavelengths of varying intensities.

Polycystic kidney is the most common inherited disorder. There is enlargement of both kidneys due to focal cystic dilatation of tubules. There may be accompanied hepatic cyst and mitral valve prolapsed. Grossly kidneys are huge but maintain shape. Cysts contain clear yellow fluid to gelatinous red or brown material in case of hemorrhage. Infantile polycystic kidney is rare.

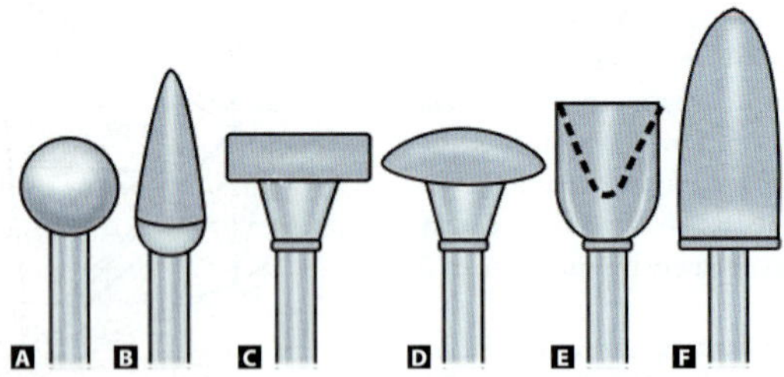

FigsA to F: *Polishing instruments (A) Huey Mandrel; (B) Moor mandrel; (C) Pinhead mandrel; (D) Polishing brushes; (E) Abrasive rubber cups and discs for Huey Mandrel; (F) Mounted fine abrasives*

Polycythemia is a condition where there is an abnormal increase in number of circulating all blood cells. It is manifested as headache, dizziness, tinnitus, visual disturbances and mental confusion. Skin is flushed or reddened. Spleen is enlarged. Gastric belching is common. Oral mucosa becomes deep purplish red. Cyanosis in a few cases may be present. Submucosal petechiae are also common. RBC count may go above 10000,000 cells per cubic millimeter. Bleeding and clotting time remains normal. Oral mucosa becomes deep red to purple and gingiva can be edematous. Gingiva may bleed easily. There can be excessive bleeding after oral surgical procedures. No specific treatment is available.

Polycythemia vera is a neoplastic proliferation of bone marrow stem cells resulting in high number of circulating red blood cells. Production of RBCs is uncontrolled. Cause of this is unknown. Disease has a gradual onset. Patient complains of headache, dizziness, tinnitus and pruritus. Some feel fatigue, impaired mental ability and visual disturbance. Face becomes reddish purple. The RBC count goes as high as 8-12 million/ mm^3 of blood. Total blood volume rises and blood viscosity increases. Platelet count is increased. Serum uric acid level goes up very high. Complications may lead to myocardial and cerebral infarctions. Patients may develop thrombophlebitis. Over production of uric acid produces gout. Acute leukemia is the terminal stage of polycythemia disease leads to impaired blood flow, vascular stasis and poor circulation.

Polymorphonuclear leukocytes (PMNS) *see* neutrophils.

Polymyositis: Dermatomyositis is an acute or chronic inflammatory disease of muscle and skin that may occur at any age.

Polyneuropathy is carcinomatous and myelomatous polyneuropathy that develops even before detection of primary tumor. Presenting features include motor weakness, muscle atrophy and sensory loss in limbs.

Polyols are artificial sweeteners, the most commonly known polyols namely sorbitol, mannitol and xylitol have the same caloric content as sucrose although less sweetness. Products sweetened by polyols have been described as sugar-free.

Polyphyodont is possessing several sets of teeth during a lifespan.

Polysaccharide is a large carbohydrate polymer formed by linking many monosaccharides in a sequence.

Polysulfide was the first rubber impression material developed. It has many useful properties such as accuracy of detail; lead dioxide is the catalyst giving strong odor and results in staining of clothes.

Pontic is an artificial tooth, i.e. it is the component of a bridge that replaces the missing teeth.

Population at risk is also known as defined risk and is crucial in epidemiological studies. It provides the denominator for calculating rates which are essential to measure the frequency of disease and study its distribution and determinants.

Porcelain veneer-ultra-thin shells of ceramic material bonded to the front of the tooth.

Porcelain jacket crowns are the oldest type of tooth colored crown. It consists of an even layer of porcelain of 1-2 mm thick covering the entire crown. Conventional dental porcelain is more like a glass than what is used for domestic purposes. It is relatively brittle and can be broken easily before cementation. It has following advantages, i.e. esthetics, brittleness, dimensional stability, economical and resistance to plaque accumulation. disadvantages include the marginal fit and compromise of tooth substance.

Porokeratosis here the plaques are surrounded by raised border of epidermal proliferation. Plaques are produced by mutant clones of epidermal cells. On section, oral lesions show characteristic cornoid lamella.

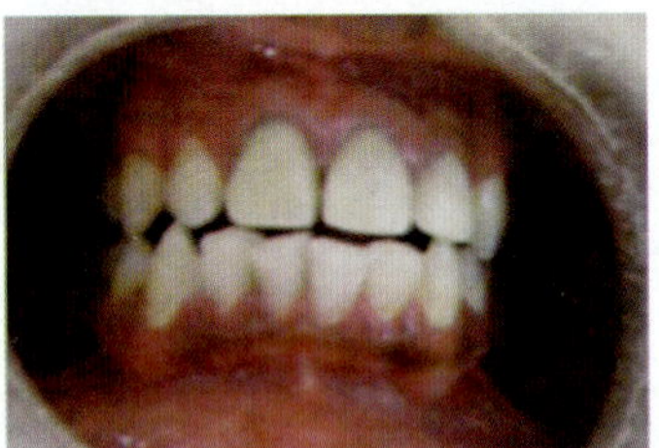

Fig.: *Porcelain jacket crowns*

Porosity is a state in which there are voids in a solid.

Porous bones are said to have occurred when adults achieve peak bone thickness around age 20-30 years. After middle age bones become thin and brittle. X-ray may show wider, thin trabeculation known as osteoporosis.

Portal hypertension is said to have occurred where portal vein pressure more than 5 mm Hg above inferior cava pressure is termed portal hypertension. It may be caused by portal vein occlusion. Cirrhosis and veno-occlusive disease may predispose it. It may produce esophageal varices and hemorrhoids.

Positioner is a soft plastic appliance used immediately after the fixed orthodontic appliances are removed.

Positive health implies the notion of complete and perfect functioning of body and mind.

Positive reinforcement is a behavior management technique applied to children to obtain desired positive behavior. Occurs if a pleasant consequence follows the response, e.g., a child rewarded for good behavior following dental treatment.

Post-crown is generally used when root has been filled. Natural crown is cut off and a post is fitted down the root canal. Artificial crown is made on this post. Post may be gold casting or of stainless steel.

Post-herpetic neuralgia pain manifested in the distribution of affected area. In younger patients, pain generally revolves within a few weeks but in older people, pain may continue for years. Even powerful analgesics fail.

Post is an endodontic pin which can be made with different materials such as metal or carbon and placed in the root canal. Its function usually is to provide support for a grossly decayed tooth. It is available in prefabricated form; can be customised also according to the morphology of the canal.

Postmortem caloricity occurs where body instead of coming down to normal temperature after death, shows a rise of temperature which persists for an hour or so. It is due to action of microorganisms in living body. It may happen in tetanus, cholera, rheumatic fever, abscess and strychnine poisoning.

Postmortem eye changes: There will be loss of lusture in the eyes. One will notice loss of papillary corneal and conjuctival reflexes. Cornea becomes opaque, hazy or cloudy. It becomes soft and pits on pressure. Shape of pupil may change from roundness to oval.

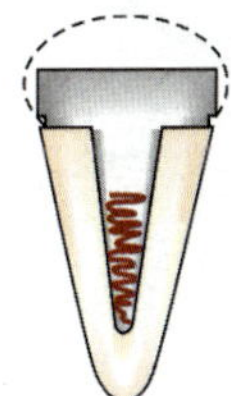

Fig.: *Post-crown*

Postmortem finding of mercury poisoning: Postmortem will show erosion in mouth and esophagus. The mucus membrane of stomach becomes salty gray with multiple cracks and fissures. Kidneys are found enlarged and deeply congested with minute hemorrhagic spots. Liver and heart show fatty degeneration.

Postmortem findings of carbon monoxide poisoning: Body surface especially lips and fingers appear to be bright red or cherry color. Irregular patches of bright red color are found over anterior surface of body. Blood becomes fluid and bright red. Lungs are edematous. Petechial hemorrhages are seen on brain and meninges.

Post mortem lividity is a reliable sign of death and gives information about the position of the body at the time of death. It helps to estimate the time since death and its color may suggest the cause of death.

Post-syncope phase the patient may demonstrate pallor, nausea and weakness and sweating which can last from a few minutes to several hours.

Post-traumatic neuralgia is the unremitting, bright burning pain which suggests painful neuritis. It may be accompanied with neuritic manifestation. Neuritic pain is interrupted by paroxysms of typical neuralgic pain.

Post-tussive tongue ulcer occurs where the child having whooping cough presents with an ulcer of tongue. It is situated on the undersurface near frenulum linguae. It is round and edge is sloping. Yellowish or greyish slough is present at floor. It is soft in consistence and regional lymph glands are not enlarged.

Posterior bridge: Bridges replacing back teeth usually have full veneer crowns on abutment teeth.

Posterior cerebral artery occlusion arises from basilar artery and supplies occipital lobe. On occlusion visual cortex is affected. When thalamus is affected contralateral sensory loss may develop.

Posterior cranial base length (S-A) the magnitude of posterior cranial base length depends on posterior face height and the position of the fossa. Short posterior cranial bases occur in vertical growth patterns and skeletal open bites and gives poor prognosis for functional appliances therapy.

Posterior cranial fossa is the most posterior part of the base of the skull. The most prominent landmark is the foramen magnum. Anterior to the foramen magnum the wall of the fossa is formed by the basilar part of the occipital bone. Between the jugular foramen, laterally, and the anterior part of the foramen magnum, medially, there is a rounded elevation called the jugular tubercle.

Posterior superior nerve is a nerve that descends from the main trunk of the maxillary nerve just before it enters the infraorbital canal; the branch provides sensory innervations to the pulpal, gingival and osseous tissues.

Posterior teeth are the back teeth, i.e. Premolars and molars.

Posterosuperior alveolar nerve block used for posterosuperior alveolar nerves. It is given for anesthetizing the maxillary third, second and first molar (sometimes mesiobuccal root is not anesthetized) and overlying structures (buccal mucosa and bone).

Post-eruptive phase takes place after the teeth are functioning to maintain the position of the

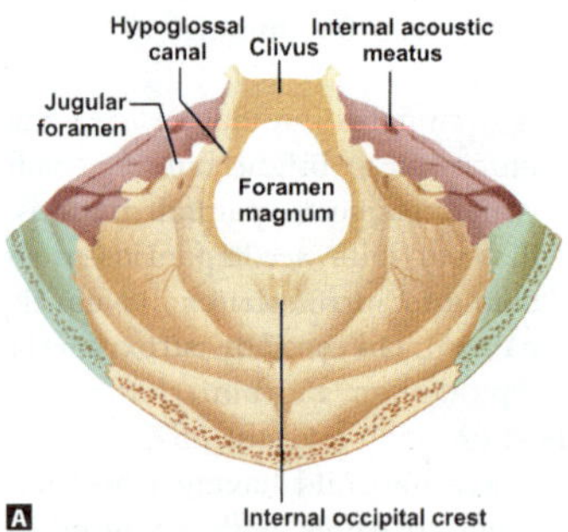

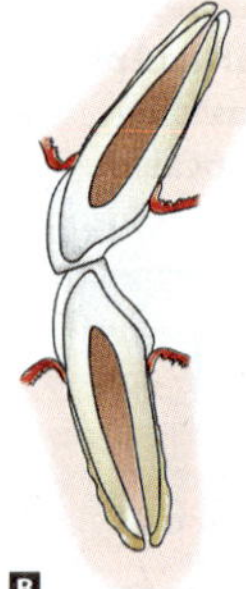

Figs: *(A) Posterior cranial fossa; (B) Post-eruptive phase*

erupted tooth in occlusion while the jaws are continuing to grow and compensate for occlusal and proximal tooth wear.

Post-lingual deafness is hearing impairment that is sustained after the acquisition of language, which can occur as a result of disease, trauma, or as a side-effect of a medicine. Typically, hearing loss is gradual and often detected by family and friends of affected individuals long before the patients themselves will acknowledge the disability. Common treatments include hearing aids and learning lip reading. Post-lingual deafness is far more common than pre-lingual deafness. Otosclerosis is a hardening of the stapes in the middle ear and causes conductive hearing loss.

Postnatal history refers to the history of a newborn child that includes the type of feed child is taking, vaccination or immunization status or any type of deleterious habit.

Postprandial is following a meal.

Postural hypotension is also known as orthostatic hypotension is a leading cause of transient loss of consciousness. Postural hypotension is defined as disorder of autonomic nervous system in which syncope occurs when patient assumes upright position.

Potassium is a chmical element depicted as K is present mostly intracellular. Diet generally contains 2 to 4 gram of potassium daily. Requirement is more during active growth. About 90% of excreted from body goes out through kidney. Death in potassium deficiency may result from respiration or cardiac failure.

Potency is the strength of a drug in terms of its ability to have a particular result.

Pott's disease is the most common manifestation of bone and joint infection by tuberculous bacilli. Tuberculous bacilli reach the spine by blood route. Lesions are rarely detected within six months of onset of symptoms. Symptoms include dull growing pain, anorexia, low-grade fever. It may start involving in the intervertebral disc producing narrowing of disc space. Anterior collapse results in kyphosis.

Powdered gold to consists of small appropriate particles blended with an organic indicator, compressed into small spheres and wrapped in gold foil. Powdered gold has greater mass than gold foil. It can be used both internally and on surface. Because of density it fills cavity rapidly. It may be overlaid with gold foil.

Poxviruses are the largest viruses to infect humans or animals. Small pox was the example of it.

P-Pronasale is the most prominent or anterior point of the nose (tip of the nose).

Pre-eclampsia and eclampsia is a complication of pregnancy characterized by hypertension, edema and proteinuria. Seizures may begin. There will be swelling of hands, face and legs. Headache and visual disturbance with altered mental status will be there. Petechial and bruising may be noted.

Pre-functional eruptive phase starts with initiation of root formation and made by teeth to move from its position within bone of the jaw to its functional position in occlusion. Has an intraosseous and extraosseous compartment. It has four stages: Root formation, movement, penetration, occlusal contact.

Premedication to anesthesia is given prior to anesthesia in order to alleviate anxiety, to enhance narcotic effect of general anesthetic agent and to minimize undesirable side effects of general anesthesia. Benzodiazepines are commonly used. Usual regime is to begin tranquilizing drug the day before the dental operation and continue a day after. Hypnotics are good to ensure a good night's sleep prior to dental surgery.

Pre-syncope is a condition where patient in sitting position complains of a feeling of warmth in neck and face, loses color (pale or ashen gray skin color). Patient may feel nauseous. Blood pressure at this time is at baseline level or lower, whereas heart rate increases and presyncope continues, yawning, increased depth of respiration and coldness in hands and feet are noted.

Precodial pulsations are a parasternal lift usually indicate right ventricular hypertrophy, pulmonary hypertension or left atrial enlargement.

Predentin (dentinoid) is a narrow band of uncalcified predentinal matrix. It is 20–25 mm in width. It is situated between the

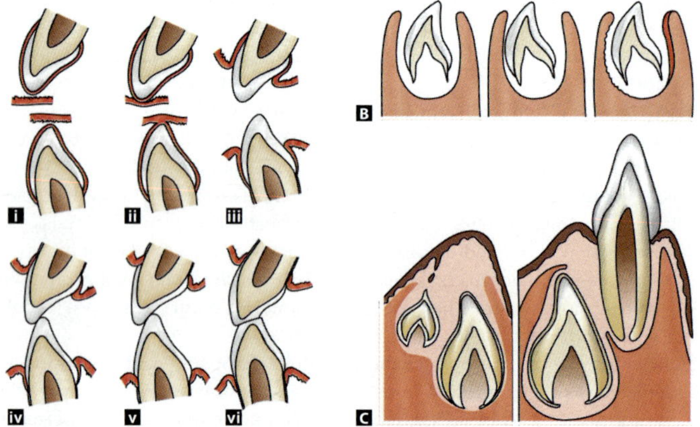

Figs A to C: *(A) Pre-eruptive phase; (B) Pre-eruptive phase–bodily movement; (C) Pre-eruptive-eccentric movement*

odontoblast layer and the mineralized dentin. It signifies a lag period in the mineralization of the dentin matrix. It is always present as long as odontoblasts are present. It is equal to osteoid in composition.

Predictive theory that is used to make predictions based on relationship between variable.

Predictive validity is the ability of a measurement made at one point in time to predict future status.

Pre-eruption bulge is a bulge present in the gingiva before the eruption of the crown into the oral cavity; the bulge is firm, slightly blanched due to the pressure of the erupting tooth and conforms to the contour of underlying crown.

Pre-eruptive phase is a phase of tooth eruption where all movements of primary and permanent formation to the time of crown completion end with early initiation of root formation.

Pregnancy associated enlargement may be marginal or gingival or may occur as a single or multiple tumors like masses. Enlargement is mainly related to elevated hormonal level during pregnancy which not only increases vascular permeability but also the subgingival microform with a predominance of p. intermediate.

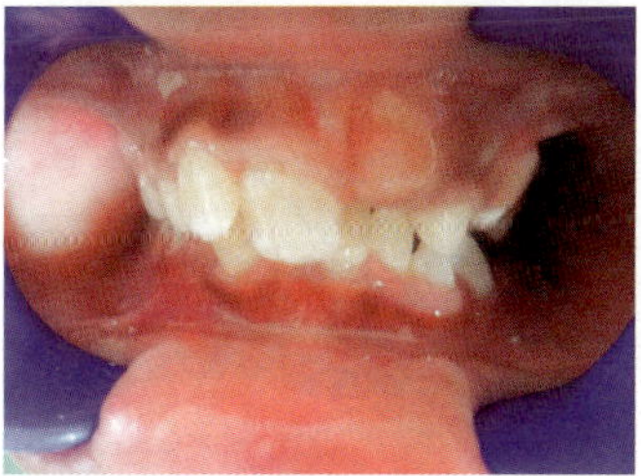

Fig.: *Pre-eruption bulge*

Pregnancy epulis is a soft swelling on the gum which bleeds easily and may be painful on ulceration. Onset is usually at the end of third month. It is reddish purple colored swelling on the gum more frequently seen in anterior region. It usually regresses after birth of a child.

Pregnancy granuloma is a hyperactive inflammatory response due to bacterial plaque mediated by systematic condition, it usually occurs during the 1st and 3rd trimester of pregnancy. *Clinical Features:* It usually appears as a mushroom like flattened spherical mass that protrudes from the gingival margin or interproximal space and attached by a sessile or pedunculated base. It tends to expand laterally and pressure from tongue and cheek predestined its flattened appearance. It is usually seen basically in upper anterior teeth. The granuloma appears dusky red or magenta in color (RASBERRY LIKE APPEARANCE) with numerous deep red, pinpoint markings and a smooth, glistening surface. It has a semi-firm consistency, but may be soft and friable, it does not innate the underlying bone. It bleeds spontaneously or on mild provocation. It is usually painless, but painful ulceration may occur if it interferes with occasion.

Prelingual deafness is hearing impairment that is sustained prior to the acquisition of language, which can occur as a result of a congenital condition or through hearing loss in early infancy. Prelingual deafness impairs an individual's ability to acquire a spoken language. Most prelingual hearing impairment is acquired via either disease or trauma rather than genetically inherited.

Premature death is the death during the period when otherwise a person would have been alive in normal course.

Premaxilla is the intermaxillary bone situated in front of maxilla proper.

Pre-medication is the medication needs to be taken before treatment.

Premolars are the two-cusped teeth immediately in front of molars.

P

Prenatal history generally refers to the maternal history during pregnancy, which can be linked with present condition, e.g. enamel hypoplasia, intrinsic stains of fluoride or tetracycline.

Presbyopia is impaired vision due to loss of elasticity of lens especially in old age.

Pressure is the force applied to a surface as a force per unit area.

Pressure habits are the habits caused by applying which apply pressure on the oral soft tissues and hard tissues, thus having deleterious effect on the dentition and the oral structures; these include sucking habits like lip-sucking, finger-sucking, and thumb-sucking.

Pressure syringe is an instrument with a trigger mechanism that delivers a measured dose of anesthetic solution and allows to express more easily the solution despite tissue resistance.

Pressure ulcer is caused by excessive non relieved pressure. In animals, a pressure of 60 mm Hg of pressure applied to skin for 1 hour may produce muscle degeneration/ tissue necrosis. When patient lies on hospital bed, pressure can range from 100-150 mm Hg. Muscle tissue is more sensitive to ischemia than overlying skin. Hence necrotic tissue is usually wider and deeper. Treatment includes relief of pressure with special cushions, beds and nutritional support.

Pressure welding is a form of welding in which the weld is made by pressure.

Prevalence refers to the total number of all cases who have an attribute or disease at a particular time or during particular period divided by population at risk of having the attribute or disease at this point in time or midway through the period. Prevalence refers to

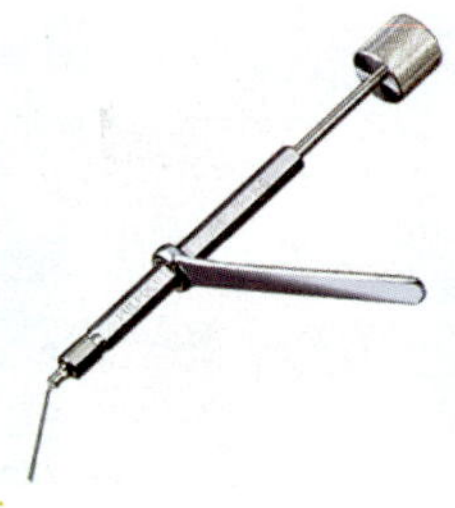

Fig.: *Pressure syringe*

specifically all current cases (old and new) existing at as given point in time or over a period of time in a given population.

Preventive a procedure performed to aid in preventing decay and/or gum disease.

Preventive dentistry is that branch of dental practice that deals with the establishment and maintenance of an oral environment conducive for the prevention of a sound and healthy stomatognathic system. The rationale is to promote optimal health of the oral tissues and to prevent damage of any sort.

Preventive orthodontics is the action taken to preserve the integrity of what appears to be normal at a specific time. This includes: Early correction of carious lesions, particularly proximal caries, early recognition and elimination of oral habits, using space maintainers in case of early loss of deciduous tooth.

Prilocaine was introduced in 1963. It is equally effective as lignocaine. It contains slight vasoconstriction properties whereas lignocaine does not. It is available in 4% solution without added vasoconstrictor.

Primary complex consists of three lesions (i) Ghon's focus (ii) caseous tuberculosis and (iii) chain of tubercles along with the lymphatic pathway between Ghons focus and mediastinum. The bacilli are inhaled into the alveoli where they are ingested by macrophages. Epitheloid cells are the hallmark of tuberculosis.

Primary culture refers to cultures prepared from tissues taken directly from animals.

Primary dentition is the first dentition which occurs in the oral cavity. It consists of twenty teeth, i.e. 8 incisors, 4 canines and 8 molars, which are exfoliated or shed naturally and replaced by permanent dentition.

Primary displacement is the process of physical carry that takes place in conjunction with a bone;s own enlargement.

Primary herpetic gingivostomatitis caused by herpes simplex virus I and II. There is abrupt onset of fever; malaise and lymphadenopathy of cervical chain of glands, vesicles rupture soon forming painful ulcers, lesions are highly infectious,

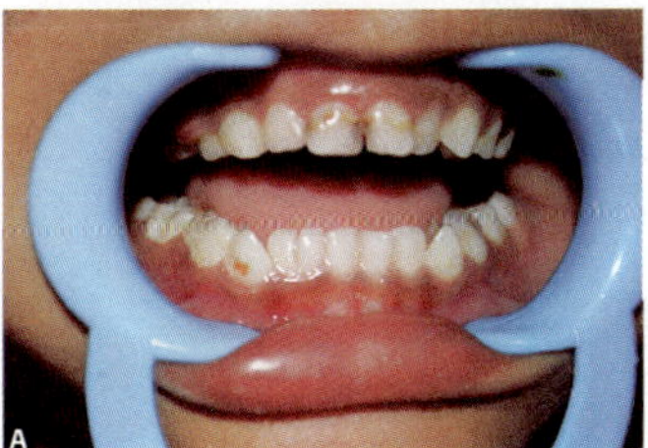

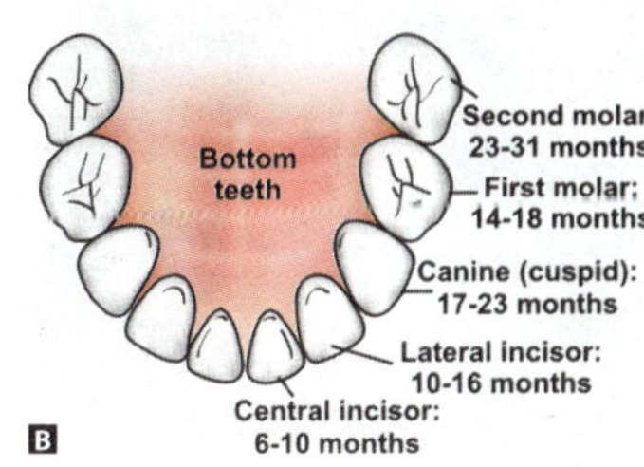

FigsA and B: *Primary dentition*

gingiva is erythematous, ulcerated and enlarged, lesions resolve automatically within 10-14 days.

Primary lymphoid organs are thymus for the T cells, bone marrow for the B cells (in fetal liver and avian bursa fabricius). These are the major sites of lymphopoiesis. Lymphocytes differentiate from lymphoid stem cells, proliferate and mature into functional cells. Lymphocytes acquire them repertoire of specific antigenic receptors in order to cope with the antigenic challenge the individual receives during life. Learn to discriminate between self-antigens, which are tolerated and non-self antigens, which are not tolerated.

Primary lymphoma of bone develops rarely in jaws but mandible is affected more. Oral mucosal lesion is ulcerated. Teeth become loose, maxilla may be expanded, X-ray shows radiolucency of alveolar bone. In some cases periosteal reaction may be seen. Biopsy confirms the tumor. Radical surgical excision is helpful.

Primary neuritic leprosy disease presents with nerve thickening and loss of sensation without any skin patches and skin smear examination is negative. Histological examination of the involved nerve shows many L. laprae with infiltration by lymphocytes and histiocytes.

Primary pain is the source of hyperexcitability that, in turn, produces secondary or referred pain. It is mostly deep somatic or visceral origin. More continuous, more server, the longer the duration the more likely are secondary pains to occur. Referred pains occur most frequently in structures innervated by same branch that mediates the primary pain.

Primary parathyroidism is due to adenoma of one of the four parathyroid glands. Pathological fracture may be the first sign. Cyst of jaw may be seen. Generalized osteoporosis develops. Lobulated lesion of mandible is to be differentiated from ameloblastoma. Small cystic areas may be seen in calvarium. Jaw may give ground glass appearance. Excision of parathyroid tumor will treat the patient.

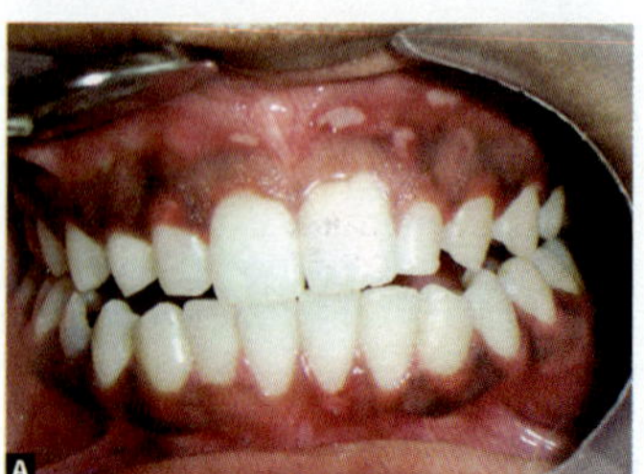

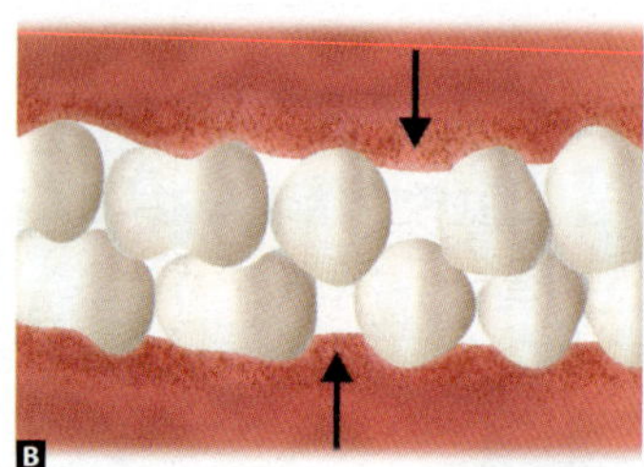

Figs A and B: *(A) Primary herpetic gingivostomatitis; (B) Primary spacing*

Primary prevention is the intervention of disease before it develops. It includes techniques, designed to prevent the onset of disease, reverse the initial stages of disease. It includes arrest of a disease before treatment is needed.

Primary syphilis is the first stage in the natural history of the disease. The incubation period is 10–90 days (average 2–4 weeks). The characteristic primary lesion of syphilis is called 'chancre' and is a solitary, painless, indurated, ulcerated or eroded lesion. To start, it develops as a dull red macule which becomes eroded. Regional lymph nodes are enlarged, painless and are rubbery.

Primary teeth are also known as the baby teeth or the primary dentition.

Primary trauma from occlusion is said to have occurred if trauma from occlusion is the prime etiologic factor in periodontal destruction, e.g. high filling, faulty prosthetic appliance, drifting and orthodontic movement which are functionally unacceptable positions.

Primate spacing is the normal physiological spacing present between primary anterior teeth.

Primer is a solution applied to the acid-etched surface of tooth. It acts as a wetting agent. It enhances the adhesive quality of bond agent.

Primordial cyst develops through cystic degeneration and liquefaction of stellate reticulum. It may be associated with a retained erupted deciduous tooth. Unless infected, it is not painful. On X-ray, it is seen as round or ovoid well-demarcated radiolucent lesion. It will show as a sclerotic border. Wall of cyst is made up of parallel bundles of collagen fibers. Surgical removal is the remedy.

Principal fibers are the most important element of the periodontal ligament which are collagenous in nature and are organized in the form of bundles.

Provitamins substances are not vitamins themselves but capable of conversion into vitamins in course of digestion. Carotenes are provitamins of vitamin A and to some extent, at least, the amino acid tryptophan can be converted to niacin.

Probes: Small occlusal cavities are found with a blunt pointed instruments called probe. Mesial and distal cavities can be found with a special double ended probe called Briault probe.

Probing depth *see* clinical pocket depth.

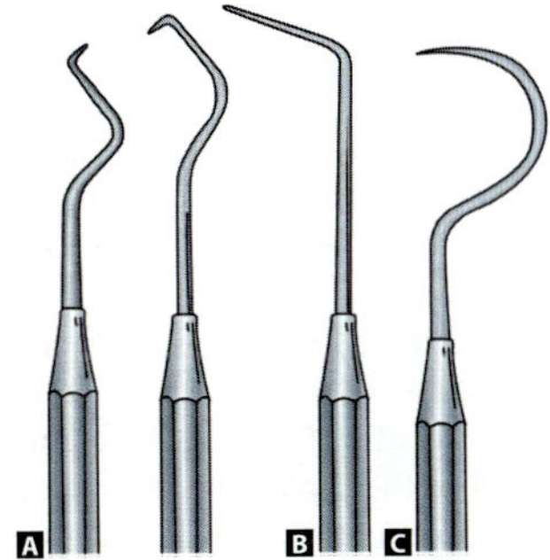

FigsA to C.: *Probes (A) Ends of Briault probe; (B) Right angle probe; (C) Sickle probe*

P

Prodrome is an early symptom of a disease.

Prodrug is the drug that undergoes metabolism in the body generally in liver.

Productive cough is produced when the active respiratory efforts expel the excessive tracheobronchial secretions. Commonly it results from infections. About 100 mL of mucus is produced in the tracheobronchial tree on daily basis. It is treated by antibiotics, steam inhalations and the drugs which cause softening of sputum.

Professional misconducts can be described as unethical acts which should not be precticed ideally. These include to issue certificate which are untrue, misleading or improper. One should not employ an unqualified assistant. You are not permitted to canvass directly or indirectly to promote practice or keeping touts to improve your clientage. One should not disclose the secrets of patients. Improper relations with patients of opposite sex are not allowed.

Professional responsibility is the obligation to fulfill specific requirement to maintain expertise and knowledge associated with profession.

Profile GT (Greater taper) technique Buchanan started that it is an instrument to flare out the coronal third of the canal. This means that this instrument is an ISO size 20 at the tip, but the taper is 0.10 mm/mm. It is used in a twisting motion, first counterclockwise and then clockwise with apical pressure, before retraction. A lubricant should be used along with it. Then next smaller-size GT file is used, number 0.08, in the same manner—counterclockwise, twist clockwise, and retract. One continues down the canal using the 0.08, and 0.06 taper instruments until the apical constriction is reached. This constitutes the "second shaping wave." It is followed by the "third shaping wave," in which ISO instruments are used to enlarge the apical canal diameter beyond size 20, the tip diameter of the GT files. Begin with fine instruments, and then step back 1 or 2 mm with instruments, up to size 35 or 40, the apical region is "rounded out." The final shaping is done with the last GT file used in the canal. Size of GT instrument and recommended canal shape is 0.06 GT file—recommended for "extremely thin or curved roots" and 0.08 GT file—lower anterior teeth, premolars, and buccal roots of maxillary molars.

Prognosis is a prediction of a course, duration and outcome of a disease once the disease is present. The prognosis can be described in various forms such as excellent prognosis, good prognosis, fair prognosis, poor prognosis, questionable prog-nosis and hopeless prognosis.

Progressive systemic sclerosis refers to scleroderma.

Prolactin is called lactogenic hormone. It promotes milk production in women. Its target organ is breast.

If the lactating mother continues to breastfeed, hormone level remains high.

Prolonged anesthesia is a condition where patient experiences numbness for many hours or days following a local anesthetic injection. It may result due to irritation to the nerve after injection of a contaminated anesthetic agent. The ensuing edema places pressure on the nerve. Persistent anesthesia also results from trauma to the nerve sheath.

Promyelocyte is larger than myeloblast. Chromatin is coarser but nucleoli are present. Cytoplasm is basophilic with a small number of prominent large red granules.

Propanidid epontal is a yellowish oily viscous liquid. It is a derivative of eugenol. It is less potent and is available for injection in 5% solution. Dose varies from 5–7 mg per kg body weight. It brings rapid unconsciousness and maintains anesthesia for 2–3 minutes. There becomes a transient fall of BP for 2-3 minutes. Its period of narcotic activity is short.

Prophy *see* prophylaxis.

Prophy paste is an abrasive agent usually made from floor of pumice that is used to remove plaque and polish the tooth.

Prophylaxis is a general meaning to clean the teeth, also known as a prophy. It is a procedure designed to prevent the onset of disease.

Propionic acid is an NSAID. Ibuprofen is the main drug. These are better tolerated as compared to other NSAIDS like phenyl butazone. It is better tolerated than aspirin in terms of GIT disturbances. It is one of the safest drugs. Its half-life is 2 hours similar to paracetamol. Abdominal dyspepsia may be a side effect.

Proprioceptive fibers are some afferent fibers; carry impulses from muscles, tendons, ligaments or joints and are important for maintenance of posture and for proper control of movement. Such impulses are referred to as proprioceptive.

Proprioreceptors are those receptors located in muscles, tendons and joints. These allow body to recognize the position of the body. Proprioceptors are also the pain receptors involved in automatic functioning and perceive movement, pressure and position free nerve endings: Deep somatic pain and other sensations. Golgi tendon organs are the mechano-receptors in muscle tendon. Muscle spindles are mechano-receptors. Pacinian corpuscles: perception of pressure. Periodontal receptors perception of tooth movement.

Propranolol is a widely used beta receptor antagonist. It blocks all beta adrenergic receptors. It reduces heart rate and cardiac output. The forces of myocardial contraction and blood pressure are reduced. Response of heart to exercise and exertion is diminished. It is used in angina, cardiac arrhythmias and hypertension. It can also be used in hyperthyroidism.

Prosopagnosia is an agnosia for faces. It has an acute onset and is due to involvement of cerebral artery. He cannot recognize face but recognizes person from voice and movements. Prosopagnosia which persists beyond a month is due to bilateral lesions at the level of lingual and fusiform gyri.

Prostaglandin E2 (PGE2) is a vasoactive eicosanoid produced by monocytes and fibroblasts, induces bone resorption and matrix metalloproteinase secretion. Evidence that prostaglandin could mediate bone resorption was first reported by Klein and Raisz in 1970 and a role for prostaglandin in periodontal bone loss soon followed (Goldhaber 1971)-Prostaglandin E2 exhibits a broad range of pronflammatory effects. It contributes to the flare and weal effects by inducing vasodilatation and increasing capillary permeability, and these effects are enhanced by synergism with other inflammatory mediators. Prostaglandins sensitize nociceptors to different types of stimuli, thus lowering their pain thresholds to all types of stimulation. Prostaglandin E increases the response of slowly adapting admethane receptors to non-noxious stimuli.

P

Prosthesis is a replacement of a missing body part.

Prosthodontics is a specialy that is concerned with restoration of natural teeth and contiguous oral and maxillofacial tissues with artificial substitute. Specialist is known as prosthodontist.

Protamine zinc insulin is a result of combination of protamine and insulin. Addition of zinc produces depression of blood sugar. Little effect is observed for 3–4 hours and is 12 hours before the maximum and activity is produced. It may be active even 24 hours after injection.

Protaper is a file that was introduced by D Cliff Ruddle, Dr Johan West, Ben John and Dr Pierre. Protaper means progressively taper. A unique feature of the ProTaper files is each instrument has changing percentage of taper over the length of cutting blades. This progressively tapered design improves flexibility, cutting efficiency and the safety of these files. Recommended speed is 150 to 350

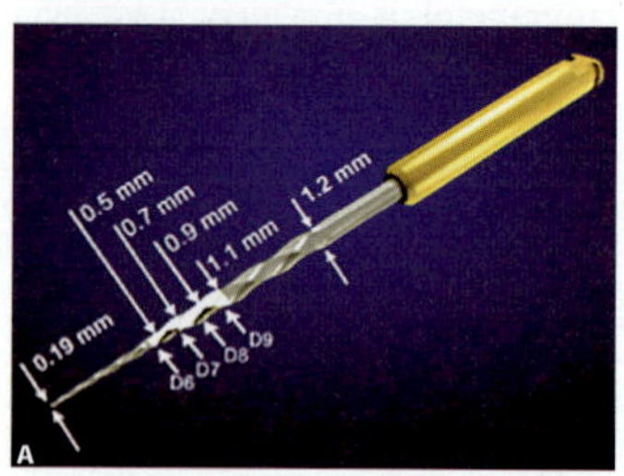

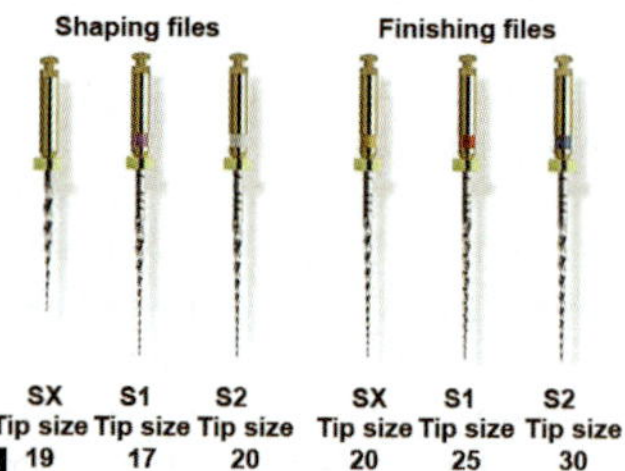

Fig.: *Protaper files*

rpm. ProTaper file has a triangular cross-section and is variably tapered across its cutting length.

Proteins are building blocks of our life because vital parts of nucleus and protoplasm are made up of proteins only. One sixth of body weight is made up of proteins. Proteins contain 16% nitrogen. Daily requirement is 1 gm per kilogram of body weight.

Proteolysis chelation theory: According to this theory, decalcification is mediated by a variety of complexing agents, such as acid anions, amines, amino acids, peptides polyphosphates, and carbohydrate derivatives. Oral keratinolytic bacteria are thought to be involved in the process. Differences in the keratin content of the enamel in children with high caries and low caries experience are considered important. It should be noted that only a small fraction of the protein of enamel bears any resemblance to the keratin of hair. Schatz and Martin challenged the chemo-parasitic theory advocated the proteolysis-chelation theory and stated that acid may prevent tooth decay by interfering with growth and activity of proteolytic bacteria.

Proteolytic theory: According to this theory, the organic component is most vulnerable and is attacked by hydrolytic enzymes of micro-organisms, this precedes the loss of the inorganic phase. Gottlieb (1944) maintained that the initial action was due to proteolytic enzymes attacking the lamellae, rod sheaths, tufts and walls of the dentinal tubules. He suggested that a coccus, probably *Staphylococcus aureus*, was involved because of the yellow pigmentation that he considered path gnomonic of dental caries. Frisbie (1944) also described caries as a proteolytic process involving depolymerization and liquefaction of the organic matrix of enamel. The less soluble inorganic salts could then be freed from their "organic bond" favoring their solution, by acidogenic bacteria that secondarily penetrate along widening paths of ingress. Pincus (1949) contended that proteolytic organisms first attacked the protein elements, such as the dental cuticle and then destroyed the prism sheaths. The loosened prisms would then fall out mechanically. He also suggested that sulfatases of Gram-negative bacilli hydrolyzed "mucoitin sulfate" of enamel or chondroitin sulfate of dentin and produced sulfuric acid. The released sulfuric acid could combine with the calcium of the mineral phase. It should be noted that the composition of the organic components of enamel does not resemble that of connective tissue and an abundance of sulfated polysaccharides has not been demonstrated. The Pincus' theory remains, therefore, without experimental support.

Prothrombin time is a test done to measure the patient's ability to form a clot. It is performed by measuring the time it takes for a clot to form when calcium and a tissue factor are added to plasma. It is between 11 and 16 seconds. Prolonged prothrombin time is associated with postoperative bleeding.

Proton is a positively charged particle.

Protrusion refers to the movement of the mandible anteriorly from ICP.

Provisional: Temporary.

Provisional diagnosis refers to the term where the diagnosis is based on clinical impression without any investigations.

Provisional prognosis is that stage where it allows the clinician to start with the best available treatment that has questionable prognosis and at the same time hopes for the favorable response which may shift the balance and helps in controlling the disease.

Provitamins are vitamin-related compounds that can be converted to active vitamins in body such as tryptophan can be converted to vitamin niacin, carotene to vitamin A and cholesterol to vitamin D.

Proximal is the nearest point of attachment; the mesial or distal surface of the tooth.

Proximal caries are the caries that affect the proximal wall of teeth. Generally occurs below the contact point. Susceptible zone. This region extends from the contact point down to the height of the free gingival margin. It increases with the recession of the alveolar bone and gingival tissues.

Proximal half crown is a ¾ crown that is rotated 90°, and distal rather than buccal surface left intact. It can be a retainer on a tilted mandibular FPD abutment. This design can be used only in mouth and excellent hygiene and low incidence of interproximal caries. It is contraindicated if there is blemish on distal surface. Mesial surface parallels path of insertion of mesial abutment preparation clearance of 1.5 mm is obtained from occlusal reduction that terminates at distal may ridge, and a little or no reduction of mesial cusps. Grooves paralleling mesial surfaces are placed in buccal and lingual axial walls. A heavy channel and occlusal offset connects the grooves to strengthen disto-occlusal margin. An occlusal isthmus augments retention and rigidity.

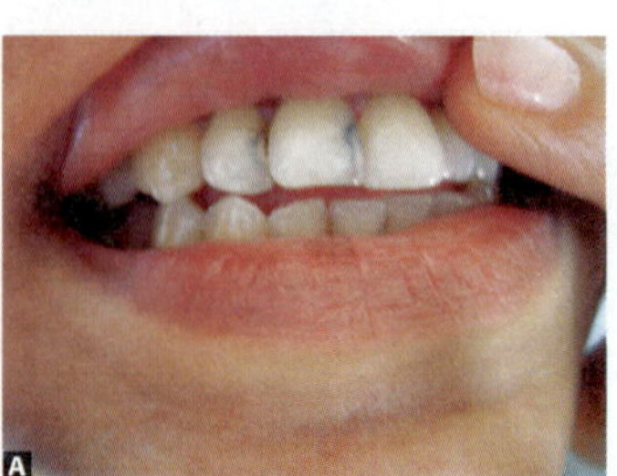

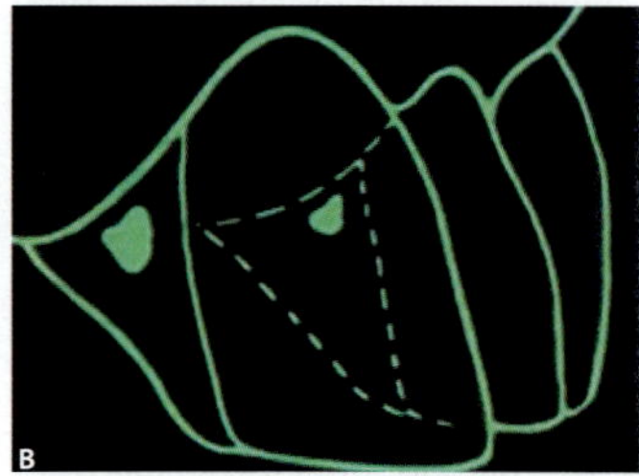

Figs A and B: *(A) Proximal caries; (B) Proximal surface*

Proximal surface is the surface of the tooth adjacent to the next tooth; refers to the mesial and distal surfaces.

Pseudoallergic reactions *see* Anaphylactoid.

Pseudocysts are that cysts that do not have epithelial lining and hence are not true cysts.

Pseudopocket refers gingival pocket.

Pseudomembrane is a membranous layer of exudates. It contains precipitated fibrin, organisms, necrotic cells produced by an inflammatory reaction on the surface of tissue.

Psoriasis: There is formatics small, sharply delineated, dry papules, each covered by silvery scales like mica. On removal of these scales bleeding points may be seen. Cutaneous lesions are painless. Papules enlarge and become raised. New lesions slowly arise over weeks/months. Oral mucosa is rarely involved but lips may be involved. On treatment may subside for sometime then may reappear. Long term cortisone is used. Uric acid levels are raised. Lithium, betablockers, chloroquine aggravate psoriasis. One has to hydrate the skin. Severe scalp involvement needs coal tar occlusive shampoo at night followed by corticosteroid lotions.

Psuedomembranous candidiasis is a fungal infection also known as thrush that may persist intermittently for months using corticosteroids topically or aerosol in HIV infected individuals. It has white membrane on the surface of oral mucosa, tongue and elsewhere. Confluent plaques can be scrapped leaving a raw erythematous bleeding base. White patches consist of necrotic material and desquamated epithelium.

Psychic seizures manifest as sudden emotions such as fear, anxiety, depression, or happiness. This type of seizure can also make patients feel as if they have lived through this moment before (*deja vu*), familiar things seem foreign to them (*jamais vu*), or the world is not real.

Psychoanalytical theory: According to this theory oral habits are the product of pleasure, a child derives from stimulation the oral erogenous zone. The pleasure

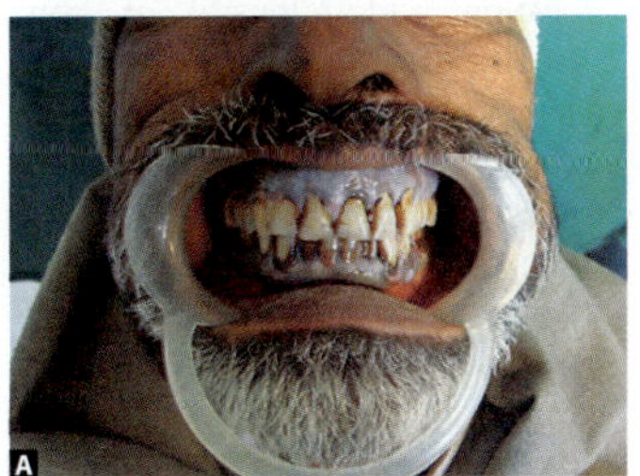

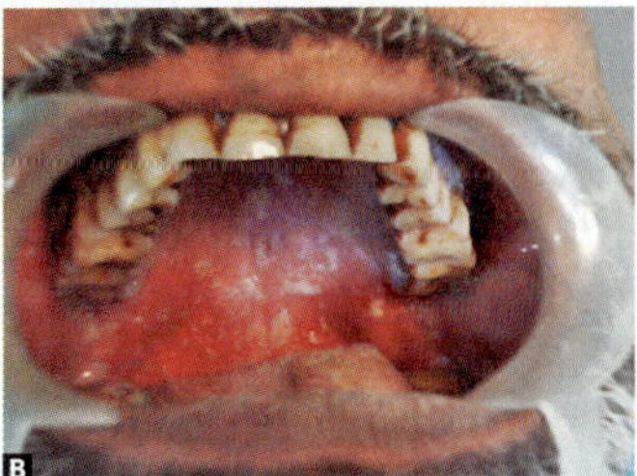

FigsA and B: *Psuedomembranous candidiasis*

derived may be sexual or escape from a painful situation, as in case of infant who sucks when he is hungry. The habit is associated with pleasurable stimuli early in life but is not discarded at the usual time due to some underlying psychological disturbance. Proponents of this theory reason that if the habit is taken away from such an emotionally disturbed child, the child may substitute an even less desirable one in its place. One of the concepts of thumb-sucking that is brought about by the psychoanalytic theory is that humans possess a biologic sucking drive. This concept is supported by the observation of intrauterine sucking and by the neonatal reflex of rooting and placing, as described by Benjamin (1967). In the rooting reflex, if a well-defined area around the mouth is touched by an object and opens the mouth. The placing reflex is the sucking activity that occurs with the object making contact with the infant's mouth.

Psychodynamics is psychoanalysis. It includes motivations, perceptions and emotions.

Psychogenic headache occurs in neurotic, hypochondrial or hysterical individual. The character is like a sense of pressure or like a tight constricting band.

Psychogenic malodor is a group of patients who are by no means have no evidence of halitosis, can be detected even with objective testing and the halitosis may be attributable to a form of delusion of monosymptomatic hypochondriasis (self-halitosis; halitophobia). Such patients rarely wish to visit a psychological specialist because they fail to recognize their own psychological condition and may have latent psychosomatic tendencies.

Psychogenic pain is a psychic and emotional states influence pain perception and its expression. These patients are emotionally disturbed and are very common in young women. Such pain can continue for days together.

Psychogenic toothache is a category of mental disorders in which a patient may complain of physical condition without the presence of any physical signs. In these cases, always think of psychogenic toothache. No damage to local tissue is typical in heterotrophic pain entities. It must be noted that psychogenic pain is rare. So, all other possible diagnoses must be ruled out before making the diagnosis of psychogenic pain. Pain is observed in multiple teeth. Precipitated by severe psychological stress. Frequent changes in character, location and intensity of pain. Response to therapy varies which can include lack of response or unusual response. Usually referred to psychiatrist for further management.

Psychological dependence is characterized by intense craving and compulsive perpetuation of abuse to repeat the desire of the drug. But not necessarily everybody taking the drugs may be an addict or drug dependent.

Psychology is the science dealing with human nature, function and phenomenon of his soul in the main.

Psychophysiological is a measurement of physiological process in an effort to draw conclusions about psychological states.

Psychosexual theory: Sigmond Freud in the year 1905 was the originator at psychoanalytical approach. He thought that personality development from biological roots, as a result of satisfaction of a sex of instincts of which sexual instinct was the most important. He categorized it into different psychosexual stages. At each stage sexual energy is integrated in a particular part called erogenous zone. Two categories in concept of Freudian theory first describe level of consciousness (or) awareness; the second function component is personality. He proposed 3 basic psychic structures for personality of individual. There are three levels of consciousness. They are: (1) conscious part of personality which individual is aware of, e.g. thought feelings for basic activities; (2) Preconscious-part of personality of which individual is not aware at the moment, however, able to recollect into awareness without great difficulty; (3) Unconscious-part of personality of which individual is unaware, which generally cannot be able brought into awareness without help of assistant.

Psychosocial theory: In Erickson's view "Psychosocial development proceeds by critical steps–'critical' are characteristics of turning points, of moments of decision between progress and regression, integration and retardation. Each stage represents a "psychosocial crisis" which is influenced by social environment. Chronological ages are associated with Erickson's developmental stages as in physical development, the chronological age varies among individuals but developmental stage remains constant. Unlike Freud, Erickson emphasised the conscious-self as much as unconscious instincts.

Psychosomatic is pertaining to mind-body relationship.

Pterygium is a triangular fold of conjunctiva encroaching the cornea in the horizontal meridian. It may come from single or both sides of conjunctiva. It may be thick, fleshy and vascular associated with opaque spots in the cornea.

Pterygomaxillary fissure is a cleft that separates the lateral pterygoid plate and maxilla.

Pterygopalatine ganglion is located in the pterygopalatine fossa and is suspended from the maxillary nerve by two ganglionic branches. The fibers passing through the ganglion. Functionally, the ganglion is autonomic and is a peripheral ganglion of the cranial parasympathetic outflow.

Puberty is the period between the ages of 12–15 years in girls and between 13–16 years in boys.

During which secondary sexual characteristics develop and become expressed.

Public health is defined as 'the organized application of local, state, national and international resources to achieve 'Health for all', i.e. attainment by all people of the world by of a level of health that will permit them to lead a socially and economically productive life.

Puddings are customary in formal dinners to serve the pudding and ice creams as the finishing item. In the process of eating food, one loses certain amount of energy that is why certain people start sweating after food. To compensate lost energy, it easily absorbs readymade glucose/fructose/levulose. That is why after 15 minutes of taking puddings one feels energetic.

Pulmonary hypertension is the counterpart in the lungs of systemic hypertension. There is hyperplasia of medial coat of vessels. Second feature is ventricular hypertrophy.

Pulmonary infarction is an infarct in an area of coagulation necrosis produced by a sudden cut off of arterial supply but in the lungs there may be vascular occlusion without infarction and there may be infarction without vascular occlusion. The infarct is always a red infarct because of dual blood supply. It is a wedge or pyramid shaped.

Pulmonary tuberculosis (TB) is bacterial infection in humans. Around one-third of the world population is infected with *M. tuberculosis*. It is still a significant cause of morbidity and mortality in the developing countries. There is an increase in the incidence of tuberculosis because of HIV infection.

Pulp is soft tissue of mesenchymal origin located in center of a tooth. It consists of specialized cells, odontoblasts arranged peripherally in direct contact with dentin matrix. This close relationship between odontoblasts and dentin is known as "pulp-dentin complex". The pulp is connective tissue system composed of cells, ground substance, fibers, interstitial fluid, odontoblasts, fibroblasts and other cellular components. Pulp is actually a microcirculatory system consists of arterioles and venules as the largest vascular component.

Pulp calcifications are discrete pulp stones and diffuse calcification. Diffuse calcification is seen in the canals of teeth known as calcific degeneration. It is an amorphous, unorganized linear strand.

Pulp canal is a portion of pulp cavity located in root area in the pulp canal. The constricted opening at root apex is known as apical foramen through which nutrient and nerve supply enter.

Pulp capping is a procedure done when vital pulp is exposed, either root filling or pulpotomy is done to conserve the tooth. It cannot be done immediately so pulp capping is a valuable temporary measure. The exposed part is covered with calcium hydroxide paste and cavity paste and cavity is filled with temporary cement.

Pulp chamber is the largest enlarged portion of pulp cavity found in coronal portion of tooth and has pulpal norms. It reflects the external form of enamel at the time of eruption, but anatomy is less sharply defined. The roof of pulp chamber consists of dentin covering the pulp chamber occlusally.

Pulp degeneration is generally present in old age. It may be the result of persistent mild irritation in young age. Usually, pulp degeneration is induced by attrition, abrasion, erosion, bacteria, operative procedures, caries, pulp capping and reversible pulpitis.

Pulp dentin complex is the close relationship between odontoblasts and dentin, sometimes referred to as the pulp-dentin complex, is one of the several reasons why dentin and pulp should be considered as a functional entity. Not only do the two tissues have a common embryonic origin, but they also remain in an intimate relationship throughout the life of the vital tooth. Anything that affects dentin will affect the pulp and vice-versa. In other words, pulp lives for the dentin and the dentin lives by the grace of the pulp.

Pulp horn is the portion of the pulp chamber that extends towards the cusp.

Pulp oximetry is a noninvasive device for determining pulp vitality. The principle of this technology is based on modification of Beer's law and the absorbency characteristics of hemoglobin in red and infrared range. It has a oxygen saturation monitor in which liquid crystal displays oxygen saturation, pulse rate and plethysmographic wave form readings. The probe consists of red and infrared light-emitting diodes opposite a photoelectric detector. Clinically the detection of a pulse should be enough to establish pulp vitality or necrosis.

Pulp testing is often referred to as vitality testing. Pulp vitality tests play an important role in diagnosis because these tests not only determine the vitality of tooth but also the pathological status of pulp. Pulp testers should only be used to assess the vital or nonvital pulp as

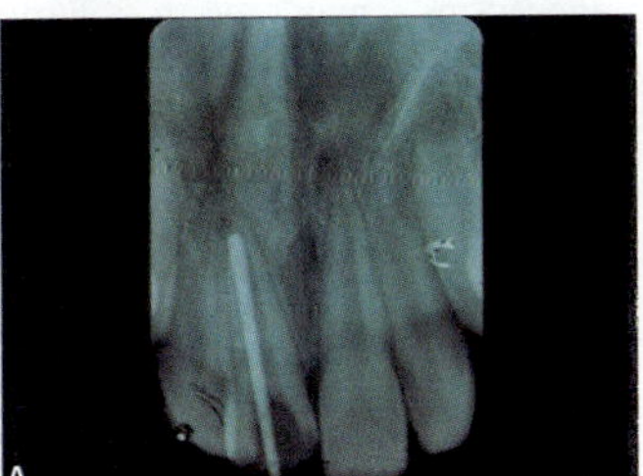

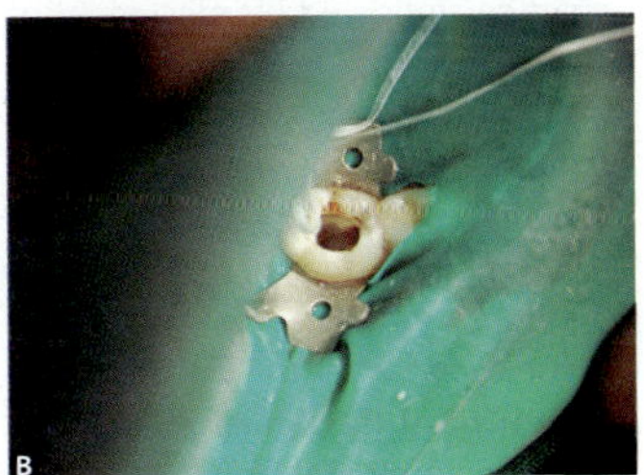

Figs A and B: *(A) Pulp canal; (B) Pulp chamber*

they do not quantify the disease, nor do they measure the health and thus, should not be used to assess the degree of pulpal disease.

Pulpectomy is the removal of the whole pulp inside a tooth.

Pulpitis irreversible is an inflammation of the dental pulp in which pulp will not recover and will require endodontic treatment.

Pulpotomy "amputation of the affected or infected coronal portion of the dental pulp preserving the vitality and function of all or part of remaining radicular pulp"(AAPD 1996).

Pulpotomy can be defined as procedures involving removal of vital, partially inflamed coronal pulp tissue and placing a dresser over the amputated pulp stumps and then place the final restoration". (DB Kennedy 1986).

P

Pulpotomy is complete removal of the coronal portion of the dental pulp followed by placement of a suitable dressing or medicament that will promote healing and preserve the vitality of the tooth" (Finn 1995).

Pulpotomy is defined as "the amputation of vital pulp from the coronal chamber followed by placement of a medicament over the radicular pulp stumps to stimulate repair, fixation or mummification of the remaining vital radicular pulp" (Braham and Morris 1985).

Pulpotomy is the removal of the coronal potion of the pulp and the treatment of the remaining radicular pulp in an attempt to maintain the tooth and its supporting structure in a state of health" (Heilig 1984).

Pulsating exophthalmos is a condition in which the eyeball becomes prominent and pulsates with each heart beat (pulsating exophthalmos). Because of the peculiar relationship of the cavernous sinus to the internal carotid artery a communication between the two may occur as a result of injury. When this happens the arterial pressure is communicated through the sinus to veins of the orbit (which open into the sinus).

Pulse is the tactile palpation of heart beat that can be felt by placement of finger in the wirst; is produced by the force imparted to arterial blood each time the left ventricle contracts and expels blood into aorta. Pulse travels to wrist taking 0.1 to 0.2 seconds after the contraction. Pulse wave depends on the stroke volume, the force of expulsion and rigidity of blood vessels.

Pulseless disease also known as Takayasu's disease is rare of unknown cause. In branches of aorta stenosis, occlusion and aneurysms may occur. Early disease is accompanied by fever, myalgias, arthralgias and pain over involved artery. There may be syncope, dizziness, stroke, angina and claudication.

Pulses are the rich source of proteins. Price-wise the proteins of pulses are cheaper than proteins of animal origin per unit. Hence pulses are known as poor man's meat.

Pulses contain 20-25% of protein. Pulse proteins are class II proteins. It contains fair amount of calcium and iron. Pulses are rich in lysine but poor in methionine. If taken with wheat rotis, it compensates. During sprouting, concentration of vitamin C increases.

Pulsus alternans is a physical finding when the left ventricle is severely diseased, it characteristically develops alternate strong and weak beats.

Pumice is a ground volcanic ash used for polishing.

Punched out papillae is a cratered papillae characteristic of acute necrotizing ulcerative gingivitis.

Punctate resembles or marked with dots/points.

Punishment involves introduction of an aversive stimulus into a situation to decrease the undesirable behavior, e.g., use of parental rake in correction of tongue.

Pupil is the term given to an aperture present at the center of the iris. It appears black because the interior of the eye (which we see through the pupil) is dark. It regulates the amount of light passing into the eye. In bright light the pupil contracts, and in dim light it dilates. In this way, the optimum amount of light required for proper vision reaches the retina, within a considerable range in intensity of illumination.

Pure culture is a culture of a single cell species, without presence of any contaminants.

Purple lesions are some vascular lesions. Some appear blue while some other may appear purple. Purple color is due to basic bluish color being modified by normal pink mucosa. Purple vascular lesions are bullae while purple lesions resulting from deposition of pigments are usually nodules or tumors.

Purpura is the extravasations of small amount of blood into mucus membrane. *Clinical Features:* It generally develops in young adults. Bleeding spots on skin or mucosal surfaces. Epistaxis, hematuria and hematemesis are common. Intracranial hemorrhage may produce hemiplegia. Bleeding in joints may limit its movements. Spleen is not enlarged. *Oral manifestations:* Gingival bleeding, palatal ecchymosis is seen, bleeding in temporomandibular joint result in pain, trismus may develop. Muscle bleeding may result in closing and opening of mouth. Steroid therapy and repeated transfusions help.

Putrefaction one of the seven stages of decomposition that starts immediately after death at cellular level. It is due to action of many enzymes. Chief destructive bacterial agent is *Clostridium welchi* which causes marked hemolysis. First sign is greenish discoloration of skin over caecum where the content of bowel is more fluid and full of bacteria Putrefaction starts above 10°C and optimum at 21°C to 38°C. Organs containing water decompose early. Fat and flabby bodies decompose early.

Pyelitis is more commonly known as pyelonephritis refers to kidney infection. There may be high fever and acute severe rigor. Several bouts of fever may come in a day. There will be frequency, urgency and burning micturition. Pain may be radiated to lumbar region. Kidney area becomes tender. Urine will show pus cells. RBCs and albumin. *E. coli* is the causative factor.

Pyknodysostosis is a bone dysplasia transmitted by an autosomal recessive trait with increased bone density, dwarfism and skeletal fragility. Patient is short statured. Dentition is anomalous and palate is high and arched. Hands and feet are stubby and finger clubbing osteosclerosis is most prominent in long bones. Facial bones and sinuses are hypoplastic. Mandibular hypoplasia with an obtuse angle results in receding jaw.

Pyogenic granuloma is a tumor like nonspecific conditioned enlargement as repose to minor

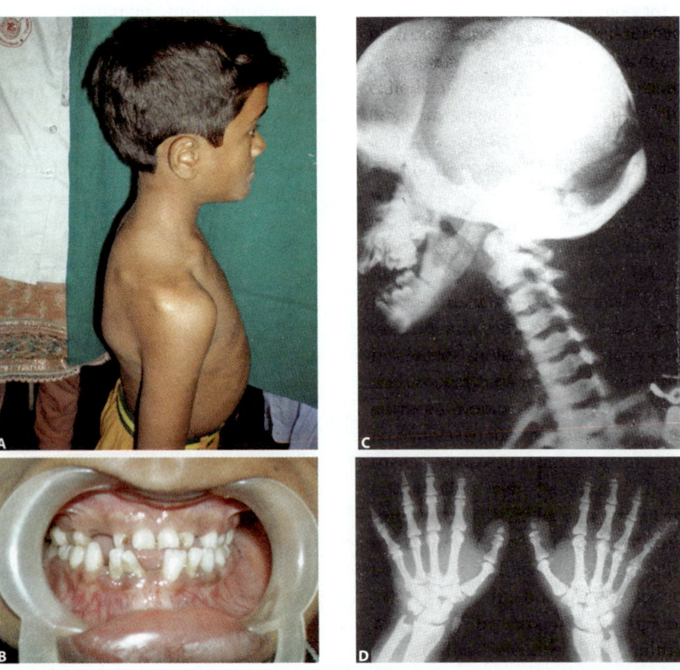

Figs A to D: *Pyknodysostosis (A) Midfacial hypoplasia; (B) Congenitally missing teeth (C) Dense bones, wide open sutures and absent angle of mandible; (D) Symmetrical increase in density of bones and typical hypoplastic distal phalanges*

P

plasma. *Clinical Features:* It is usually seen on gingival, but may also arise from lips, tongue and buccal mucosa. Lesion varies from a discrete spherical tumor-like mass to a flattened, keloid-like enlargement with a broad base. It is usually bright red or purple in color with a friable or fruits consistency and which bleeds on slight promulgation surface may show ulceration and purulent exudates may be present. It is painless. Surgical excision is the treatment.

Pyorrhea is a purulent discharge of pus.

Pyostomatitis vegetans is an uncommon inflammatory disease. There develops large number of broad-based papillary projections with tiny abscesses. Tongue is involved more. Buccal mucosa gives a cobble-stone appearance.

Pyramidal fracture *see* Lefort II.

Pyrazolones is a most potent NSAID but the adverse effects are serious. It may cause agranulocytosis. It relieves pain of rheumatoid arthritis. It has unusual sodium retaining power hence has to be avoided in hypertension and renal disease.

Pyridoxine vitamin B_6 was discovered by Gyorgyi in 1936. Vitamin exists in three forms pyridoxine, pyridoxal and pyridoxamine. It plays a vital role of metabolism in amino acids. Liver, meat, fish, whole cereals are rich source of it. Treatment INH and oral contraceptives may cause its deficiency. If diet is containing 100 gm of protein, the requirement is 1.25 mg. Its deficiency may cause glossitis, dizziness and vomiting. Morning sickness of pregnancy also responds to it. Daily requirements depend upon consumption of total quantity of protein. *Oral Manifestations include:* Angular cheilitis, glossitis, stomatitis, and Atrophy of papillae on dorsum of tongue.

Pyrogen is a substance or agent producing fever. Paget's disease—It is a disease of middle age. Most of patients are asymptomatic. There will be pain with multiple fractures. Milkman's syndrome indicates local areas of demineralization within the bone. Pseudofractures may also be seen. Spinal cord and nerve root compression may be seen.

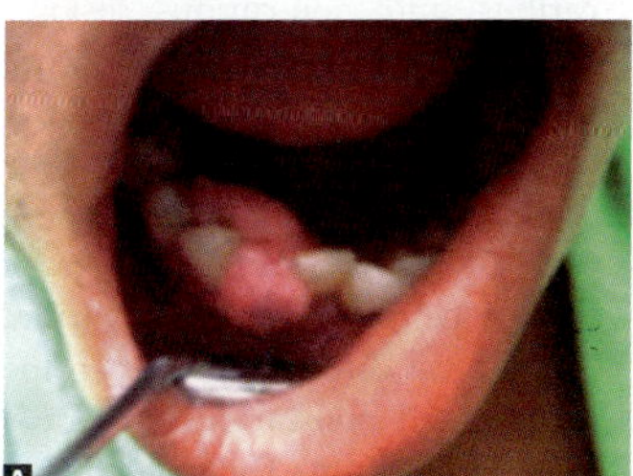

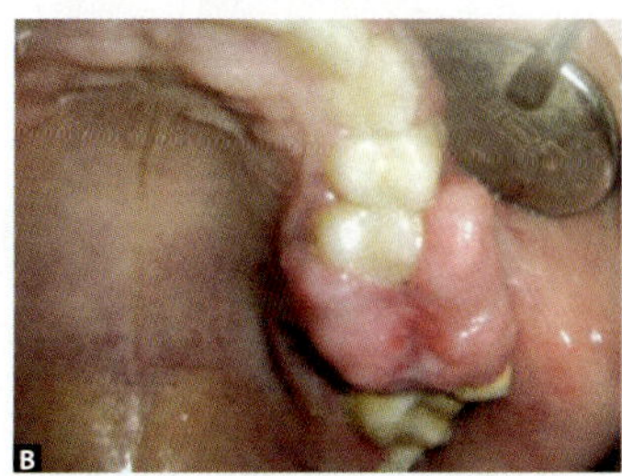

FigsA and B: *Pyogenic granuloma*

Q-sort is a survey research technique in which respondents generate forced choice ranking of many alternatives.

Quadrant denotes one of four equal sections in the mouth. The upper right, upper left, lower right or the lower left.

Quadriplegia means paralysis of all the four limbs and trunks and muscles that control the mouth, tongue and pharynx are affected. It is the resultant of spinal cord disease or fracture. There will be clumsiness of leg movements or unsteadiness of gait and other walking problems. Quadriplegia is due to cervical cord lesion. The ipsilateral to lesion is involved first followed in sequence by weakness of ipsilateral leg, the contralateral leg and finally the contralateral arm. Peripheral neuropathy produces symmetrical distal muscle weakness. Cerebral dysfunction is more extensive, and the prognosis is worse. Quadriplegics have severe motor impairment and other signs and symptoms of CNS dysfunction, such as cognitive impairments, seizures, speech and swallowing difficulties. Primitive reflexes persist lifelong, and extrapyramidal signs are common.

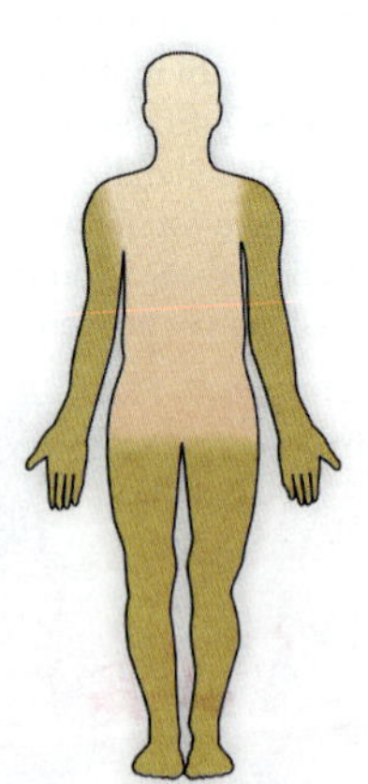

Fig.: *Quadriplegia—Involvement of all limbs*

Qualitative research is a research paradigm based in part on assumption of multiple constructed realities. There is independence of investigator and participant and time and context dependency information.

Quantitative light induced fluorescence is the technique used for caries detection. The use of fluorescence for the detection of caries dates back 1929, when Benedict observed that normal teeth fluoresce under ultraviolet illumination and suggested that fluorescence might be useful in the determination of dental caries when monochromatic light is used at 350 nm, 410 nm and 530 nm on carious and non-carious lesions. Additionally, he noted a difference in fluorescence between sound and caries enamel. In the carious lesions the emission spectra-shifts to more than 540 nm or the red range of the electromagnetic spectrum. The largest difference between the carious and non-carious spectra is found at 600 nm. They stated that when the enamel is illuminated with light in the blue-green range, the observable fluorescence occurs in the green-yellow range.

Quartan fever: When two days intervene between consecutive attacks.

Quasi experimental is a form of experimental research characterized by nonrandom assignment of subjects to groups or repeated treatments to the same group.

Questionnaire is a written self-report instrument used in survey research.

Quotidian fever: When a paroxysm of intermittent fever occurs daily.

Rabies encephalitis is a disease that spreads along peripheral nerves to reach CNS. One may develop severe anxiety, speech and psychomotor overactivity. Dysphagia and spasm of throat muscles may take place. Coma follows and death is due in 4-7 days.

Radiation is the emission and propagation of energy through space or material in the form of waves or stream of particles.

Radiation scatter is a form of secondary radiation, results from an X-ray beam that has been deflected from the path.

Radicular atrophy of pulp teeth are symptomless and respond normally to vacuolated spaces. Odontoblasts start disappearing. It may result due to improper fixation of tooth and pulp after extraction.

Radicular dentin dysplasia is inherited as autosomal dominant trait. It is characterized by teeth with normal crowns and abnormal tooth-roots. X-ray will show partial lack of pulp chambers and root canals. Color of tooth is normal. Roots are short. Pulp chamber of permanent teeth are not obliterated.

Radioisotopes are *in vivo* markers of certain elements or compounds when injected into tissue to get incorporated in the developing bone. The radioisotopes can later be detected by tracking down the radioactivity they emit.

Radiosurgery is a surgical technique that uses radio waves to produce a pressureless, boodless incision.

Radiograph refers to an X-ray picture.

Radiographic apex is "tip or end of root determined radiographically".

Radioimmunoprecipitation assay (RIPA) is mainly a research technique because it is expensive, time consuming, requires radioisotopes and requires maintenance of infected cell lines. The principle is that HIV infected cells are exposed to a radioactive isotope, lysed and centrifuged in an ultracentrifuge to obtain a cell lysate containing radiolabeled viral proteins. Patient's serum is pre-absorbed with protein A–sepharose beads, then mixed with cell lysate. An immunoprecipitate is formed by boiling in buffer, and is separated by electrophoresis. The banding patterns are seen similar to those of Western blot and interpretation is made.

Radioimmunoassay (RIA) used detection of anti-HIV antibodies in patient specimens. It uses the principle of competitive binding and isotope-labeled conjugate for detection. Radioactivity labeled anti-HIV antibodies compete with antibodies in patient's serum for binding sites on a solid phase. The quality of HIV antibodies in patient's serum is inversely proportional to the number of radioactive counts measured.

Rake angle is the angle formed by leading edge with the radius of file. Acute angle is considered as a negative rake angle and obtuse angle is considered as a positive rake angle.

Ramford index teeth is a periodontal index where six index teeth often used when evaluating periodontal health, maxillary right, first molar, left central incisor, left first premolar, mandibular left first molar, right central incisor and right first premolar.

Ramon syndrome patient develops gingival and alveolar enlargement, micro-ophthalmia. Cornea becomes cloudy. Hypopigmentation results with athetosis. Mental retardation is rare.

Rampant means spreading unchecked.

Ramsford teeth are teeth 3, 9, 12, 19, 25 and 28. These teeth are used in clinical trial research as a representation sample of entire dentition.

Randomization is a statistical procedure by which the participants are allocated into groups called study and control groups. It is an attempt to eliminate the bias. It is a 'high' point of control trial.

Randomized clinical trial is a clinical research in which subjects are randomly assigned to treatment and control groups.

Ranula is a special type of mucocele which occurs on floor of the mouth from trauma of submandibular or sublingual gland. It is slowly enlarging painless mass on one side of the floor. A lesion is deep seated and mucosa over it is normal. Some prefer to excise entire sublingual gland.

Raphe is a union of soft tissue.

Rapid cell growth occurs in most malignant tumors grow in rapid and invasive fashion while benign tumors grow in a slow, expansile manner. Most neoplasms arise from a single stem cells.

RCT *see* root canal therapy.

Reaming means use of sharp-edged tool for enlarging holes. In endodontic practice, reaming is commonly done by use of reamers, though files can also be used. It involves clockwise rotation of an instrument to generate a cutting effect.

Recession is the exposure of root surface by an apical shift in the position of the gingiva. The recession may be of two types: one,

R

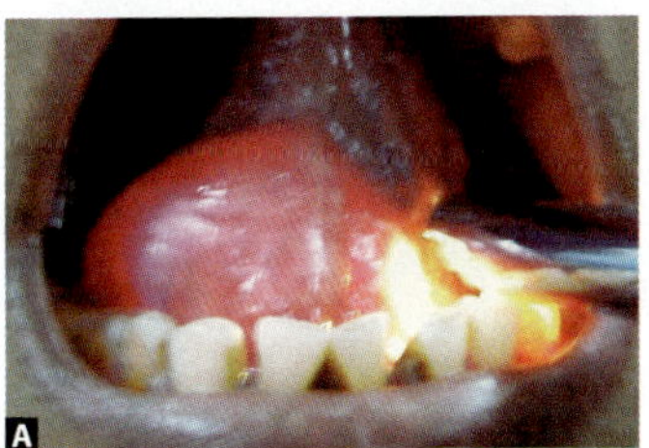

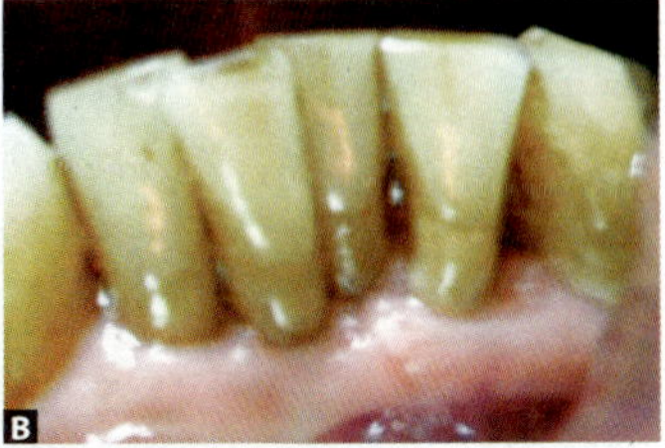

Figs A and B: *(A) Ranula showing transillumination; (B) Clinical and line diagram showing gingival recession*

which is clinically apparent and other, the hidden one, which can be determined only by the insertion of probe. Recession may also be localized to one tooth or a group of teeth.

Recovery period is the illness that subsides and patient returns to health during this period.

Recurrent aphthous stomatitis (RAS) refers to the condition where there is development of painful, recurring solitary or multiple recurring ulcers confined to oral mucosa with no other signs of disease. These have been classified as recurrent aphthous minor and major. These ulcers begin as a single or multiple superficial erosion covered by gray membrane. It is well-circumscribed by erythematous halo. Lesions are very painful and person is not able to eat. In one outbreak number of ulcer may go up to 100. Size may vary from 2-3 mm. Size of the minor ulcers is less than 1 cm. These ulcers heal without scar formation. They may start after trauma, menstruation or contact with certain foods. Within hours, a small white papule forms, ulcerates and gradually enlarges over the period of next 72 hours. Lesions are round, symmetric and shallow. Multiple lesions are present. Lesions heal slowly and leave scars.

Recurrent gingivitis can be described as the recurrence of disease after it has been eliminated.

Recurrent herpes simplex is a viral infection where there is a prodromal period of tingling or burning. oedema is followed by clusters of small vesicles of 1 to 3 mm. Bigger lesions may cause discomfort. Large, frequent, painful or disfiguring lesions require consultation. Oral acyclovir is effective.

Red blood cells carry hemoglobin and has a lifespan of 120 days. The cell is flexible, biconcave disc. Majority are disc form and minority are bowl shaped, normocytic are of normal size and normochromic are having normal amount of hemoglobin. RBCs carry O_2 from lungs to the tissues and return in venous blood with CO_2 to lungs. Lack of RBCs count may result in anemia.

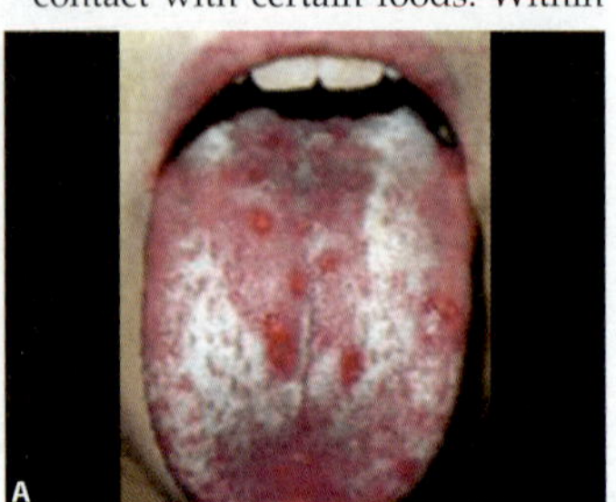

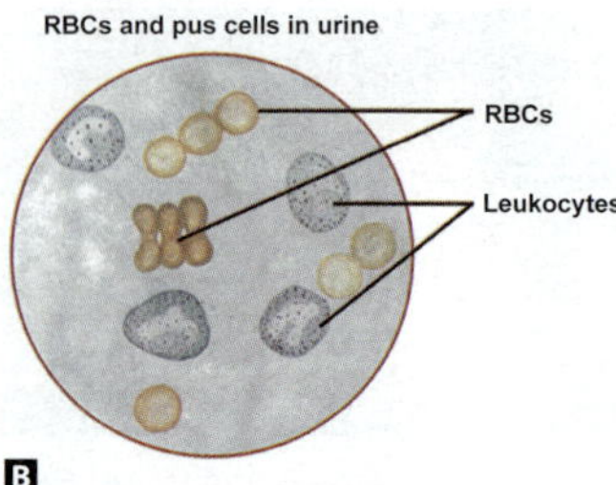

Figs A and B: *(A) Stomatitis; (B) RBCs and pus cells in urine*

Red-green color blindness: When a single group of color receptive cones is missing from the eye the person is unable to distinguish some colors from others. When person is lacking either red or green types of cones, person is known as red-green color blind.

Reduction of a fracture means the restoration of a functional alignment of the bony fragments.

Reference point refers to that site on occlusal or the incisal surface from which measurements are made. It should be stable and easily visualized during preparation. Usually it is the highest point on incisal edge of anterior teeth and buccal cusp of posterior teeth. It should not change between the appointments. Therefore in case of teeth with undermined cusps and fillings, they should be reduced considerably before access preparation.

Referred pain is generally described when there is generally a close segmental relationship between the primary initiating pain and secondary effects of noxious stimulus. Most secondary symptoms occur in structures innervated by the same major nerve that mediates the primary pain. Sensory effects resulting in referred pain and secondary hyperalgesias. (e.g. Angina pectoris radiates to the top of the left shoulder). The exact mechanism is unclear but appears to depend on convergence of afferent inputs onto central neurons from both the source and the referred sites, in addition to central summation.

Reflex sympathetic dystrophy is a minor form of causalgia involving face/mouth. It has all the features of autonomic reflex pain. It may follow trauma, surgery or infection.

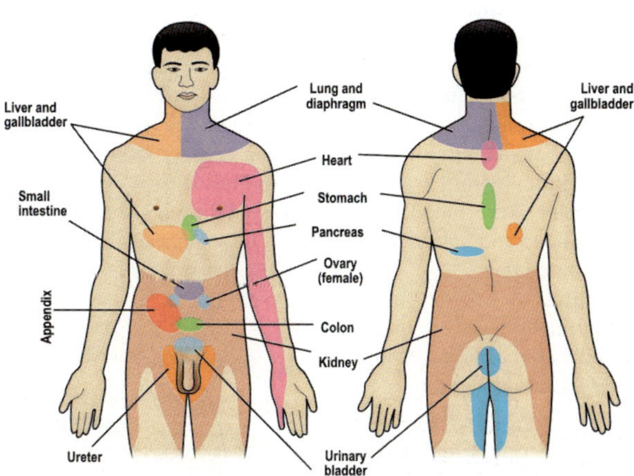

Fig.: *Referred pain regions*

R

It is a dull, persistent, diffusely located burning symptom. It is arrested by a diagnostic analgesic block of the stellate ganglion.

Refractory periodontitis has been defined as disease in which patients are unresponsive to any type of treatment provided.

Refractory refers to a heat resisting material capable of resisting high temperature.

Regeneration is the growth and differentiation of new cells to form new tissues or parts of the body.

Regional odontodysplasia maxillary teeth are affected more. Etiology is unknown. There is either a delay or a total failure in eruption. Shape is irregular with defective mineralization. Tooth assumes a ghost appearance. There is marked reduction in dentin. Reduced ena-mel shows many irregular calcified bodies.

Regulated waste sharps contaminated with blood saliva, nonsharp solid waste with liquid, blood and saliva are defined as regulated waste.

R

Regulation of body temperature: Body temperature is maintained at 98°F. Hypothalamus controls it. Three structures within skin assist in body temperature, blood vessels, sweat glands and arrector pili muscles contraction.

Rehabilitation is the combined and co-ordinated use of medical, social, educational and vocational measure for training and retraining the individual to the highest possible level of functional ability. It includes all measures to reduce the effect of disability.

Reiter's syndrome is a clinical tetrad of nonspecific urethritis, conjunctivitis and uveitis, mucocutaneous lesions and arthritis. Arthritis is asymmetric and involves weight-bearing joints. It is totally confined to man between 20-30 years. Oral lesions are painless, red, elevated areas with a white border on buccal mucosa, lips and gingiva. The palatal lesions appear as small, bright red pupuric spots. Antibiotics and corticosteroids help. Disease may undergo spontaneous remission.

Relative humidity is the percentage of moisture present in the air, complete saturation being taken as 100. Greater the relative humidity nearer the air to saturation. If relative humidity is more than 65 in a room person feels sticky and uncomfortable. Better ventilation lowers down the humidity.

Relative polycythemia is a condition occurring due to decreased plasma volume and not to increase in RBCs. It can be caused by diuretic use, diarrhea and excessive sweating.

Remittent fever: When daily fluctuation of fever varies more than 2°C, and it is known as remittent fever.

Remodeling is the major pathway of bony changes in shape, resistance to forces, repair of wounds and

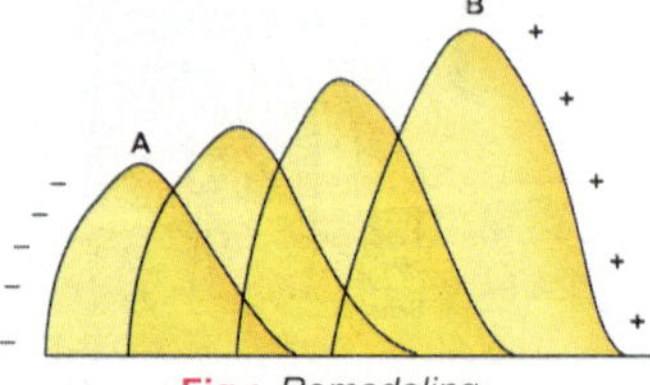

Fig.: *Remodeling*

calcium and phosphate homeostasis in body.

Remodeling of callus is always overabundance of new bone produced to strengthen the healing site because it may contain a dead bone also. These fragments are slowly resorbed and replaced by mature type of bone. External callus is remodeled to give a shape.

Removable functional appliances are the Myofunctional appliances that can be removed and inserted into the mouth by patient themselves, e.g., activator and bionator.

Removable habit breakers are passive removable appliance that consist of a crib and anchored to the oral cavity by means of clasps on the posterior teeth.

Renal amyloidosis kidneys become white enlarged. They have smooth surface and widened pale cortex. Microscopically amyloid deposits are seen in glomeruli appearing in meningeal region. Deposits obliterate capillary lumina. Amyloidal deposits are seen in blood vessels.

Renal artery stenosis is produced by atherosclerotic occlusive disease. It may cause renovascular hypertension and ischemic nephropathy.

Renal calculi refers to stones in kidney. Renal calculi may be of various types. Pain travels from cost vertebral angle to flank. Pain may excruciate if it is horny and travels down the ureters. If stones are in renal pelvis, it causes constant dull pain. In bladder, it may cause hematuria.

Renal cell carcinomas are usually solitary, unilateral tumors. It is seen at upper pole in elderly age group. These are solitary, unilateral tumors, a golden yellow circumscribed mass. Large areas of hemorrhage, necrosis and cystic changes give variegated appearance. It spreads by blood stream.

Renal cortical adenomas are small 0.5 to 3 cm grey or greyish yellow nodule in cortex. There may be scars of atherosclerosis. Microscopically these show clear cells. Cells show uniform nuclei and no mitosis. Less than 3 cms are benign.

R

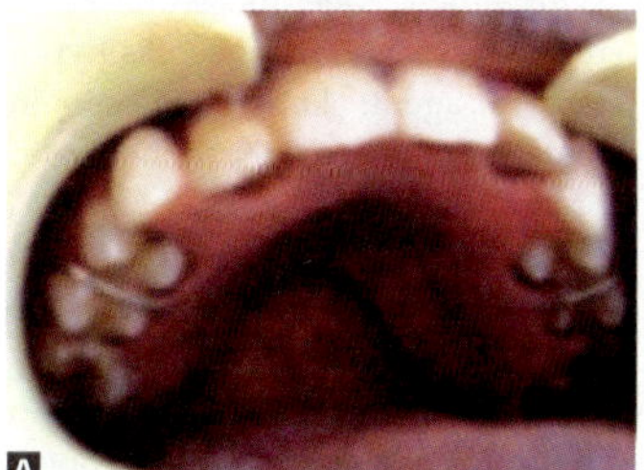

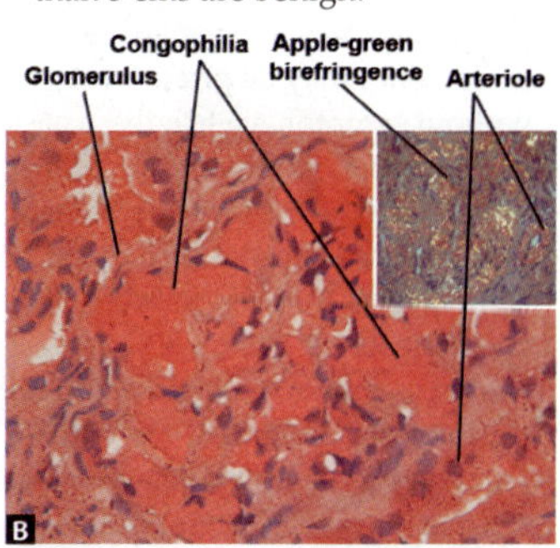

Figs A and B: *(A) Removable appliance; (B) Renal amyloidosis*

Renal cortical necrosis refers to diffuse bilateral cortical necrosis with sparing of medulla is very uncommon. When present, it is an evidence of renal failure. Renal cortical necrosis may be seen in Gram-negative endotoxic shock and hemolytic uremic syndrome. In some lesion may be patchy. Patient may develop sudden oliguria, anuria or hematuria.

Renal edema refers to edema of kidney. Acute glomerulonephritis edema is due to retention of sodium and water due to fall in glomerular filtration rate. Distribution of edema is in loose tissues, face and around the eyes. Fluid is transudate.

Renal hamartomas are often bilateral. It shows mixture of irregular fibrous and fatty tissue blood vessels and smooth muscle cells. It may be associated with fibromas and lipomas.

Renal stone crystals are mixed. 70-75% of renal stone are purely calcium oxalate or calcium oxalate + calcium phosphate. 15% of calculi consist of magnesium ammonium phosphate. 10% stones are of uric acid. Stones may be present with or without symptoms when these pass down to ureters; may produce renal colic. There develops hematuria. Urinary infection causes dysuria. About 60% small stones pass spontaneously.

Renal transplant is an accepted modality of treatment of chronic renal failure and end-stage renal disease. In order to suppress the rejection, immunosuppression with a single or combination of drugs is achieved.

Renal tuberculosis refers to tuberculous lesion affecting kidneys. It is common in India. Person develops urinary symptoms and abacterial acid pyuric recurrent cystitis IVP will show irregularity, cavitation, calcification and diminished renal function. Demonstration of tubercle bacilli is the most specific test. It results from hematogenous seeding of renal cortex to form small caseous foci and spreads to medulla. Eventually loss of function with hydronephrosis develops.

Repair is the process which restores the continuity of the disease and reestablishes a normal tissue.

Reproductive system in male's reproductive system includes testes, prostate and seminal vesicle while in females, it includes ovaries, fallopian tubes, uterus and vagina.

Research hypothesis is a statement that makes predictions about the expected outcome of study, contrast and null hypothesis.

Reserpine is a rauwolfia alkaloids. It blocks postganglionic sympathetic nerve endings. It reduces peripheral symptathetic tone. Its central effect reduces anxiety. It is used as hypotensive agent. Long-term use in females may cause carcinoma of breast.

Residual volume is the volume of air in the lungs which cannot be expelled.

Resilience is the energy needed to deform a material to the proportional limit.

Resilon: A new material has been developed to replace gutta-percha and traditional sealers for root canal obturation. It offers solutions to the problems associated with gutta-percha—shrinkage of gutta-percha on cooling and gutta-percha does not bind physically to the sealer, it results in gap formation between the sealer and the gutta-percha. It consists of a resin core material (Resilon) composed of polyester, difunctional methacrylate, bioactive glass and radiopaque fillers and a resin sealer. Resilon is nontoxic, nonmutagenic, and biocompatible.

Resin filling *see* composite filling.

Resin-modified glass ionomers (RMGIs) resin-modified glass ionomers were developed to overcome the problems of moisture sensitivity and low initial mechanical strength of GICs. They consist of a GIC with an added resin system that allows light setting followed by the acid-base reaction of the glass ionomer. This occurs within the light-polymerized resin framework. The resin increases fracture strength and wear resistance. Adhesion is enhanced by the use of enamel and dentin-conditioning agents before placement.

Resorb is to dissolve into the tissue.

Resorption litterally means breakdown of substance of teeth in addition to deciduous teeth the roots of permanent teeth may undergo resorption. External resorption may be due to periapical inflammation, reimplantation of teeth, tumors or cysts, impaction of teeth and idiopathic.

Respiratory acidosis occur due to affected CO_2 washout because of any cause. Alveolar hypoventilation leads to in increase $PaCO_2$ and there by decreased $HCO_3^-/PaCO_2$ ratio further leading to decreased pH. It may be caused by depression of respiratory centre by drugs affecting cerebellum. Patient may feel anorexia, confusion, mental disturbance.

Respiratory exchange ratio is the ratio of oxygen uptake to CO_2 output at rest and during exercise.

Respiratory failure is defined as a condition in which lung function is inadequate to meet the metabolic requirement of the individual. The dysfunction can be in one or more components of the respiratory system such as airways, respiratory muscles, alveolar units and pulmonary vessels. Respiratory failure manifests as hypoxemia (PaO_2 <60 mmHg) and/or hypercapnia ($PaCO_2$ >50 mmHg).

Resting "plaque" refers to plaque 2–2.5 hours after the last intake of dietary carbohydrate as opposed to starved "plaque" which has not been exposed to carbohydrate for 8–12 hours. Resting plaque pH is

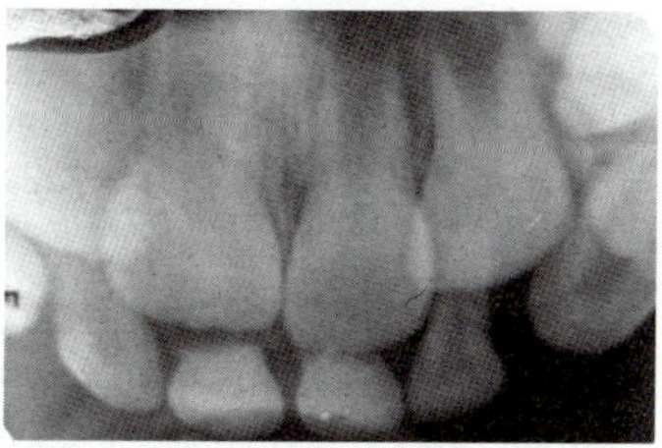

Fig.: *Resorption*

R

usually between 6 and 7 whereas the starved plaque pH is normally between 7 and 8. A large range of plaque ph values seem to be compatible with oral health, but due to the multifactorial nature of dental caries, what may be healthy for one individual may be unhealthy for another. Resting plaque contains relatively high concentrations of acetate compared with lactate. The predominant amino acids are glutamate and proline, with ammonia also found at significant level. The presence of elevated levels of acetate is due to the accumulation of end products of amino acid breakdown as well as those of carbohydrate metabolism. These metabolic products are present at much higher concentrations than in saliva.

Restoration is any replacement for lost tooth structure or teeth, (i.e. Bridges, fillings, crowns and implants).

R

Restorative dentistry is a branch of dentistry that deals with the process of restoring missing, damaged or diseased teeth to normal form and function.

Resuscitation: Bringing back to life.

Retained infantile swallowing is a pattern that is seen due to persistent presence of this swallowing reflex even after arrival of permanents teeth. The tongue lies between the teeth in front and on both sides, particularly noticeably are the contractions of the buccinator muscle. In expressive faces since the 7th cranial nerve muscles are not being used for the delicate purpose of facial expression. Modification often occurs between the tongue tip and palate because of the inadequate occlusal contact.

Retainer is a removable appliance used to maintain teeth in a given position (usually worn at night). Retainer can also be referred as root stump or an implant used for the retention of a fixed or removable prosthesis.

Retention cysts of maxillary sinus; these are mostly asymptomatic and are found on radiography jaw. Discomfort on maxilla/cheek may be present. Upper lip may become numb. Pain and soreness of head and face may be present. X-ray shows well-defined radiopacity which is well defined. These cysts may persist or disappear automatically.

Retention grooves are the markings in the surface of the tooth that enhance placement and retention of restoration.

Retinal migraine manifests as episodes of unilateral transient visual disturbance such as prolonged visual blacking and brainstem symptoms such as vertigo, double vision and loss of consciousness. Headache and vomiting are usual.

Retro fill amalgam is the sealing of apex of tooth with amalgam following an apicoectomy.

Retroviruses are large, spherical enveloped RNA tumor viruses. These have unique enzyme, genome and mode of replication.

Retrocuspid papilla is a small, elevated nodule located on lingual mucosa of mandibular cuspid. It is a soft, well-circumscribed, sessile, mucosal nodule. It is bilateral and is common in children. It regresses with age and does not require any treatment.

Retrograde amnesia refers to failure to remember up to the time of injury.

Retrograde pulpitis is a condition where the bacterial and the inflammatory products of periodontitis gain access to the pulp via the accessory canals, dentinal tubules or apical foramina, the reverse of effects of necrotic pulp on periodontal tissue is known as retrograde pulpitis.

Retrusion refers to movement of the mandible posteriorly from ICP.

Rett syndrome is a severe neurological disorder which affects females within the first 2 years of life. After approximately 2 years of apparently normal development, the child suffers from the loss of speech and the ability to walk normally, and begins to exhibit autistic-like behaviors (repetitive hand movements such as clapping, body rocking). There is no cure for the disease. Approximately 80% of children who have Rett syndrome also have epilepsy.

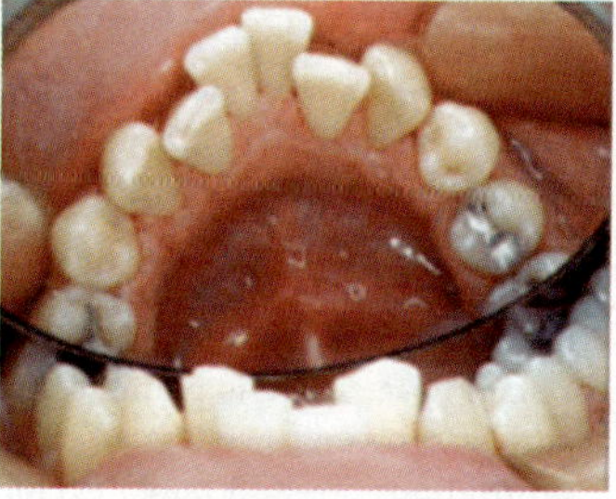

Fig.: *Retrocuspid papilla*

Reverse three-quarter crown is used on mandibular molars to preserve an intact lingual surface. It is useful on FPD abutments with severe lingual inclination, preventing destruction of large quantities of tooth structure that could occur if a full veneer crown were used. The grooves at lingual proximal line angles are pointed on the occlusal offset on buccal slope of lingual cusps. This preparation closely resembles a maxillary ¾ crown preparation because axial surface of nonpenetration cusp is uncovered.

Reversed architecture is a bony defect produced by the loss of interdental bone that includes facial and lingual plates, thereby reversing the normal architecture.

Reversible index: Index that measures conditions that can be changed. Reversible index scores can increase or decrease on subsequent examinations, e.g. Indices that measure periodontal conditions.

Reversible pulpitis is mild-to-moderate inflammatory condition of the pulp caused by noxious stimuli in which the pulp is capable of returning to the normal state following removal of stimuli. It is an indication of peripheral A delta fiber stimulation. Determination of reversibility is the clinical judgment which is influenced by history of patient and clinical evaluation.

Rh classification: Rh factor is an antigen located on the surface of RBC. If an RBC contains Rh factor, the blood is said to be Rh positive; and if RBC lacks Rh factor, it is said to be Rh negative.

Rhabdomyoma is benign neoplasm of striated muscles. Tongue and floor of mouth are usually involved. It is a slow growing. It is well-circumscribed, painless mass. Lesion is often deep-seated. Rhabdomyoma is a benign tumor of striated muscle origin. It is a well-circumscribed tumor of unknown duration. Tumor is composed of large, round cells with eosinophilic cytoplasm.

Rhabdomyosarcoma is the malignant tumor of striated muscle. It may be pleomorphic, alveolar, embryola or botryoid. It contains spindle cells in a haphazard arrangement. Tongue and palate are usually affected. *Clinical Features:* It is rapidly growing lesion. It causes swelling, pain and extensive tissue damage. These are fixed, ulcerated and hard. It has a poor prognosis even after surgery/chemotherapy followed by radiotherapy. Nuclei are ovoid or elongated. Prognosis is poor.

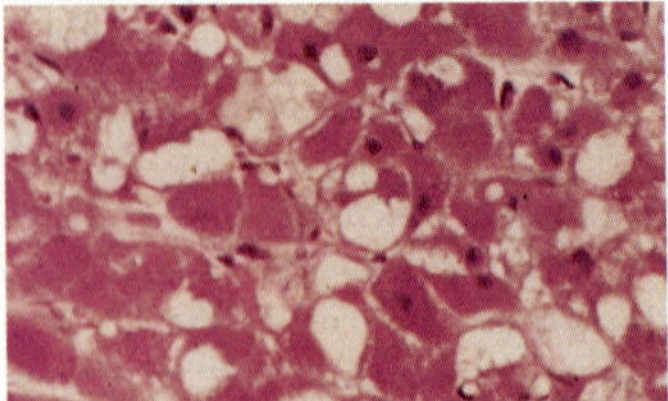

Fig.: *Rhadbomyosarcoma—histological sechar*

Rheumatoid arthritis is a chronic recurrent systemic inflammatory disease primarily involving the joints. Begins in small joints of hands and feet and progresses in centripetal and symmetric fashion. Its exact cause is not known. Onset is insidious with pain, swelling and stiffness of joint usually proximal interphalageal joints are involved. It is polyarticular and symmetrical. It presents exacerbations and remissions. TM joint is not commonly involved. Person develops fever, loss of weight and fatigue. Movement of jaw causes stiffness. Clicking and snapping is not common. It is also associated with vasculitis, skin and muscle atrophy, subcutaneous nodules, lymphadenopathy, splenomegaly and leukopenia. Hemorrhagic infarcts in nail fold and finger pulp are due to vasculitis. Over years, ankylosis may develop. Malocclusion develops. Rh factor is positive in 75% of cases.

Rheumatoid nodule in 25% of cases subcutaneous/intracutaneous nodule is present. These are discrete, firm, nontender swellings on extensor surfaces of forearm. Wrist and ankle are also involved. Some nodules may even break.

Rhinitis refers to common cold.

Rhinophyma is also known as potato nose. There is painless and slowly growing swelling of nose of insidious onset. It may develop due to longstanding rosacea but may develop as a complication of acne also. There develops irregular thickening of nose. Distal part of nose swells and becomes irregular with many shallow pits. Swelling is of bluish red color and a few dilated capillaries are seen. Hypertrophy of nose leads to lobulated and purplish masses. Face, cheeks and forehead may be affected.

Rhinosporidiosis is caused by rhinosporidium seeberi, a fungus. Skin lesions are like wart with peduncle. Oral lesions are soft, red polypoid growth of a tumor like nature which spread to the pharynx. Lesion bleeds easily. There is no specific treatment.

Riboflavin is a yellow green fluorescent compound soluble in water. It is soluble in water being part of Vitamin B complex and is decomposed by heat and on exposure to light. Liver, meat, milk, eggs are good source of it. Cereals don't remain rich source as milling of grains removes it. Daily dose is 1.7 mg in adult man. Deficiency of it affects eyes and nerves. Lips are cracked at corner of mouth and tongue gets swollen. Therapeutic dose is 5 mg.

Rickets is the disease occurring in children due to the deficiency of Vitamin D. The infant with rickets often receiving sufficient calories may appear well nourished but

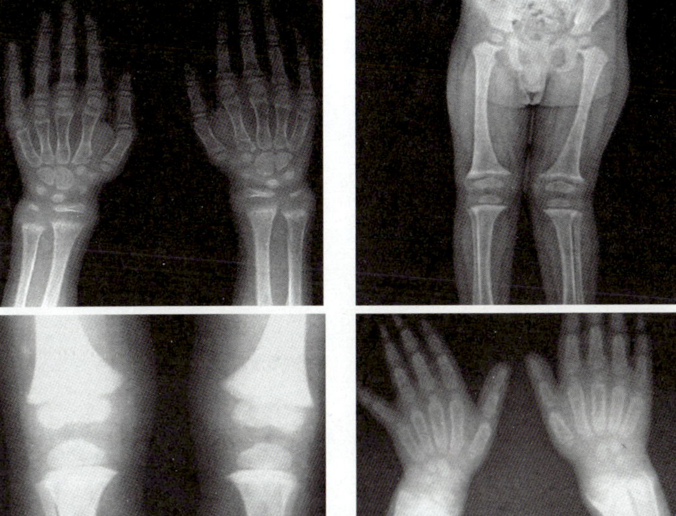

Fig.: *Rickets before treatment shows cupping and fraying*

will be restless, fretful and pale with flabby muscles. Sweating of head is common. Abdomen distends. Sweating of head is common. Development of child is delayed and teeth erupt late. Infant becomes prone to develop respiratory disease. In some cases knock knee and bow legs are seen.

Rickett's E-line *see* E-line.

Ridge is a linear elevation.

Rifampicin is a drug that is used against tuberculosis. It is metabolized in liver and excreted in bile. Urine is stained red.

Rigidity: Increased muscle tone.

Rigor mortis starts after a gap of 2 hours. Once body becomes stiff, it remains for 20 hours. It first appears in involuntary muscles of the heart and then spreads to the voluntary group of muscles. It develops due to coagulation of muscle plasma and formation of lactic acid. It develops early in feeble, fatigued and exhausted muscles in warm and moist air.

Ringworm lesion is a fungal infection. Lesions are red, annular round, scaling which develops suddenly. Ringworm lesion may be single or, if multiple, may not be symmetrical. Acute infective disorder may be confused with psoriasis.

Risk is the probability, that an individual will get a specific disease in a given period of time. The risk of developing a particular disease varies from an individual to individual.

Risk factors are that factors which, when present, increase the likelihood that an individual will get a disease. These factors include environmental, behavioral and biologic factors.

Risk indicators are probable risk factors that have been identified in cross-sectional studies but not confirmed by longitudinal studies.

Roane file refers to Flex-R-file.

Rodent ulcer occurs due to basal cell carcinoma. It is over face near the medial canthus of eye. It is a large, irregular having a well-defined, raised and beaded eye. It is indurated. Regional lymph nodes are not enlarged.

Roentgen is the traditional unit of exposure for X-rays, the quantity of X-radiation that produces an electrical charge of 2.58×10^{-4}.

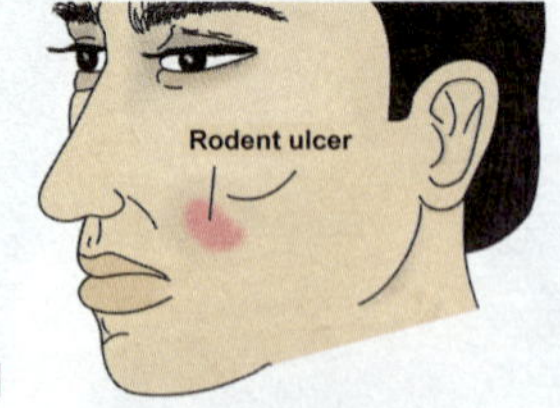

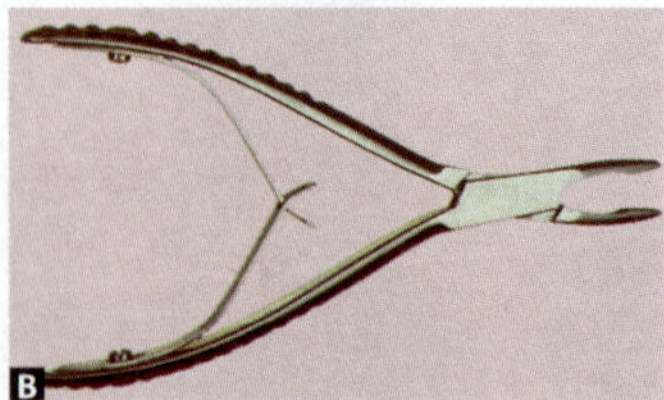

Figs A and B: *(A) Rodent ulcer; (B) Rongeur*

R

Rongeur forcep is a nipper-like instrument to trim alveolar bone.

Root amputation is to remove one or more roots of a tooth.

Root canal is that portion of pulp cavity which extends from canal orifice to the apical foramen. The shape of root canal varies with size, shape, number of the roots in different teeth. A straight root canal throughout the entire length of root is uncommon. Commonly curvature is found along its length which can be gradual or sharp in nature. In most cases, numbers of root canals correspond to number of roots but a root may have more than one canal.

Root canal files are hand instruments resembling reamers and made in standard length but in different width. Their job is to smoothen and clean the walls of enlarged root canals and remove debris. After inserting in canal, they are used in up and down filing action against canal wall. These are used in increasing sizes.

Root canal pluggers are the endodontic hand instruments that have a long tapered smooth point. Their aim is to fill any gap that is existing. They have a long handle with a small head.

Root canal reamers these enlarge the root canal. These are having set length but different width. Each one is numbered to indicate its size. First small reamer is inserted with hand rotation with successively wider reamers until canal becomes large enough for filling.

Root canal therapy (RCT) is a clinical procedure used to save an abscessed tooth in which the pulp chamber is cleaned out, disinfected, and filled with a permanent filling.

Root caries index is the epidemiological index that is best choice for evaluating caries prevalence in the senior population of the community. Old generation is more prone to root caries.

Root filling object is a procedure to where inflamed or dead pulp from a tooth is removed and replace it with a sterile nonirritant, insoluble root canal filling. It is generally done in two stages. First is to prepare the canal and second is to insert the root filling. In first stage, pulp is removed then canal is enlarged and cleaned to prepare

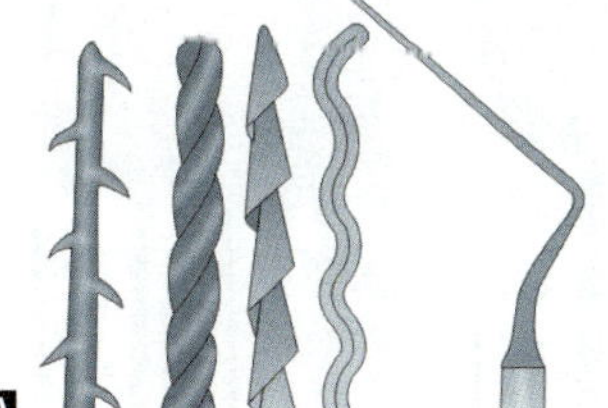

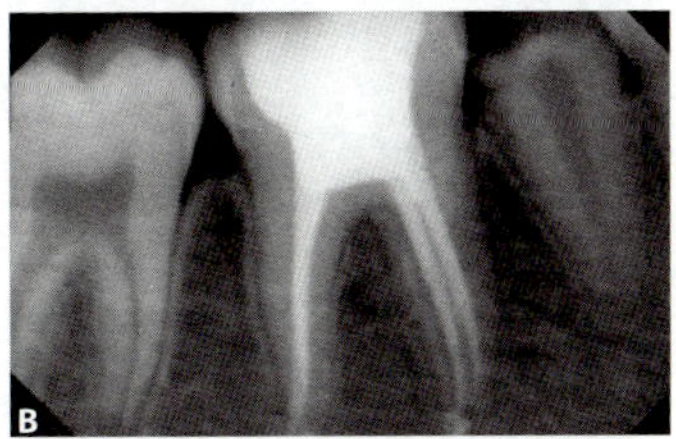

Figs A and B: *(A) Root canal file; (B) Root canal therapy (RCT)*

a dry, smooth empty canal tapering from pulp chamber to apex. Then temporary filling is done to cover entrance of empty root canal. In second stage temporary filling is removed and if canal is clean and dry, it is filled to seal off the entire canal to within a millimeters of an apex.

Root forceps are the forceps used to extract root portions that are left behind for any reason. These have blades with rounded ends. There are different patterns available. Different angles are made with handle. Lower root forceps are used for all lower teeth, straight forceps for upper incisors and canine. Reade's forceps for premolars and molar, bayonet forceps for upper premolars and molars.

Root planing stroke is a moderate to light stroke used for planing or final smoothening of root surface or the removal of plaque embedded calculus and altered cementum from the roots of teeth.

Root trunk is that portion of the root that is not bifurcated or trifurcated.

Rooting reflex and sucking reflex is a reflex when the full term infant sucks vigorously, when the breast is brought into contact with the infant's cheeks, he/she seeks the nipple. Stimulation of the upper and lower lip produces movements of the lip and tongue in the direction of the stimulus. Rooting reflex is week, not synchronized with swallowing at 28 weeks of gestation. It is stronger and well-synchronized at 32 weeks of iu life.

Rotary scrub method of tooth brushing is a method of tooth brushing in which circular strokes are used.

Rotatory root canal paste fillers are instruments for inserting paste into root canal. It is made up of spiral wire with handpiece which propels the required material to fill the full length of root canal.

Rothera's test 10 mL of urine is saturated with an excess of ammonium sulfate crystals, 3 drops of strong freshly prepared sodium nitroprusside and 2 mL of strong ammonia solutions are added. A deep permanganate

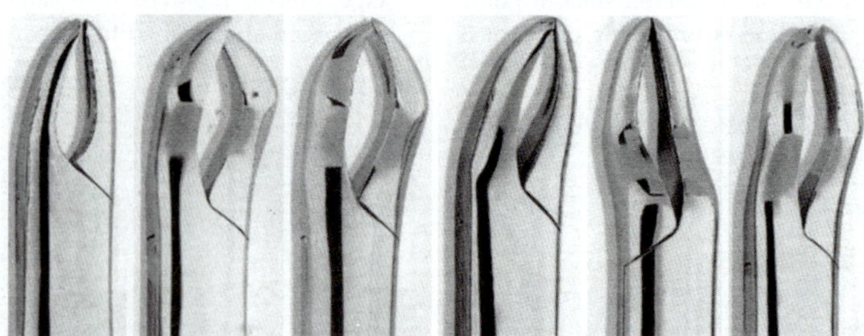

Fig.: *Root forceps*

R

color is produced by acetone and acetoacetic acid. Positive test confirms presence of ketone bodies.

Rubber cups are the polishing instruments which consist of a rubber shell with or without webbed configurations in the hollow interior; they are placed in handpiece with a special prophylaxis angle.

Rubber dam is an isolation kit used in dentistry. Introduced by Barnum, a New York Dentist in 1863. Improves accessibility, visibility, gives clean and dry aseptic field, and protects patient from inhalation of instruments and medicaments. Contraindicated in asthmatic patients, mouth-breathers, and third molar cases. Rubber dam can be defined as a flat thin sheet of latex/non-latex that is held by a clamp and frame which is perforated to show the tooth/teeth to protrude through the perforations while all other teeth are covered and protected by sheet.

Rubber dam forceps are instruments used to carry the clamp to the tooth. They are designed to spread the two working ends of the forceps apart when the handles are squeezed together.

Rubber dam punch is used to punch holes in the rubber dam to be placed over tooth.

Rubella is also known as German measles. It is caused by RNA virus of togavirus family. Child of 3 to 10 years is mostly affected. It is transmitted directly. Incubation period is 2 to 3 weeks. 50% patients are asymptomatic. There develops low-grade fever and lymphadenopathy. Rash is an inconstant feature. The infection spreads through droplets. Incubation period is 14–21 days. Skin, joint and placenta are mainly involved. Patients are infective from up to a week before two weeks after the onset of the rash.

Ruddle's solution is a new experimental irrigating solution, introduced in the endodontics in an attempt to visualize the microanatomy of the canal system.

Rule of 5 is the simplest method for calculation of TBSA (total body surface area) is to subtract 1% from head and neck and adding 1% to lower limb for every year after 1 year of age. This charting technique has been described by Lund and Browder. Rule of 5 has also been used though

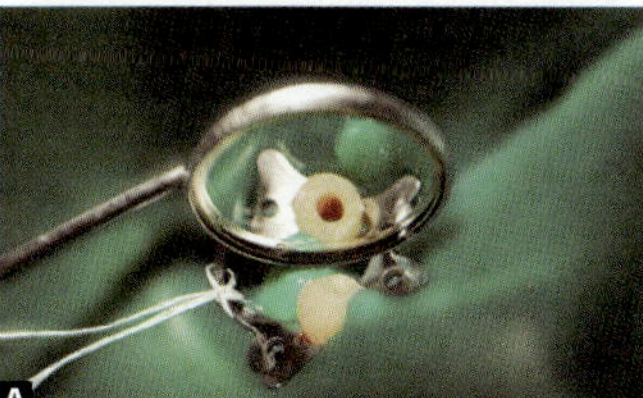

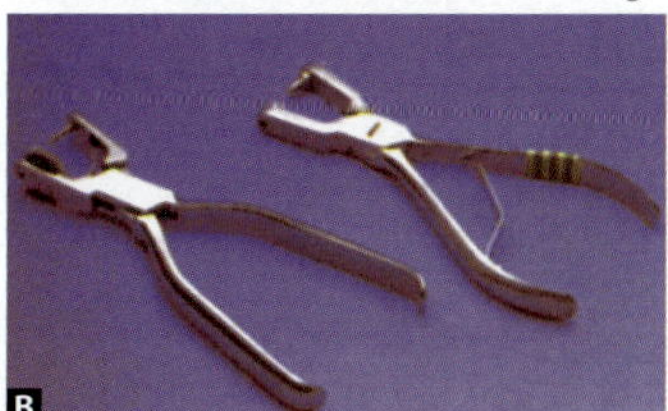

Figs A and B: *Rubber dam (A) Clamps; (B) Forceps*

infrequently. According to this rule, the body is divided into 20 areas of 5% each by dividing the body into coronal and sagittal planes.

Rule of nine is a frequently used method to determine the extent of burn injury. The body is divided into 11 areas of 9% each to help estimate the amount of skin surface burned in an adult.

Rutherford syndrome: There are con-genitally enlarged gingiva, delayed tooth eruption and superior curtain-like corneal opacities. Person may have mental retardation, aggressive behavior and dentigerous cysts.

RVG a digital radiography machine. Imaging which uses photostimulable phosphor is also called as an indirect digital imaging technique. The image is captured on a phosphor plate as analog information and is converted into a digital format when the plate is processed.

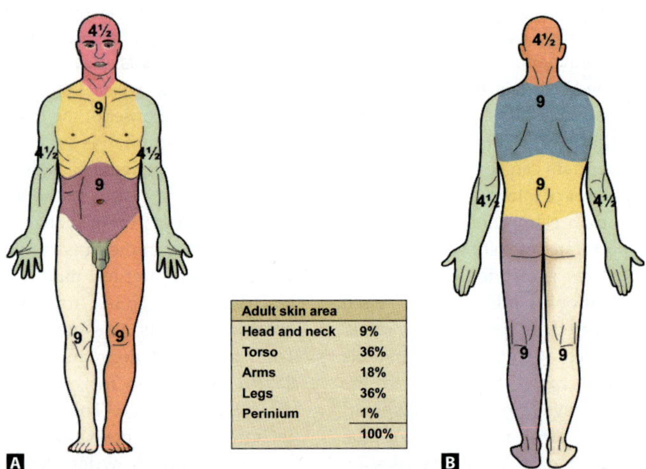

Adult skin area	
Head and neck	9%
Torso	36%
Arms	18%
Legs	36%
Perinium	1%
	100%

Figs A and B: *Rule of nine for body areas; (A) Front; (B) Back*

S

S refers to sella is the midpoint of hypophyseal fossa.

Saccharine is an artificial sweetener that is 500–600 times sweeter than sucrose, is stable in aqueous solution and is compatible with most food and drug ingredients. Its major disadvantages is its metallic aftertaste.

Sacroiliac strain refers to a pain that may radiate to buttock, hip and lateral aspect of thigh. There may be tenderness over symphysis pubis and person may limp.

Saddle angle (n-s-a) refers to the angle formed by joining these three points provides a parameter for assessment of the relationship between anterior and posterior lateral cranial bases. Thus a large saddle angle usually signified a posterior condylar position and a mandible that is posteriorly positioned with respect to the cranial base and maxilla.

Safe period is the period of menstrual cycle when conception is least likely to result from intercourse without use of contraceptive device.

Sagittal plane is an imaginary longitudinal vertical plane that divides the mouth into two halves (left and right).

Sealant is the application of a clear resin over the biting surfaces of teeth to prevent decay.

Second transitional period is characterized by the replacement of the deciduous molars and canines by the premolars and the permanent canines respectively. The combined mesio-distal width of the permanent canines and premolars is usually less than that of the deciduous canines and molars. The surplus space is called leeway space of Nance. The amount of leeway space is greater in the mandibular arch than in the maxillary arch. It is about 1.8 mm (0.9 mm on each side of the arch) in the maxillary arch and about

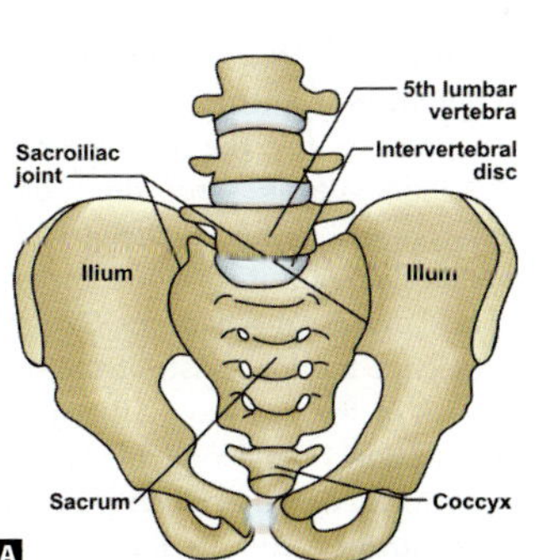

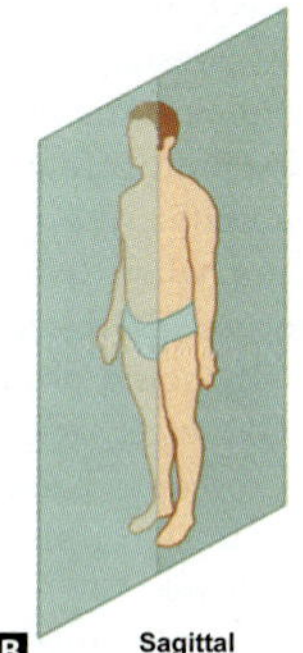

Figs A and B: *(A) Sacroiliac joint; (B) Sagittal plane*

3.4 mm (1.7 mm on each side of the arch) in the mandibular arch. This excess space available after the exchange of the deciduous molars and canines is utilized for mesial drift of the mandibular molars to establish class I molar relation.

Salad is a roughage and best to start a meal with fresh raw salad. Common vegetables used for salad are salad leaves, onions, cucumber, green chillies, carrots and turnip. All these contain minerals and Vitamin C. On cooking, these nutri-ents are being lost hence should be used in raw form but before consumption these should be properly washed in fresh water. Most of these contain cellulose which is not digested but does not allow constipation to develop. Salad is having negative calorific value.

Salicylate e.g. aspirin is the widely used analgesic and was first used in medicine by Dreser in 1899. It is an antipyretic, analgesic and anti-inflammatory drug. Pain is relieved by peripheral and central nervous system effect. It inhibits the synthesis of prostaglandins which occurs in inflamed tissue. It reduced the sensitization of pain receptors to local stimuli. Antipyretic effect only occurs when temperature is above normal. It dissipates body heat also. It should not be used in cases of GIT ulcer/acidity. It may cause microscopic hemorrhage. It may result in skin rashes, urticaria and angioedema.

Saliva is the glandular secretion, which constantly bathes the teeth and the oral mucosa. It is constituted by the secretions of the three paired major salivary glands, the parotid, submandibular and sublingual, the minor salivary glands and the gingival fluid. Saliva is armed with various defense mechanisms, such as the immunological, enzymatic and other organic and inorganic defense system. In addition, saliva has the ability to protect the mucosa against mechanical insults and to promote its healing via the activity of the epidermal growth factors. The involvement of the oral tissues in diverse functions such as mastication and deglutition of food, taste sensations, speech; and initial digestion of carbohydrates would not be possible without salivary secretions. The interface between saliva and oral tissues is the site of many dynamic reactions, which affect the integrity of both the soft and hard tissues of the mouth, and saliva constitutes one of the main natural defense systems of the oral cavity. Salivary organic, inorganic and physical factors are indispensable for the control of different oral microorganisms and its product for the maintenance of homeostasis in the oral environment. The challenges to homeostasis are met with a variety of host defense mechanisms. Several protective barriers exist for the soft tissues of the oral cavity. Bacterial penetration of the oral mucosa is first impeded by the salivary barrier. This barrier confronts the bacteria with a variety of antibody mediated and innate immune components (e.g., mucin, lactoferrin, lysosome, lactoperoxidase) that can mediate protective effects in several ways.

Salivary amylase is a digestive enzyme found in saliva that begins chemical digestion of carbohydrates.

Salivary duct stones are the calcareous concentrations in salivary duct. There is severe pain just before during meals and after it. There is no free flow of saliva. Swelling is due to obstruction of saliva. Occasionally stone present may not show any symptoms. Stone may measure from a few mm to a cm. Small calculi may be sometimes removed manually, bigger stones require surgery.

Salivary hypofunction there are three main causes of salivary hypofunction, dehydration, damage of salivary glands or interference with the neural transmission.

Salt and milk fluoridation is a method of providing systemic fluoride by adding fluoride to salt, i.e. by spraying a concentrated solution of NAF2 or KF on salt on a conveyor belt another method is by adding premixed granules of caf2 and PO_4 to salt. Salt fluoridation first started in Switzerland in 1955 and subsequent tests revealed a 20–25% decrease in caries experience by using salt with 90 ppm of F. In 1967, Muhlensen found that 300 mg F/kg salt yielding 1.5 mg, Zeigler (1956) first explored that possibility of fluoridating milk. In 1959, Inamura (Japan) reported a 33.3% caries reduction in school children served daily with milk containing 2.5 mg F. In India, since there is no central milk supply regulating this method, caries prevention would be a daunting task. Moreover, socio-economic religious and ethnic factors affect the quantity of milk consumed.

Salt-restricted diet refers to low-salt diet due to certain systemic condition normal consumption of 5 gm daily in salt restricted diet only 2 gram of it is permitted. Sodium restricted diets are advised in congestive cardiac failure. It reduces edema. In renal disease, it reduces edema while in toxemia of pregnancy, it prevents fluid retention. During act and cortisone

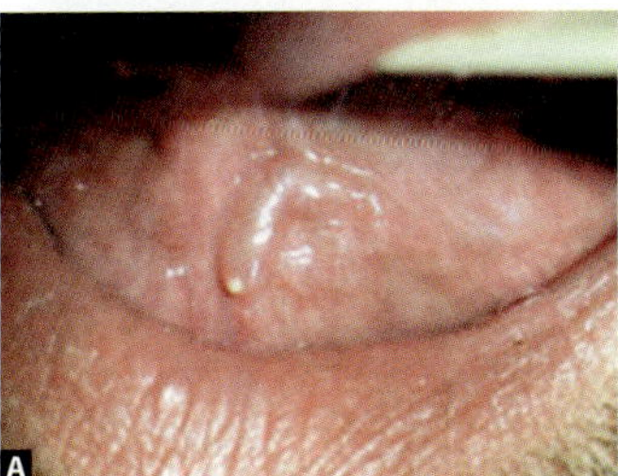

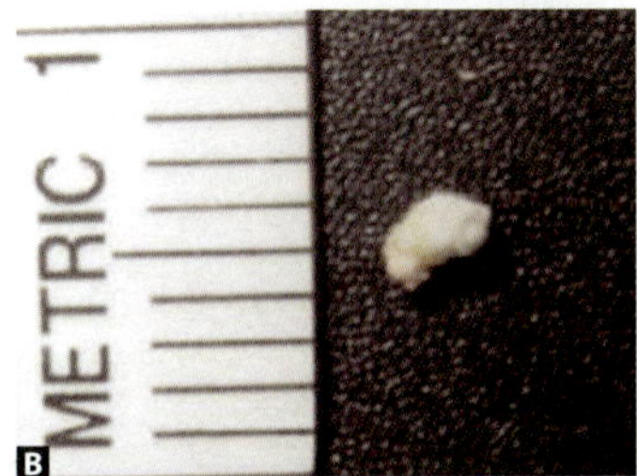

Figs A and B: *(A) Salivary duct stone; (B) Salivary stone*

therapy also it has to be avoided. Person should avoid all salted and canned vegetables, pickles, salted butter, cheese and salted nuts.

Sampling distribution is a distribution of sample means formed by drawing repeated samples from the same population.

Sanguinarine is a herbal root extract of the plant Sanguinaria Canadensis; it is a mixture of benzophenanthridine alkaloids. Evidence from studies Loesche (1976), Southard et al (1984), and Walker (1990) supports the claim of its antibacterial properties, anti-plaque effects, and anti-inflammatory activity. Sanguinary can reduce the acid-producing ability and affect the adherence of bacteria. Since it contains alcohol (11.5%), it may produce a burning sensation and is contraindicated with the use of Metronidazole/ Tinidazole.

Sarcoid sialadenitis is bilateral, firm, painless enlargement. Decreased or absent salivation is present in 5% cases. Parotid is involved in 3rd or 4th decade. Biopsy helps in diagnosis. Treatment is symptomatic. Corticosteroids are effective.

Sarcoidosis is a chromic glaucomatous disease which involves lymph nodes, lungs, lines, speech, seen in 2nd and 3rd decade of life and more in blacks. It is a disease of unknown cause. It generally affects hilar lymphadenopathy pulmonary infiltration and skin. Symptoms are not severe enough to cause an alarm. Mild malaise and cough may be the features. Oral manifestations are sarcoid granuloma, sarcoid gingivitis, gingival tissues are hyperplastic with a granular appearance; they are red in color and bleed on probing, painless enlargement. Lesions of lips are manifested as small, popular nodules or plaques on palate and buccal mucosa lesions are bleb like. Kveim–Siltzbach test is an important aid. Histopathologically, connective tissue shows destruction,

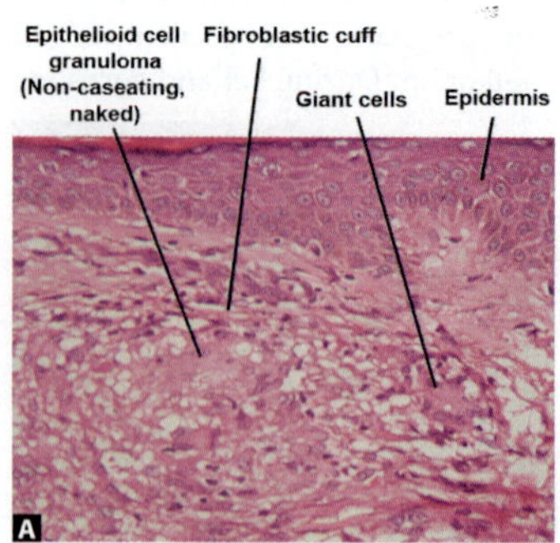

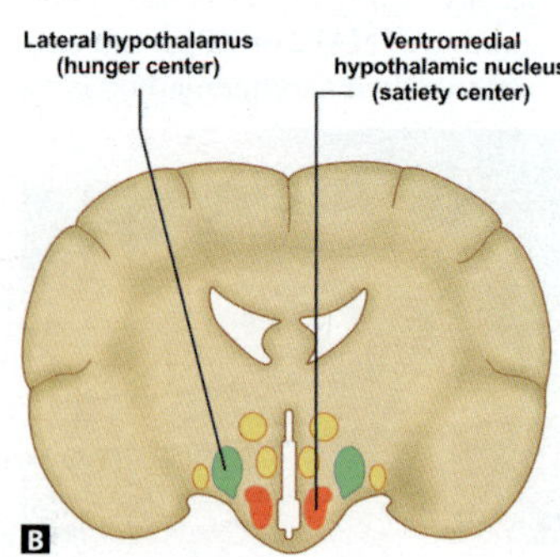

Figs A and B: *(A) Sarcoidosis of skin; (B) Satiety center*

noncaseating epithelial cells and multinucleated foreign body type giant cells with peri-pheral mononuclear cells. In some cases, Severe and rapid periodontal destruction can occur.

Satiety centers are centres that cause satification while eating, sends the signal to stomach for fullness. Stimulation of lateral hypothalamus causes to eat voraciously while stimulation of ventromedial nuclei of hypothalamus causes complete satiety and person will refuse to eat.

Scabies is a dermatological disease caused by sarcoptes scabei. Transmission is by direct personal contact or through linen towels, etc. The most frequent areas involved are interdigital folds, penis, scrotum and hypothenal eminence on genitalia lesions are firm 5 mm red nodules. Intense pruritus especially is worse at night. 1% gamma benzene hydrochloride is effective to skin for 12–24 hours, re-application is required after 5–7 days to kill newly hatched nits. Antihistamines may be given if itching is more.

Scalds are moist heat injuries produced by application to the body of a liquid at or near boiling point or by steam. Scalds are not as severe as burns and produce hyperemia or vesiculation.

Scaling is the process of removal of plaque and calculus from the crown and root surfaces of the teeth. Curettes and scalers are used for this.

Scaling stroke is a powerful stroke which can be used in a pull motion to remove hard and tenacious calculus.

Scalp is the term applied to the soft tissues covering the vault of the skull. This region extends anteriorly up to the eyebrows, posteriorly up to the superior nuchal lines, and laterally up to the superior temporal lines. It has five layers; **S**—is the most superficial layer in skin. It contains numerous sebaceous glands. The skin is closely adherent to underlying tissues; **C**—the superficial fascia is represented by dense connective tissue that is firmly united to the skin and to the underlying epicranial aponeurosis; **A**—the third layer of the scalp is partly muscular and partly fibrous. The greater part of this layer is formed

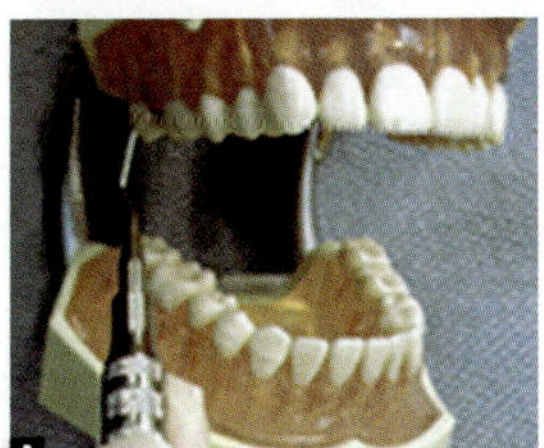

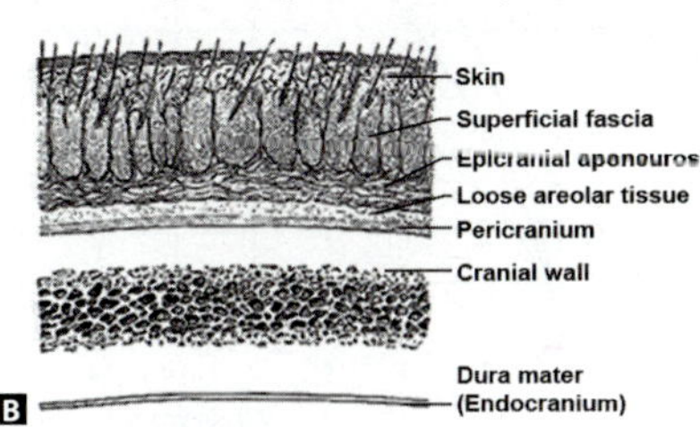

Figs A and B: *(A) Scaling stroke; (B) Scalp*

by the epicranial aponeurosis (or galea aponeurotica). The muscular part is formed by a muscle called the occipitofrontalis; **L**—the three layers of the scalp described above are firmly united to one another. All the three layers move together over the fourth layer that is made up of loose areolar tissue. This layer contains emissary veins passing from the scalp to intracranial venous sinuses; **P**—is the deepest layer of the scalp is the pericranium/periosteum over the bones of the vault of the skull.

Scammon's growth curve explains that different tissue systems of the body grow at different times and rate. The four important tissue systems that show characteristic growth pattern are: lymphoid, neural, general, genital. As the graph indicates, the growth of neural tissue is nearly complete by 6 to 7 years of age. General body tissue including muscle, bone and viscera show "S" shaped curve with a definite slowing of the rate of growth, during childhood and acceleration during puberty. Lymphoid tissue proliferates far beyond adult amount in late childhood and then undergoes involution. At the same time, the

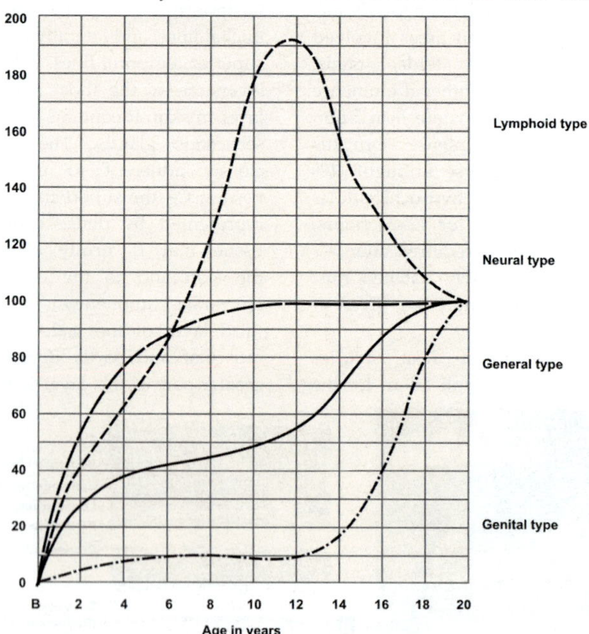

Fig.: *Scammon's growth curve*

S

growth of genital tissue acculturates rapidly.

Scarlet fever is caused by streptococcal organisms of beta hemolytic type producing erythrogenic toxin. It looks like tonsillitis. Throat is generally involved. Throat becomes red and there is moderate edema of pharynx. Typical strawberry tongue is seen. Tonsils are enlarged and show patchy exudate. Cervical group of glands become tender. After 24 hours, rash tends to spread all over. Rash is smooth with minute punctate spot on axilla, groin and dorsum of feet. Rash disappears in 2–5 days. Number of different strains of streptococci produces the disease. Incubation period is 3–5 days. Oral manifestation is 'stomatitis scarlatina, mucosa of palate is congested and throat becomes red. Tonsils are swollen. Tongue becomes strawberry. Tongue shows coating, papillae become edematous with small red knobs. Later tip of tongue becomes clean and then lateral borders. At last tongue becomes smooth and glistening.

Scheffe test multiple comparison procedure.

Schistosomiasis is caused by schistosomiasis hematobium; cercariae are the infective stage of parasite. Adult worm resides in portal vein and in bladder venous plexuses. Hemorrhage can occur due to erosion of blood vessels. Urticaria, fever anaphylactic reaction may be seen.

School water fluoridation started as an alternative therapy in community water fluoridation. The recommended concentration is 4–5 ppm. It is shown to reduce caries experience by 40%. The disadvantage is that children start receiving the advantage of fluorides only when they start school.

Schwannoma is a benign tumor These are derived from Schwann cells. Intraorally, dorsum of tongue is most favored location. Buccal mucosa floor of mouth, gingiva, and lips can also be involved. *Clinical Features:* It clinically presents a slow enlarging lesion. It is painless, nodule of different size. Sometimes small, lobulated, firm growth may occur in gingiva. It has a true capsule. Surgical excision is the line of treatment.

Schwartz periotrievers are the set of two double ended, highly magnetized instruments that are designed for retrieval of periodontal instrument from the deep periodontal pockets and the furcation areas.

Scientific misconduct is fabrication, falsification and other defilations

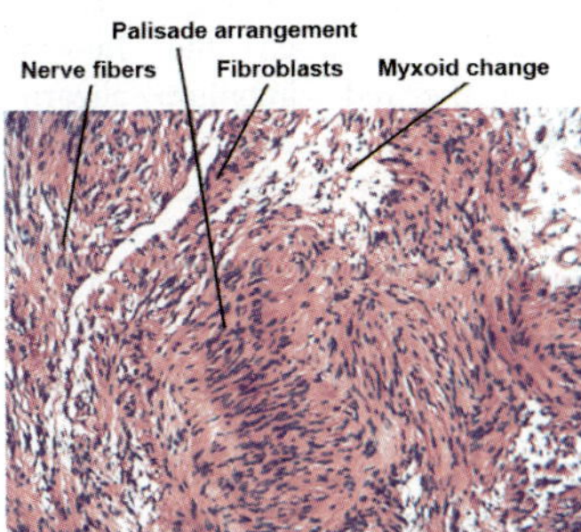

Fig.: *Schwannoma (Neurilemmoma)*

S

from accepted practice in carrying out of reporting results from research.

Scissors and nippers are the surgical instruments which are used for removing tabs of tissues, trimming of flaps, enlarging the incisions and for removing muscle attachments.

Sclera is made up mainly of fibrous tissue. Its external surface gives attachment to the extrinsic muscles of the eyeball.

Scleroderma is a disease of unknown cause characterized by an increased collagen deposition in skin. Crest/ limited pseudoderm, localized sceleroderm–skin.

Sclerotic bone is a well-defined radio- opacity seen below the apices of vital noncarious teeth.

Sclerotic cemental masses are multiple, symmetric lesions producing pain and localized expansion.

Scope of pedodontics refers to the range of activities or range of therapeutic treatment to be considered in a pediatric dental practice.

Scot Sanchis method for estimation of fluoride in water. This fluoride estimation test is based on the reaction between the fluoride and the red zirconium alizarin. The fluoride forms a colorless complex ion ($ZrI F^6$) and liberates free alizarin sulfuric acid, which is yellow in acid solution. As the amount of fluoride increases, the color produced varies from yellow to red. The fluoride level in the test material is determined by comparing the color thus produced with the standards.

Scott's hypothesis (cartilaginous theory) cartilage grows actively, bone later replaces it. Thus cartilage has innate growth potential. Transplantation and extripation experiments prove that some innate potential is evident though results are equivocal, e.g. mandibular growth has been explained that the condyle acts as diaphysis of a long bone with growth occurring at both ends. Recent studies have proven that growth at the condyle is mostly reactive and not of primary nature and maxillary growth can be explained due to translation of nasomaxillary complex as a unit.

Scratched film is a film handling error a scratched film showing white lines from which emulsion has been removed by a sharp object.

Scrotal tongue is also known as fissured tongue. It shows many small furrows on dorsal surface. It is a painless condition unless infected material is lodged in fissures.

Scurvy is due to long-term deficiency of Vitamin C. Children between the age of 4 and 18 months are affected. Bleeding gums and hematuria may be presenting symptom. Cartilage cells don't proliferate at normal rate. X-ray will show osteopenia, white line of Frankel, Wimberger sign and Pelkan's spur.

Se is the midpoint of the line connecting the posterior clinical process and anterior opening of the sella turcica.

Sebaceous glands are associated with hair follicles. These secrete an oily substance called sebum. Sebum lubricates and helps waterproof hair and skin. Sebum inhibits the growth of bacteria on surface of skin. It inhibits the growth of bacteria.

Seborrhoeic dermatitis is an inflammatory scaling disease of scalp, face generally. Composition of sebum remains normal. Onset in adults in gradual and dermatitis is apparent only as dry. There may be diffuse greasy scaling of scalp. Marginal blepharitis and dry yellow crusts and conjuctival irritation may be present. It does not cause hair loss. Seborrheic dermatitis is common at all ages. Flexures of face are mostly involved. Rash is red and scaly, a few papules and pustules may develop.

Second branchial arch refers to the cartilage of the second or hyoid arch (Reichert's cartilage) appearing at the 45th–48th days influence, is the basic of the greater part (head, neck and crura of the third ear ossicles, the stapes and contribute to the malleus and incus, the styloid process of the temporal bone, the stylohyoid ligament, and the lesser horn and cranial part of the body of the hyoid bone. Reichert's cartilage attaches to the basicranial otic capsule, where it is grooved by the facial nerve it provides the remaining cartilaginous circumference to the labyrinthine and tympanic segments of the facial canal. The muscles of the hyoid arch subdivide and migrate extensively to form the stapedius, the stylohyoid the posterior belly of digastric all the mimetic muscle of the face and levator veli palatine muscle all of which are innervated by the vii cranial or facial nerve, serving the second arch. The path of migration of these muscles is traced out in the adult by the distribution of branches of facial nerve. The special sensory component of is nerve for taste, known as chorda tympani nerve, invades the first arch as a pretrematic nerve and thus comes to supply the mucosa of the anterior two thirds of the tongue. The artery of this arch forms the stapedial artery which disappears during the fetal period

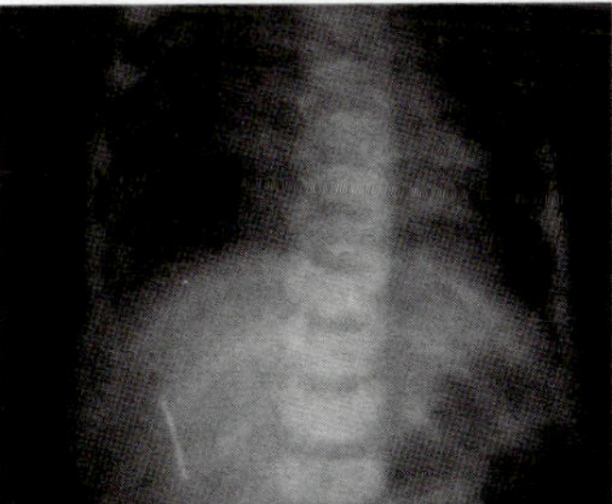

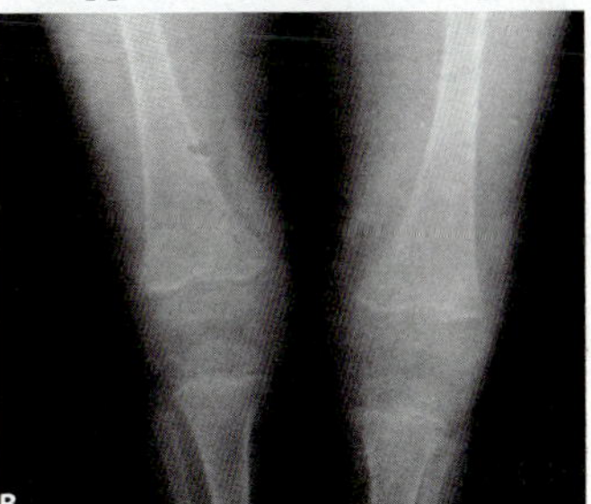

Figs A and B: *Scurvy*

leaving the foramen in the stapes. The Stapedial artery, derived from the second aortic arch, is significant in the development of the stapes ear ossicles. The stapedial blastema grows around the stapedial arch forming a ring around the centrally placed artery. The mid-portion of the stapedial artery involutes, leaving the foramen in the stapes. Stapedial arterial branches persist, to become part of the internal carotid artery proximally and the external carotid artery distally.

Second degree burns are those which involve epidermis and varying depths of dermis. These have been further divided into superficial and deep second degree burns.

Second pharyngeal pouch is part of pharyngeal arches. It lies between 2nd and 3rd pharyngeal arches. The ventral portion of this pouch is obliterated by the developing tongue. The dorsal portion of this pouch persists in an attenuated form as the tonsillar fossa, the endodermal lining of which covers the underlying mesodermal lymphatic tissue to form the palatine tonsil.

Secondary culture refers to a subculture derived from a primary culture.

Secondary dentin is a dentin that is formed after the deposition of primary dentin. Physiologically, it happens in old age. Pathologically, it results from abnormal irritation. It develops due to dental caries, abrasion, attrition and erosion. Dentin forms an additional insulting layer of calcified tissue between the pulp and the pathological process. On X-ray size of pulp is decreased.

Secondary displacement is said to have occurred when the movement of the bone is not directly related to its own enlargement, e.g.: anterior direction of growth by the middle cranial fossa and the temporal lobe of the cerebrum displaces the maxilla anteriorly and inferiorly.

Secondary effects are related to drug administration but not directly attributable to drug action. For example, during broad spectrum

S

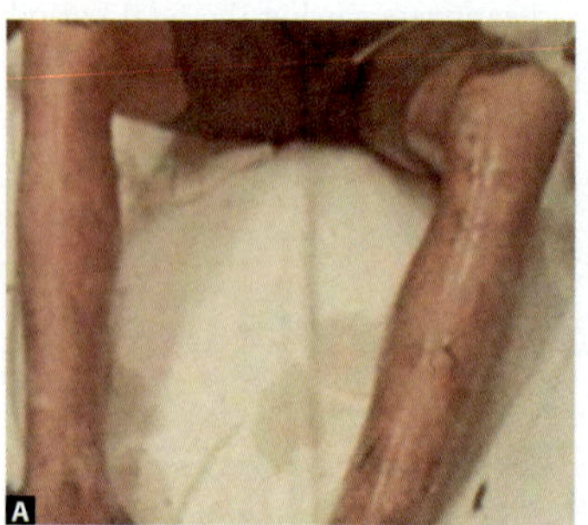

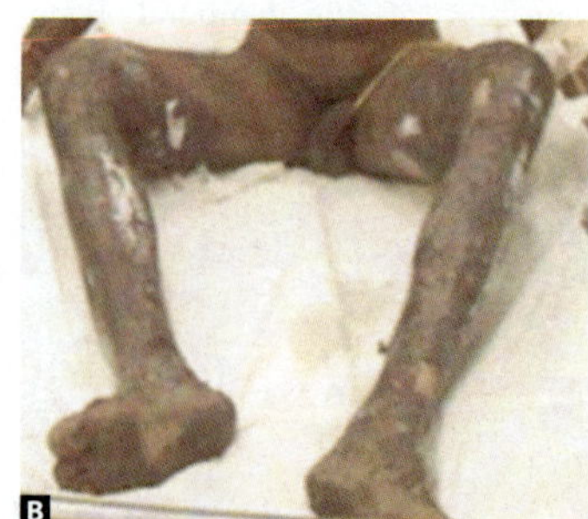

Figs A and B: *Second degree burns*

antibiotic therapy, superinfection with *Candida Albicans* may cause thrush.

Secondary hyperparathyroidism is a clinical condition that can be seen in rickets, osteomalacia and chronic renal failure. Brown tumors are less frequently seen. Calcification of arteries and soft tissue occurs.

Secondary lymphoid organs include the lymph nodes, spleen, and MALT: mucosa associated lymphoid tissue, e.g. tonsils. *GALT:* gut associated lymphoid tissue, e.g.: Payers' patch. SALT: skin associated lymphoid tissue. These organs create an environment where lymphocytes can interact with each other and with antigen and disseminate the immune response once generated.

Secondary polycythemia occurs When number of RBCs increases due to decreased oxygen. Decreased oxygen in blood triggers in increase in erythropoietin by kidneys which results in increase in RBCs. Pulmonary disease, high altitude and elevation of carbon monoxide may cause it.

Secondary prevention includes techniques designed to terminate disease and restore tissues to near normal function. Secondary prevention is done to diagnose the proliferation of a disease in its early stages and retard or stop the progress so that the damage is minimized and the subsequent repair is facilitated.

Secondary spacing was initially described by Baume, 1950. In closed dentitions the permanent mandibular lateral incisors emerge and the primary mandibular canines are moved laterally. Thus a space is created that causes the permanent maxillary lateral incisors to emerge into a favorable alignment.

Secondary syphilis is a clinical stage that occurs 6–8 weeks after the development of chancre. The manifestations are due to the dissemination of *Treponema pallidum* to distant site. **Secondary syphilis** usually appears in about 6–8 weeks after the appearance of primary chancre. It is characterized by skin and mucosal lesions. There will be generalized lymphadenopathy. Skin lesions may be macular, papular, follicular or lenticular. Coin-like lesions are

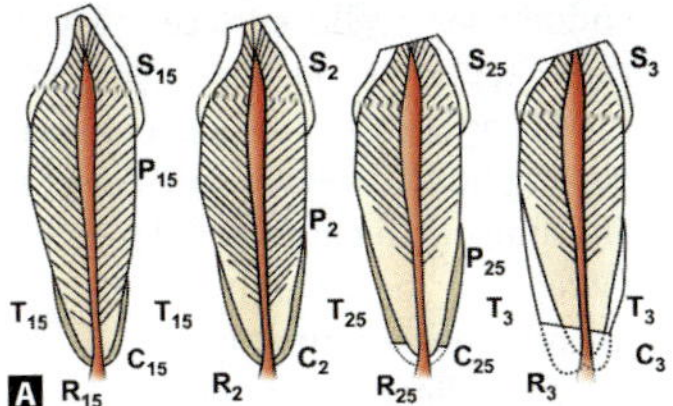

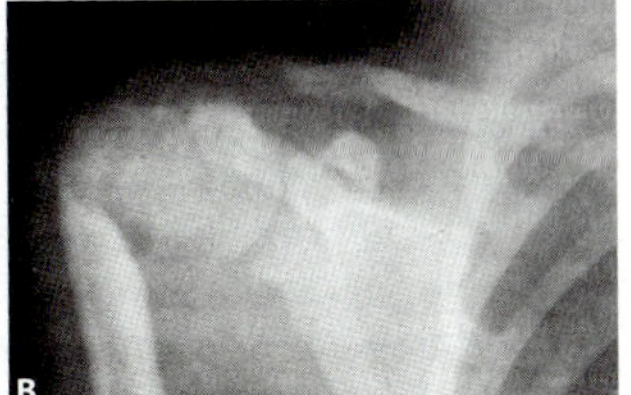

Figs A and B: *(A) Secondary dentin;*
(B) The 'rotting fence post' sign of secondary hyperparathyroidism

S

common on face. Areas of hyperpigmentation can be seen on soles and palms. Lymph nodes are painless, discrete and not fixed to the surroundings. With or even without treatment, lesions heal in 2–4 weeks. **Secondary syphilitic oral ulcer** appears 3–12 weeks after primary lesion. Oral lesions are rarely seen without rash appearing. Ulcers are painless. Palate tongue and lips may be affected. Shape is flat and irregular ulcer covered by grey membrane. They coalesce to form rounded areas known as mucus patches. Patient will have fever and malaise. There may be skin rash on palms and ulcers are serologically positive and highly infective.

Secondary trauma from occlusion is said to have occurred when the adaptive capacity of the tissues to withstand occlusal forces is impaired due to bone loss.

Secretomotor fibers are those efferent fibers end in glands and their stimulation produces secretion. They are, therefore, called secretomotor fibers.

Secretomotor nerves are the nerves to glands.

Sedation is a technique that refers to allaying stress, irritability, excitement or calming a person with the help of drugs.

Sedative is a drug that subdues excitement and calms the subject without inducing sleep but drowsiness may be produced. Sedation refers to decreased responsiveness to any level of stimulation and is associated with some decrease in motor activity and sedation. At higher doses sleep may occur.

Seizure is a transient clinical event due to abnormal paroxysmal excessive discharges from a group of central nervous system neurons. The seizure may present in form of motor, sensory, autonomic or psychic manifestations.

Selected polishing is a term given to polishing of only those teeth affected with stain and plaque.

Selectin is a class of adhesion proteins that recognize specific oligosaccharide residues displayed on cell surface glycoprotein called mucin. Mucin refers to any heavily glycosylated protein with a polypeptide backbone of amino acids, serine and threonine residues. Selectin binds to sugar residues in mucin chains, e.g.: mucin CD34 HSC surface marker.

Selectin mediated phase is a phase where the neutrophils collide with vessel wall, allowing P selectin and E selectin molecules on activated endothelial cells to bind neutrophil surface mucin. L selectin which is expressed on neutrophil, binds to its own set of target mucin on endothelial cell surface. These three types of selection establish initial adhesive contact between neutrophil and vessel wall. Selectin and mucous ligands are elongated molecules located at the tip of microvillus. Selectins binds tightly to their ligands in less than a millisecond so that even momentary contact can tether a moving neutrophil firmly to the wall. Neutrophil continues to roll or skip intermittently along vessel wall due to the force of the flowing blood. The rolling exposes neutrophil to a diverse group of substances leukocytic chemotactic factors expressed by activated endothelium or diffuse into blood from injured tissue.

Selective anesthesia is given to rule out which tooth is paining. If specific tooth is involved, pain will disappear on anesthesia.

Selective dorsal rhizotomy (SDR) is a procedure that is done by sectioning of the dorsal column rootlets to interrupt the spinal reflex arc, inhibiting afferent input from the muscle and tendons, and reducing efferent activity at the level of the spinal cord. There is a general muscle tone reduction in the lower extremities with loss of superficial and deep sensation.

Sella turcica is a depression present on the superior surface of the body of the sphenoid bone also known as the hypophyseal fossa.

Semi-critical instruments don't cut soft tissues or cut bones but remain in contact of oral tissues like mirror, plastic instruments, burs, etc. These should be sterilized after each use. Some may be kept in disinfection solutions for 6–10 hours.

Semicircular fibers are the group of fibers which are attached at the proximal surface of tooth below the CEJ, go around the facial or lingual margins of the tooth and attach on the other proximal surface.

Semiconductor lasers sometimes, called diode lasers, are not solid-state lasers. These electronic devices are generally very small and use low power. They may be built into larger arrays, such as the writing source in some laser printers or CD players.

Semi-longitudinal method is a method adpted to monitor age-groups or subgroups at different level of development only for a period which separates one group from the next.

Senile caries are those that occur during old age. This may be due to reduction in salivary secretion or exposure of roots following gingival recession.

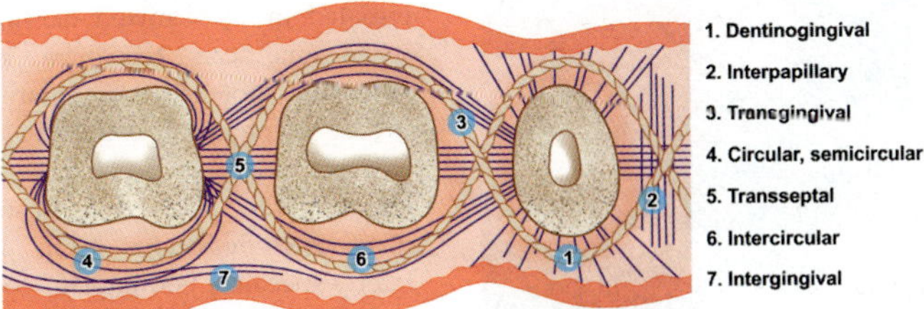

Fig.: *Semicircular fibers*

Senile cataract refers to cataract due to aging. There will be gradual impairment of vision. In immature cataract, lens appears greyish, iris shadow is present. Finger counting at a short distance may be present. In mature cataract, lens appears partly white and iris shadow is absent. The vision is reduced to perception of hand movement. There is no red fundal glow when examined in dark room.

Senile gait in old age senility looses speed and balance. Gait is slow, stiff with decrease in length of stride. Skeletal deformity and joint abnormality affects gait.

Sensorineural hearing impairment results from dysfunction in the inner ear, especially the cochlea where sound vibrations are converted into neural signals, or in any part of the brain that subsequently processes these signals. This dysfunction may be congested due to genetic or developmental abnormalities, or acquired through trauma or disease during the lifetime. Few of the unusual sensorineural hearing impairments vestibulo-cochlear nerve or, auditory cortex.

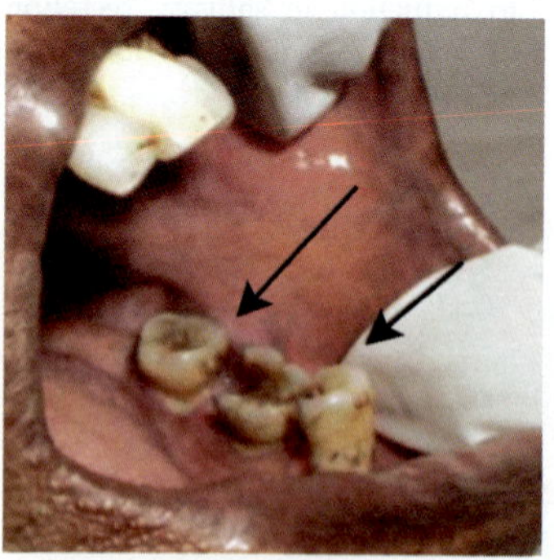

Fig.: *Senile caries*

Sensory ataxia lesions occur in posterior column of spinal cord, posterior roots or peripheral nerves causes sensory ataxia. Patient clears the ground abruptly. He walks in a flexed positive. Romberg sign is positive.

Sensory interaction theory contended that pain results from the interaction of both nociceptive and non-nociceptive afferent fibers on central neurons, the resulting excitatory or inhibitory interactions determining whether or not pain was perceived.

Septic arthritis of TMJ commonly results from blood-borne bacterial infection. It may involve joint by direct trauma or infection may extend from infection of maxillary sinus or parotid.

Sequestrum is a piece of necrosed bone that has become separated from the surrounding as seen in chronic osteomyelitis.

Serial extraction is an interceptive orthodontic procedure usually initiated in early mixed dentition when one can recognize and anticipate potential irregularities in the dentofacial complex and is corrected by a procedure that includes the planned extraction of certain deciduous teeth and later specific permanent teeth in an orderly sequence and pre-determined pattern to guide the

S

erupting permanent teeth into a more favorable position.

Serotonin is 5 hydroxy tryptamine derived from tryptophan. It is commonly associated with feeling of well-being is associated with vascular pain syndromes as an algogenic agent, an im portant endogenous anti-nociceptive mechanism.

Setting time is the time calculated from the very beginning of mixing of the cement to the development of a hard and rigid state in mouth.

Severe internal hemorrhage can be manifested when the patient becomes pale and restless. Patient may develop thirst and visual black outs. Skin becomes cold and moist. Pulse becomes thread and rapid. Body temperature comes down and BP falls. Subcutaneous vein collapses and it becomes difficult to locate vein.

Severe periodontitis is said to have occurred when the periodontal destruction is severely affected, i.e. when 5 mm of clinical attachment loss has occurred.

Sex drive is the primary instinctual urge of sexual gratification. It reaches its peak in late teens in males and mid-thirties among females. In contrast of animals the human sex drive is less seasonal, less dependent upon an oestrous cycle, more varied in expression and aroused by a wide range of stimuli.

Sexual abuse is said to have occurred when there is an exploitation of the child for the sexual gratification of an adult.

Sexual apathy is a negative attitude towards sexual relations, ranging from indifference to listlessness to active repulsion. Apathy is often based on distasteful or painful experiences and monotonous and unimaginative approach to the partner.

Sexual ecstasy is the peak of pleasure, excitement and euphoria experienced at the moment of orgasm.

Sexual flush is the rushing of blood during sexual excitement, especially in women. Flushing begins with rash-like discoloration of lower chest and spreads to breast, rest of chest, neck, reaching a peak during the late plateau phase.

S

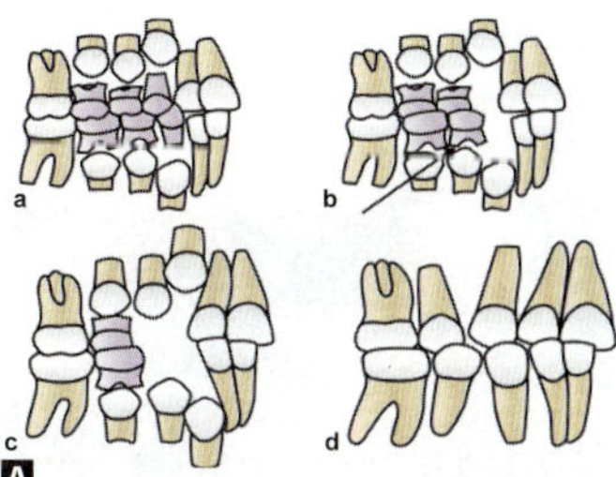

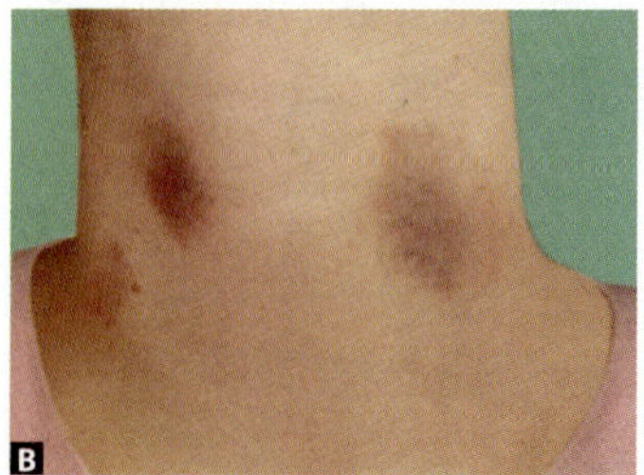

Figs A and B: *(A) Serial extraction; (B) Sexual abuse*

Shaken baby syndrome also known as abusive head trauma results from extreme rotational cranial injuries is a severe form of child abuse caused by accelerated violent shaking of an infant or child. The incidence of the syndrome is one in a million or 2.81 in 100,000 children. In 1972, the term whiplash shaken baby syndrome was coined by John Caffey, a pediatric radiologist to describe the constellation of clinical findings that include; (i) Cerebralhemorrhages, (ii) Retinal hemorrhages, (iii) Encephalopathy. With little or no evidence of extracranial trauma. This occurs due to rupture of cortical bridging veins.

Shape memory is a property of certain wires that will permit shaping at a higher temperature, followed by deformation at a lower temperature and a return to the original shape by reheating.

Shaping refers to the establishment of a specifically shaped cavity which performs the dual role of three-dimensional progressive access into the canal and creating an apical preparation which will permit the final obturation instruments and materials to fit easily.

Sharpey's fibers can be described as a terminal portion of principal fibers that gets inserted into cementum and bone.

Shelf-life is the period of time during which a compound retains its useful characteristics.

Shigellosis ***Shigella sonnei*** is the leading cause. Illness starts abruptly with abdominal cramps and diarrhea. Fever, chill, loss of appetite and headache develop. Patient becomes more dehydrated. Abdomen is tender. Stool culture is positive. Stool will contain red cells and leukocytes.

Shovel-shaped incisors is a develop-mental anomaly where affected incisors demonstrate prominent lateral margins creating a hollowed lingual surface resembling shovel. Typically the thickened marginal ridges converge at the cingulum, not uncommonly there is a deep pit or dens invaginatus at this junction. Maxillary incisors are more commonly affected.

Shunt: To divert from one location to another.

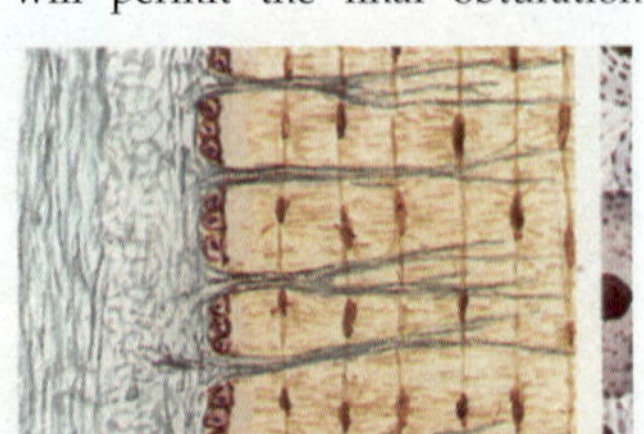

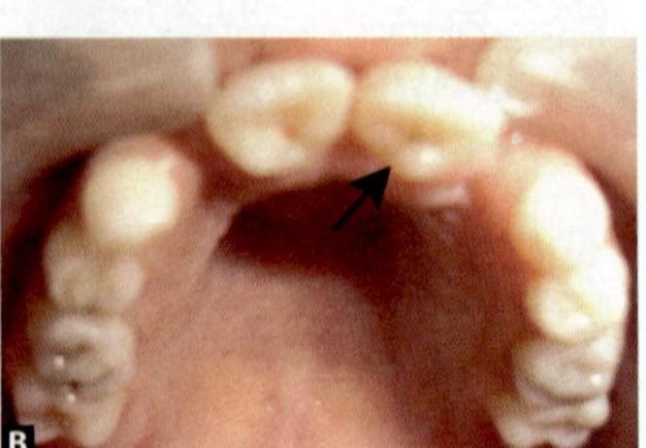

Figs A and B: *(A) Sharpey's fibers; (B) Shovel shape incisors*

Sialadenosis is a non-neoplastic, non-inflammatory enlargement of salivary gland. There develops recurrent, painless enlargement. Parotid glands are affected. There is significant elevation of salivary potassium and decrease in sodium in saliva is seen.

Sialolithiasis refers to salivary calculi or salivary stones that result in painful intermittent swelling in area of a major salivary gland. Pain worsens while eating food. Stasis of saliva leads to infection, fibrosis and atrophy of parenchyma. Sialography remains the best method to diagnose. Acute infections secondary to stasis should be treated with antibiotics.

Sickle cell anemia is a hereditary type of chronic hemolytic anemia. It is more common in females. On dental X-rays mild to moderate osteoporosis is seen. Trabecular change is prominent in alveolar bone. Hair on end appearance of skull may develop. Outer table appears absent and diploe thickened. Hemoglobin level is decreased. No specific treatment is available except blood transfusion. One may live a normal lifespan.

Sickle scalers are the instruments used to remove plaque, supra-gingival calculus from the crown of the tooth. These scalers are bulky with a flat surface and two cutting edges that converge to form a pointed tip. The tip is used primarily to remove the hard deposits present on the crown.

Side effects are those unwanted effects that are due to normal pharmacological actions of drug.

Sigmoid sinuses are continuations of the corresponding transverse sinuses. As indicated by the name each sigmoid sinus is S-shaped. It first runs downwards and medially in a deep groove on the mastoid part of the temporal bone, and then across the jugular process of the occipital bone. Finally, it runs forwards to reach the jugular foramen where it ends by becoming continuous with the upper end of the internal jugular vein.

Sigmoid volvulus there is generalized lower abdominal distension. X-ray will show a greatly distended loop of bowel.

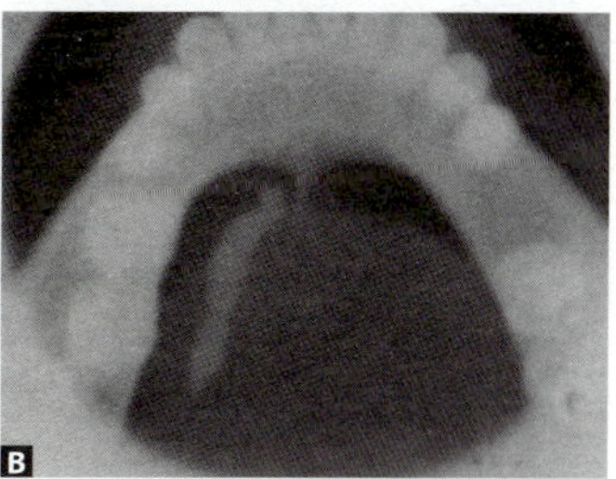

Figs A and B: *Submandibular sialolith; (A) Clinical; (B) Radiological*

There is loss of haustral markings. On barium enema a bird's beak deformity with spiral narrowing of the upper end of lower segment is pathognomonic. Laparotomy is the ultimate answer.

Significant caries index: In 1981, WHO declared that the global goal for oral health by the year 2000 should be that the DMFT for the 12-year-old should not exceed 3. DMFT describes the amount—the prevalence—of dental caries in an individual and is obtained by calculating the number of decayed (D), missing (M) and filled (F) teeth. A new index, the significant caries index, was introduced by Bratthall (2000) in order to bring attention to the individuals with the highest caries values in each population under investigation. The significant caries index is calculated as follows: Individuals are sorted according to their DMFT values, one-third of the population with the highest caries scores is selected, and the mean DMFT for this subgroup is calculated. This value is the sic index.

Signs are the effects of disease noticed by doctor.

Silicate cement is a dental cement which was previously used for esthetic temporary restorant because of its porcelain look.

Silicone rubber is a polymer resulting from the formation of silicone-oxygen-silicone bonds.

Silver + Copper amalgams these are currently in clinical use because of their resistance to corrosion and their higher creep. At 5 weeks, they elicited only slight response.

Simple caries *lesions* are involving only one surface of the tooth.

Simple fracture refers to the closed linear fracture.

Simple index is the index that measures the presence or absence of a condition.

Simple partial seizures "Simple" means consciousness is not impaired and "partial" means only part of the cortex is disrupted by the seizure. They manifest as auras or symptoms a patient experiences at the beginning of the seizure. Such symptoms may be the only manifestation of the seizure or it may progress.

Simple tongue thrust is a thrust with teeth together swallows, usually

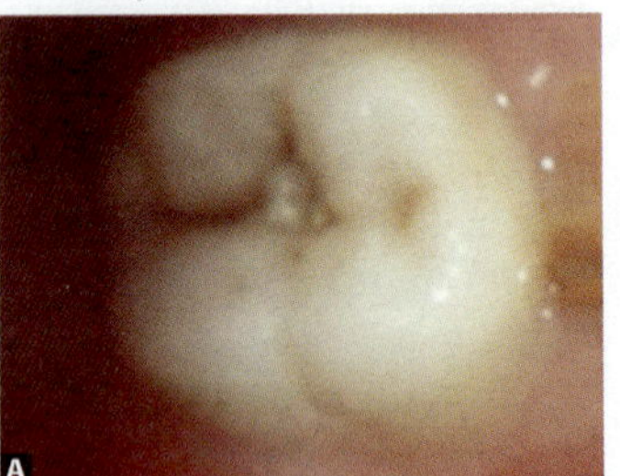

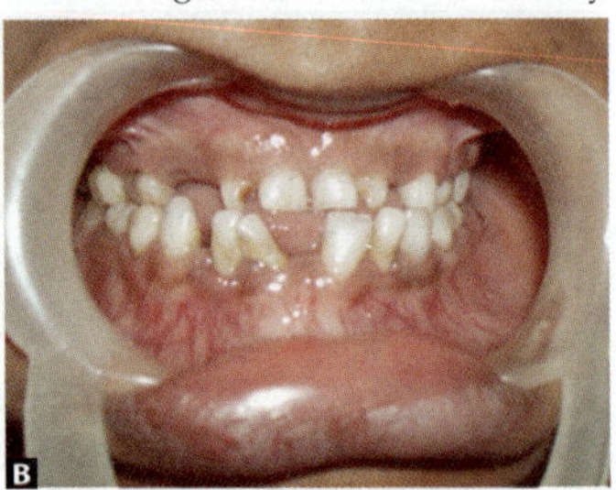

Figs A and B: *(A) Simple caries; (B) Simple tongue trust*

presents with a malocclusion which demonstrates a well-circumscribed anterior open bite and posterior teeth in a stable inter-digitations. Associated with a digit habit and may persist after the digit habit has subsided. Once the malocclusion is resolved, the tongue will usually change its swallow pattern and adapt to a new tooth alignment (Peterson, 1991). Complex tongue thrust occurs with a teeth apart swallow. There is generalized open bite and poor posterior occlusal fit and during swallowing, contraction of the lip, mentalis and facial musculature, mandibular and maxillary teeth not in contact and the tongue held between the teeth. It is often associated with chronic airway problems such as mouth breathing, tonsillitis, pharyngitis or nasorespiratory distress.

Simplified fluoride mottling index (FMI) the simplified fluoride mottling index (FMI) was introduced by Rahmatulla M and Rajasekhar A in 1984. The FMI is based on enamel opacities/lesions present on facial surfaces of the six upper and lower anterior teeth, which are esthetically important. The scoring is based on a hypoplastic facial surface which may range from opaque white spots to grayish-yellowish discolored surfaces. The weighing score assigned is restricted to four.

Simplified indices are those indices that measure only a representative sample of the dental apparatus, e.g. Greene and Vermillion's oral hygiene index-simplified (OHI-S).

Simplified oral hygiene index (OHI-S) proposed by Greene and Vermillion in 1964 as a modification of the OHI. Assess oral cleanliness by estimating the tooth surface covered with debris or calculus. The OHI-S has two components, the simplified debris index and the simplified calculus index. The two scores may be used separately or may be combined for the OHI-S.

Single visit endodontic therapy is defined as the conservative, non surgical treatment of an endodontically involved tooth consisting of complete biomechanical preparation and obturation of the root canal system in one visit.

Single visit endodontics implies to cleaning, shaping and disinfection of a root canal system followed by obturation of the root canal at the same appointment.

Sinter consolidating particles into a more dense agglomerate without melting. It takes place during manufacture and during heating to drive off impurities.

Sintering is a densification process in which solid particles are fused together at high temperature.

Sinusitis is a generalized inflammation of paranasal sinuses mucosa. Cause may be allergic, viral or bacterial. It causes blockage of drainage and thus retention of sinus secretion. It may be caused by extension of dental infection. Sinusitis is divided into three types: **(i) Acute sinusitis**—It is of less than two weeks; **(ii) Subacute sinusitis**—Up to three months;

(iii) Chronic—When it exists for more than three months. *Clinical Features:* Presence of common cold, nasal discharge, allergic rhinitis, pain and tenderness over the sinus involved, pain may be referred to premolar and molar teeth, fever, chills and malaise. *Radiological Features*: Secretions reduce air and make sinus radiopaque, mucosal thickening at floor and later on may involve whole sinus, thickened mucosa may be uniform or polypoid, air fluid level may also be present due to accumulation of secretions. It is horizontal and straight, chronic sinusitis may result in opacification of sinus.

Sixth branchial arch: The cartilage of this arch probably forms the cricoid and aryteroid cartilages of the larynx. The mesoderm forms the intrinsic muscles of the larynx, which are supplied by the nerve of the arch, the recurrent laryngeal branch of the 10th cranial or vagus nerve. Because the nerve of this arch passes caudal to the fourth arch artery in its recurring path from the brain to the muscles it supplies, the differing fate of the left and right fourth arch arteries, when migrating caudally into the thorax accounts for the different recurrent paths of the left and right laryngeal nerve. The right recurrent laryngeal nerve recurves around the aorta (fourth arch artery), the dorsal part of the sixth aortic artery and the entire fifth aortic artery having disappeared. The sixth arch arteries develop in part into the pulmonary arteries. The remainder disappears on the right side and forming on the left side of the temporary ductus arteriosus of the fetal circulation that becomes the ligamentum arteriosum.

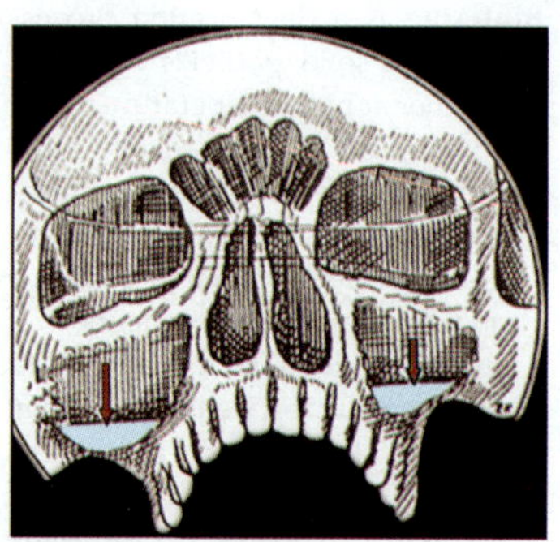

Fig.: *Sinustitis*

Sjogren's syndrome is a triad consisting of keratoconjunctivitis sicca, xerostomia and rheumatoid arthritis. It is an autoimmune disorder of exocrine glands which may be associated with neuropathy and lymph proliferative disorder. Histological hallmark is focal lymphocytic infiltration of exocrine glands. Epstein—Barr or a type a retrovirus is the causative organism. Xerostomia is a major complaint in most patients with parotid gland enlargement. Enlargement of submandibular gland may be there. There may be symptoms of rheumatoid arthritis. Kidney involvement is noted. Generally women are affected above the age of 40. Due to hypofunction of salivary and lacrimal glands, dryness of mouth and eyes results.

There will be intense lymphocytic infiltration of gland or there may be atrophy of gland. There is no satisfactory treatment.

Sjogren's syndrome tongue is typically red with atrophied papillae. Dorsum becomes lobulated with a cobblestone appearance. Amount of saliva is reduced.

Skewed distribution that is not symmetrical. It is with a long tail at its upper or lower end.

Skin is a largest sensory organ of our body. It has two layers. An outer layer called epidermis and an inner layer is dermis. Epidermis has five layers. The stratum germinativum is the layer in which cells division takes place. New cells produce keratin and die and are pushed towards surface. Dermis is the true skin. It lies on subcutaneous tissue. Color of skin depends on amount of melanin.

Skin nasion is the point of max convexity between the nose and forehead.

Skull refers the cranium that encases brain. The bone forming the lower jaw is called the mandible. The other bones of the skull are firmly united to one another at joints called suture bones collectively form the cranium. That has two main parts; (i) Its upper is a large cranial cavity in which the brain lies, (ii) The part of the maxilla that bears the teeth is called the alveolar process.

Slant culture is made on the surface of solidified medium in a tube which has been tilted to provide a greater surface area for growth.

Sleep is a periodical physiological depression of function of parts of brain controlling consciousness. As sleep deepens there is a transition from normal alpha waves to a phase of bursts of more rapid wave and then development of slow random waves. It is known as non-REM sleep. It has four stages. Insomnia in elderly is associated with awakening and with a reduced proportion of paradoxical sleep. Pulse rate, BP and respiratory rate fall.

Sleep apnea are bouts of breathing cessation during sleep due to closing of upper airway associated with obesity due to deposition of fat.

S

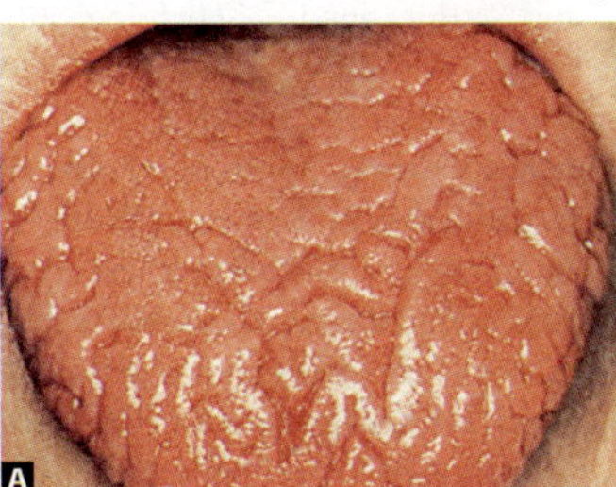

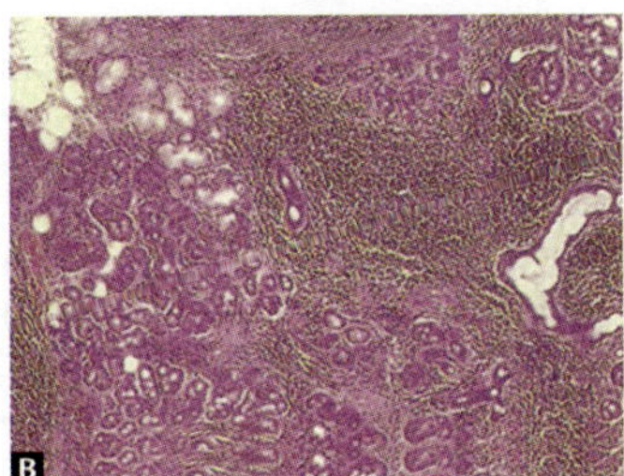

Figs A and B: *Sjogren's syndrome (A) Clinical; (B) Histological*

Sleep paralysis is a condition in which the patient when falling asleep or more often on walking finds himself unable to move a muscle.

Slide agglutination tests are the diagnostic tests used for detecting presence of HIV antibodies or antigen has recently developed. These are used widely in field work to detect HIV antibodies in blood products.

Slight periodontitis is said to have occurred when the periodontal destruction is generally considered slight where 1 to 2 mm of clinical attachment loss has occurred.

S-line or Steiner line is a line drawn from soft-tissue pogonion to the midpoint of the S-shaped curve between subnasale and nasal tip. Lips lying behind this reference line are too flat; those lying anterior to it are too prominent.

Sling ligation is the suture used for flaps on one surface of the tooth that involves two interdental spaces.

Slough is a mass of dead tissue.

S

Slow-rising pulse is an arterial pulse in aortic stenosis. The pulse is of small volume with a late systolic peak. There is a drill in carotid pulse.

SLS (superior labial sulcus) is the point of greatest concavity in the midline of the upper lip between subnasale and labrale superius.

Slurry is a mixture of pumice and water used to remove plaque and debris from crown of tooth.

Small bench top automatic autoclaves are very popular in dentistry. There is downward displacement of air because steam enters at the top of chamber. It requires 136°C at 32 pound pressure for 5 minutes.

Smoke tar is a brownish liquid which is obtained when tobacco smoke is cooled or condensed. It contains polycyclic aromatic hydrocarbon compounds. Actually these are produced as a result of incomplete combustion of tobacco. When the cigarette of 85 mm length is smoked, having a butt of 30 mm, total quantity of tobacco smoke or effluent formed is about 500 mg in weight. Tobacco tar formed is 17–40 mg is weight. Dry tobacco gives more tar than tobacco containing moisture.

Smoker's melanosis diffuse macular melanosis of the buccal mucosa, lateral tongue, palate and floor of the mouth is noted in smokers. Lesions are brown, flat and irregular/map-like configuration.

Smoker's patch is a specific lesion which develops on palate in heavy cigarette, pipe and cigar smokers. Lesions are more prominent on keratinized hard palate. To start mucosa is red but later on becomes greyish white, fissured and thickened. Histologically epithelium shows acanthosis and hyperkeratosis.

Smoker's throat: There is number of constituents in tobacco smoke in sufficient concentration to produce irritation to throat. The delicate mucous membrane becomes inflamed which induces cough of a persistent nature. As long as person smokes his cough persists.

Smooth surface caries is the carious lesions located on surface other than pits and fissures are classified as smooth surface lesions. Smooth surface lesions may be further subdivided as inter-proximal, occurring on mesial or distal contact points, cervical, occurring on buccal or lingual surface near the dentin-enamel junction.

Sn (subnasale) is the point at which the columella (nasal septum) merges with the upper lip in the midsagittal plane.

SNA is the angle S-N-A expresses the sagittal relationship of the anterior limit of the maxillary apical base to the anterior cranial base. It is the large in prognathic maxilla and small in retruded maxilla. In class ii division malocclusion caused by prognathic maxilla in which SNA angle is larger than normal, the use of an activator is contraindicated. Mc Namara (1981) in his study should that the SNA angle does not vary much among the different types of malocclusion nor does it change much with functional appliance treatment. The growth increments are small for this criterion, and the difference between growth direction types is insignificant.

Snake venom is highly concentrated digestive juice of snake. Venom on drying forms fine needle like crystals which are easily soluble in water. Its toxic properties are due to proteolytic enzyme. Phosphatidase causes hemolysis and toxic effect on heart and circulation. There is hemorrhage from lungs due to damage of capillary endothelium. Neurotoxin produces curare-like effects as well as paralysis.

SNB expresses the sagittal relationship between the anterior extent of the mandibular apical base and anterior cranial base with a prognathic mandible. It is large, and with a retrognathic mandible. It is small. Functional appliance treatment is indicated if the mandible is retrognathic and has a small SNB. This angle provides information only on the anteroposterior direction of the mandible, not on its morphology or growth direction. A posteriorly located mandible can be large or small, if it is small; the prognosis for anterior posturing in the mixed dentition is good because a larger

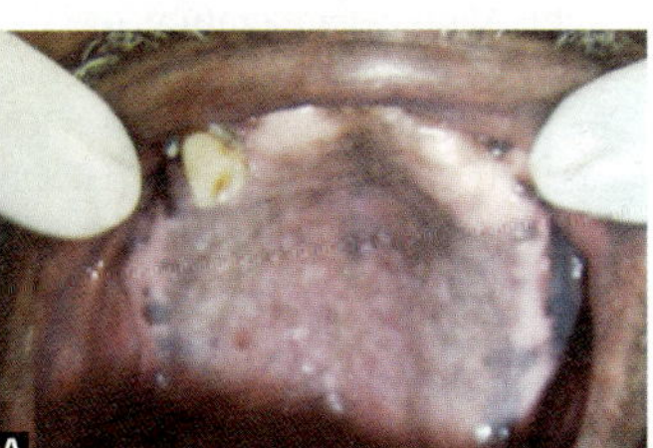

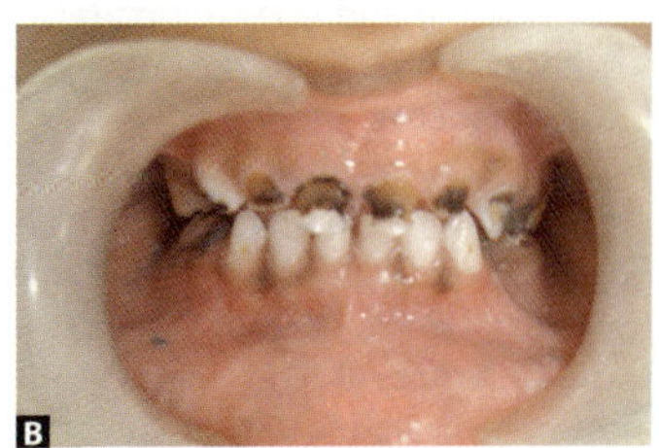

Figs A and B: *(A) Smoker's patch; (B) Smooth surface caries*

growth increment can usually be expected.

Snow-capped teeth is a type of amelogenesis imperfecta, inherited defect in enamel matrix apposition and characterized by teeth having normal enamel thickness but have low value of radiodensity and mineral content. The problem is related to the persistence of organic content in rod sheath resulting in poor calcification, low mineral content and a porous surface that becomes stained. Defect is due to altered matrix apposition (or) large amount of poorly calcified enamel matrix, which results in enamel, which is relatively soft and becomes discolored. Enamel is soft and vulnerable to attrition. Hard tissue is neither structurally weakened nor more susceptible than normal tooth structure to caries. It manifests as a white, chalky, opaque discoloration of the incisal and occlusal 3rd of the crown. The opaqueness may be solid or freckled, appears to involve only the surface of the enamel. The junction of the opaque white and translucent enamel is very sharp. The pattern of affected teeth has a distinct anteroposterior relationship and does not correlate with chronologic order of tooth development.

Social learning theory was given by Bandura in the year 1963. Social learning theory is thought to be the most complete. It is clinically useful and theoretically a sophisticated form of behavior therapy. *Advantages:* Less reductionist, provides more explanatory concepts, encompasses a broader range of phenomena. The learning of behavior is affected by 4 principle elements. **(1) Antecedent determinants**: The conditioning is affected if the person is aware of what is occurring; **(2) Consequent determinants**: Person's perception and expectances (cognitive factors) determine behavior; **(3) Modelling: learning through observation eliminates the trial-error search**: It is not an automatic process but requires cognitive factors and involves four processes which are: Attentional processes, retention processes, reproduction processes; **(4) Self-regulation**: This system involves a process of self-regulation judgment and evaluation of individual's responses to his own behavior.

Socket wall can be described as dense, lamellated bone which is partially arranged in the Haversian system and partially in bundle bone.

Sodium hypochlorite is a clear, pale, green-yellow liquid with strong odor of chlorine. It is easily miscible with water and gets decomposed by light. At body temperature, reactive chlorine in aqueous solution exists in two forms—hypochlorite (OCl) and hypochlorous acid (HOCl). State of available chlorine depends on pH of the solution. At acidic and neutral pH, chlorine acts as HOCl. HOCl is antibacterial. It dissrupts vital function of bacterial cell resulting in cell death.

It's an excellent disinfectant and is bactericidal. It is corrosive to aluminium, nick, steel and other metals. Items may be disinfected for 20 minutes. Gloves can be disinfected thoroughly by rinsing gloved hands and then rinsing with soap and water. It is effective against biofilms containing *P. intermedia, Peptostreptococcus micros, Streptococcus intermedius, Fusobacterium nucleatum* and *E. faecalis* as it disrupts oxidative phosphorylation and inhibits DNA synthesis of bacteria. Dunavant et al (2006) concluded that both 1 percent NaOCl and 6 percent NaOCl were more efficient in eliminating *E. faecalis* biofilm than the other solutions tested.

Sodium there is some sodium in practically every food. It is an extracellular fluid maintaining the osmotic equilibrium between the extracellular fluid and tissue cells. It maintains the pH of blood within normal limits. It is also concerned with the conduction of nervous impulses, muscle contractility and control of sodium is lost if vegetables are boiled in water and water is discarded. When tissues are lacking, potassium, sodium may substitute for it. It regulates the heart's contraction. 5 gram is the daily requirement. Heart patient should take 2 gm/daily ideally.

Sodium valporate is drug that controls petit mal epilepsy and psychomotor epilepsy. Patient becomes more alert. It generally doesn't produce side effects.

Soft acrylic liners are the denture lines with the softness of silicone that provides adequete seal to denture. Its advantages include high peel strength to acrylic denture base and high rupture strength. It has reasonable resistance to damage by cleaness. Disadvantage of it is of poor resilience and some buckle in water.

Soft lasers (low-level energy): A thermal low energy lasers emitted at wavelength, which are supposed to stimulate cellular activity. Example: He-Neon; Ga-arsenide.

Soft liner a soft polymer used as a thin layer on tissue bearing surface of a denture.

Soft palate is attached to the posterior margin of the hard palate. In its normal relaxed position, it has one surface directed upwards and backwards, and another surface directed forwards and downwards. The soft palate consists of two layers of mucous membrane (continuous with those lining the upper and lower surfaces of the hard palate). Between these layers of mucosa there is a fibrous basis called the palatine aponeurosis. Several muscles are present in the soft palate.

Soft tissue cysts are commonly occurring masses in musculoskeletal system. On MRI, these show a uniform low and high signal on T_1 and T_2 weighted images.

Soft tissue sarcoma arises from mesenchymal tissue. Many soft tissue sarcomas are poorly differentiated. These include

S

malignant fibrous histiocytoma, liposarcoma and leiomyosarcoma. Large heterogeneous painless mass within a deep compartment should be regarded with a high suspicion of malignancy.

Solar cheilitis refers to sun exposure resulting in degeneration of tissue of lips. Condition is related to the total cumulative exposure to sunlight and amount of skin pigmentation. Lower lip is generally involved. Vermillion border of lip is affected and not specific treatment is required.

Soldering refers to surfaces to be joined should be without contamination. A metal or ally with lower melting point should be brought to the solder's melting temperature. Then ports and shoulder is being brought to the solder's melting temperature. If molten metal wets the solid metal, it will spread between the flux and the metal part providing good contact. Solder penetrates joints by capillary action.

Solid-state lasers have lasing material distributed in a sold matrix (such as the ruby or neodymium: yttrium-aluminium garnet "YAG" lasers). The neodymium-YAG laser emits infrared light at 1,064 nanometers (nm).

Solitary bone cyst *see* traumatic cyst.

Soluble insulin: It is standardized to contain 20, 40 per mL. It is normally given subcutaneous route and full effects come in 2–3 hours. Duration of action is 5–8 hours.

Somatic is the nerve that supplies muscles.

Somatic efferent fibers supply skeletal muscle of the limbs and body wall. They also supply the extrinsic muscles of the eyeball and the muscles of the tongue.

Somatic efferent nuclei supply skeletal muscle that is derived from somites.

Sonicare is an electric toothbrush. It vibrates at over 31,000 brush strokes per minute. Most models offer a 3 minute timer to let you know when you're done.

Spillway *see* embrasure.

Stain, extrinsic is a stain located on the outside of the tooth surface originating from external

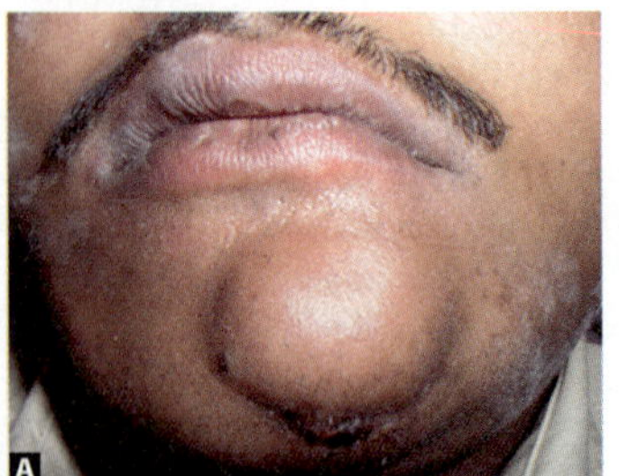

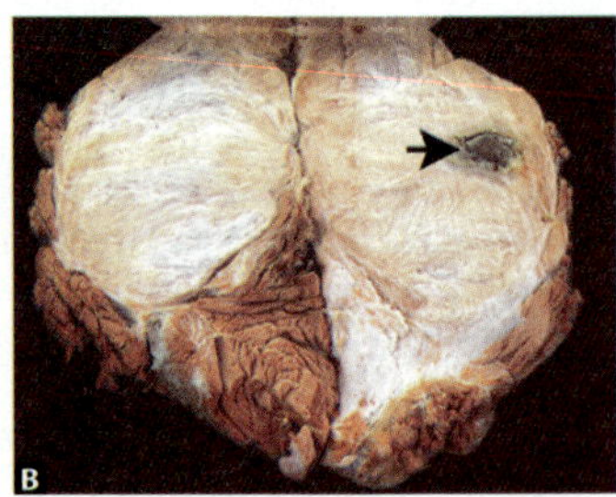

Figs A and B: *(A) Soft tissue cysts; (B) Soft tissue sarcoma*

substances such as tobacco, coffee, tea or food; usually removed by polishing the teeth with an abrasive prophylaxis paste.

Stain, intrinsic is a stain originating from the ingestion of certain materials or chemical substances during tooth development, or from the presence of caries. This stain is permanent and cannot be removed.

Somatic pain often reflects a pathological lesion in a specific organ or tissue.

Somatic structures are those present in relation to the body wall (or soma); they include the tissues of the limbs thus the skin, bones, joints and skeletal muscle of the limbs and body wall are classified as somatic.

Sonants are voiced sounds which include all vowels and vowel-like sound. They are produced by vibration of some portion of vocal folds. In this the vocal tract is relatively open above the glottis.

Sorbitol is a sugar alcohol made from glucose. These also give 4 calories per gram as sucrose but don't promote cavities because these are not easily metabolized by bacteria in mouth. ***Sorbitol*** was isolated in 1872; sorbitol is mainly used in chewing gum. Intra-oral trials have indicated that plaque pH does not drop below 5.7 after chewing sorbitol sweetened gum and the need for further studies is emphasized, more so by the fact that *S* mutans is known to metabolize sorbitol.

Sore mouth refers to the inflamed mucosa that may be red, smooth, swollen and granular. It is painful. Severe burning sensation is common. Condition is not due to allergy.

Space regainer is an appliance that is used to regain lost space, e.g. rapid maxillary expansion appliance and jackscrews. The appliance consists of a split acrylic plate with a jackscrew in relation to the edentulous space and is retained using Adam's clasp.

Space regaining is a procedure that is performed due to premature loss of deciduous teeth. Results in the migration of adjacent teeth into the edentulous space and interferes in the eruption of the succedaneous permanent teeth, due to inadequate space. Space regainers are used in such situation to regain the lost space due to migration and to provide space for the eruption of permanent teeth. Space regaining can be done using springs distalized of molar.

Spacing usually exists between the deciduous teeth. These spaces are called physiological spaces

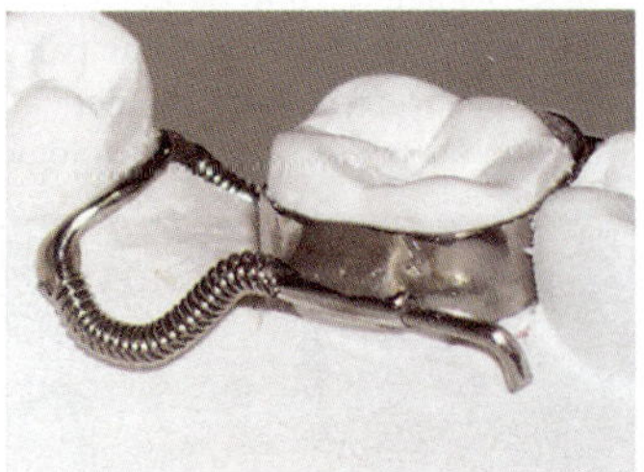

Fig.: *Space regainer*

S

or developmental spaces. The presence of spaces in the primary dentition is important for the normal development of the primary dentition. Absence of spaces in the primary dentition is an indication that crowding of teeth can occur when the larger permanent teeth erupt. The spacing is invariably seen mesial to the maxillary canines and distal to the mandibular canines. These physiological spaces are called leeway space of Nance.

Spasmodic dysphonia is a chronic phonatory disorder of adulthood without any obvious cause. It results from intermittent spasmodic hyper-adduction of vocal folds leading to jerking, effortful strained sounds with laryngeal discomfort.

Spasmodic torticollis: When head is flexed, it is known as antecollis, extended it is known as retrocollis. It may be tilted, twisted and rotated. Some may show head tremor; muscles involved are sternocleidomastoid, trapezius and scalenus.

Spastic cerebral palsy is the most common form of cerebral palsy. Approximately 70 to 80 percent of children who have cerebral palsy are spastic. Spasticity is defined as an increase in the physiologic resistance of muscle to passive motion. It is characterized by hyperreflexia, clonus, extensor plantar responses, and primitive reflexes.

Spastic gait refers to when patient walks on a narrow base, has difficulty in bending his knees. Actually patient drags his feet. Foot is raised by tilting the pelvis and leg is swung forward. It is seen in spinal cord disease.

Special somatic afferent fibers carry impulses of vision, hearing, and equilibrium (from the vestibular apparatus).

Special visceral afferent fibers carry the sensations of taste.

Special visceral efferent nuclei supply skeletal muscle derived from branchial arch mesoderm.

Specific gravity is the ratio of the mass of a material to an equal volume at 4°C.

Specific heat is the ratio of thermal capacity of a material to that of water at 15°C.

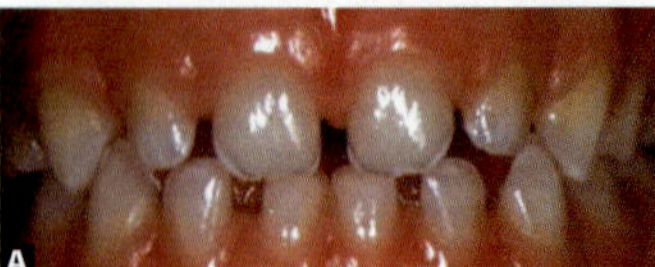

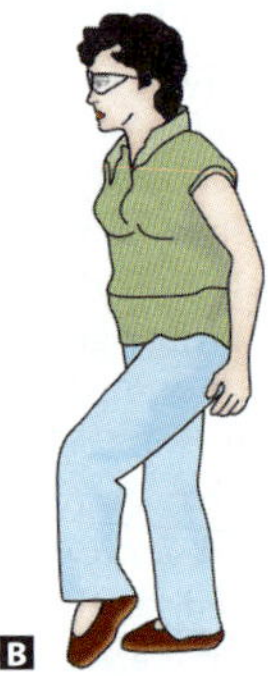

Figs A and B: *(A) Spacing; (B) Spastic gait*

Specific plaque hypothesis (Walter Loeshe – 1976) states that only certain plaque is pathogenic and its pathogenicity depends on the presence of or increases in specific micro-organisms. According to this hypothesis, plaque harboring specific bacterial pathogens results in periodontal disease. These organisms produce substances that mediate the destruction of host tissues. Acceptance of the specific plaque hypothesis was confirmed by recognition of AA comitans as pathogens in localized aggressive periodontitis. An increased risk for periodontal breakdown is observed in sites colonized by same potentially pathogenic organisms.

Specific plaque hypothesis revisited states that the disease is associated with specific strains of a given species. It's likely that most, if not all, recognized periodontal pathogens demonstrated difference in phenotypic properties related to their ability to cause disease, i.e. genetic (molecular) basis for variability in virulence properties among pathogenic strains to cause periodontal diseases.

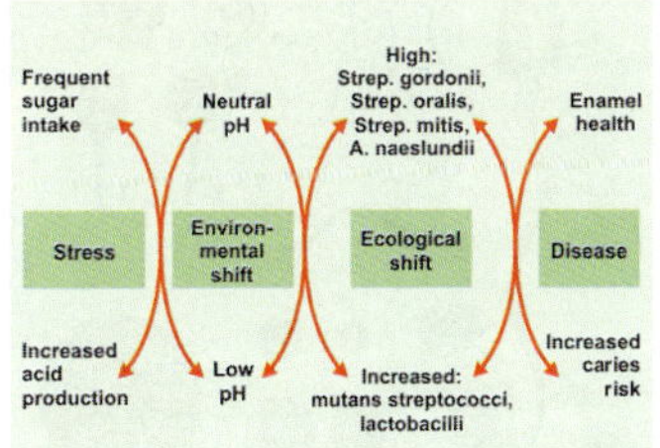

Fig.: *Specific plaque hypothesis*

Specificity theory of pain was considered a specific sensation with its own anatomically distinct receptors, primary and cortical reception areas. This theory contended that only free unmyelinated nerve endings in the orofacial area were activated by noxious stimuli. More recently, the anatomical specificity of receptors has been discarded as most receptors, if sufficiently stimulated can respond to noxious irritation.

Speech is the skilled, willful and elaborate movement of muscle used for initiating sounds plus the moulding of these sound into meaningful oral communication. Speech is the most complex and highly organized voluntary activity, in which a number of mechanisms also served. More vital physiological purposes are made use i.e. breathing, swallowing and hearing. The roles of speaker and listener are combined in each individual that is the process of generation and reception of speech.

Speech or language impairment means an impairment of speech or sound production, fluency, voice or language which significantly affects a child's educational performance or his social, emotional or vocational development.

Spermatid refers to the cell derived from the secondary spermatocyte by fission, and develops into a mature spermatozoon.

Sphenoid bone is large bone, extending across the entire width of the

S

base of the skull and extending also onto the lateral wall of the vault. It is made up of the body, the right and left greater and lesser wings, and the right and left pterygoid processes.

Sphenoidal sinuses are spaces present in the body of the sphenoid bone. Each sinus opens into the corresponding half of the nasal cavity through an aperture on the anterior aspect of the body of the sphenoid. The part of the nasal cavity into which the sinus opens lies above the superior nasal concha and is called sphenoethmoidal recess.

Sphygmomanometer is an instrument used in conjunction with a stethoscope to measure blood pressure. It consists of cloth cuff, a pressure bulb, a measuring gauge and a release valve. These are of two types—mercury and aneroid one.

Spinal cord is a continuation of brain stem. It is a tube like structure located within the spinal cavity. It is 17 inches long and extends from foramen magnum of occipital bone to L1 level.

Spinal cord syndrome refers to a typical type of analgesia with thermo anesthesia bilaterally in several dermatomes. It extends in a cap-like fashion over arms, back and shoulder. Spastic weakness of legs may develop. When brain stem is involved facial analgesia may develop. Atrophy of tongue results in dysarthria. Person may develop dysphagia.

Spinal tuberculosis: There will be variable loss of pain and temperature sensation and motor function. It also causes spasticity, bladder incontinence and absent abdominal reflexes.

Spindle cell carcinoma is an unusual form of poorly differentiated squamous cell carcinoma consisting of spindle-shaped epithelial cells. *Clinical Features*: Lesion develops pain, ulceration and swelling. There is fleshy but polypoid growth pattern. Histologically tumor cells often exhibit marked nuclear hyperchromatism. There is a minimum degree of epithelial dysplasia with little or no keratin formation. This tumor is less

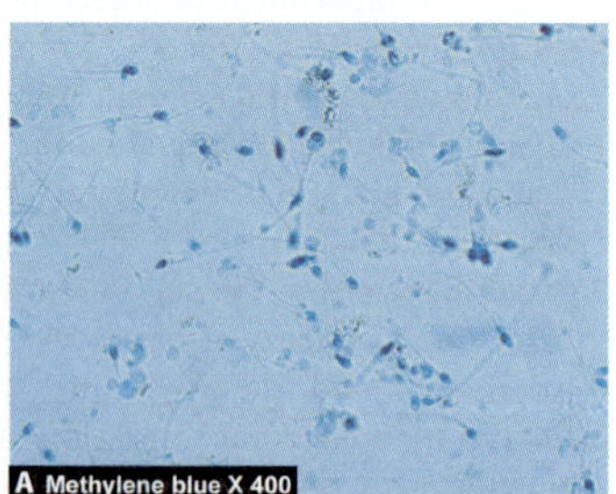

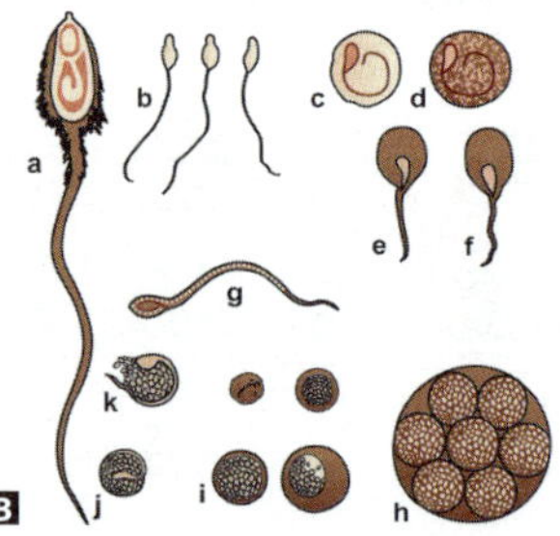

Figs A and B: *(A) Spermatozoa in semen; (B) Spermatozoa*

aggressive hence wider surgical excision serves the purpose.

Spirometry is a test done to measure lung volumes. This is most useful in differentiating obstructive from restrictive lung diseases. In obstructive lung diseases such as COPD, asthma, and bronchiectasis, the FEV1/FVC ratio is reduced. The ratio is unaltered in restrictive lung diseases such as pulmonary fibrosis. Forced vital capacity (FVC) is the total amount of gas which can be forcefully exhaled following a maximal inhalation.

Spleen is a secondary lymphoid organ located in the upper left of abdomen behind stomach, close to the diaphragm. It has a collagen capsule. Histologically, it contains a red pulp, where destruction of RBCs takes place along with venous sinuses and cellular chords. White pulp contains lymphoid tissue arranged around a central arteriole, periarteriolar lymphoid sheath (pals). It is also organized into distinct 'b' cell areas and 't' cell areas or follicles. Primary unstimulated follicles and secondary stimulated follicles with germinal center containing follicular dendrite cells, phagocyte and macrophages, principally the antigen presenting cells.

Split thickness flap refers to partial thickness flap.

Split tooth or incomplete fracture is a tooth that is split or cracked but not yet fractured. The tooth may be uncomfortable only occasionally during mastication. Pain may be like unbearable stab. This is when there is crack in the dentin and suddenly spreads as the cusp is separated from the remainder of tooth. Pulp may remain hypersensitive for years. Most frequent complaint is of pain while biting or contracting cold fluids. If the pulp is involved in fracture any exciting agent will bring on discomfort.

Spongy bone *see* trabecular bone.

Sporotrichosis is caused by Sporothrix schenckii and develops after exposure to animals. It involves skin, oral, nasal and pharyngeal mucosa. Regional lymph glands are enlarged. Lesions are healed by soft, pliable scars even though causative organism may be present. There is no specific treatment.

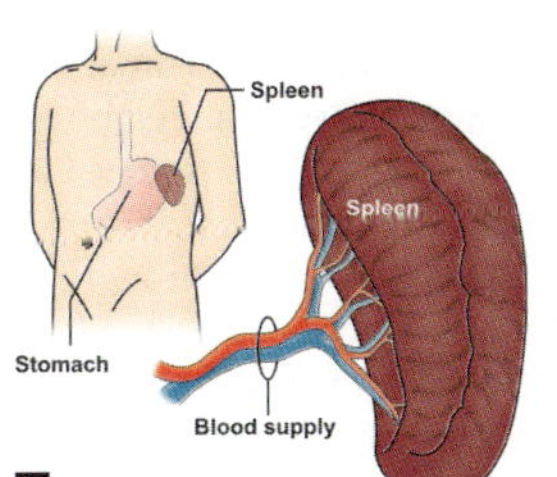

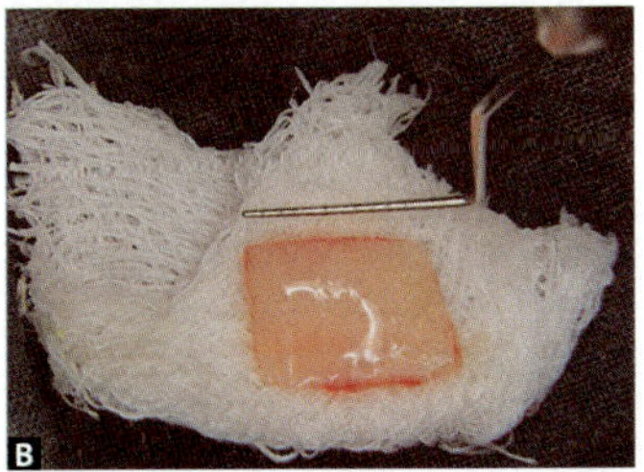

Figs A and B: *(A) Spleen; (B) Partial thickness flap*

S

Spot welding is used to join orthodontic bonds and brackets and to join orthodontic wires. Work is pressed together between two copper electrodes and electric 2 to 6 V for 1/25 to 1/50 seconds at 250 to 750 ampere.

Sprain is an injury limited to ligament. Sprain is a stretching injury to a muscle or its tendinous attachment. First degree sprain is a tear of only a few fibers of a ligament. There is minimal swelling and localized tenderness. In second degree sprain all the fibers of a ligament are disrupted. There is pain, swelling and inability to use the limb. In third degree sprain there is a complete tear of ligament. Often pain is minimal. It requires immobilization of 4–6 weeks.

Spreading pains is due to development of painful muscle spasms. The secondary myogenous pain may occur some distance from the site of its mother primary pain. But its location bears a segmental relationship to the nerve which mediates the primary pain.

Spring catarrh patient is usually a young boy who presents with marked itching in the eyes which becomes worse in summer. There develops flat cobblestone like papillae in the upper tarsal conjunctiva.

Sprue is a part of malabsorption syndrome. There develops glossitis, large pale, foul stools. The disease starts with intestinal problems. Excessive amount of fats is passed in stool. There may be severe glossitis and atrophy of filiform papillae. Painful burning sensations of tongue are common. Blood findings are similar to pernicious anemia. Vitamin B_{12} helps. Gluten wheat and rye flour should be avoided.

Squamous acanthoma has no distinctive clinical appearance and can develop at any site of oral mucosa. It is a small, flat or elevated white or sessile or pedunculated lesion.

Squamous cell carcinoma is the most common neoplasm of oral cavity. It is derived from stratified squamous epithelium; commonest sites involved are lower lip, lateral borders of tongue and floor of mouth. Tobacco, betel nut chewing, alcohol, AIDS, lichen planus and nutritional deficiencies are the important causative factors. *Clinical Features*: It may appear as extended oral leukoplakia and erythroplakia. It may be symptomless, white or red variegated patch. It is painless. Advanced lesion is fast-growing irregular and large tumor mass. Ulcer has indurated borders with everted margin. Secondary infection may result in pain. It bleeds on touching. Tumor is fixed to tongue. Regional lymph nodes are tender, fixed and enlarged. Untreated case may destroy oral tissue and extend through cheek. Patient may not be able to eat food as pathological fracture of jaws may take place. Such cancer may also be present in intestine and lung. In an oral cavity itself two or more separate malignant lesions may be seen. Tongue lesions are more vascular and start bleeding even on slightest touch. Tongue may be fixed to mouth and patient may be unable to talk or swallow. Carcinomas originating on or near the crest of mandibular ridge or on the posterior hard palate are the tumors to cause destruction of bone. Such tumors can be of two types—peripheral or mucosal. In peripheral type, patient may complain of worsening oral ulcer. Person may be alcoholic or smoking heavily. Other complaints are foul odor and taste. There may even by anesthesia of lip. While in central type patient will complain of pain and swelling. There may be anesthesia also. In peripheral type lytic effects of two types are seen. Semicircular or saucer shaped erosion into bony surface with ill-defined borders. Mandibular lesion with advanced horizontal resorption is seen. Tooth may be migrated, loose and resorbed. Regional lymph glands will be enlarged. Glands will be enlarged, painless and very firm. Histologically lip carcinoma is well-differentiated. Tobacco, alcohol and nutritional deficiency are the predisposing factors. Highly anaplastic lesions do occur. Metastases from intraoral carcinoma of different sites involves submaxillary and deep cervical glands are seen. Prognosis is good before the metastasis occurs. Radiographically bone involved shows large, irregular and ill-defined radiolucent area and appears as of 'moth-eaten' type. In addition to histopathology, exfoliative cytology is helpful. Toluidine blue test is needed to detect dysplastic lesions.

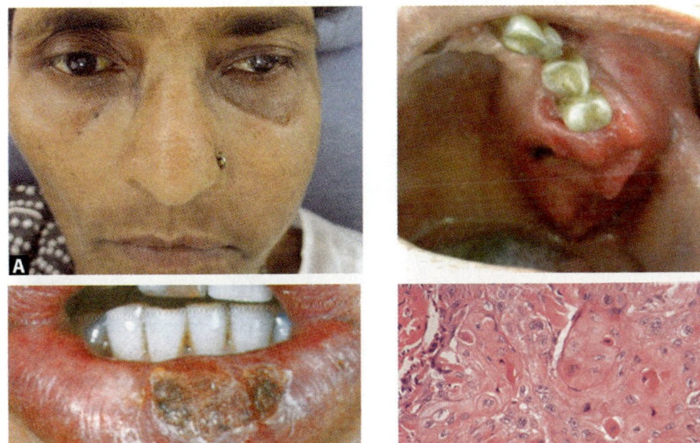

Figs A and B: *Squamous cell carcinoma of oral cavity*

S

Squamous odontogenic tumors in maxilla, lesions are centered on the incisor cuspid area while in mandible lesions had a predilection for bicuspid molar area. Lesions are asymptomatic. On X-ray, it looks as triangular or semicircular translucent area with or without sclerotic areas. It is made of squamous mature epithelium. Peripheral layer is flattened. Post-surgery, there is no recurrence.

Squint (Strabismus) is a condition in which the two eyes do not look in the same direction. The squint becomes obvious when the eye movement involves a muscle that is paralyzed or weak, because the weak muscle cannot keep up with the muscle of the normal side. Trigeminal nerve is so called because it consists of three main divisions: (1) Ophthalmic nerve; (2) Maxillary nerve; (3) Mandibular nerve. These nerves arise from a large trigeminal ganglion. The trigeminal nerve also has a motor root which emerges from the pons medial to the sensory root. The trigeminal nerve contains both afferent and efferent fibers.

Stab culture in this culture, the medium is inoculated by thrusting a needle deep into its substance.

Stab wound is one in which depth of wound is more than length of skin. It is caused by sharp, pointed object like knife, spear, dagger, etc. Edges of object may be sharp or blunt. If sharp, the wound will be incised and if blunt, wound will lacerated penetrating.

Stability of Vitamins carotene is destroyed by heat in presence of air and copper. It can withstand boiling in alkaline solution. Thiamine is unstable in alkaline condition. Riboflavin is stable to air and destroyed by excessive heat and light. While nicotinic acid most stable of B-vitamins being unaffected by light, heat, air, acid or alkali. Only losses are during washing. Vitamin C is destroyed by enzyme present in leafy vegetables. Vitamin D is stable to all normal storage and processing conditions.

Stafne bone defect is a sharply defined cyst-like area of radiolucency seen near the angle of mandible.

S

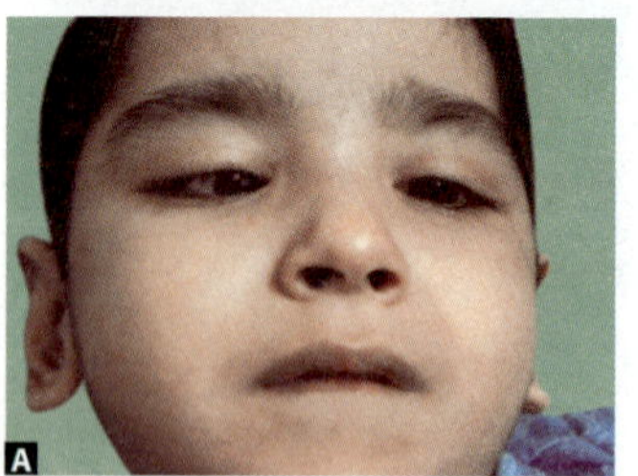

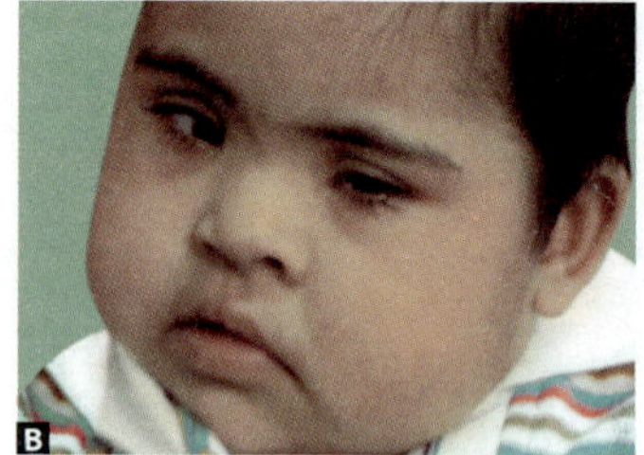

Figs A and B: *Squint (Strabismus)*

Staggering gait is common to alcohol and barbiturate intoxication. Base is wide and steps are irregular.

Stain, extrinsic is a stain located on the outside of the tooth surface originating from external substances such as tobacco, coffee, tea or food; usually removed by polishing the teeth with an abrasive prophylaxis paste.

Stain, intrinsic is a stain originating from the ingestion of certain materials or chemical substances during tooth development, or from the presence of caries. This stain is permanent and cannot be removed.

Stainless-steel crowns (SSCs) are preformed extracoronal restorations that are particularly useful in the restoration of grossly broken down teeth, primary molars that have undergone pulp therapy, and hypoplastic primary or permanent teeth. They are also indicated when restoring the dentition of children at high risk of caries, particularly those having treatment under general anesthesia.

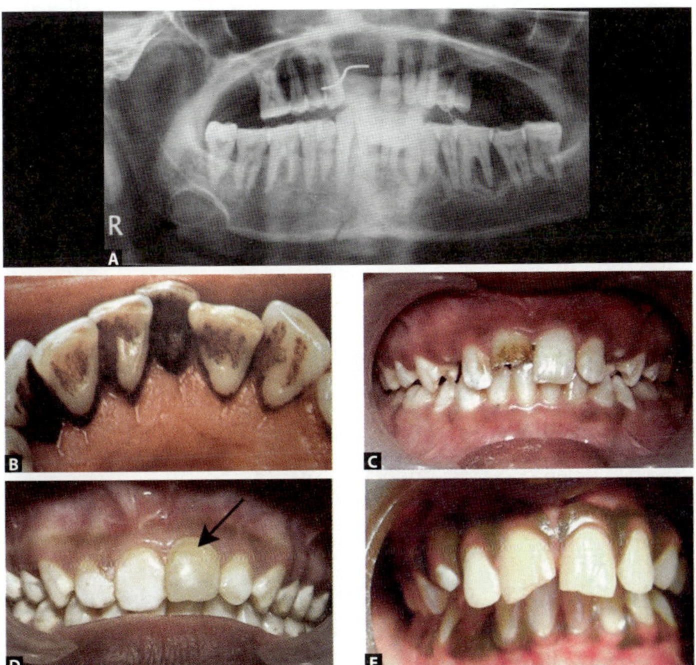

Figs A to E: *(A) Stafne bone defect; (B) Staining of teeth; (C) Stain occuring due to trauma; (D) Stains occuring post-composite restoration; (E) Stains occuring due to obturating material*

SSCs are very durable restorations and should be the restoration of choice in the high-caries mouth.

Stainless-steel wire has good combination of mechanical properties and corrosion resistance in oral environment. Cost is reasonable. Modulus of elasticity ranges from about 160 to 180 gpa. The yield strength of these wires ranges from 1100 to 1500 mpa. Austenitic stainless steel alloys can be rendered susceptible to intergranular corrosion when heated 400°C to 900°C due to formation of chromium carbides at grain boundaries.

Stammering is a disorder of articulation by repetition of sounds or syllables and by prolonged pauses in speech. Facial grimacing may accompany. It is not a result of acquired organic disease.

Stamping gait is seen in sensory ataxia. Patient raises his feet very suddenly often abnormally high and then jerks forward and bringing to the ground with a jerk. It is seen in tabes dorsalis.

Standard deviation refers to the square root of the variance expressed in units of original measure.

Standard error of measurement is a measure of absolute reliability. It represents the standard deviation of measurement errors.

Standard normal distribution is a normal distribution with a mean of 0.0 and a standard deviation of 1.0.

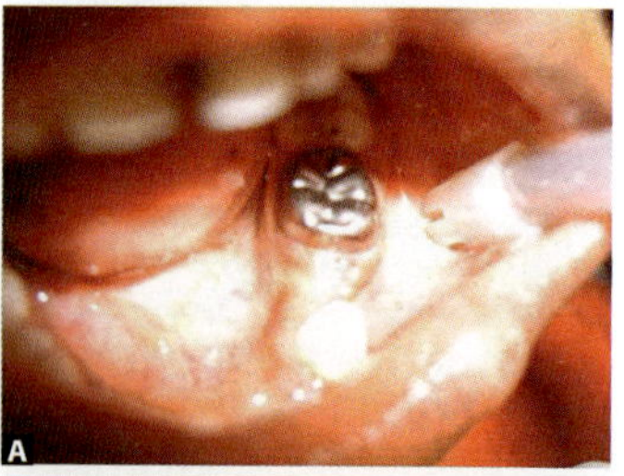

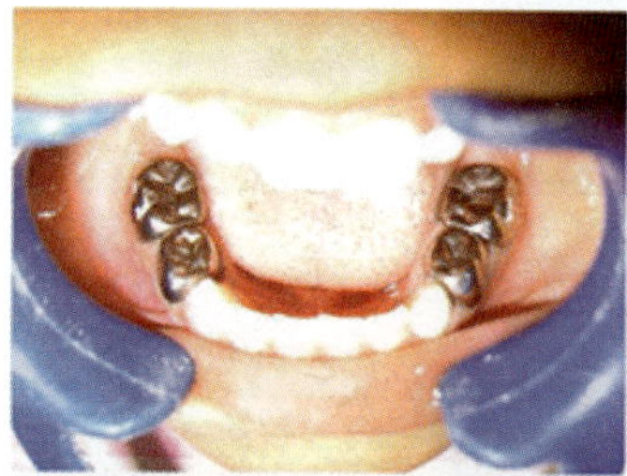

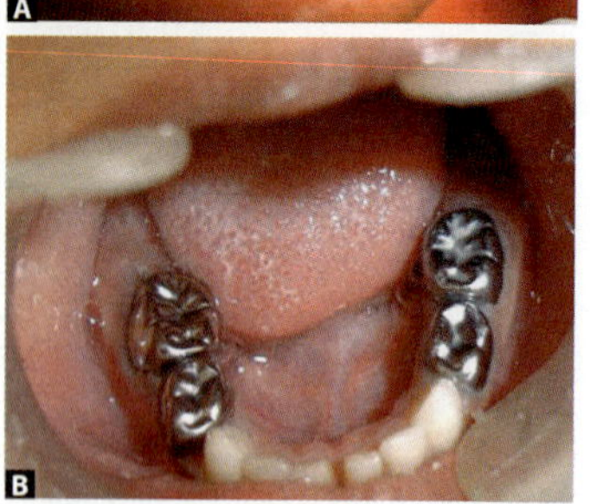

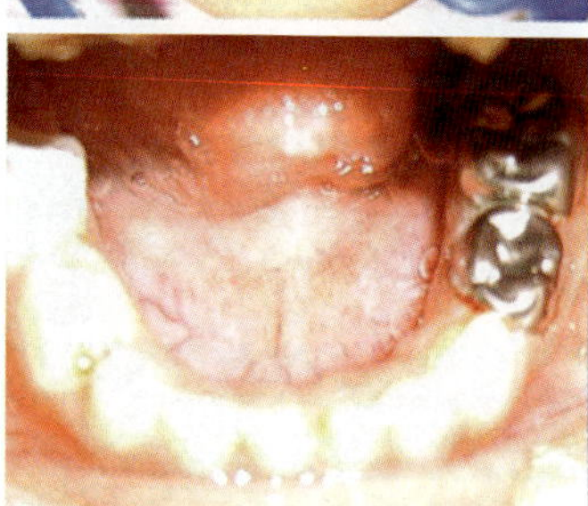

Figs A and B: *(A) Permanent stainless steel crown; (B) Primary stainless steel crown (SSCs)*

Stapes refers to the bone of the middle lobe ear; is shaped like a stirrup. It has a head, that is connected by two limbs or crura (anterior and posterior), to an oval plate called the base. The constricted part adjoining the head is called the neck.

Staphylococcal pneumonia refers to pneumonia of *Staphylococcus* origin. It needs a separate description. It may cause a confluent bronchopneumonia in children. Due to appreciable tissue necrosis, produces thin fluid pus. Small cystic cavities contain thin pus and air. It responds to antibiotics.

Staphylococcal scalded skin syndrome: It is an illness which is caused by exfoliative endotoxins produced by *S. aureus*. Symptoms include rash, fever, malaise and irritability. There develops diffuse, tender, red rash with a sand paper texture. Bullae and vesicles may appear and exfoliation of large sheets of epidermis is seen.

Startle reflex is similar to Moro reflex, but it is initiated by a sudden noise stimuli. In this reflex, the elbows are flexed and the hands remain closed and there is a less outward and inward movement of the arms.

Starvation is when necessary food has been suddenly withheld. Feeling of hunger lasts for 36–48 hours. It is succeeded by pain in epigastrium relieved by pressure. After 4–5 days, eyes appear sunken and glistening pupils are widely dilated. Cheeks become hollow. Lips become dry and cracked. Tongue becomes dry and coated with thick fur. Voice becomes weaker.

Static bone cyst is not a true cyst since it is lined by epithelium. Hence it is known as pseudocyst. On X-ray, it is a well-defined cyst like radiolucency in mandible inferior to mandibular canal. It may not require any treatment.

Static stretching is stretching a muscle in a stationary position.

Status epilepticus refers to continuous seizure activity or intermittent seizures with impaired consciousness in interictal period. This can be convulsive (tonic clonic) or non-convulsive type. Practically seizure activity lasting for more than 5 minutes should be managed as status epilepticus.

Steam sterilization refers to steam under pressure; kills all bacteria, spores, fungi and viruses. Steam is produced in autoclave and is kept at temperature of 134°C for at least 3 minutes. Whole process may take 20 minutes. Steam is suitable for metal instruments, diamond and tungsten, rubber, swab, cotton and most plastics.

Stepping reflex *see* walking.

Sterility *see* impotence.

Stethoscope is an instrument used to ampliy and listen soft internal sounds of the body, e.g. heart sound and lung sound.

Stevens Johnson syndrome is a very severe bullous form of erythema multiformae with widespread involvement skin, genitals and eyes. Suddenly patient may develop fever, photophobia and eruption of mucosa of oral cavity, skin and genitalia. Oral lesions may be so severe that mastication becomes impossible. There is no specific treatment. Sometimes cortisone helps.

Sticky wax is a brittle wax containing resin used to hold metal parts in investment of soldering. It fractures instead of deforming under stress.

Stillman's tooth brushing method is a method of tooth brushing provides gingival stimulation. Bristles are placed partly on cervical portion of tooth and partly on gingiva. Strokes are completed in each region and bush is moved to another area. Bristle ends are not directed into sulcus so can be recommended for clients with progressive recession. It is considered less traumatic to gingiva.

STMI (Stomion inferius): The median point in the vermilion of the lower lip.

STMS (Stomion superius): A point indicating the mucocutaneous border of the upper lip. The most anterior point of the upper lip.

S

Stomach is a dilated portion of alimentary canal and has 3 functions. It stores food having a capacity of 1500 mL. Then it mixed the food with gastric secretion to form a semisolid chime and thirdly it regulates the rate of delivery of the chime to small intestine. It has two openings—cardiac and pyloric, two curvatures greater and lesser.

Stomatitis is also known as leukokeratosis. Smoker's patch develops on palate in heavy smoker. Lesions are limited to smoke area. To start with mucosa is reddened but becomes greyish white. It is thick and fissured. Histologically epithelium shows acanthosis and hyperkeratosis. There is chronic inflammation in the subepithelial connective tissue. If smoker stops, smoking changes are reversible. Lesion has no precancerous potential.

Stomatitis medicamentosa is the term given to the eruptions occurring in the oral cavity due to the sensitivity of the drugs which has been consumed orally.

Stomatitis venenata is term given to the local reaction caused due to the use of medicament in the oral cavity, e.g. Aspirin burn.

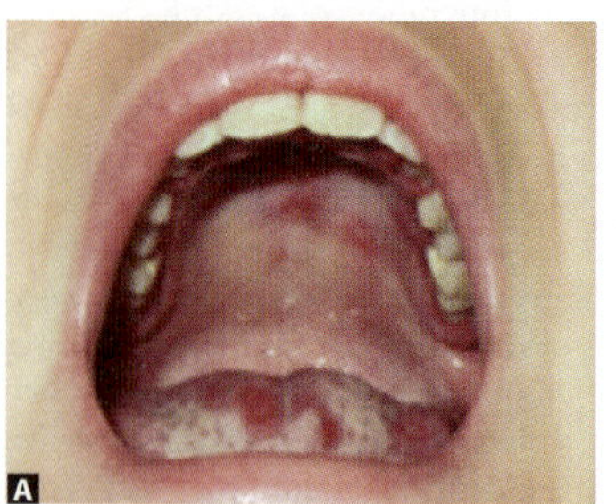

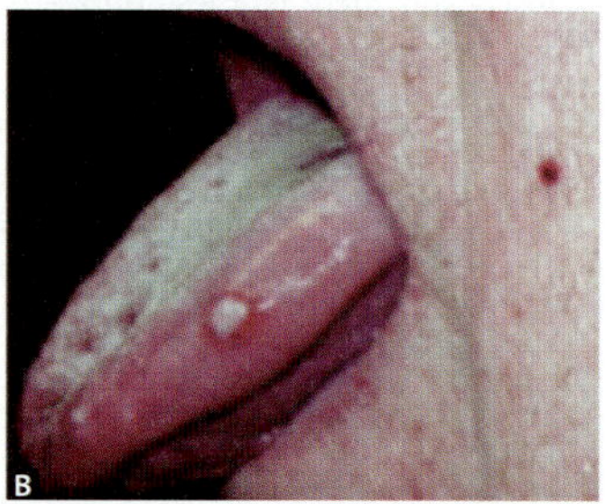

Figs A and B: *Stomatitis*

Stone's index was introduced by Stone HH, Lawton FE, Bransby ER and Hartley HO in 1949. The scoring is done as follows: (1) One point of one or more cavities in the same tooth detectable by sharp probe where the lesion has not penetrated through the enamel to involve the dentin; (2) Two points to one or more cavities in the same tooth where the dentin is involved, where a total of less than a quarter of the crown is estimated to have been destroyed; (3) Three points to one or more cavities in the same tooth resulting in a total destruction of more than a quarter of the crown.

Stops ***refers to small,*** round, sterile pieces of rubber/plastic that are placed on endodontic instruments to mark the working length.

Storage phosphor screen technology: This screen contains embedded phosphorus crystals that luminesce when stsimulated by light at a specific wavelength. The energy released results in a latent image that is stored in the screen rather than on conventional film. *Advantages:* no darkroom/day light loader required. No processing chemicals needed. Less image resolution. Less radiation required. The image detector is generally larger. The image is immediately available. Image may be electronically transferred. Image may be enhanced. Image is easily altered. Image is easily copied. No duplicating film equipment needed. Image large enough to be seen by patient.

Strabismus please *see* squint.

Straight sinus lies in the triangular interval where the lower edge of the posterior part of the falx cerebri joins the tentorium cerebelli.

Strain is defined as the deformation or the length/dimension of a dental material that results from applied stress. The stiffness of an object determines its ability to resist dimensional change or strain.

Streak culture refers to the culture in which the medium is inoculated by drawing an infected wire across it.

Streptococcal gingivostomatitis is a rare condition characterized by presence of diffuse erythema of gingiva and other parts of oral mucosa, sometimes, it may also appear as marginal erythema, studies indicate that group A beta-hemolytic streptococcus may be a main cause to this lesion.

Streptococcus mutans**:** In 1924, Clarke isolated a *Streptococcus* that predominated in many human carious lesions and that he named *Streptococcus mutans* because of its varying morphology. Clarke noted that *S. mutans* adhered closely to tooth surfaces in artificially induced caries for the next 40 years; *s. mutans* was virtually ignored, until the 1960s when it was "rediscovered" and its prevalence in plaque confirmed. Characteristics of this group of streptococci have been described as nonmotile, catalase-negative, Gram-positive cocci in short or medium chains. On mitis-salivarius agar they grow as highly convex to pulvinate (cushion-shaped) colonies. These colonies are opaque; the surface resembles frosted glass. These *S. mutans* variants also posse caries-inducing properties, and when re-isolated from infected animals they may resume the original rough colonial form.

Streptomycin is bactericidal and acts against Gram-positive and Gram-negative bacteria. It is active against tuberculosis. In high doses toxicity is marked of eighth cranial nerve, vestibular damage is first noted. Auditory division is less vulnerable but tinnitus and deafness can occur. It is given IM and is painful.

Stress is when an external force is applied to a specimen an internal force equal in magnitude but opposite in direction is set up. Stress = f/a, where 'f' is the applied force and 'a' is the cross-sectional area.

Stridor is a respiration produced by turbulent air flow, narrow air passage. Inspiratory stridor is produced in obstructive lesions of supraglottis while expiratory stridor is produced in lesions of thoracic trachea and bronchial foreign body and tracheal stenosis.

Stroke is an abrupt loss of neurological function. It may be caused from atherosclerosis, aneurysm and malformations, decreased perfusion pressure and hemorrhage. Atherosclerosis is the most common cause of cerebral infarction. Hyperviscosity, hypercoagulability by producing cerebral venous thrombosis can impair cerebral blood flow. Smoking, diabetes mellitus, hypertension and hyperlipidemia with obesity are the predisposing factors.

Stroke or cerebrovascular accident are characterized by abrupt onset of symptoms and neurologic deficits attributable to focal vascular cause. Ischemia may be transient and there may be recovery from the neurological deficit within few hours but always within 24 hours. This is known as transient ischemic attack (TIA). TIAs are usually embolic. TIA is a risk factor for future stroke. A reversible ischemic neurological deficit (RIND) is similar to TIA but persists for >24 hours but resolves within a week. In some patients, the deficit continues to worsen after about 6 hours of the onset (stroke-in-evolution).

Strokes are referred as the vertical or oblique movements performed during instrumentation.

Structural spinal disorder pain disc degeneration results in pain which is aggravated by activities. Staying in one position for long may also result in pain. Partial relief may

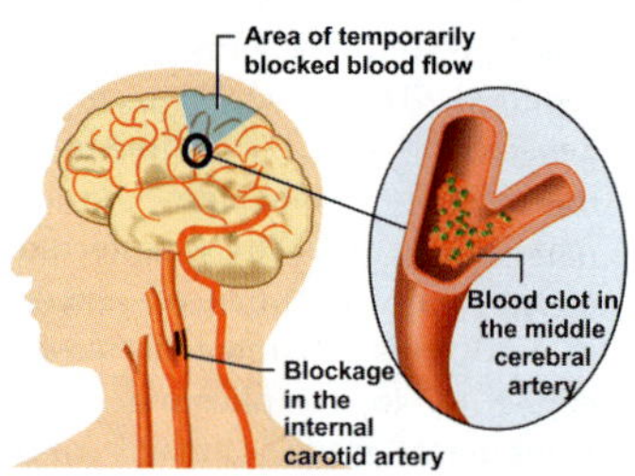

Fig.: *Stroke*

be got by rest. Disc pain becomes worse with sitting, bending, lifting and straining activities. Facer type pain is worst with extension type activities.

Strychnine poisoning: These are poisonous, flat, circular disc, concave on one and convex on other side. They are 2 cm in diameter and ¼″ thick. Ash gray in color have shiny surface. These are too bitter. It acts within 5 to 10 minutes. Choking sensation in throat and stiffness of neck, face and stretching of face start convulsion are first clonic and then become tonic.

Sturge-Weber syndrome is an abnormality of blood vessel formation occurring early in the development of the fetal face and brain. Children with this disease are born with a red birthmark (port-wine stain) on the forehead and, at times, extending over the eye and lower face. In this disease blood vessel formation causes atrophy (shrinking) of the underlying brain, leading to seizures and paralysis of the opposite side of the body. The seizures are usually one sided and may be difficult to control with medication. Children with Sturge Weber may be of normal intelligence but are often progressively handicapped by mental retardation, seizures and paralysis. Surgery to remove the affected portion of the brain is sometimes possible and should be done early in treatment.

Sub-phrenic abscess is due to intra-peritoneal infection, appendicitis or perforation of GI Tract may result in it. Pus may track from one compartment to another compartment. General symptoms are more marked than any local symptoms. There will be unexplained fever, right upper abdominal tenderness and pain. Liver is pushed down and diaphragm is elevated. Chest movement is slowed down. Surgical drain under antibiotic cover helps.

Subarachnoid hemorrhage can be caused by rupture of a cerebral aneurysm or rupture of arteriovenous malformation. Early diagnosis and surgery has a significant future. Symptoms include worst headache of life, neck pain and back and radicular pain. Focal or generalized neurological abnormalities may be seen. Its causative factors are saccular aneurysm, ruptured AV malformation and hypertension. Saccular aneurysms are congenital thin sac-like protrusion from circle of Willis. It develops in anterior circulation. Mycotic aneurysms occur at distal ends of cerebral vessels. Person will develop orbital pain/occipital headache. CSF study shows blood. Xanthochromia and RBC in CSF disappears after 2 weeks of blood.

Subclavian arteries: The right subclavian artery is a branch of the brachiocephalic trunk and begins behind the right sternoclavicular joint. The left subclavian artery is a direct branch of the aorta. It has a thoracic part. Thereafter, the course and relations of the right and left subclavian arteries are similar.

Subclinical is without clinical manifestation.

Subdural manifests after subdural hematomas. There will be decreased level of consciousness involving head injury. Seizures may develop with focal neurologic symptoms. Confusion and personality change results. Pupil will dilate with hemiparesis.

Subgingival biofilm: Subgingival plaque residing in a more protected location is not subject to the same degree of intraoral abrasion or salivary host defense components. The main determinants limiting its growth are physical space and the innate defense system of the host. One result of subgingival plaque accumulation is a continual increase in the space available by reducing epithelial cell attachment levels and increasing pocket depth. The innate host defense system limits this spread by maintaining an intact epithelial cell barrier. GCF, although a rich source of nutrients, contains a potent array of antimicrobial activities. It contains innate components which include lysozymes, complement and a variety of vascular permeability enhancers such as bradykinin, thrombin and fibrinogen and adaptive components including antibodies and lymphocytes.

Subgingival calculus is the one which is located below the crest of the marginal gingiva and is, therefore, not visible in the oral cavity. The calculus is hard, dense and frequently dark in color. Such calculus is less extensive, flatter and more brittle and darker in color. These are deposited at irregular intervals throughout life.

Sublingual gland is a salivary gland that is present in relation to the floor of the anterior part of the oral cavity. It is placed just deep to the oral mucous membrane and is responsible for raising up the sublingual fold. Inferiorly, the gland rests on the mylohyoid muscle. Laterally it is in contact with the anterior part of the mandible above the mylohyoid line. Sublingual gland produces 2–5% of total salivary volume. It lies above the mylohyoid, below the mucosa of the floor of the mouth, medial to the sublingual fossa of the mandible and lateral to the genioglossus. About 15 ducts emerge from the gland. Most of them open directly into the floor of the mouth on the summit of the sublingual fold. A few of them join the submandibular duct. Sublingual glands lie just below the mucosa on

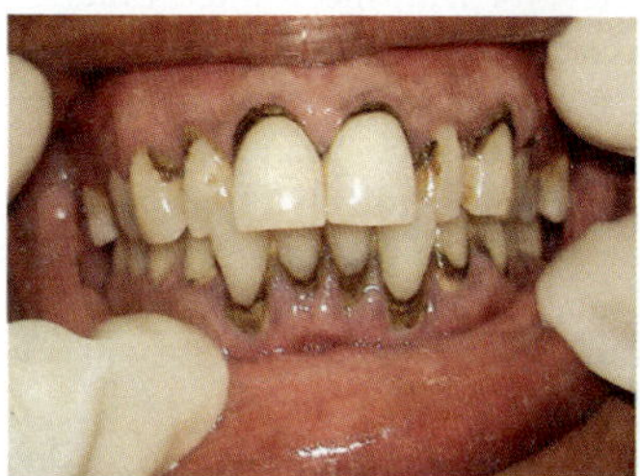

Fig.: *Subgingival calcus*

the floor of the mouth. Each gland raises a ridge of mucosa which starts at the sublingual papilla and runs laterally and backwards. This ridge is called the sublingual fold. The hard palate has a skeletal basis formed by the palatal processes of the right and left maxillae, and the horizontal plates of the palatine bones. This bony basis is covered by periosteum. The lower surface of the palate is lined by mucous membrane of the mouth and its upper surface by mucous membrane of the nasal cavity.

Sublingual keratosis develops as white lesion on the floor of mouth and ventral tongue. Malignant changes have been noted. It is a white soft plaque wih a finely wrinkled surface. There is an irregular but well-defined outline. There is no associated inflammation.

Sublingual plaque is a plaque that forms under the gum line.

Sublingual space refers to the space existing below the oral mucosa in the anterior part of the floor of the mouth and contains sublingual gland, its excretory ducts, submandibular duct which is traversed by lingual nerve and hypoglossal nerve. Infection to this area raises the floor of the mouth and displaces tongue, resulting in pain and difficulty in swallowing.

Submandibular duct is an excretory duct that allows the passage of the saliva from gland to the sublingual papilla. It emerges from the medial surface of the submandibular gland near the posterior margin of the mylohyoid. It is also known as Wharton's duct.

Submandibular ganglion is an autonomic ganglion connected with the cranial parasympathetic outflow. It lies over the hyoglossus muscle, suspended from the lingual nerve by two or more roots. The fibers passing through the ganglion is concerned with the secretomotor innervation of the submandibular and sublingual salivary glands. These fibers are parasympathetic.

Submandibular gland this is a paired muco-serous gland lying in the submandibular space salivary

S

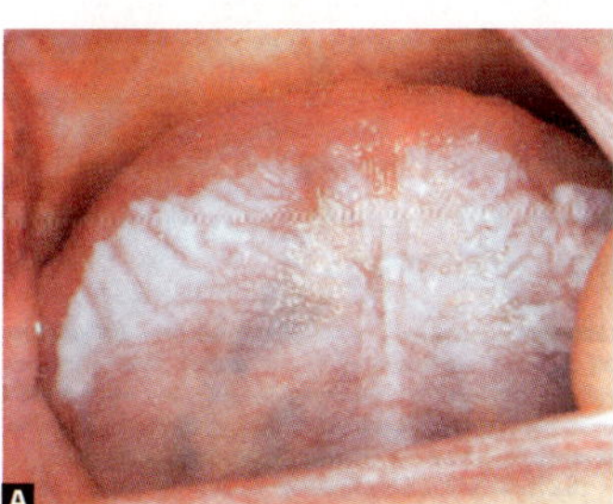

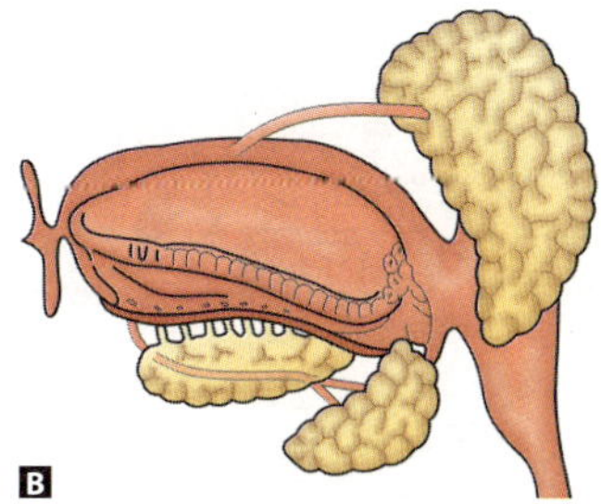

Figs A and B: *(A) Sublingual keratosis; (B) Submandibular gland*

gland that is located partly below, and partly deep to the body of the mandible. The part below the mandible lies in the digastric triangle. The inferior surface is covered by skin, platysma, and submandibular lymph nodes. Lateral surface is related to, submandibular fossa of mandible and medial surface is related to the extrinsic muscles of tongue and mylohyoid muscle. Secretions are discharged into the oral cavity through Wharton's duct which runs forward from the anterior border of the upper part, raising a fold of mucous membrane in the floor of the mouth and opens on little papilla to the side of the lingual papilla just behind the lower incisor teeth. The submandibular duct is approximately 5 cm long. The submandibular gland is enclosed by two layers of fascia formed by splitting of the investing layer of deep cervical fascia.

Submandibular space refers to the space existing external to the sublingual space, below the mylohyoid and hyoglossus muscle. The space contains the submandibular gland, which extends slightly above the mylohyoid muscle thus communicating with sublingual space.

Submental space refers to the space existing between the mylohyoid muscle superiorly and the platysma inferiorly, bounded posteriorly by hyoid bone and laterally by mandible, it is traversed by anterior belly of digastrics muscle. Infection results in swelling of submental region.

Submerged teeth these are generally deciduous teeth specially second molar which undergo variable degree of root absorption. It becomes ankylosed with bone. X-ray confirms it.

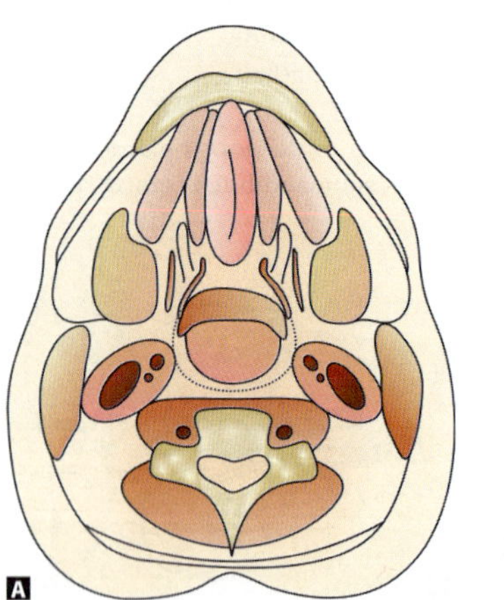

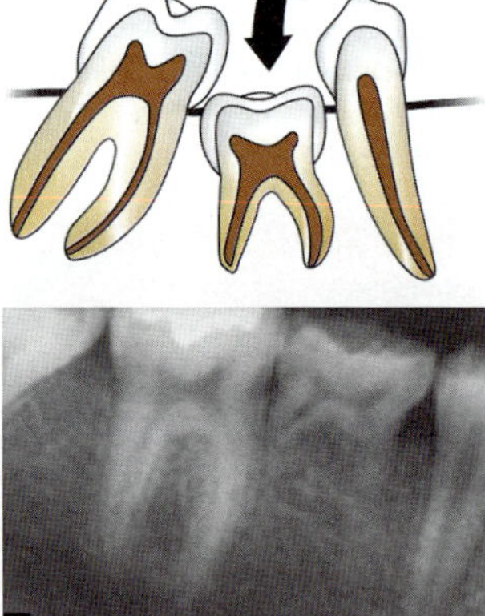

Figs A and B: *(A) Submandibular space; (B) Submerged, ankylosed teeth*

Substance P polypeptide acts as an excitatory neurotransmitter. It is released from spinal cord cells by A δ and c fiber afferent stimulation and excites dorsal horn neurons.

Substrate is the material being abraded.

Subzygomatic fractures *see* Lefort II.

Succedaneous is a tooth that replaces or succeeds another.

Sulcus is a broad depression on the chewing surfaces of your back teeth.

Supragingival is the area above the gingival margin.

Supernumerary teeth are the extra teeth, in addition to the development of the normal 32.

Suture is a joining of two bones, also stitches.

Succedaneous teeth are permanent teeth which replace or succeed the primary teeth. While permanent molars are nonsuccedaneous teeth they don't replace primary teeth.

Suckling is a specialized form of ingestion where mother's nipple is drawn deep in mouth. Everted lips form a seal lingual muscular activity; generate a peristathic wave moving posteriorly which milk the nipple and propel it toward the pharynx.

Sucralose is 600 times sweeter than sucrose derived from sucrose. It is claimed not to be hydrolyzed nor dechlorinated in the body.

Sucrose is a disaccharide composed of glucose + fructose, i.e. table sugar.

Suicidal wounds are located inside the mouth, over temple, under chin or on left side of chest. Firearm may remain grasped in cadaveric spasm. Wound is directed from below upwards. Wound is single. Due to close range of wound scorching or blackening of area is found. There will be no signs of struggle. Room may be locked from inside and farewell note may be found.

Sulcular epithelium lines the sulcus of the gingiva and can be described as thin, nonkeratinized stratified squamous epithelium which extends from the coronal limit of the junctional epithelium to border of marginal gingiva.

Sulcular fluid is the tissue fluid that seeps into the gingival sulcus through the wall of sulcus.

Sulcus is a long depression in the surface of a tooth between ridges and cusps.

Sulphonamide in 1900 first sulphonamide para-amino-benzene-sulphonamide was synthesized.

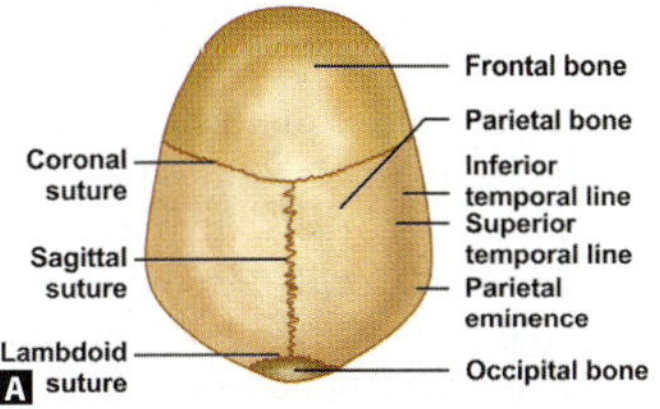

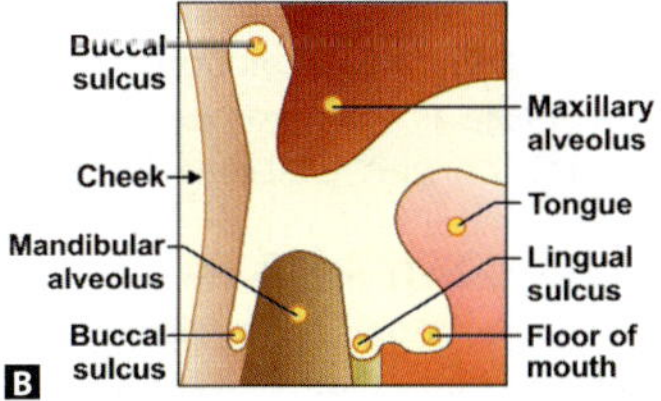

Figs A and B: *(A) Suture; (B) Sulcus*

It is generally bacteriostatic rather than bactericidal. It acts by interfering with the utilization of para-amino benzoic acid bacteria. It is extensively used in gonorrhea. Kidney excretes it. Occasional occurrence of agranulocytosis may develop. Mostly these are used in respiratory and urinary tract infection.

Summation theory is an alternative theory postulates that pain does not depend on specific pathways but on excessive stimulation involving all types of receptors with the resultants central neural summation or convergence of activity.

Superego ***is prohibition*** learned from environment more from parents and authorities. Acts as censor of acceptability of thoughts, feelings and behavior. It is determined by regulation imposed on the child by parent's, society and culture. It is internalized control that produces a feeling of shame guilt. The expression of discomfort (anxiety-/fear) by the child is as the result of conflict between the three components as the psychic structure.

S

Superficial dermal is the one which involves the epidermis and the papillary dermis. These also heal on their own by epithelial growth from the abundant skin appendages but slower than epidermal burns because as we go deeper the number of epithelial cells decreases and amount of connective tissue increases. Therefore the healing in these burns is by regeneration and repair that leaves a scar. These usually heal in 14 days.

Superficial partial thickness burns refer to superficial dermal burns.

Superficial temporal artery is the second terminal branch of the external carotid artery. It begins behind the neck of the mandible in the substance of the parotid gland. It runs upwards behind the tempero-mandibular joint and ramifies in the scalp over the temporal region. The artery is accompanied by the auriculotemporal nerve.

Superior alveolar neuritis involves maxillary dental plexus and is the direct extension of inflammation of antral mucosa. There may be burning neuritic pain. No muscle or autonomic symptoms are present.

Superior levator labii alaeque nasi ***arises*** from frontal portion of maxilla. It passes obliquely downwards and divides into two medial and lateral slips. The lateral slip raises and everts the upper lip, the medial slip acts as a dilator of nostril.

Superior orbital fissure is a prominent cleft that separates the posterior parts of the roof and lateral wall. It is bounded above and medially by the lesser wing of the sphenoid, and below and laterally by the greater wing.

Superior sagittal sinus occupies the triangular space produced by the reflection of the inner layer of dura mater to form the falx cerebri. It begins anteriorly in front of crista galli. It then runs backwards deeply grooving the frontal bone (in the midline); the two parietal bones (where they join at the sagittal suture); and the occipital bone (again in the midline).

Supernumerary cusps *see* cusp of carabelli, dens evaginatus and talons cusp.

Supernumerary roots refer to development of increased number of roots on a tooth compared with that classically described in dental anatomy. Both deciduous and permanent can be involved. Detection of supernumerary root is critical when endodontic therapy and exodontia is undertaken. Otherwise no specific treatment is required.

Supernumerary teeth occur more frequently in the permanent dentition. 90% of the cases occur in the maxilla with strong predilection for the anterior region. The most common region is the maxillary central incisor followed by maxillary 4th molar. Most supernumerary teeth are unilateral. Supernumerary tooth located between maxillary central incisors is termed mesiodens. Supernumerary 4th molar is called distomolar. A supernumerary tooth situated lingually or buccally to a molar is called paramolar. Supernumerary teeth are morphologically classified as either supplemental or rudimentary. Supplemental teeth duplicate the typical anatomy of posterior or anterior teeth. Rudimentary supernumerary teeth are dysmorphic and can assume conical or tuberculate form. The eruption of supernumerary teeth is variable and depends on the space available. 70% of supernumerary teeth in the anterior maxilla fail to erupt. In such situation midline diastema is common. Whenever there is a large midline diastema, radiographic evaluation to detect presence of supernumerary tooth is essential. Supernumerary teeth can also prevent eruption of adjacent teeth, displacement or rotation, crowding. Unerupted supernumerary teeth can be associated with cyst. At times, they can erupt into nasal cavity as well. Meticulous clinical and radiographic examination is required to detect supernumerary teeth. Horizontal tube shift technique where two periapical radiographs are taken at different horizontal angulation is helpful in detecting the position of the unerupted teeth.

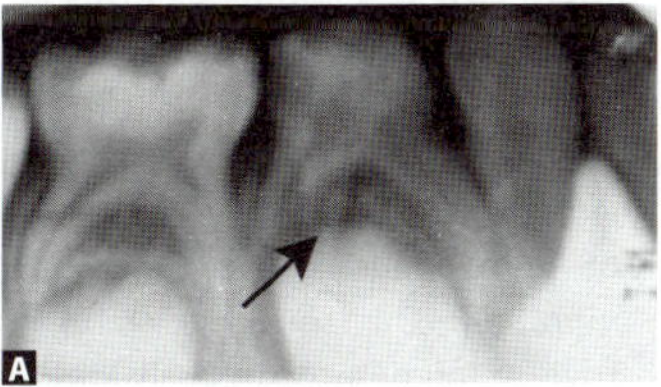

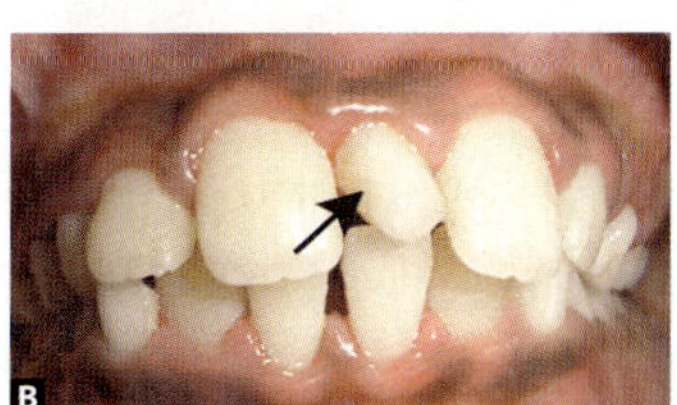

Figs A and B: *(A) Supernumerary root; (B) Supernumerary teeth*

Suppurations refer to lung abscess, brain abscess, pyocele and perpural sepsis. Similarly common infection can also give rise to rigors such as tonsillitis, sinusitis bronchiectasis.

Suppurative arthritis of TM Joint local manifestations consist of spasm of masseter muscles, difficulty of opening of mouth. There can be fever, leukocytosis and general malaise. X-ray may show normal findings.

Suppurative inflammation damage to vessels is severe. Plenty of neutrophils are killed in inflammation. Dead neutrophil and degraded products, necrosed tissue with inflammation is called purulent inflammation.

Suprabony pocket is the term used where the base of the pocket is coronal to the underlying alveolar bone.

Supraclavicular nerves arise (as a single ramus) from the third and fourth cervical nerves. The origin lies deep to the sternocleidomastoid. The nerve trunk runs downwards and backwards deep to the muscle and appears at its posterior border.

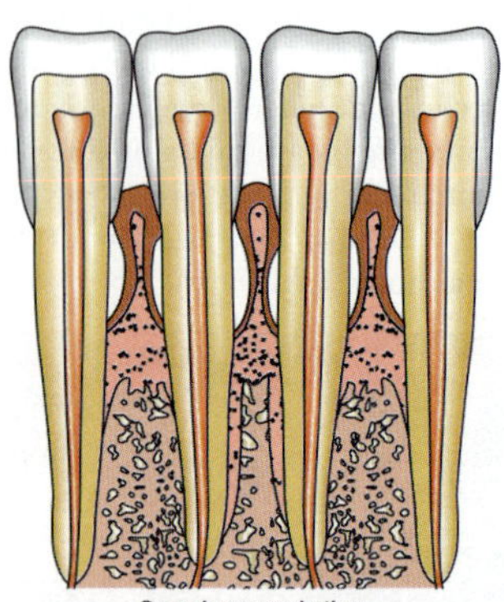

Fig.: *Suprabony pocket*

Supracontact *see* interference.

Supragingival biofilm forms above the gingival margin. Supragingival plaque growth, being located in contact with the oral cavity, is subject to much more intraoral abrasion which restricts its net accumulation. In addition, this biofilm is subject to flow characteristics of saliva and its host defense components. Saliva contains secretory IgA, lactoferrin, lysozymes and peroxidases that display a wide spectrum of antimicrobial activity and serve to limit both colonization and spread of the supragingival bacterial biofilm.

Supragingival calculus is the calculus which is present coronal to the gingival margin and is visible in the oral cavity. It is usually whitish yellow in color, clay-like consistency and easily detached from the oral cavity. It mainly occurs on the lingual aspect of the lower incisors and the buccal aspect of the maxillary molars.

Supragingival plaque is a plaque located above the gingival margin.

Suprazygomatic fracture *see* Lefort III.

Surds refer to any voiceless sound and is produced by separation of vocal folds without marginal vibration. This sound is made by friction of airstream as it passes through the appropriate cavities.

Surface anaesthetics are the agents that anesthetize the surface of mucous membrane so that syringe needle can be inserted painlessly. It is used as spray, solution/paste. It is applied a few minutes before the injection. 5% lignocaine generally used.

Surface coat is the first coating applied to a wax pattern or the surface of mould that comes in direct contact with a cast metal.

Surface energy is an extra energy that atoms or molecules on the surface of a substance have over those in the interior. The surface energy of a liquid is referred to as surface tension expressed in erg/cm^2.

Surface tension force acting parallel to the boundary surface, generally expressed in dynes/cm.

Surgical chisels and hoes are the instruments used during the periodontal surgery for removing and reshaping the bone. The hoe has curved shank and blade whereas the chisel is straight shanked. The surgical hoe has flattened fishtail shaped blade with a pronounced convexity in its terminal portion. It is used for detaching pocket walls after the gingivectomy incisions; also it is helpful for smoothening root and bone surfaces.

Surgical ciliated cyst of maxilla develops after surgical entry into maxillary sinus. Patient complains of nonspecific poorly localized pain and tenderness. Swelling is evident. X-ray will show radiolucent area closely related to maxillary sinus. Filling defect of cyst can be seen; treatment includes enucleation.

Surgical crown lengthening is the process where clinical crown height of teeth can be increased by surgically repositioning the gingival margin with alveolar bone recontouring. This procedure creates longer teeth but maintains the existing vertical dimension.

Surgical files are the those surgical instruments which are mainly used for smoothening of bony ledges and to remove all areas of bone.

Surgical length burs are long 32 mm burs. They are useful in teeth which present problems with access and visibility. With these burs, visibility of cutting tip of instrument is increased because of displacement of handpiece away from incisal or occlusal surface of tooth.

Surgical mallet is a special nylon tipped hammer used with a surgical chisel to remove bone.

Surgical scissors are sharp bladed scissors used to trim soft tissues and cut suture material.

Surgical scrubbing is a mechanical procedure to eliminate the bacterial flora on the skin. After the scrub has begun, contamination should be avoided.

Surgical stent is a clear acrylic template placed over the alveolar ridge to assist in locating the proper placement for dental implants.

Survey is a research method based on self-reported information from participants rather than observations.

Susceptible host is the one who is unable to resist infection by the pathogens. Host is in poor health and has compromised immune system.

Suspension culture refers to a culture in which cells multiply while suspended in a suitable medium.

Sutural dominance theory was put forward by Sicher and says that proliferation of sutural connective tissue causes appositional growth. Genetic factor was accepted and the membranous bones were considered as growth centers.

Suture an immovable joint.

Suture instruments include dissecting forceps, needle holders, suture needle, spencer wall forceps and scissors.

Suture needle is a curved needle used with suture material to close the surgical site.

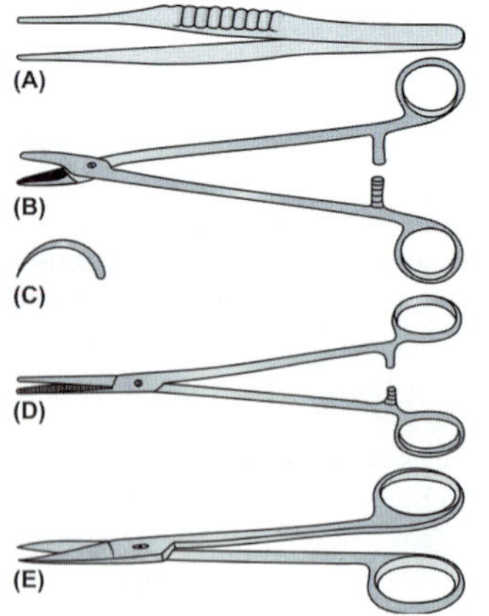

Figs A to E: *Suture instruments (A) Dissecting forceps; (B) Needle holders; (C) Suture needle; (D) Spencer wells forceps; (E) Scissors*

Swallowing is complex muscular act which prevents the ball of food entering nasal cavity or larynx. It is propelled by the tongue from mouth to the back of throat. From here it goes down to esophagus.

Sweat retention syndrome is an extravasation of sweat in the tissue with subsequent inflammation, keratin plug formation in sweat glands.

Symmetry as close to identical from one side of the mouth to the other. Ideally, the incisal edges of your teeth should follow the contour of the upper lip.

Sympathetic nervous system is the part of autonomic nervous system which arises in the thoracic and first three lumbar segments of spinal cord.

Symptoms are defined as signs of departure from the normal. They are indicator of illness. These are effects of disease noticed by patient himself.

Symptoms of nicotine poisoning are nausea and salivation occurs quickly and is followed by pain and severe diarrhea. Cold sweet is prominent. Headache, dizziness, disturbed hearing and vision, mental confusion are experienced. Respiration is stimulated and blood pressure may be elevated. Pupils first constrict and later on dilate.

Synchondrosis refers to movements of joints are absent or minimal. Examples include intercostals joint and a joint between diaphysis and epiphysis.

Syncope is transient loss of consciousness without prodromal symptoms that is followed within seconds to minutes (<30 minutes) by resumption of consciousness. Although many causes do exist, a closer examination reveals 3 factors when present, increase the likelihood that a patient may experience an alteration or loss of consciousness. These factors include stress, impaired physical status, administration or ingestion of drugs. It is a complicated problem frequently encountered in clinical practice. It describes a loss of consciousness, usually from a sudden decrease in cerebral blood flow. Brain can with-stand only a few seconds of total interruption of blood flow without loss of consciousness.

Syndesmoses in these joint bones are held together by an intraosseous ligament. Example includes inferior tibiofibular joint and radioulnar joint.

Synergistic–acting jointly: Adding the effect of another drug.

Synovial ball and socket joint a multiaxial joint having movements around more than 2 axes. Examples include hip and shoulder joint.

Synovial chondromatosis contains multiple cartilaginous nodules of synovial membrane and loose calcified bodies in joints. Part of the synovium calcifies and breaks off into the joint space.

Synovial condylar joints are biaxial joints and movement include flexion, extension, abduction and adduction. Examples are wrist joint, metacarpophalangeal joint atlanto-occipital and metatarso-phalangeal joint.

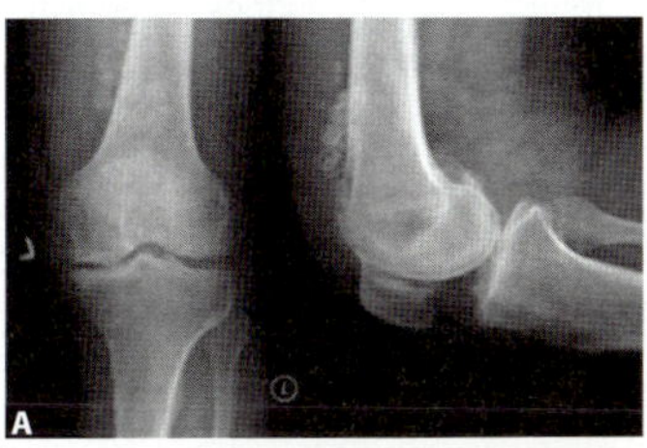

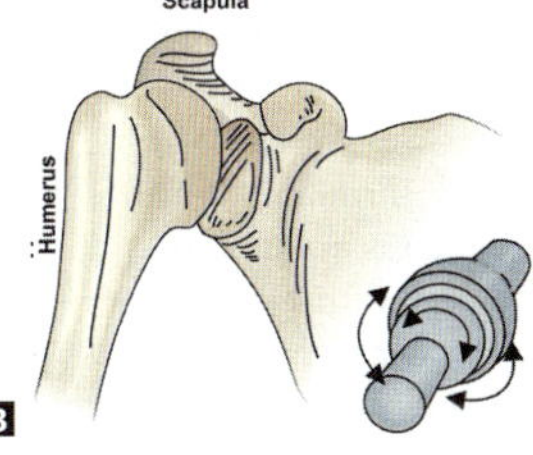

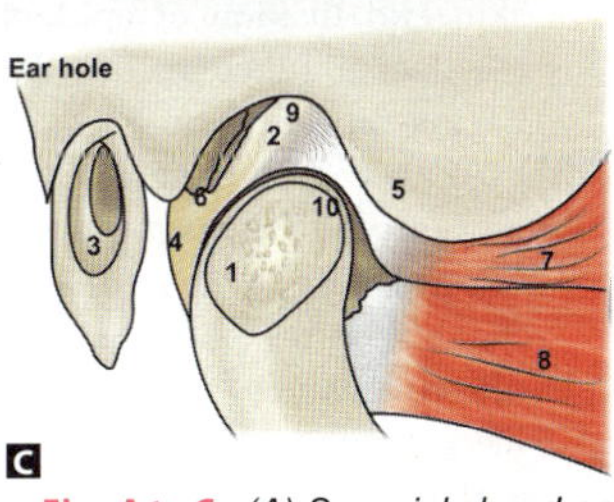

Figs A to C: *(A) Synovial chondromatosis; (B) Ball and socket joint; (C) Closed mouth TMJ anatomy*

Synovial hinge joint: There is movement around one joint, flexion and extension. Elbow joint and interphalangeal joints are its example.

Synovial pivot joint is a uniaxial joint and rotational movement. Examples of joint include superior and inferior radioulnar joint.

Synovial sarcoma is malignancy arising from articulate or para-articular site, bursae or tendon sheath. It develops in young people. In oral cavity cheek, tongue, floor of mouth and soft palate are involved. There may be fibrosarcoma like proliferation of cells with collagen and reticulin. Early radical excision gives better results.

Synthetic phenols are compounds with broad spectrum disinfecting action.

Syphilis is the sexually transmitted chronic systemic infection caused by *Treponema pallidum*. It is transmitted during sexual contact through abrasions in skin or mucous membranes. It can be transferred from mother to fetus via placenta (congenital syphilis). Transmission may also occur by blood transfusion, kissing and percutaneous injury. The clinical features of syphilis are broadly classified as early and late syphilis. Early syphilis includes primary syphilis, secondary syphilis and latent syphilis. Late syphilis includes "Late" latent syphilis and tertiary syphilis (benign tertiary syphilis, cardiovascular and neurosyphilis).

Syphilitic oral ulcer is painless until secondarily infected. Lip or tip of tongue is affected. Size may vary from 5 mm to several cms. Edges of ulcer are raised and indurated. It is highly infectious and heals without scar. Regional lymph glands are enlarged, rubbery and discrete.

Systemic lupus erythematosis was described by Sir William Osler in 1895. He described the systemic manifestations of this chronic systemic inflammatory disease with alternating exacerbations and remissions. It is characterized by multiorgan involvement including polyarthritis (polyarthralgia, avascular bone necrosis). Skin butterfly rash, which is an erythematous rash involving areas of body, chronically exposed to UV light, mucosal ulceration, oral and genital mucosa in 15% cases; kidney (nephritis, glomerulitis either diffuse, membranous, sclerosing); vascular: with small vessel vasculitis, splinter hemorrhage, periungual occlusion, finger pulp infarctions.

Systemic sclerosis is a progressive fibrosis of skin and multiple organs. There is induration of skin and fixation of epidermis to the deeper subcutaneous tissue. It begins on face, hands and trunk. Skin becomes yellow, gray or ivory white waxy appearance. Tongue, soft palate and larynx are the structures involved. Tongue often becomes stiff and board like. Gingival tissues are pale and unusually firm. Lips become thin, rigid and partially fixed.

Dysphagia and chocking sensation also develop. There is no adequate treatment.

Systemic therapy: Treatment that reaches and affects cells through out the body.

T-cells is a component of white blood cells and plays a vital role in immune system. It does not express Ig but detects presence of foreign substances by way of surface protein called T-Cell receptor (TCR). TCR is a heterogeneous clan of membrane proteins on T-cells consisting of a pair of transmembrane polypeptides of alpha and beta chains. TCR shares structural and functional properties with Ig and are closely related to each other in evolution. TCRs are never secreted; hence, T cells lack the ability to strike their targets at long distance. They exert their protective effects through direct contact with a target or by influencing activity of other immune cells. They are the principal cells involved in cell-mediated immunity. T cells can detect foreign substances only in specific context; can recognize a foreign particle only if first cleaved into small peptides and displayed on the surface of second host cell 'antigen presenting cell (APC)'. Antigen presentation depends on specific protein *'Major Histo-compatibility Complex (MHC)'* in surface of APC and this combination is recognized by a T-cell receptor.

Tactile is pertaining to touch.

Tactile sensitivity is the ability to distinguish relative degrees of roughness and smoothness on the surface of tooth.

Talons cusp is a cusp-like structure projecting from the cingulum of incisors. In shape, it resembles an eagle's talon. It can be considered as dens evaginatus, of anterior teeth. It is predominately seen on maxillary permanent lateral incisors and very rarely seen on deciduous teeth. Like dens evaginatus talon cusp is composed of enamel, dentin and pulp extension. Talon cusp is common in Chinese, Caucasians and African-Americans. Incidence of talon cusp is high in patients with Rubinstein–Taybi syndrome and Struge-Weber syndrome.

Tardive dyskinesia is a repetitive uncontrolled activity of head, jaw, tongue and lips. It may follow long-term use of phenothiazines. Symptoms include rapid repetitive movements of lips.

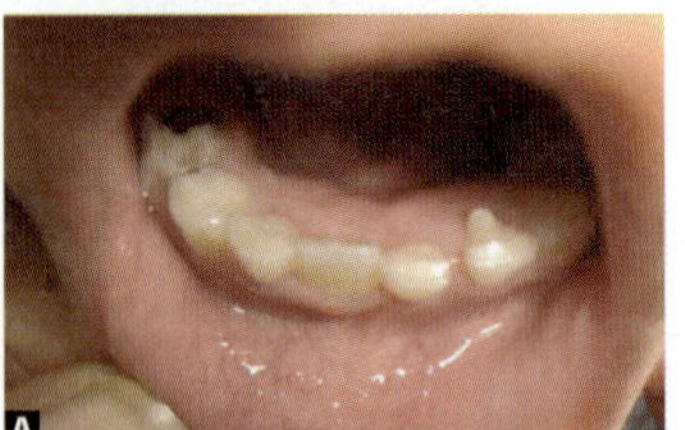

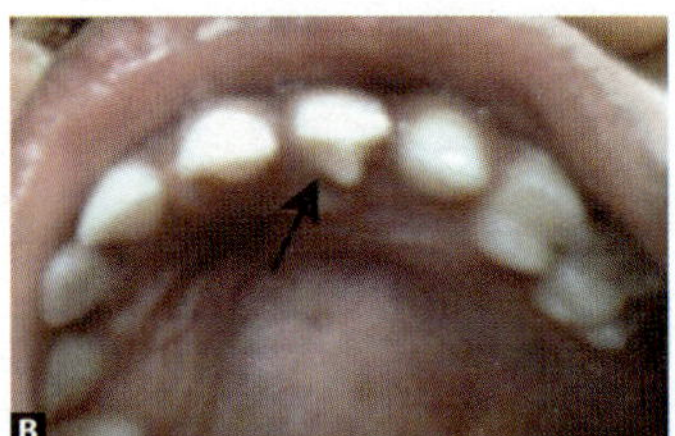

Figs A and B: *Talon cusp*

Tarnish is a chemical reaction between a metal and its environment that results in discoloration of the surface of metal.

Tartar *see* calculus.

Taste refers to perception of food as butter, sweet, sour, urnami. It may be deformed in many ways. Ageusia is a complete loss of taste while hypogeusia is decreased taste for all taste stimuli. Dysgeusia is a perversion of taste. Hypergeusia is an increased sensitivity for all tastes, while gustatory agnosia is a loss of ability to distinguish and identify different tastes.

Taurodontism is an enlargement of the body and pulp chamber of a multirooted tooth with apical displacement of the pulpal floor and bifurcation of the roots. Affected teeth tend to be rectangular in shape and a bull-like appearance. There is an increase inch apico-occlusal height of pulp chamber and furcation is close to the apex. The diagnosis is made from the radiographic appearance. Depending on the degree of apical displacement of the pulpal floor taurodontism can be mild, moderate or severe. If endodontic treatment is required in such tooth, the shape of the pulp chamber increases the difficulty of locating, instrumenting and obturating the pulp canals.

Teething is a process where the baby teeth are emaging through gums.

Temper refers to a degree of hardness and elasticity of metal or sled. The spring character of an orthodontic wire, which is related to the mechanical properties of yield strength and resilience.

Temporal arteritis is a rare, febrile or inflammatory disease of variable

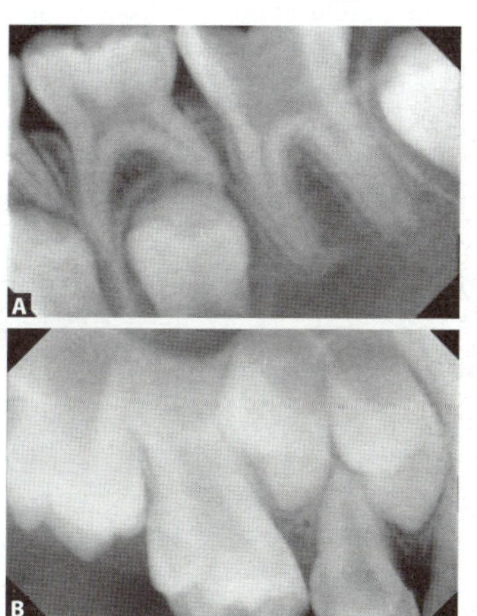

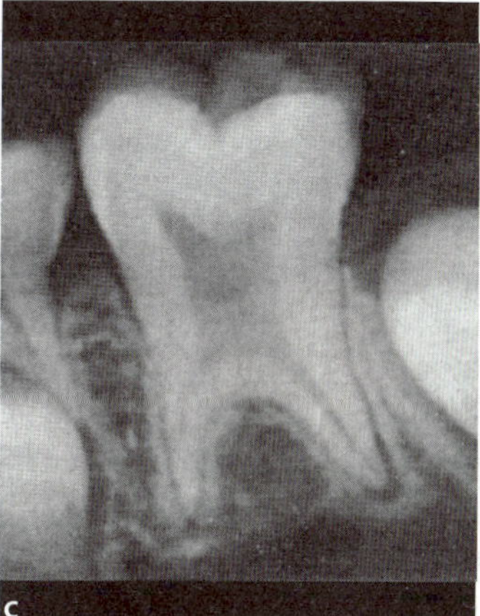

Figs A to C: *(A) Mild taurodontism; (B) Taurodontism; (C) Severe taurodontism of maxillary molar*

duration. Distended arteries are extremely tender on palpation. Headache, scalp hyperalgesias and painful mastication are present. It is a type of immunologic vasculitis and is a self-limiting disease of many days.

Temporal lobe tumor produces expressive aphasia and impaired performance of hearing. Auditory illusions, hallucination psychomotor seizure or visual hallucination develop.

Temporalis muscle is one of the muscles of mastication. It has 2 fibers that run anteriorly and posteriorly. The anterior fibers of the muscle run vertically downwards; the posterior fibers run horizontally forwards; while the intermediate fibers run obliquely to converge in a tendon. The tendon passes deep to the zygomatic arch.

Temporary bridges are the provisonal or interim restoration/ bridges that are necessary between visits to prevent closure and enable chewing.

Temporary fillings are interim restoration that are given during the healing period or when the teeth is going through treatment of multiple visits. Zinc oxide, zinc phosphate and gutta percha are used. These are soft and soluble and will not remain for long hence are not to be used for permanent filling.

Temporomandibular disorder is a deviation from normal function which includes restricted movement of mandible ≥2 mm deviation of mandible on opening, pain on palpation of masticatory muscles. There may be sound in temporomandibular joint and pain during chewing and swallowing.

Temporomandibular dysfunction involves both muscle and joint derangements. Physical therapy and relaxation technique are beneficial. Intraoral splints provide relief.

Temporomandibular joint (TMJ) is a synovial joint of the condylar variety. It is a complex joint as its

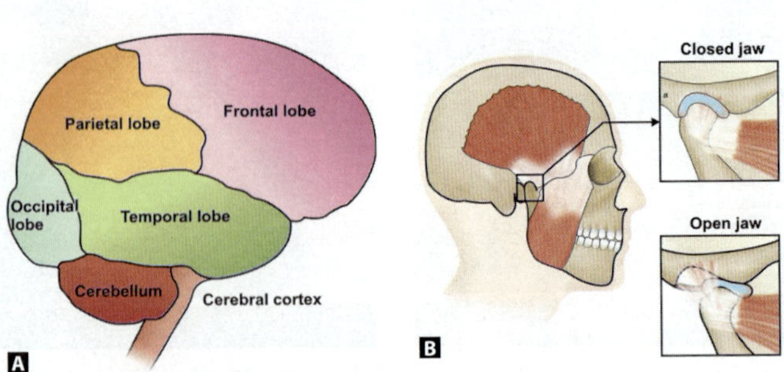

Figs A and B: *(A) Brain: Temporal lob; (B) TMJ-Image*

cavity is divided into upper and lower parts by an intra-articular disc. The upper articular surface of the joint is formed by the mandibular fossa of the temporal bone. Inferior articular surface of the joint is formed by the head of the mandible. Articular disc is made of fibrocartilage.

Temporomandibular joint arthritis occurs during periods of severe psychic stress, clenching and bruxism may become exaggerated and lead to severe mandibular joint and muscle pain. Marital problems, menopause and fatigue all may cause it. X-ray may show evidence of bone resorption or irregularity of head of condyle or anterior slope of glenoid fossa.

TENS stands for transcutaneous electrical nerve stimulation has been used in the treatment of phantom limb pain; peripheral nerve injury joint pain, etc. electrical stimulus is typically generated from a portable battery operated device. Mode of action is not very well-understood. It blocks pain signals carried over to small unmyelinated 'C' fibers.

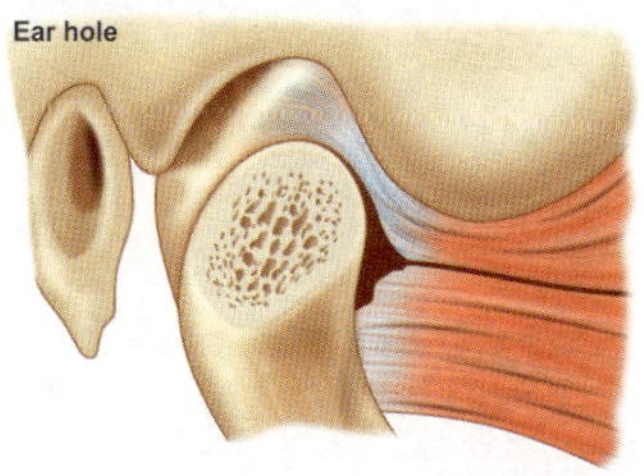

Fig.: *Temporomandibular joint (TMJ)*

Tension headache is bilateral and diffuse. It is felt as a sense of tightness, pressure in head and band-like constriction. Onset is gradual and may persist for a few days. During worry and anxiety headache is worst. These responses best to anxiolytics and antidepressants.

Teratogenesis is the development of organic defects due to certain drugs used in pregnancy.

Teratoma is the neoplasm composed of multiple tissues including those which are normally not found in the organ in which it arises. It is a heterotopic collection of various forms. Benign tumors are cystic lesions. Walls of lesion are thickened. These contain hair, sebaceous material and teeth. Teeth are uncommon in malignant form of teratoma. Teeth resemble bicuspid.

Tertian fever: When fever comes on alternate day.

Tertiary health care offers super-specialized care. It is provided by regional and central level of institutions.

Tertiary prevention is a post-pathogenic prevention. It includes techniques designed to replace lost tissues and rehabilitate a normal function. It is done to prevent any further damage and maintain homeostasis.

Tertiary syphilis: Benign tertiary syphilis may develop between 3–10 years of infection and can involve skin, mucous membrane, bone, muscle or viscera. Gumma can be single or multiple and most commonly involved sites are the skin, bone, mouth, upper respiratory tract, liver, and the stomach. It develops after 5-10 years of primary lesion affecting every organ of the body. It mainly affects CNS and CVS. Typical lesion is 'gumma'. It is a localized chronic granulomatous lesion having either nodular or ulcerated surface. Ulcer is a punched out ulcer having vertical walls. Base is dull, red granulomatous with irregular outline. Skin lesions leave tissue paper-like scars.

Tertiary syphilitic oral ulcers are very rarely seen after the invent of penicillin. It is known as gumma, a destructive granulomatous process. It is painless. Usually palate, tongue and tonsils are affected. Shape is round with punched out areas. Floor is depressed with a pale appearance. Edges are punched out.

Test cavity method should be used only when all other test methods are inconclusive in results. Here a test cavity is made with high speed number 1 or 2 round burs with appropriate air and water coolant. The patient is not anesthetized while performing this test. Patient is asked to respond if any painful sensation occurs during drilling. The sensitivity or the pain felt by the patient indicates pulp vitality. Here the procedure is terminated by restoring the prepared cavity. If no pain is felt, cavity preparation may be continued until the pulp chamber is reached and later on endodontic therapy may be carried out.

Testes is a gland where sperm and testosterone is produced. It forms the part of male reproductive system and located in scrotum. Testosterone is a steroid secreted on the stimulation of luteinizing hormone. It helps in maturation of sperm and is responsible for sex characteristics. It helps in growth and development of male reproductive organs, musculoskeletal growth, growth and distribution of hair and enlargement of larynx accompanied by voice changes.

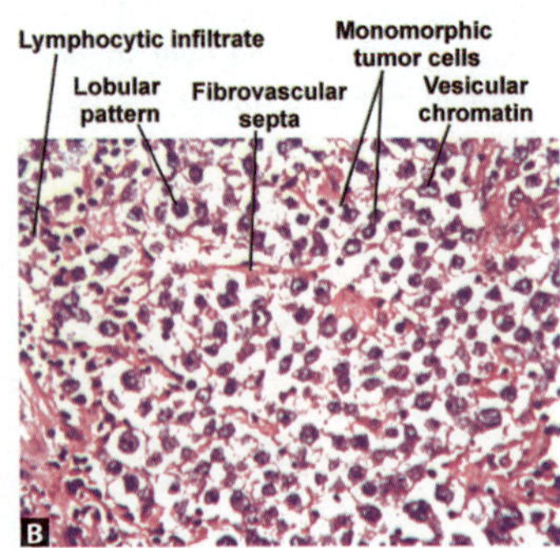

Figs A and B: *Seminoma testis*

Tetanus is a serious bacterial disease and the causative organism is a Gram-positive, actively motile anaerobic spore bearing rod called *Clostridium tetani*. It is found in soil and horse dung. Organism may enter through injury. Clinical features develop within 14 days. Symptoms appear once toxins fix to cell bodies of motor nerves. Incubation period is 5 to 15 weeks. Short duration indicates serious disease. Titanic spasm follows within 24–72 hours of lock jaw. Diagnosis is clinical and does not require clinical confirmation. Convulsion becomes less frequent after 10 days and survivors recover completely by 4 weeks. There develops pain and stiffness in jaws and neck muscle. It results in dysphagia. After stimuli reflex spasm develops. Cranial tetanus paralyses 7th nerve.

Tetany refers to a clinical condition. Due to low extracellular calcium, condition develops with marked muscle cramps, twitching and convulsions.

Tetracycline is a broad spectrum antibiotic drug which forms complex with calcium and deposits on tooth. Tetracycline has a wider range of activity. Spectrum includes most species of Gram-positive and Gram-negative bacteria and spirochetes. These are absorbed slowly from GIT. Larger the dose, less of proportion is absorbed. Peak levels in blood occur after 3 hours hence 6 hours interval between two doses is sufficient. All tetracyclines are chelating agents. In fetus or growing child, permanent staining of teeth may occur. The degree and color of staining varies with different tetracycline in different doses. Retardation of fetal growth is noted down when given during pregnancy.

Tetracycline stains are the intrinsic stains that are seen on the dentition when consumed by mother during the intrauterine life. The drug was widely used once upon a time to fight variety of infections. At that point little was known about the side effects of the drug. The antibiotic has an affinity towards the mineralized tissue and gets absorbed by the hard tissues of the body. Since the drug also has a capability to pass across the placenta of fallot and enters the fetal circulation, so when the expecting mother is administered this drug during the third trimester, the drug gets deposited in the forming bones

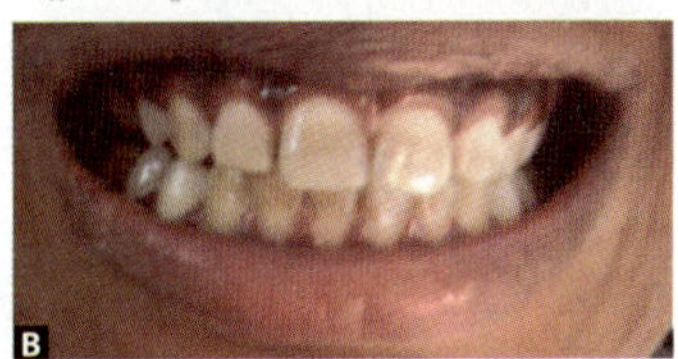

Figs A and B: *Tetracycline stains*

and teeth of the fetus. Discoloration can also occur when the drug is administered to the child in infancy and early childhood.

Tetralogy of fallot is a type of congenital heart disease that consists of following four components: (1) Ventricular septal defect; (2) Pulmonary stenosis, (3) Overriding of VSD by aorta, (4) Right ventricular hypertrophy. This is the most common cause of cyanotic CHD. The pulmonary flow is reduced due to RV outflow obstruction. This results into shunting of desaturated blood from RV to LV across the VSD leading to cyanosis, clubbing and polycythemia. The cyanosis increases during feeding or crying while it may reduce in squatting posture. There is ejection systolic murmur in the pulmonary area.

Tetraplegia refers to the involvement of all four limbs but three limbs are more severely affected than the fourth one. It is also accompanied with neck and head paralysis.

Th refers to CD_4.

Thalamic pain is a characteristic widespread pain due to spinal cord lesions affecting spinothalamic tracts producing pain in limbs. Similarly a lesion of thalamus itself may cause severe pain in the contralateral face and arm/leg. Thalamic pain is intense, burning and continuous. It is felt around angle of mouth and cheek.

Thalassemia is a bleeding disorder with defective synthesis of α or β globulin chain of hemoglobin. Severe form develops within 2 years of life-skin becomes pallor. Face is mongoloid due to prominence of cheek bones. There is unusual prominence of premaxilla. Buccal mucosa becomes pallor. There is no treatment for this disease. It is a group of chronic hemolytic anemia. It produces thin, fragile erythrocytes. In this condition, there is insufficient synthesis of alpha and beta chains of hemoglobin. Disease is inherited as autosomal dominant trait. *Clinical Features:* It is detected in first two years of life. There may be jaundice,

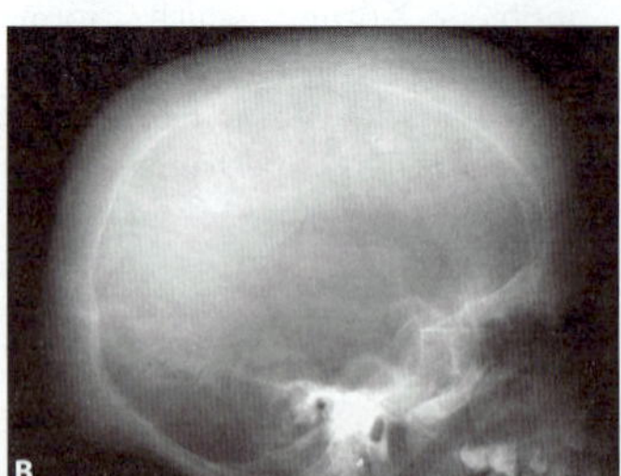

Figs A and B: *Thalassemia (A) Histological section; (B) Radiological: Sun ray appearance*

fever with chills. Marked anemia and malaise. Spleen is enlarged. Mongoloid face. Death often occurs during puberty. *Oral Manifestations:* Spacing of anterior maxillary teeth. Pallor of oral mucosa. Bimaxillary protrusion. Prominent molar bones. Delayed pneumatization of sinuses. Discoloration of teeth due to iron. Anemia is of microchromic microcytic type. WBC count is high. Bone marrow shows cellular hyperplasia with large number of immature, primitive and stems form of red cells. *Radiological Features:* Skull bones will show "hair on end" appearance. Jaw bones may show "salt and pepper effect".

Thelarche is faster breast development in absence of additional signs of sexual maturation. Exact cause is not known.

Therapeutic occlusion is said to be present where the specific interventions are designed to treat the disease.

Therapy refers to the treatment of a disease.

Thermal conductivity is a measure of speed at which heat travels in calories per second through a given thickness of 1 cm when one side of material is maintained at a constant temperature, i.e. 1°C higher than the other side. Thermal conductivity is expressed in units of cal/sec/cm/ sec°C. Thermal conductivity depends on the distance the heat travels, area through which heat travels and the difference of temperature between source and destination.

Thermal diffusivity is a measure of heat transfer of a material in the time dependant state.

Thermogenic refers to the process that creates heat.

Thermometer is the devices used to measure temperature.

Thermoplastic is the property of softening on heating and hardening on cooling.

Thermoset is a polymer which is not able to undergo softening upon heating.

Thiamine was the first of the Vitamin B complex discovered. Thiamine B_1 vitamin is water soluble and is destroyed by refining, exposure to alkalies such as baking power. It is destroyed by refining, exposure to alkalis such as baking powder. Up to 50% is lost in cooking water and 15% during baking. Toasting of bread destroys further 15% for thick slice or up to 30% for thin slice. Recommended daily intake is 0.4 mg/1000 kcal or about 1.2 mg in adult man. Limited amount is synthesized by microorganisms in GIT. Normally, about 25–35 mg is stored in the body. Deficiency of it leads to accumulation of pyruvic and lactic acid in tissues and body fluids. Severe deficiency may lead to neurological and mental deficiency.

Thiazides are derivatives of sulphonamides and are used as weaker diuretics. These exert their diuretic effect by inhibiting the Na^+ CL^- transport in early distal convoluted tubules. These cause increased loss of K^+ and Mg but reduce calcium excretion. These are indicated in hypertension, mild heart failure, and idiopathic hypercalciuria.

Thiopentone has largely been superseded in outpatient dental practice by short-acting methohexitone. Thiopentone is freshly prepared to produce 2.5% solution by dissolving powder in sterile distilled water. Dose is 4 to 7 mg/kg body weight. It is a powerful myocardial depressant.

Third branchial arch also known as third pharyngeal arch. The cartilage of this small arch produces the greater horn and caudal part of the body of the hyoid bone. The remainder of the cartilage disappears. The mesoderm forms the stylopharyngeal muscle, inverted by the IX nerve (glossopharyngeal) supplying the arch. The mucosa of the posterior third of the tongue is derived from this arch, which accounts for its sensory innervations by the glossopharyngeal nerve. The artery of this arch contributes to the common carotid and part of the internal carotid arteries. Neural crest tissue in the third arch forms the carotid body which first appears as a mesenchymal condensation around the third aortic arch artery. This chemoreceptor body thus derives its nerve supply from the glossopharyngeal nerve.

T

Third degree burns refer to the burn involving entire epidermis and dermis and all dermal appendages so there is no spontaneous healing of the wound, leaving an ulcer. Since the entire thickness of skin is burned with no tissue left for repair and regeneration, these will require skin grafting or will close by contractures wherein two raw surfaces fuse together.

Third molar *see* wisdom tooth.

Third pharyngeal pouch: The ventral diverticulum endoderm proliferates and migrates from each side to form two elongated diverticular that grow caudally into the surrounding mesenchyme to form the elements of thymus gland. The two thymic rudiments meet in the midline but do not fuse, being united by connective tissue. Lymphoid cells invade the thymus from hemopoietic tissue during the 3rd month of IU. The dorsal diverticulum endoderm differentiates and migrates caudally to form inferior parathyroid gland. The gland derived from the endodermal lining of the pouch loses the connection with the pharyngeal wall when the pouches become obliterated during later development. The lateral glossoepiglottic fold represents the third pharyngeal pouch.

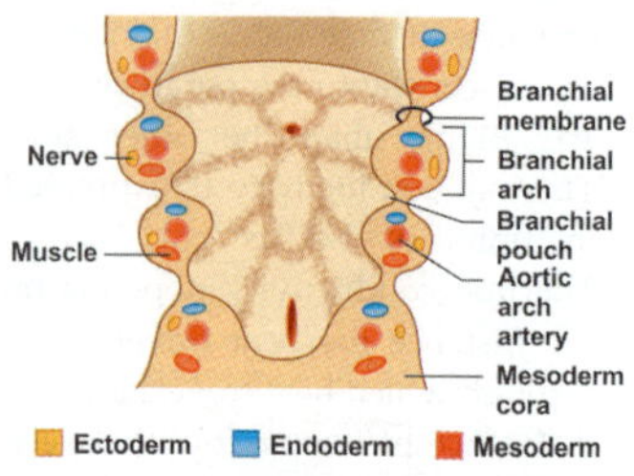

Fig.: *Third pharyngeal pouch*

Three-quarter crowns refer to the one that covers four-fifths of the tooth surface—mesial, distal, occlusal, lingual or palatal. They are always made up of cast metal and are used when the buccal surface of the tooth is intact. The advantage of these types of crowns is that they are more conservative of tooth tissue than complete crowns and the margin does not approach gingival margin buccally.

Thromboangitis obliterans is an inflammatory occlusive peripheral vascular disease of unknown etiology affecting arteries and veins especially of lower limbs. Smoking is the risk factor. Small and medium sized arteries are more involved. There is proliferation of intima and thrombosis. There develops digital ulceration or pain from ischemia. Arteriography and biopsy are confirmatory.

Thrombocythemia is increased number of circulating blood platelets. Etiology is not known. Epistaxia and intestinal bleeding exists. Hemorrhage into skin is found. There may be spontaneous gingival bleeding. After dental extraction also excessive bleeding takes place. Radioactive phosphorus and blood transfusion helps.

Thrombocytopenia is very low quantity of platelets in circulatory system. These patients have tendency to bleed from small capillaries while in hemophilia bleeding is from larger vessels. As a result, large punctate bleeding develops over skin. For bleeding count should fall below 50,000 per cu/mm Level below 10,000 becomes lethal.

Thromboplastin is a plasma protein that aids blood coagulation by converting prothrombin to thrombin.

Throttling refers to the constriction produced by pressure of fingers and palm, finger marks may be found on either side of front of neck, i.e. wind pipe. Marks are obliquely downwards and outwards one below the other.

Throwing power is a measure of the uniformity in plating thickness of irregular surface.

Thrush is an infection of mouth due to overgrowth of fungus. *Candida albicans*. Cream—white curd like patches are seen in mouth. On scrapping, a raw bleeding surface is left. Lesions may be found over buccal mucosa, tongue or fauces. It involves upper layers of mucosal epithelium and produces white flecks. Surrounding mucosa may or may not be reddened. On scrapping, area of erythema or shallow ulceration may be seen. Bad taste and loss of discrimination of taste develops as a prodromal symptom. Thrush has to be differentiated from flecks of milk and other debris. Thrush develops as pearly white pin head sized flecks scattered all over dorsal surface consisting of large number of yeasts pseudomyelia. Constant use of corticosteroids and cholinergic drugs may cause it. Antifungal drugs are helpful. In infants, lesions are soft, white or bluish. It is adherent to oral mucosa. Intraoral lesions are painless and removed with difficulty, it leaves a raw bleeding surface. Any mucosal area of mouth may be involved. Constitutional symptoms are not present but in adults rapid onset of a bad taste may develop. Some may feel burning of mouth also. It occurs in both yeast and mycelia forms of oral cavity and infected tissue. Candidate species are normal inhabitants of the oral flora. Concentration is 200–500 cells per mL of saliva. Carrier state is more in diabetics. The wearing of removal prosthetic appliances may also become asymptomatic carrier. Predisposing factors include – After administration of antibiotics, irritant dentures, long-term consumption of cortisone, pregnancy, old age, AIDS and low immunity.

Thumb and digit sucking is defined as placement of the thumb or on or more fingers in varying depths into the mouth. Thumb and digit sucking is one of the commonest seen habits in children. Recent studies have shown that thumb sucking may be practiced even during intra-uterine life. The presence of this habit until the age of 2–4 years is considered normal. Persistence of the habit beyond this age can lead to various malocclusions.

Thymol is a derivative of phenol obtained from thyme old. It is relatively a weak antiseptic and antifungal agent. It is widely used as mouthwashes. It has a good flavor.

Thymus is a primary lymphoid organ, bilobed structure located in the thorax anterior to the sternum. Histologically, each lobe contains lobules separated by connective tissue trabeculae; each lobule is made up of an outer cortex with immature cells, inner medulla, epithelial cell network-differentiation from bone marrow skin cells to T-cell, interdigitating cells, which are bone marrow derivatives, rich in MHC II antigen and enable learning to recognize self-antigen. Hassau corpuscles in thymic medulla containing degenerating suspected cells.

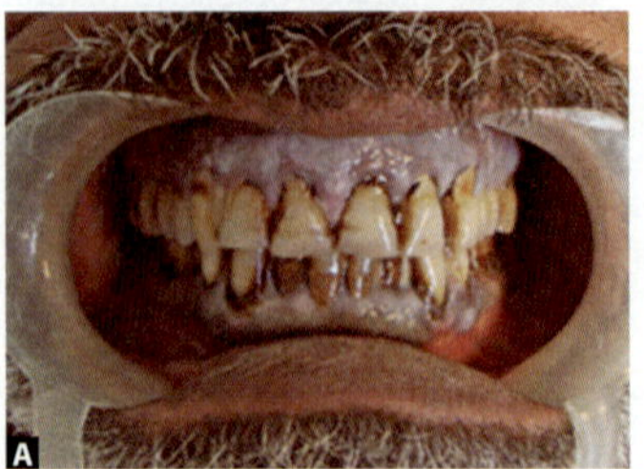

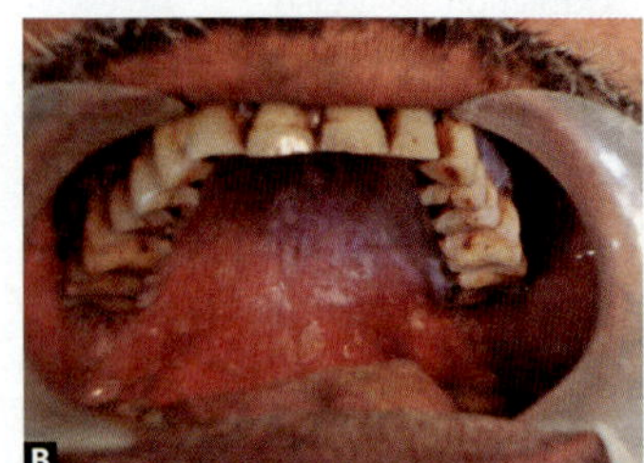

Figs A and B: *Oral thrush*

Thyrocervical trunk is a short artery that arises near the junction of the first and second parts of the subclavian artery. On the left side, it usually arises just medial to the scalenus anterior muscle, i.e. from the first part of the subclavian artery. On the right side, the trunk usually arises deep to the scalenus anterior, being a branch of the second part of the subclavian artery.

Thyroglossal tract cyst arises from remnants of thyroglossal duct and may develop anywhere along the embryonic thyroglossal tract between the foramen cecum of tongue and thyroid gland. It consists squamous and glandular epithelium. It generally develops in young person. It raises from a few mm to a few centimeters. It is asymptomatic and grows slowly. If large, it may cause a dysphagia. Occasionally fistula may form.

Thyroid gland is a butterfly-shaped gland that lies in front of the neck, in front of the lower part of the larynx and the upper part of the trachea. It consists of right and left lobes that are joined, across the midline, by an isthmus. The vertical diameter of each lobe is about 5 cm (2 inches) and that of the isthmus is about 1 cm (half inch). The anteroposterior diameter of each lobe is about 2 cm. The transverse diameter of the entire thyroid is about 8 cm. Thyroid is seen to have three surfaces—lateral, medial and posterior. A finger-like projection of thyroid tissue frequently arises from the upper border of the isthmus. This is called the pyramidal lobe. It secretes T^3 and T^4. One hormone containing three atoms of iodine in each molecule is called tri-iodothyronine or T3. Another hormone containing four atoms of iodine is called tetraiodothyronine or T^4.

Thyroid storm is a medical emergency. Fever may go up to 41°C with anxiety, tremor, weakness, heat intolerance, sweating and weight loss. Sinus tachycardia is always present. Atrial fibrillation develops. Reflexes become brisk.

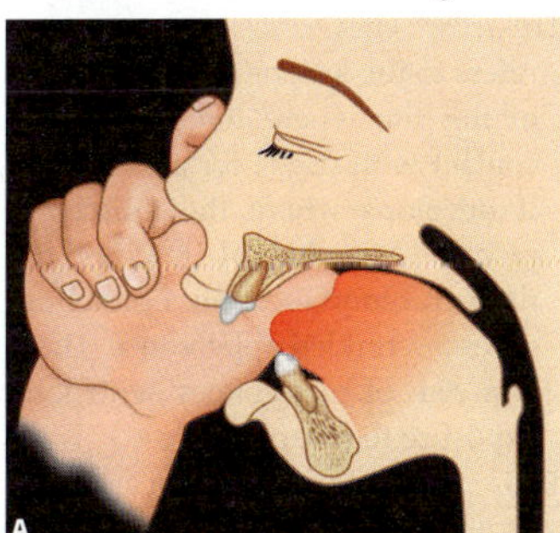

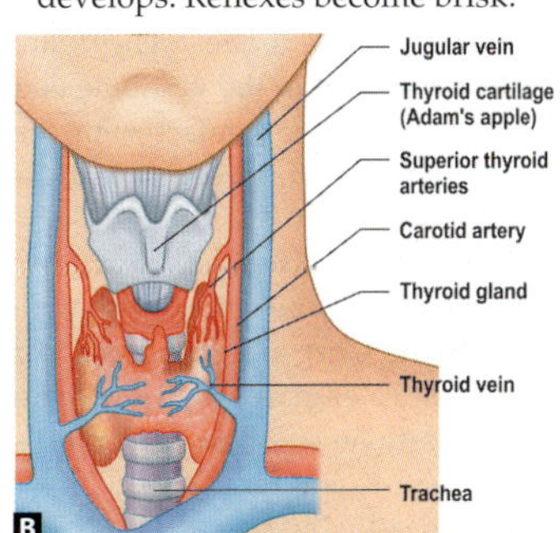

Figs A and B: *(A) Thumb sucking; (B) Thyroid gland*

Tic douloureux literally means tic spasm and dolor is the Latin word for pain. As trigeminal neuralgia pain comes as electrical shock, each pain spasm is called tic douloureux.

Tics are a sudden rapid twitch-like movements always of same nature and same type. These are generally common in childhood and disappear in adult life. All forms of tics can be suppressed clinically.

Tin oxide is a pure white powder that is used as a final polishing agent. Tin oxide is mixed with water, alcohol or glycerine and is used as a paste. Finishing abrasives are coarse, hard particles and polishing abrasives are fine articles.

Tissue repair is a process following inflammation white cells repair by filling the breach with a temporary repair called granulation tissue. New capillaries are formed, but repair cannot take place in presence of pus. Hence tooth requires extraction or root treatment to drain off pus.

Tissue-borne passive appliance refers to the appliances that are contact with tissue. They are mostly located in the vestibule and have little or no contact with the dentition, e.g. functional regulator or frankel.

Tissue culture refers to the culture in which maintenance or growth of tissue, organ primordia, or the whole or part of an organ in vitro is done so as to preserve its architecture and function.

Tissue health index was also developed by Sheiham A, Maizels J and Maizels A, at the second alternative indices, which is a modification of the DMFT index. In the THI, selective weighing is given for decayed, filled and sound teeth, (i.e. '1' decayed, '2' filled and '4' sound).

Titanium is a material of choice because of its good biocompatibility, mechanical properties and in implantology, its proven ability to achieve osseointegration.

T-lymphocytes once developed from bone marrow stem cell, the T-lymphocytes travel to the thymus where they mature. Thymus is large in children and shrinks as an individual matures. Different types of T-cells have different functions. Some are memory cells. Some are T-helper cells increasing the function of B-lymphocytes and increase the antibody response. Others are called T-suppressor cells decreasing the function of B-lymphocytes. T-killer cells are active in vigilance against tumor or virally affected cells.

Tobacco chewer's white lesion refers to the lesions that are formed in the site where the tissue is in contact with tissue for a long time. It develops where the tobacco is placed. Mucobuccal fold is the most common location. Epithelium gives a wrinkled appearance. There is a risk of malignancy with long exposure to tobacco.

Tobacco stains appear as light brown to dark brown or black. They may appear in various forms such as - Narrow crest following the gingival contour, wide band extending from the cervical third to the middle third of the tooth and diffuse. They are primarily present on the cervical third of the tooth but may involve any surface including pits and fissures and the lingual surface. These stains are generally formed from the smokeless tobacco and are mainly composed of tar and combustion products. The heavy deposits may penetrate the enamel and present as endogenous stains.

Tolerance refers to an ability to withstand. Immune system is constantly exposed to self-Ag (antigen) without inducing lymphocyte stimulation 'self-tolerance'. It is a result of several mechanisms designed to distinguish between lymphocytes with potential to bind to self-components and those with much higher binding specificity for antigenic determinants expressed by foreign Ag.

Tongue is a sensory organ. The tongue lies in the oral cavity. It has free upper and lower surfaces. The greater part of the tongue is attached below to the floor of the mouth. The attached part is called the root of the tongue. This part of the tongue has a free upper surface or dorsum. On either side, the tongue has lateral edges that are also free. The free surfaces of the tongue are lined by mucous membrane.

Tongue brushing is an act of cleaning of tongue that should be combined with tooth brushing. Dorsum of the tongue is a primary source of infection. Tongue brushing can reduce the number of these organisms. It improves patient's taste perception also. Tongue should remain free of coating or debris. But tongue may not be scrubbed with tooth brush.

Tongue papillae are multiple tiny bumps present on the dorsal surface of the tongue. They are of four types present on the dorsal surface of tongue: (1) Filiform papillae are numerous white hair-like projection that covers the dorsal surface; (2) circumvallate papillae on tongue in a V formation on dorsal surface. It contains bitter taste buds; (3) Foliate papillae are projection found on posterior lateral borders of tongue and consist of sour and

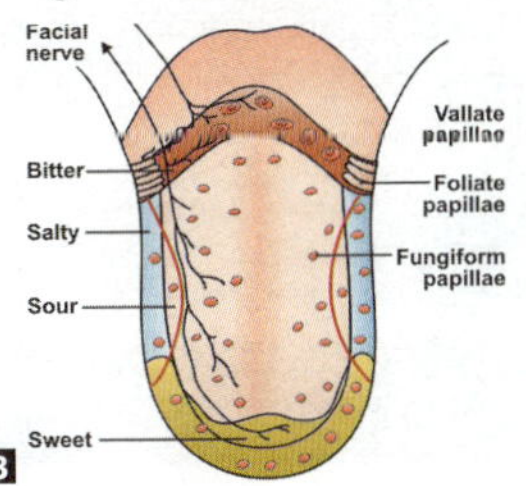

Figs A and B: *(A) Tobacco stains; (B) Tongue*

acidic taste buds; (4) Fungiform papillae among filiform papillae on the dorsal surface of tongue. These consist of sweet, sour and salty buds.

Tongue thrust habit is defined as a condition in which the tongue makes contact with any teeth anterior to the molars during swallowing.

Tongue thrusting (Schneider 1982, Profit 1990, Barber 1975, Viazis 1993) corrector appliance consists of a palatal wire that is inserted in the upper lingual molar sheaths, passes through the open-bite area, and carries over the lower incisors toward the labial vestibule, ending 1–2 mm above the labial surface. 'U'-shaped palatal loops are used to adjust the appliance in an anteroposterior or vertical direction with a three prong plier. The TCA can also be expanded, like a palatal expansion appliance, to correct the posterior crossbites that often accompany open bites. It does not contact the teeth or the soft tissue. The TCA is designed to keep the patient from inserting the thumb in the mouth, and it prevents tongue thrusting or abnormal tongue posturing during swallowing by blocking the tongue from the anterior teeth. This, in turn, helps to close the open bite.

Tonic seizure is the one where tone of muscle is greatly increased leading to stiffness. There is no tonic contraction of muscle with altered consciousness. These generally occur during NREM sleep with day drowsiness.

Tonic-clonic are general seizures that originate in all regions of the cortex. They begin with an abrupt loss of consciousness, often in association with a cry. It is not a cry from pain but rather from air being forced through the contracting vocal cords. All arm, leg, chest and back muscles become rigid. The person will fall and their back may arch, then their muscles begin to jerk and twitch. During this clonic phase the tongue or cheek can be bitten and frothy and bloody saliva may be expectorated from the mouth.

Tonsilar sinus is the depression in which the palatine tonsil lies.

Tonsillectomy is referred to surgical removal of the tonsils.

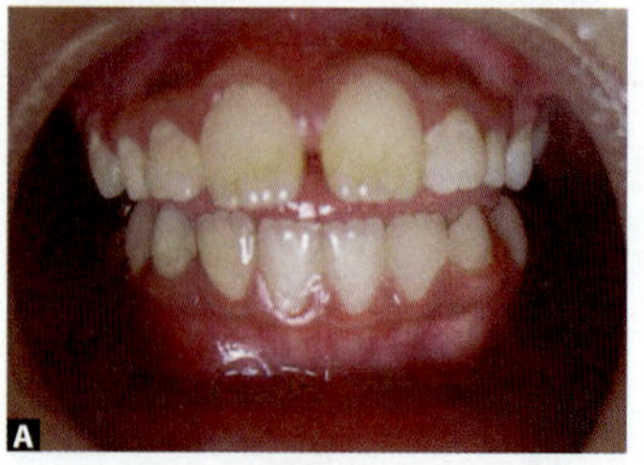

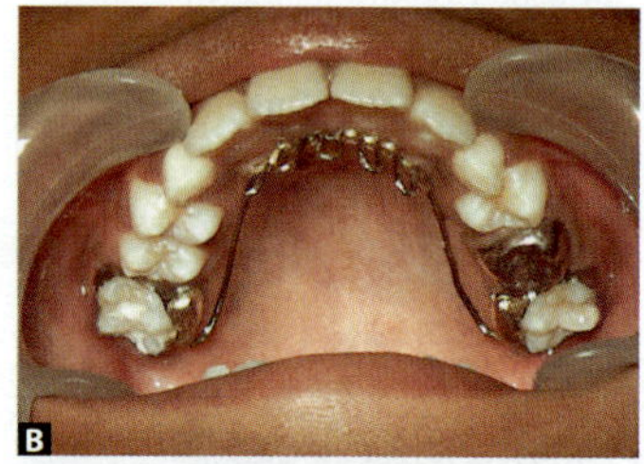

Figs A and B: *Tongue thrust*

Tonsillitis refers to infection of the tonsils. It is a bacterial infection. Patients will complain of sore-throat with dysphagia. Child is not able to eat food. Pain and fever accompanies. There develops leukocytosis. Amoxicillin and analgesic anti-inflammatory drugs help.

Tooth ankylosis can be defined as fusion of tooth root to the underlying bone more after bone injury. Periapical inflammation is a well-recognized cause of it by way of root absorption. If more of root surface is involved, it may give a dull, muffed sound on percussion instead of normal sharp sound. It may be visible on radiograph. There will be loss of normal thin radiolucent line with mild sclerosis of bone. There is no treatment. It serves well unless infected.

Tooth banks are several banks to store tooth with different techniques such as chemical coagulation, vitrification, freeze drying and regular freezing.

Tooth-borne active appliance refers to those who take support from tooth; includes modification of activator and bionator that include expansion screws or other active components like spring to provide intrinsic force to transverse or anteroposterior changes.

Tooth-borne passive appliance that has no intrinsic force generating components such as spring or screw. They depend on the soft tissues stretch and muscular activity to produce the desired treatment results, e.g. Activator, Bionator and Herbst appliance.

Tooth brush filaments are the nylon filaments superior to natural bristles made of hog or boar hair. Nylon filaments flex 10 times more than breaking. These are more resistant to accumulation of bacteria and fungi. Soft nylon filaments are less traumatic to gingival tissues. Range of nylon filament diameter is 0.15 mm to 0.4 mm. Most bristles are 10 to 12 mm long. Those with thickness from 0.007 to 0.12 mm are considered medium and 0.013 to 0.015 mm are classified as hard. End of the tooth brush filament can be cut bluntly or rounded. Round cut edges reduce gingival abrasion.

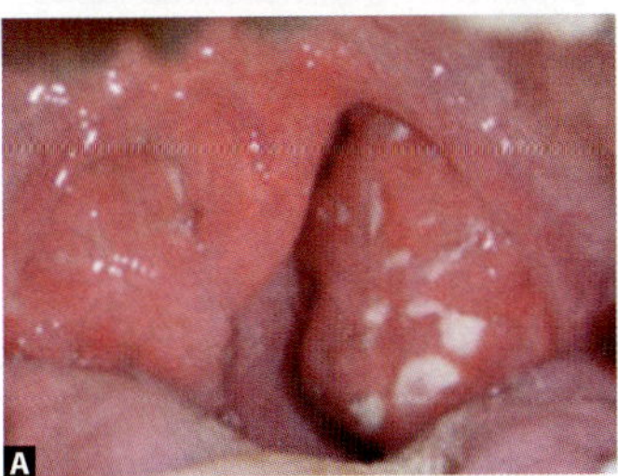

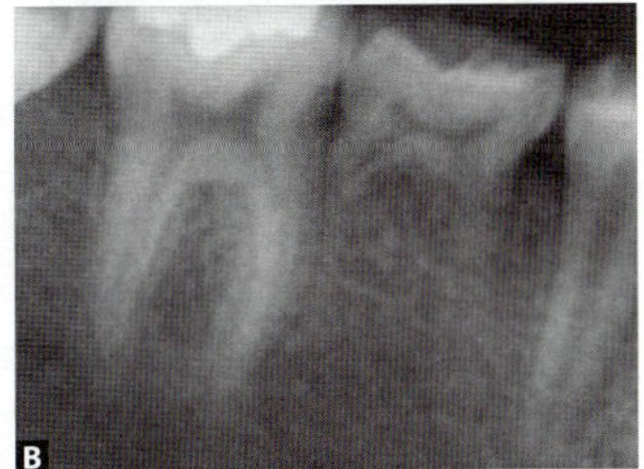

Figs A and B: *(A) Tonsillitis-mononucleosis; (B) Submerged ankylosed teeth*

Tooth brushing is an act of cleaning done domestically after meals to remove plaque. Tooth brushes with a small head and multi-tufted medium nylon bristles are most effective. Brushed in rinsed and pea size portion of fluoride tooth paste is added. Effective tooth brushing requires time, knowledge and skill.

Tooth eruption is the process by which developing teeth emerge through the soft tissue of the jaws and the overlying mucosa to enter the oral cavity, contact the teeth of the opposing arch, and function in mastication. Therefore, it is a continuous process.

Tooth fracture is a common injury of tooth due to trauma. It may occur at any age. Minor chipping is common. Fracture has been classified in many ways. Prognosis depends whether pulp is involved, or crown/root is involved. If dentin over pulp is thin bacteria may penetrate producing pulpitis. Fractured crown is a more serious problem if the pulp is exposed.

Tooth surface index of fluorosis (TSIF) The Tooth Surface Index of Fluorosis (TSIF) was developed by Herschel S Horowitz, William S Driscoll, Rhea J Meyers, Stanley B Heifeta, and Albert Knigman in 1984. TSIF was developed in order to eliminate or reduce some of the shortcomings of 'Deans Index'. TSIF was applied in a survey to assess the prevalence of dental caries and dental fluorosis in communities having optimal and above optimal concentrations of naturally occurring fluoride in the drinking water.

Tooth wear refers to a loss of tooth substance by means other than caries and trauma. It is an increasing problem in older adults due to long period of functioning. It has 3 causes—abrasion, attrition and erosion; reduction in lubricating effect of saliva may cause it.

Tooth zones refer to an area that is divided into imaginary third, named according to areas in which they are found. Root of tooth is

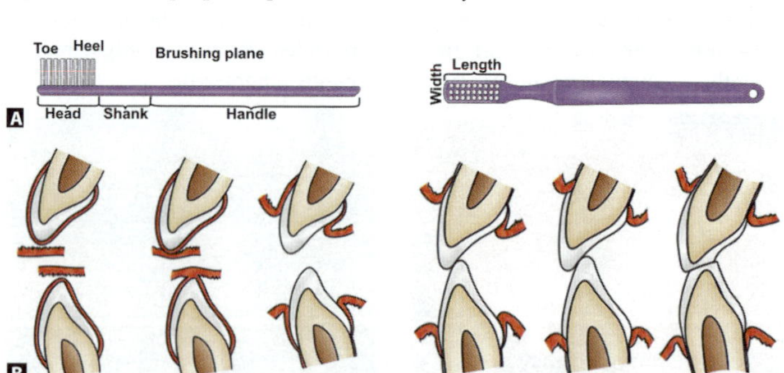

Figs A and B: *(A) Tooth brush design; (B) Tooth eruption*

divided into apical, middle and cervical third. Crown of the tooth is divided into cervico-occlusal division, mesiodistal division and buccolingual division.

Topical is application directly to an affected area for producing superficial anesthesia.

Topography is detailed description and analysis of features of an anatomic region.

Toronto automated probe is a diagnostic probe to measure clinical attachment levels. Here the sulcus is probed with the Ni-Ti wire that is extended under air pressure.

Torus mandibularis is an outgrowth of bone on the lingual surface of mandible opposite bicuspid tooth. These may be multiple and on both the sides. It may be removed surgically.

Torus palatinus is slowly growing, flat base bone protuberance. It generally occurs in midline of hard palate. Women are affected more. On trauma, it becomes ulcerated. It never becomes malignant. It is not treated.

Toxic myocarditis is a clinical condition that occurs due to drugs that cause a direct toxic injury to the myocardial fibers. Response is cumulative and dose related. In this group, drugs include arsenicals, catecholamines, lithium, cyclophosphamide, emetine, etc. Healing occurs by fibrosis.

Toxic shock syndrome is a multisystem illness caused by endotoxins produced by stains of *Staphylococcus aureus*. Symptoms include fever, chills, diarrhea, diz-ziness, headache, myalgias and sore-throat. Person may develop hypotension with desquamation of skin.

Toxic refers to poisonous.

Toxicology is the study of toxic and harmful effects of drugs and chemicals. It deals with the science of knowledge of sources, characters, properties and symptoms of poisons, their fatal effects, the lethal doses and remedies to be taken to counteract the effect.

Toxin is any poisonous substance of microbial, vegetable or animal origin that causes symptoms after a period of incubation. It can induce the elaboration of specific antitoxin in suitable animal.

Trabecular bone is a light porous bone enclosing multiple large spaces that give a spongy or honeycomb appearance.

T

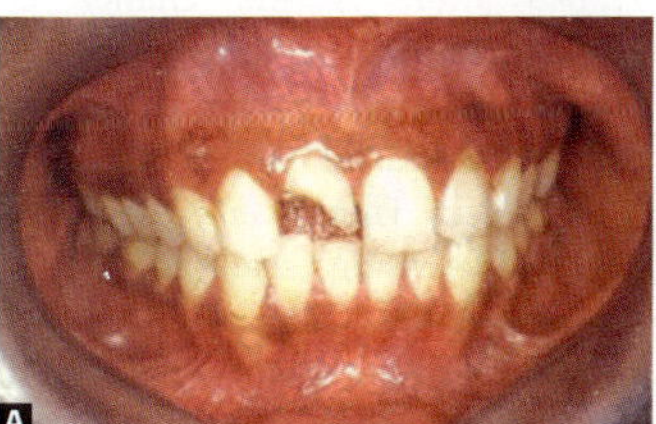

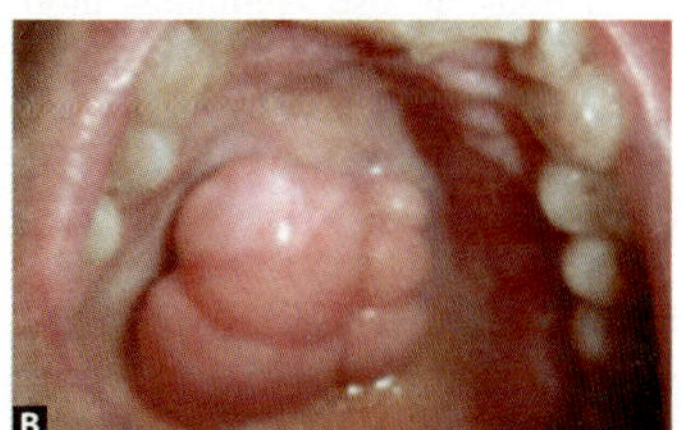

Figs A and B: *(A) Ellis class III dentoalveolar fracture; (B) Torus palatinus*

Trachea is a wide tube lying on the front of the neck more or less in the middle line. The upper end of the trachea is continuous with the lower end of the larynx. The junction lies opposite the lower part of the body of the sixth cervical vertebra.

Tracheostomy is the term given to the surgical establishment of an opening into the trachea. It is done to have alternate pathway for breathing, improves alveolar ventilation, to give anesthesia.

Traditional alloy contains silver 66 to 72% by weight, tin 25–29%, copper 2–6%. Zinc 2% and mercury 3% by weight.

Tragus is the cartilaginous projection anterior to external opening of the ear.

Tramadol is an analgesic with both opioid as well as nonopioid actions. It works like aspirin as well as like morphine. High doses of it should be avoided. It is used in the dose of 50–100 mg daily.

Tranquilizers are the drugs which decrease anxiety and tension without producing sedation. Tranquilizers do not produce sleep and serve effectively to block intolerant and overly aggressive reactions. It also eliminates more objectionable types of patient defense reactions and produce acceptable relaxation.

Transcutaneous electrical nerve stimulation (TENS) is non-invasive technique in which a low-voltage electrical current is delivered through wires from a power unit to electrodes located on the skin. TENS has been applied successfully to treat acute and chronic pain in medicine for many years and more recently in dentistry. Its use for treatment of myofascial pain is well-documented and has also been tried during simple restoration and electroanalgesia.

Transient ischemic attack (TIA) also termed incipient stroke, transient cerebral ischemia is characterized by ischemic cerebral neurologic deficits that last for less than 24 hours. These attacks rarely last more than 8 hours and often resolve within 15–60 mins. Platelet, fibrin or other atherosclerotic embolic material from the neck or heart may lodge in a cerebral vessel and interfere transiently with blood flow causing the TIA.

Transfixation is a type of method of achieving immobilization in dentulous as well as edentulous mandible using Kirschner wires, where 2 mm Krischner wire is inserted within the medullary cavity across the fracture line. The wire is cut off at skin entry point from where it can be withdrawn once.

Transitional dentition *see* mixed dentition.

Translocation is the change in position.

Translucency is the amount of incident light transmitted and scattered by that object. Translucency decreases with increasing scattered within materials. A high translucency gives a lighter color appearance. Translucency decreased with increasing scattering within a material.

Translucent lesions are those lesion demonstrating translucent quality are bullae or vesicle. Translucent pink lesions are due to accumulation at clear fluid such as serum, mucin or lymph. Blue translucent lesion indicates clear fluid or blood accumulation. Red or purple translucent lesion indicated blood accumulation.

Transmissible is the term which denotes a capacity of a lesion to maintain an infectious agent in successive passages through a susceptible host.

Transmission spreading of disease through saliva. Contacting disease through saliva is low. Herpes virus may secrete into saliva. Coxsakie virus is also a latent infection and has a risk of transmission of virus through dental clinic.

Transosseous wiring is a type of intermaxillary fixation with osteosynthesis where direct wiring is done across the fracture line in order to achieve effective immobilization of the fracture of the body of the mandible including angle. The holes are drilled in the bone ends of both the sides of the fracture line and the soft stainless-steel wire is passed through the holes across the fracture. After achieving the accurate reduction, the free ends of the wires are twisted together and tucked into a nearest hole. Achieving osteosynthesis by wiring has an advantage of requiring minimal equipment and can be used for many types of mandibular fractures.

Transplantation of organs is the procedure where a viable organ is planted into another body. The viability or transplantable organs falls sharply after somatic death such as liver must be taken out within 15 minutes, a kidney within 45 minutes and a heart within an hour. After molecular death it is not feasible.

Trans-septal fibers are those fibers which extend interproximally over the alveolar bone crest and get embedded into the cementum of the adjacent tooth. These fibers can be considered as a part of gingival fibers as they lack osseous attachment.

Transverse ridge is a linear elevation that crosses a surface (usually the occlusal surface).

Transverse sinuses are the large paired sinuses that lie horizontally as indicated by their names. They begin posteriorly at the internal occipital protuberance. The right sinus is usually a continuation of the superior sagittal sinus and the left sinus is usually a continuation of the straight sinus, but this arrangement is sometimes reversed. Each sinus runs in a curve at first laterally and then forwards, along the line of attachment of the tentorium cerebelli. The sinus produces a transverse groove on the inner surface of the occipital bone, and on the posteroinferior angle of the parietal bone. Finally, it reaches the petrous part of the temporal bone where it becomes continuous with the sigmoid sinus.

Trauma from occlusion (TFO) can be described as when occlusal forces exceed the adaptive capacity or margins of safety of the tissues, it results in tissue injury. This resultant injury is known as trauma from occlusion.

Traumatic cyst is a benign cyst of bone. The cause of solitary bone cyst is not known. Bone cysts are not true; it is not being lined by epithelium. Expansion ceases when cyst-like lesion reaches the cortical layer of bone. When roots are involved, cavity may become scalloped. A thin connective tissue lines the cavity. X-ray shows smoothly outlined radiolucent area of variable size within sclerotic border.

Traumatic fibroma refers to fibroma.

Traumatic neuroma is not a true neoplasm but is an exuberant try to repair a damaged nerve trunk. It is a hyperplasia of nerve fibers and supporting tissue. Degeneration of distal nerve after injury begins with swelling, fragmentation and disintegration of myelin sheath and axis cylinder. Oral neuroma begins with small nodule or swelling of mucosa near mental foramen. Treatment includes surgical excision of nodule along with small proximal portion of nerve involved.

Traumatic occlusion is the term used when the injury is produced by the occlusion.

Traumatic ulcer results due to physical injury such as denture irritation, on ill-fitting of denture, biting the mucosa. Traumatic ulcers are usually single or variable size and round in shape. The floor will be yellow with margins red and there will not be any induration. It is covered by a white or tan fibrin clot and generally located at lateral border. It can be painful. Recurrent trauma can make it firm and elevated with rolled borders. After removing the cause ulcer may heal within 1-2 days, occasionally ulcers persist for long. Traumatic ulcers may be accidental or deliberate biting or thermal burns from hot pasty foods.

Treatment is an act or handling of a procedure done in the best of interest of patients in order to free them from and pain discomfort and restoring quality of life.

Treatment index: The 'F (filled) portion of the DMF Index best exemplifies a treatment index. In general, there are two types of dental indices. This type of dental index measures the 'number' of people affected and the 'severity' of the specific condition at a specific time or interval of time.

Treatment manual is a written material that identifies key concepts, procedure and tactic to treat a person.

Treatment plan is known as blue-print for case management. It includes all the procedures required for the maintenance of oral health.

Tremor is the rhythmic oscillation of part of body around a fixed point. Tremors usually involve distal part of limb, head, tongue and rarely trunk. Tremors at rest even in lying supine are seen in Parkinsonism. Essential tremors occur in anxiety, fatigue and due to alcohol while intentional tremors are seen in phenytoin toxicity, multiple sclerosis and in cerebellar disease.

Tremors of Parkinsonism are of a rapid, rhythmic, alternating tremor. Pill rolling tremors are seen, which are usually unilateral.

Trench mouth refers to acute necrotizing ulcerative gingivitis.

Trephination refers to making a window in the bone. When drainage through the canal is not possible due to restorative issues, or in case of certain conditions like failing treatments or necessary correction of procedural accidents, surgical trephination can be used as a palliative measure. It involves the surgical perforation of the alveolar cortical plate over the root-end to release the accumulated exudates to release pain. However, it is not the first line of treatment because of the additional trauma, invasiveness and questionable beneficial result.

Trichloroethylene is a colorless volatile liquid with chloroform-like smell. It is colored blue to avoid confusion with chloroform. It has a poor relaxation of skeletal muscles. It has good analgesic properties but induction and recovery are poor. Bradycardia and cardiac arrhythmias may occur.

Trichodento-osseous syndrome is a rare autosomal dominant disorder that also shows enamel defects in conjunction with morphologic dental anomalies. These patients have tightly curled kinky hair with osteosclerosis of bone cortices. The enamel is hypoplastic and hypocalcified, lacking mesiodistal contact with pitting.

Triclosan is a non-cationic antibacterial agent and has been added to several dentifrices to inhibit plaque and gingivitis. It has good antibacterial activity against Gram-positive and Gram-negative organisms and is compatible with anionic component of fluoride dentifrices. Two clinical studies

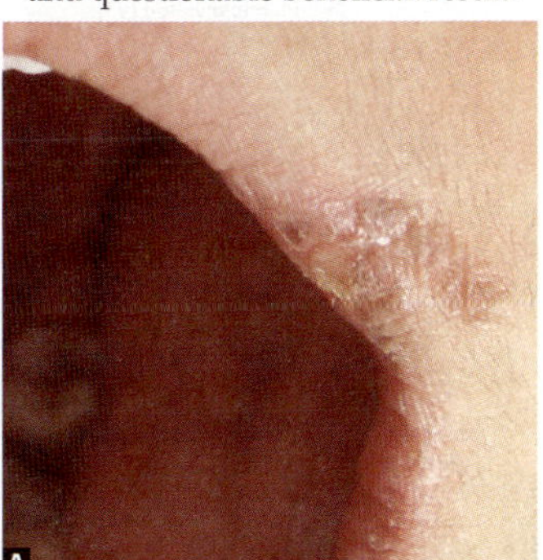

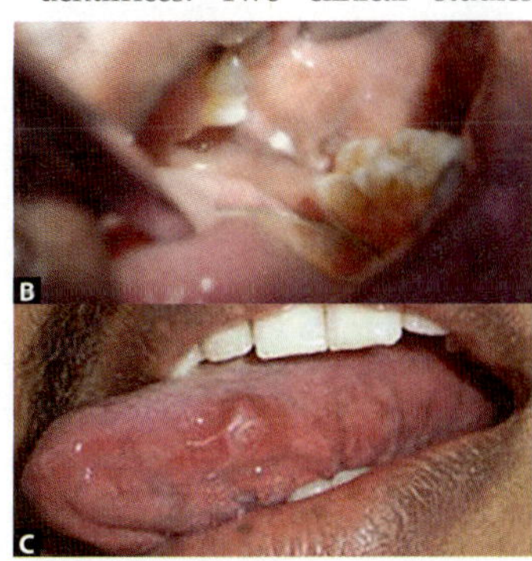

Figs A to C: *Traumatic ulcer of tongue*

over a 3-month period by Schiff et al (1990) and Lobene et al (1990) showed a statistically significant reduction of plaque formation.

Tricuspid regurgitation is a cardiac condition, may occur with right ventricular and inferior myocardial infarction. Symptoms and signs of tricuspid regurgitation are identical to those resulting from right ventricular failure of any cause.

Tricuspid stenosis is a cardiac condition that is usually rheumatic in origin. It is suspected when right heart failure is marked with liver enlargement, ascites and dependent edema. Acquired tricuspid stenosis needs valvotomy.

Trifurcation is forked or divided into three parts.

Trigeminal ganglion is crescent shaped. It has a convex border facing anterolaterally and a concave border facing posteromedially. The convex border is continuous with the ophthalmic, maxillary and mandibular nerves; while the concave posterior border is continuous with the sensory root. The ganglion is placed in a depression (called the trigeminal fossa) on the anterior aspect of the petrous temporal bone. The ganglion is enclosed within a pouch-like recess of dura mater. This recess is called the trigeminal cave.

Trigeminal nerve is the fifth cranial nerve contains both sensory and motor fibers. Fifth cranial nerve is the largest. It has 3 branches: (i) Ophthalmic nerve is purely sensory and is the smallest division. It divides into three branches lacrimal, frontal and nasociliary nerve. It supplies cornea, skin of forehead, scalp, eyelids and nose also the mucous membrane of paranasal sinuses; (ii) Maxillary branch is purely sensory. It leaves the skull through foramen rotundum. It supplies skin over, face, over maxilla and the upper lip, teeth of upper jaw, mucous

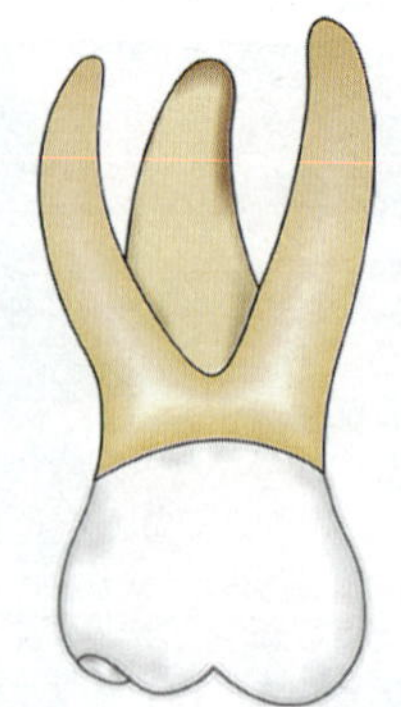

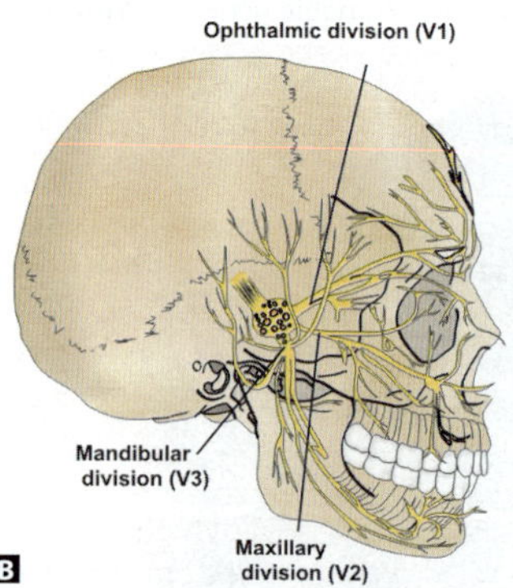

Figs A and B: *(A) Trifurcation; (B) Trigeminal nerve*

membrane of nose, maxillary air sinus and palate; (iii) Mandibular division is a mixed branch and is the largest branch. Motor part supplies muscles of mastication. Sensory supply is to skin of cheek, skin over mandible, lower lip and side of head, teeth of lower jaw, mucous membrane of mouth and anterior 2/3rd of tongue.

Trigeminal neuralgia refers to the pain along with the path of trigeminal nerve. A single branch may be affected without affecting other branch. It is an intermittent brief, laminating pain in face. It is evoked by facial movement or by touching the skin. Pain is sudden, excruciating and brief like the stabbing. Peripheral receptors are not hyperalgesic. Pain does not extend outside area supplied by trigeminal nerve. The trigger may occur from light touch or movement of same receptor areas. Pain is usually unilateral and remains in the anatomical distribution of affected nerve. Typically individual pains are paroxysms of hot, shocking, burning or electric like lasting from a few seconds to several minutes. They may be repeated so frequently that pain becomes continuous. Paresthesia and motor symptoms are generally absent. Trigeminal neuralgia primary is idiopathic while secondary results due to trauma. Idiopathic neuralgia involves maxillary and mandibular branch. Due to stimulation of trigger zones recurrent, shock like unilateral pain develops from a few seconds to a few minutes. Such trigger zones lie in the same dermatome. Normally after each episode there is a refractive period. During this period even stimulation of trigger zone will not produce pain. No sensory loss is detected. No specific cause is known. Progressive degeneration and demyelination of trigeminal ganglion is seen. Secondary trigeminal neuralgia can result due to intracranial tumor, tumor vascular malformation, CNS lesions involving trigeminal pathways. Trigeminal neuralgia due to multiple sclerosis may have bilateral facial pain. There may be hypoesthesia too. In both cases carbamazepine and GABA are used. Phenytoin in doses of 400 mg/day reduces the dose of carbamazepine.

Triple flex file is endodontic hand instrument is made up of stainless steel and are triangular in cross-section. It has more flutes then reamer but lesser than K-file. Triangular cross-section provides better flexibility and cutting efficiency.

Triplegia refers to involvement of three limbs this could be either both legs + one arm/or both arms + 1 leg.

Trismus is a spasm of the muscles of mastication that results in difficulty in opening of mouth. Intraoral injections may result in it.

Triturate is to mix together.

Trochlear nerve is the fourth cranial nerve. It is made up of fibers that arise in the trochlear nucleus located in the lower part of the midbrain. The trochlear nerve is the only cranial nerve that emerges on the posterior (or dorsal) aspect of the brainstem and the only nerve that undergoes decussation. As a result of the decussation, the left trochlear nerve is formed by fibers arising from the right trochlear nucleus and vice versa. The fibers of the trochlear nerve are classified as somatic efferent. It is a motor nerve, cranial nerve numbers four. It assists in turning eyeball downward and laterally. It emerges from posterior surface of midbrain. It enters the orbit through the superior orbital fissure.

Trochlear nucleus is situated in the midbrain. The nucleus lies ventral to the aqueduct in the central grey matter.

Tropical ulcer is a painful, non-healing ulcer. It is situated on front of leg. Floor of ulcer is covered by brownish tenacious and foul swelling slough. Surrounding skin is edematous; regional lymph nodes may be enlarged and tender. Injury may be mechanical and thermal. First and fifth metatarsals are commonly affected. There may be spontaneous blister or nodule. Ulcer may become infected. Deep tissues and bone may be involved.

True denticle is made up of dentin and is lined by odontoblasts. These are rare and are usually located close to apical foramen. Development of true denticle is caused by inclusions of remnants of epithelial root sheath within the pulp. These epithelial remnants induce the cells of pulp to differentiate into odontoblast which forms dentin masses called true pulp stones.

True oral malodor is not due to the above simple causes is most often a consequence of oral bacterial activity typically arising from anaerobes arising is due to:

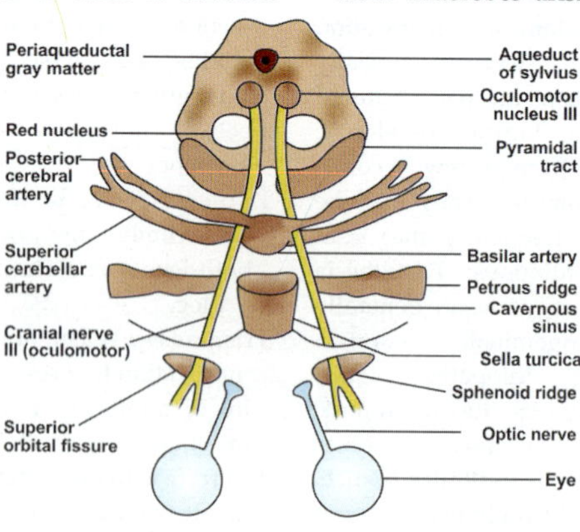

Fig.: *Trochlear nerve*

Poor oral hygiene, gingivitis (ANUG), periodontal disease, infected extraction sockets, oral sepsis, residual blood post operatively, debris under fixes or removable appliances, ulcers, dry mouth, putrefaction of postnasal mucus drip stagnating on the tongue.

Tubercle is a small, rounded projection.

Tuberculin test was discovered by Von Pirquet in 1907. A positive reaction to test is accepted as evidence of past or present infection by *M. tuberculosis*. It is done to test in population.

Tuberculin type hypersensitivity: It was originally described by Koch in patients with TB who had fever and generalized sickness, following a spontaneous injection of tuberculin, a lipoprotein antigen from tubercle bacillus. 12 hrs after intradermal tuberculosis challenge, T-lymphocytes are present at perivascular sites and this infiltrate, which extends outwards and disrupts the collagen bundles of the dermis, increases to a peak at 48 hrs. Cells of the macrophage lineage are probably the main APCs in tuberculin hypersensitivity.

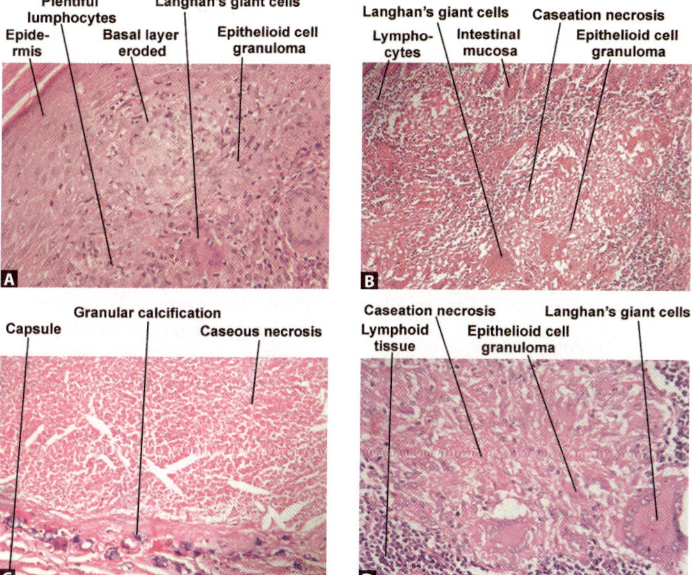

Figs A to D.: *(A) Tuberculoid leprosy; (B) Tuberculosis of small intestine; (C) Tuberculous lymph node showing dystrophic calcification; (D) Tuberculous lymphadenitis*

T

As the lesion develops, it may become a granulomatous reaction. It has well-defined skin lesions with raised margins and healing centers are characteristic of tuberculoid leprosy. These lesions are anesthetic to touch and pin prick. The leprae are usually not detected on skin smear examination. Microscopically lesion shows collections of epitheliod cells and Langerhan's type giant cell. Caseation is usually absent.

Tuberculoid leprosy is a chronic communicable disease of skin caused by *Mycobacterium leprae* characterized by a sharply demarcated, hypopig-mented macule. Temperature sen-sation is first to be affected followed by pressure, touch and pain. Margins of lesions are elevated, superficial, larger nerves closer to skin are enlarged. Neuritic pain, muscle dystrophy, contracture and trauma from pressure and burns are common.

Tuberculosis is an infectious granulomatous disease caused by acid-fast bacillus. Patient may suffer from evening fever, fatigue, malaise and loss of weight. Spread is through blood or lymph TB of submaxillary and cervical lymph nodes may progress to the actual abscess. Glands are enlarged. Lesions of oral mucosa are seldom primary but secondary to pulmonary disease. Tongue is most commonly affected. Lesion is irregular, superficial or deep, painful ulcer which increases slowly. Mucosal lesions show swelling or fissuring. Tuberculous gingivitis is an unusual form of tuberculosis which produces hyperaemic, nodular or proliferative gingiva. Diffuse involvement of maxilla or mandible may occur.

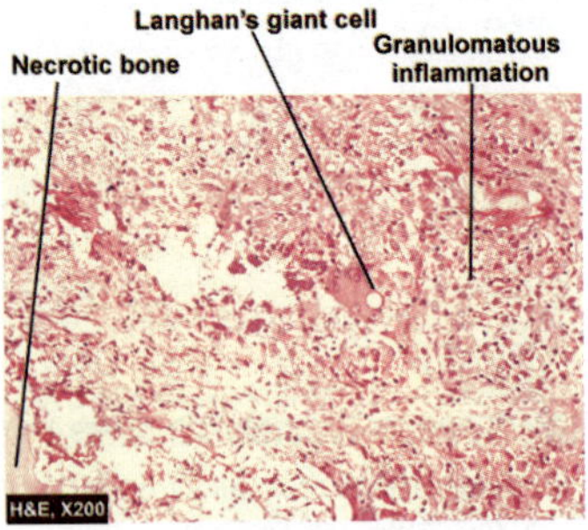

Fig.: *Tuberculous osteomyelitis*

Tuberculous lymphadenitis is caused by *Mycobacterium tuberculosis*. It is a condition where cervical glands are commonly affected. Route may be via tonsils or oral mucosa. There will be a lump in neck. It is painful. In early stage swelling is firm and mobile. Later the mass becomes fixed. Lesion may be unilateral, bilateral, single or multiple. It requires systemic therapy for 6 months. Such glands are enlarged and matted.

Tuberculous meningitis caused by *Mycobacterium tuberculosis* may develop as a consequence of military TB. Human tubercular bacilli are responsible. Prodromal symptoms include lassitude weight loss and anorexia. Diffuse headache and neck stiffness develop. Mild fever appears. Patient assumes a flexed position. CSF pressure is raised. On long-standing 'cob web' is formed. CSF sugar is low. Treatment is to begin with 3 anti TB drugs. Total duration is 12–18 months.

Tuberculous ulcer is caused by *Mycobacterium tuberculosis*. It is an aerobic, slender, non-motile, non-spore forming, rod-shaped organism. Most of the people get infection in first year of life. Primary infection usually takes place in lungs. Hemoptysis, abundant sputum and pleuritic pain are very common. Tuberculous lesions of the oral cavity are secondary to pulmonary infections. Important oral lesions are tuberculous ulcers, tuberculous gingivitis, tuberculous osteomyelitis and tuberculosis of salivary gland. For tongue ulcers, it is the most common site of occurrence. On lateral borders, these appear either single or multiple lesions. On palate, these may appear as small ulcer or granuloma. Lesions often produced are small, granulating ulcers at the mucocutaneous junction. Gingival lesions of tuberculosis usually produce granulating ulcers or erosive lesions with gingival hyperplasia.

Tuberosity is a large, rounded projection.

Tuberous sclerosis is an autosomal dominant gentic disorder of neuroectodermal orgin which affects multiple systems. It leads to formation of benign tumors i multiple organs including brain, eyes, heart, kidney, skin and lungs. Tuberous sclerosis is the largest know genetic cause of epilepsy. Seizers are caused by tubers or lesions in the brain. These lesion are smell patches of the brain that don't develop normally. The most common type of epilepsy is infantile spasm. Presenting features are autism, behavioural problems, destruction of kidneys, lungs, heart and other organs. Up to 80% of afftcted individuals experience seizure at same point of their life. X-ray shows intracranial calcification with generalized thickening and hyperostosis of cranial vault. Multiple cortical tubers are classical findings. Metacrapals and

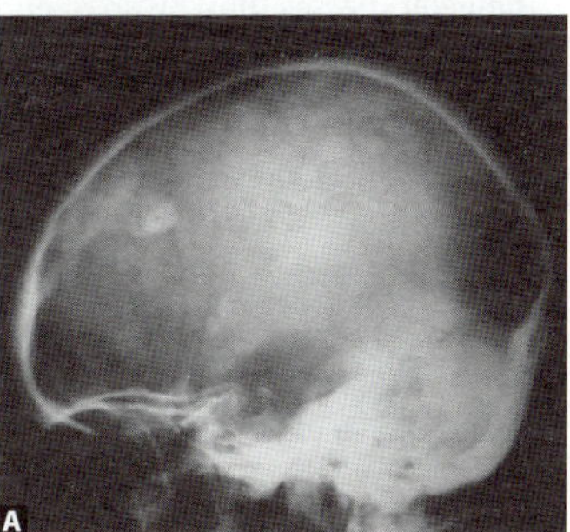

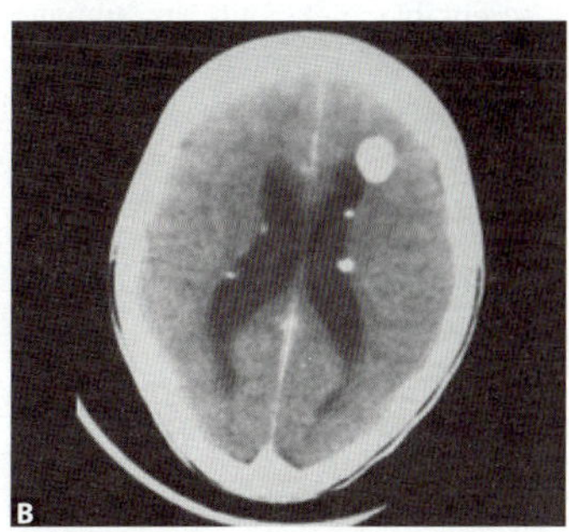

Figs A and B: *Tuberous sclerosis*

phalanges may show subperiosteal irregular new bone formation. Small well defined cysts are seen.

Tumor necrosis factor alpha refers to a substance involved in systemic inflammation. It is chiefly produced by macrophages in activated form and also belongs to a group of cytokines that stimulate acute phase reaction shares many of its biological activities (pro-inflammatory properties, MMP stimulation, eicosanoid production and bone resorption) with IL-1. In addition, its secretion by monocytes and fibroblast is stimulated by bacterial lipopolysaccharide.

Turkey tests refers to multiple comparison procedure.

Turku sugar studies were a series of collaborative studies carried out in Turku, Finland, by Scheinin, Makinen et al. They were investigated by a comprehensive program including clinical, radiographic, biochemical, and microbiochemical determinants of health. In addition to the massive data indicating that xylitol would be an acceptable metabolite in humans, there was a dramatic reduction in the incidence of dental caries after two years if xylitol consumption. Subsequently a 1-year chewing gum study was conducted on 102 subjects who consumed the xylitol or sucrose chewing gum but otherwise pursued their usual dietary and oral hygiene habits.

Turner's spot is an enamel hypoplasia of permanent tooth as a result of local trauma or infection of a deciduous tooth infection restricts work of ameloblasts and results in poorly formed enamel.

Tweed's method involves the extraction of the first molars around 8 years of age. This is followed by the extraction of the first premolars and the deciduous canine.

Twitch refers to the contraction of a muscle in response to a single action potential.

Tympanic membrane is a thin membranous diaphragm separates the external acoustic meatus from the middle ear. Anatomically, it is an oval membrane about 9 mm in long diameter, and about 8 mm in its short diameter. The long diameter passes downwards and forwards. The membrane is placed

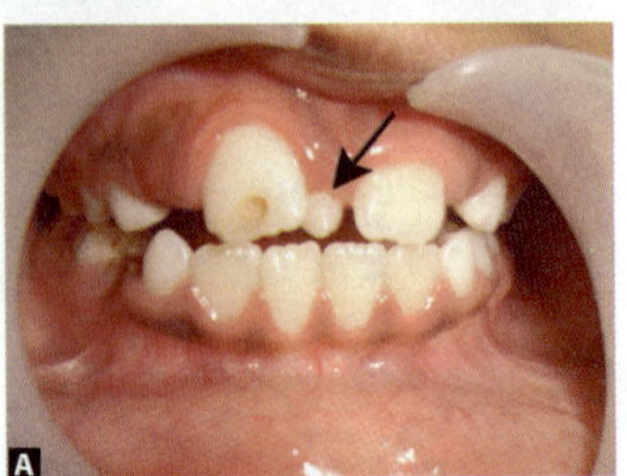

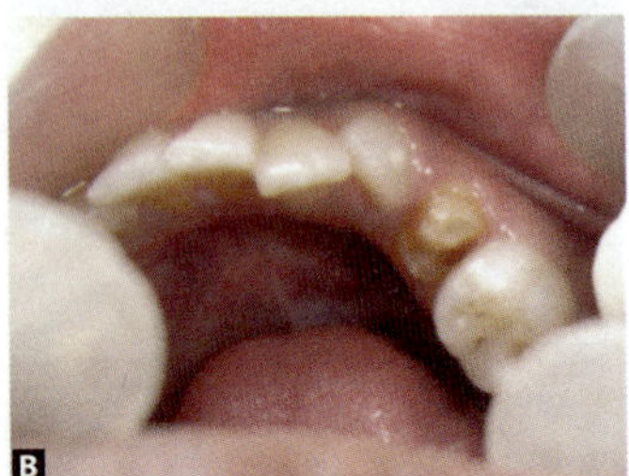

Figs A and B: *(A) Turner's tooth; (B) Turner's tooth involving premolar*

obliquely both in the vertical and anteroposterior planes. In the vertical plane its upper end is distinctly lateral to its lower end, and the membrane forms an acute angle of about 55° with the floor of the external acoustic meatus.

Typhoid fever *see* enteric fever.

Type I hypersensitivity is characterized by an allergic reaction immediately following contact with an antigen referred to as an allergen. Allergy (coined by Von-Pirquet in 1906) is defined as the changed reactivity of the host when meeting an agent. In recent years, allergy has become synonymous with Type I hypersensitivity. Dependent on the specific triggering of IgE sensitized mast cells by antigen, resulting in the release of pharmacological mediators of inflammation.

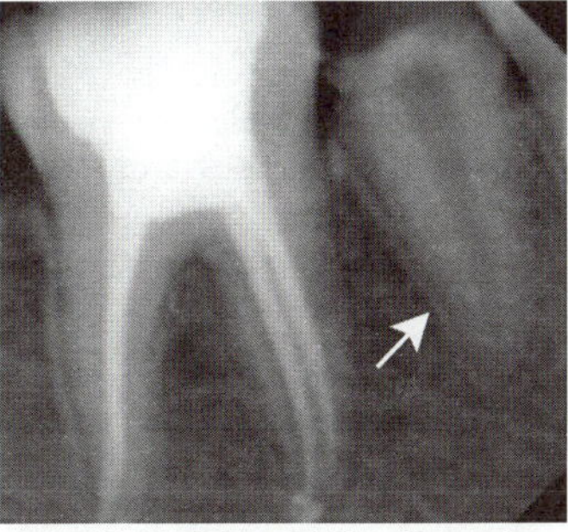

Fig.: *Turner's hypoplasia of premolars*

Typhoid is caused by *Salmonella typhi*. The infection gets localized to small intestine. To start, person may have headache, general body ache and malaise. Fever rises in step ladder fashion. Temperature increases every day especially in the evening. In morning, fever comes down but never touches normal. It happens for 7–10 days. During the second stage patient usually looks very ill. Tongue is coated with clean tip. There will be relative bradycardia. During third week patient starts looking better. During acute stage, the organisms would be positive in first week and urine, stool culture becomes positive by second week. Widal test is positive during second week.

Tzanck cells are the epithelial cells which show ballooning degeneration, consisting of acantholysis, nuclear clearing and nuclear enlargement. This is a histologic feature and can be appreciated only at a microscopic level.

Transitional dentition *see* mixed dentition.

U**Ulcer** is a pathological condition in which there is a breakdown of epithelial tissue. There is a full thickness loss of surface epithelium with exposure to underlying connective tissue. In mouth, ulcers are usually painful, except malignant one which may be initially painless. Biopsy is needed if ulcer is not responding for more than 3 weeks.

Ulcerative colitis is a disease of young people between the age of 15-25 years. Symptoms range from small amount of rectal bleeding to prominent diarrhea and colonic hemorrhage with prostration. It may manifest as spondylitis, peripheral arthritis, iritis and skin disorders. Recto sigmoid colon is commonly involved.

Ultimate strength is the maximum stress a solid can support based on its original cross-section area.

Ultrasonic is the conversion of high frequency electrical current into mechanical vibrations.

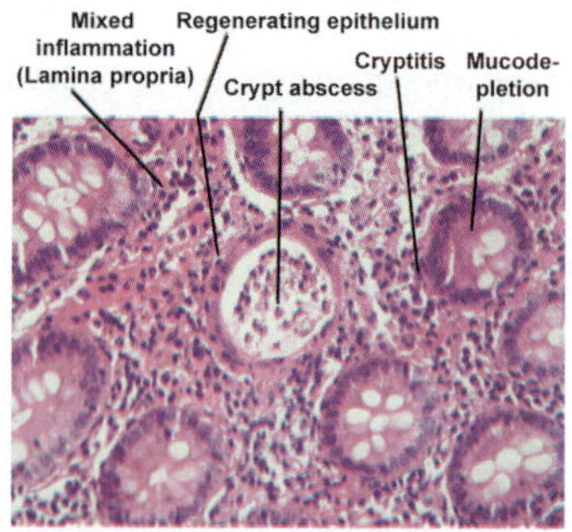

Fig.: *Ulcerative colitis*

Ultrasonic cleaning is the loosening and removal of debris from instruments by sound waves travelling through a chemical solution. It has increased efficiency in cleaning and has reduced danger of aerosolization of infectious particles released during scrubbing. Injury to instrument is lesser and is an easy process.

Ultrasonic scaler is an electronically powered device that produces vibratory motions to dislodge deposits from teeth. Commonly used scalers operate in the 5000 to 7000 cycles/second range. Most magnetostrictive ultrasonic operate at 25000–30000 cycles per seconds while Piezo electric ultrasonic operates at 40000 to 50000 cycles/second.

Ultrasonic scaling is a use of an ultrasonic scaler to remove mineralized deposits from tooth surface.

Ultrasonic's is the use of sound waves for detection and this offers considerable potential as a diagnostic instrument. Ultrasonic imaging was introduced by Ng et al. (1988) as a method for detecting early caries in smooth surfaces. With the use of this instrumentation, sonic velocity and specific acoustic impedance can be determined for the dentin and enamel as well as for the soft tissue and bone.

Ultrasound refers to an oscillating sound pressure wave with the frequency greater than human hearing range. Upper limit of hearing is 20 KHz (20,000 cycles per second). Ultrasound is very much above this therapeutic frequencies being in the region of 1 MHz to 3 MHz.

Uncontrolled diabetes is a clinical condition where the blood sugar is way above the normal range. Oral manifestations include multiple periodontal abscesses, velvety red gingival and marginal proliferation of the periodontal tissues.

Undercut is the portion of tooth lying between the height and contour of gingiva.

Underfilling is filling of the root canal system more than 2 mm short of radiographic apex.

Undermining resorption is the term used when the bone loss occurs from a healthy or viable periodontal ligament which is present adjacent to the necrotic areas.

Undifferentiated mesenchymal cells are the stem cells located in the cell-rich zone and the pulp proper which can differentiate into odontoblasts and/or fibroblasts.

Unfavorable fractures are the one where the vertical fracture or the horizontal fracture lines are opposed by the action of the muscle around them. However, these types of fractures are not so easy to reduce and stabilize.

Unicystic ameloblastoma refers to the cystic lesions of the bone. There will be localized thinning and haziness of radiopaque rim. It generally occurs before the age of 30. Lesion slowly enlarges due to expansion of cortex. On palpation, it is hard and bony.

Unilateral condylar neck fractures are the fractures involving the neck of the condyle and are of two types: low condylar neck fractures and high condylar neck fractures. If the fracture is undisplaced, no active treatment is required but in case of displaced fractures, dislocation will induce malocclusion. A low neck fracture can be treated by open reduction and a high condylar neck fracture with extensive displacement and malocclusion, intermaxillary fixation (IMF) is done for up to 3-4 weeks and maintained until bony union has occurred.

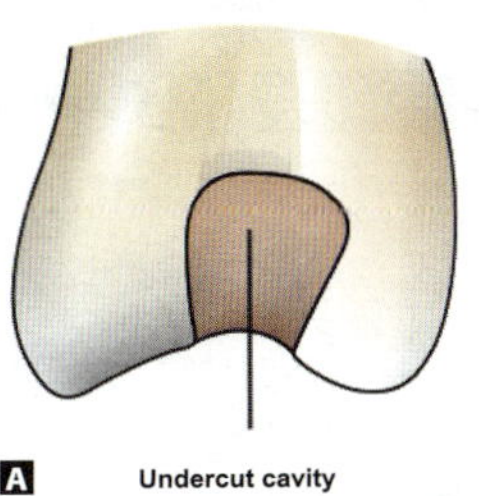

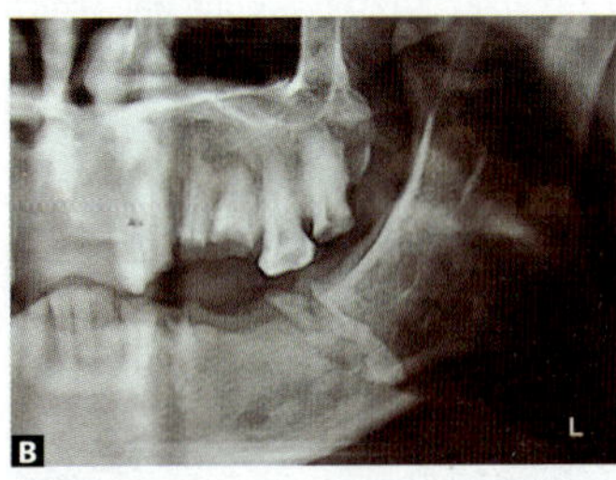

Figs A and B: *(A) Cavity preparation for plastic fillings; (B) Unfavorable fractures*

Unilateral extracapsular fractures refer to unilateral condylar neck fractures.

Unilateral fracture usually occurs on one side of the body but occasionally more than one fracture may be present. It is generally caused by direct violence.

Unilateral intracapsular fractures are the fractures occurring in the condyle. In these cases the occlusion is usually undisturbed and fracture should be treated conservatively, if malocclusion does occur, the intermaxillary fixation (IMF) for 2-3 weeks is indicated.

Universal is approved by the American Dental Association in 1968. Most commonly used throughout the United States. The permanent teeth are numbered from 1 to 32. Numbering begins with the upper right third molar, works around to the upper left third molar, drops to the lower left third molar, and works around to the lower right third molar. In the Universal Numbering System, the primary teeth are lettered with capital letters from A to T.

Universal curettes are the one which can be used in most areas of the dentition by altering and adapting the finger rest and hand position of the operator. The blades of these curettes are curved in one direction.

Upper lip prominence is a line drawn from subnasale (Sn) to soft-tissue pogonion (Pog′). The most prominent point of the upper lip (Ls) should be 3 ± 1 mm anterior to this line.

Upper lip-lower lip-chin prominence: A vertical reference line is drawn through subnasale (SnV) perpendicular to the true horizontal. The upper lip should be 1 to 2 mm ahead of this line. The lower lip should be on the line or 1 mm posterior to it. The chin (Pog′) should fall within 1 to 4 mm posterior to SnV. Alternatively the distance from soft-tissue chin to a line perpendicular to FH through soft tissue nasion can be measured. This is also known as 0-degree meridian and Pog′ is estimated to be 0 ± 2 mm from this line.

Urea is a white, odorless, crystalline powder. It was used in World War first as a therapeutic agent for infected wounds. Urea solution

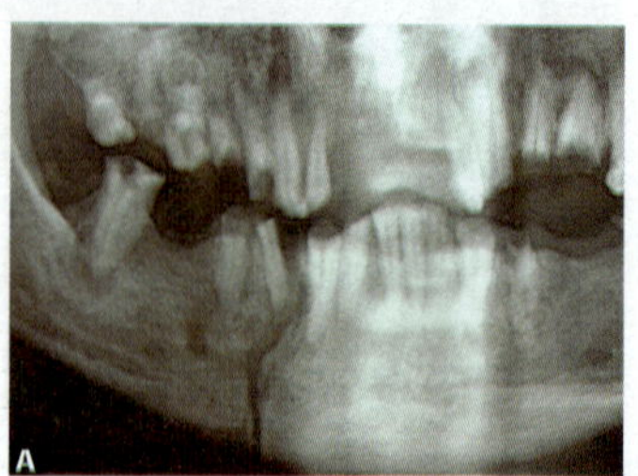

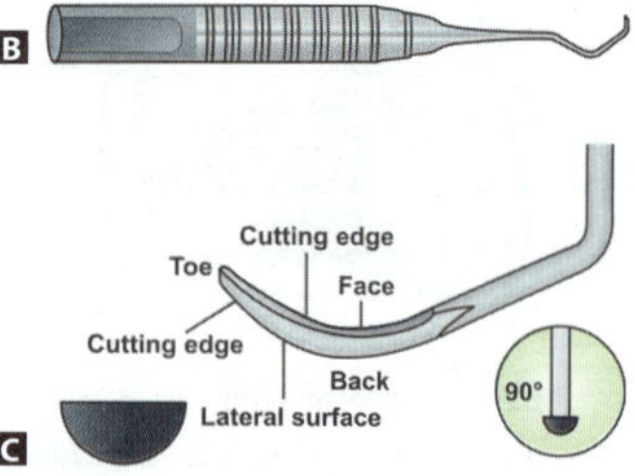

Figs A to C: *(A) Unilateral fracture; (B) Universal curette; (C) Cutting edge*

(40% by weight) is mild solvent of necrotic tissue and pus and is mild antiseptic too. In 1951, Blechman and Cohen suggested that 30% urea solution can be used as root canal irrigant in patients with vital pulp as well as those with necrotic pulp.

Urea peroxide is white crystalline powder with slight odor. It is soluble in water, alcohol and glycerine.

Uremic syndrome an early symptom of kidney failure is decreased creatinine clearance. As the disease progresses, glomerular filtration rate falls and blood urea nitrogen rises. Person may develop impaired ability to concentrate urine, nocturia and mild anemia. Advanced uremia is associated with pericarditis, pericardial effusion and neuropathies.

Ureter is a duct that transmits urine from kidney to bladder.

Urgency of urine is the sudden desire to void. It is seen in inflammatory conditions, i.e. cystitis or neurogenic bladder.

Uric acid refers to the end product of purine metabolism.

Uricosuric drugs are those drugs that block tubular reabsorption of filtered urate and reduce the metabolic pool of urates, preventing the formation of new tophi. When given with colchicines these lessen the frequency of recurrence of gout.

Urinary tract obstruction refers to a severe obstruction can produce acute anuria, burning and pain on urination, overflow in continence or dribbling, voiding of small amount and flank pain. In secondary infection fever, chills malaise develop along with foul smelling urine.

Urine pregnancy test a test done to confirm pregnancy. It depends on the presence of human chorionic gonadotropin in urine. Usually a concentration of about 2500 IV HCG per liter of urine is required to register a positive health. It usually occurs 12 days after the first missed period.

Urticaria results is a manifestation of an allergic reaction when antigen reaches specific skin areas causing localized anaphylactic reaction. Histamine on release results in red flare and increased permeability of capillaries resulting in swelling within a few minutes.

Useful habits include habits that are considered essential for normal function such as proper positioning of the tongue, respiration and normal deglutition.

Uterine fibroids are uterine leiomyoma. If large, it produces a round, multinodular mass in suprapubic region. She may feel heaviness in abdomen and pressure on surrounding organs with frequency of urine. Menorrhagia develops. Edema and varicosities of lower extremities develop.

Utilitarian ethics is in ethical theory based on the principle of the greatest good for the majority.

Uvula is a small muscular structure located on the free edge of soft palate. When you swallow the food it prevents your food from coming out of your nose. It directs the food down the throat into esophagus.

Vaccination refers to an administration of vaccine that is used to produce acquired immunity. Person can be vaccinated by injecting dead organisms which are no longer capable of causing disease but still have chemical antigen. These are used against typhoid, diphtheria and whooping cough. Secondly immunity can be achieved against toxins which have been treated with chemicals. These are used against tetanus and botulinism. Thirdly person can be vaccinated by infecting him with live organism that has been attenuated. These are used against polio, measles and other viral diseases.

Vagus nerve is a mixed tenth cranial nerve. Motor part supplies pharynx and larynx, bronchi and heart. Sensory fibers carry taste from epiglottis and vallecula. It arises from the lateral side of the medulla, by about ten rootlets that are attached to the groove between the olive and the inferior cerebellar peduncle, below the rootlets of the glossopharyngeal nerve. Thus formed nerve leaves the skull through the jugular foramen. Its position relative to other structures in the foramen. The part of the nerve within the jugular foramen shows an enlargement called the

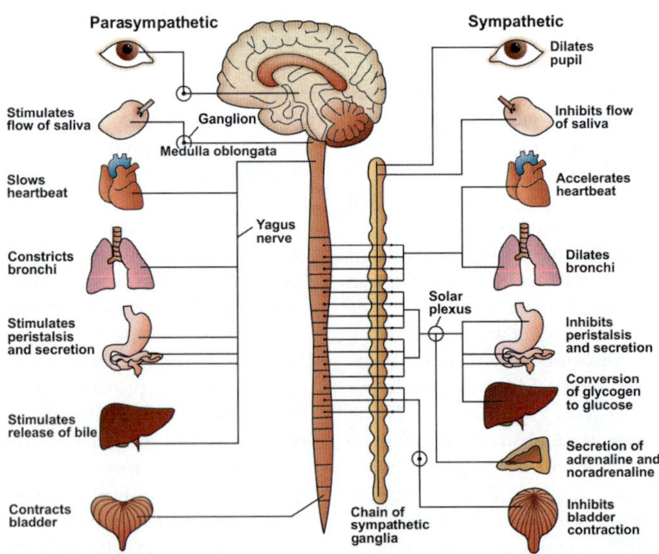

Fig.: *Vagus nerve*

superior ganglion. Just below the foramen the nerve has a much larger enlargement called the inferior ganglion.

Validity is the meaningfulness of test scores as they are used for specific tests.

Van Limborgh's theory is a multifactorial theory that was put forward by Van Limborgh in 1970. According to Van Limborgh, the three popular theories of growth were not satisfactory, yet each contains elements of significance that cannot be denied. Van Limborgh explains the process of growth and development in a view that combines all the three existing theories. He supports the functional matrix theory of Moss, acknowledged some aspects of Sicher's theory and at the same time does not rule out genetic involvement. Van Limborgh has suggested the following five factors that he believed control growth: Intrinsic genetic factors, local epigenetic factors, general epigenetic factors, local environmental factors, general environmental factors.

Vapor pressure is a measure of liquid's tendency to evaporate. Materials with high vapor pressure at room temperature tend to evaporate readily.

Varicocele is a pampiniform plexus of veins of the spermatic cord. It is a consequence to venous stasis aided by gravity forces and prolonged standing. Intra-abdominal tumor also results increased pressure on the spermatic veins.

Varicose ulcer is a chronic ulcer of leg of insidious onset. Mostly ulcer is on medial side of leg. It is solitary. It is a shallow ulcer where floor is covered by bluish granulation tissue of pale slough. Edges are irregular and sloping. It is mobile on underlying bone surrounding skin is swollen and pigmented.

Varicose veins are an abnormal dilatation and tortousity of vein especially in leg. In legs these are abnormally dilated, elongated and tortuous. Incidence increases with age. It has familial tendency. Increased intraluminal pressure leads to it. Affected veins are dilated, stretched, tortuous and nodular. There is irregular thinning and atrophy of vein. Thrombosis is common. Fibrosis results in tortuousity. Intima is thickened. Valvular defect causes an important defect. Long-standing cases may develop fibrosis, chronic edema and skin pigmentation. Person feels dull, aching heaviness or a feeling of fatigue.

Varnishes are used such as thin layers but don't provide thermal insulation. These serve to isolate the tubule contents from the cavity. Several applications are needed to prevent penetration of bacteria.

Vascular dementia is the single brain lesion that doesn't lead to dementia but affects mental function. The most common type of vascular dementia is caused by multiple supra-tentorial infarcts. Hypertensive small vessel disease produces predominant deep white matter infarcts.

Vasculitis describes a diverse group of inflammatory disorder characterized by multiorgan vessel involvement. There develops fever, malaise, weight loss and raised WBCs and ESR.

Vasoconstrictor drugs refer to drugs that have the ability to control bleeding, i.e. adrenaline and nor-adrenaline are useful when there is an access to the bleeding site. These are effective in controlling the oozing from capillaries. These are useful in controlling gingival bleeding. It is not useful in controlling heavy hemorrhage because these are diluted and washed out.

Vasodepressor syncope refers to sudden loss of consciousness that usually occurs secondary to a period of cerebral ischemia. Predisposing factors for vasodepressor syncope are psychogenic factors: Fright, anxiety, emotional stress, pain especially sudden and unexpected, sight of blood or surgical or other dental instruments. Non-psychogenic factors include sitting in an upright position which permits blood to pool in the periphery decreasing cerebral blood flow; hunger from missed meal which decreases the glucose supply to brain, exhaustion, poor physical condition and hot, humid environment.

Vasomotor syncope may be due to excessive vagal tone or impaired reflex control of peripheral circulation. Common faint is initiated by a stressful, painful or claustrophobic experience.

Vasovagal syncope is a transient attach of loss of consciousness. Person will develop low blood pressure, pallor, cold sweats bradycardia and weakness.

Vehicle is a substance possessing little or no medicinal action used as a medium to confer a suitable consistency or form.

Vein refers to a blood vessel carrying blood from periphery to heart.

Veneer is a layer of tooth-colored material (can be porcelain, composite, or ceramics) attaches to the front of the tooth to improve appearance. These are bonded to enamel by means of acid-etch technique with the help of resin.

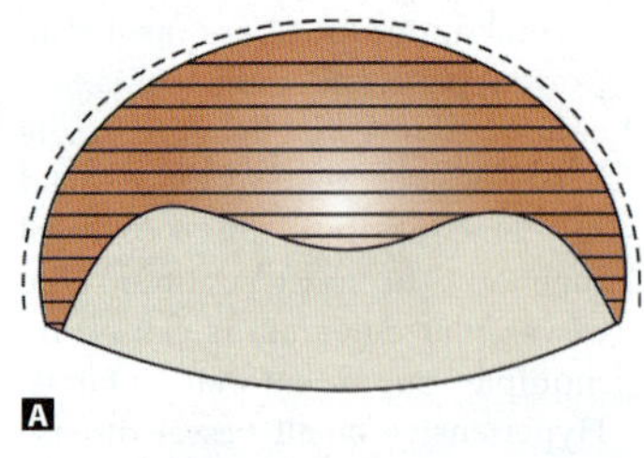

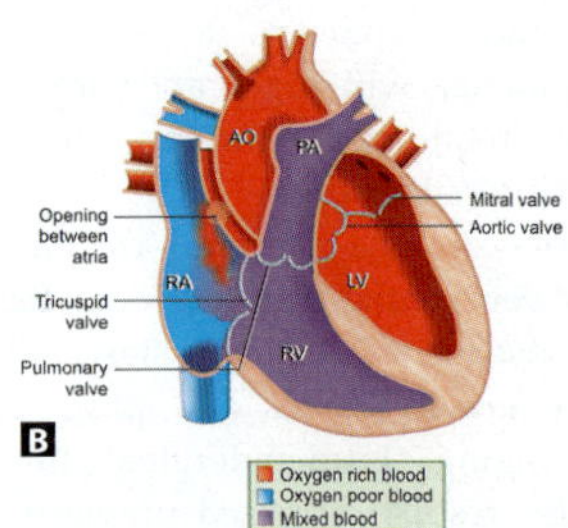

Figs A and B: *(A) Veneer; (B) Ventricular septal defect (VSD)*

Venous pressure is a diagnostic test. Clinicians' examining the cardiovascular system uses the level of blood in the external jugular vein as an indication of venous pressure. Venous pressure can be raised if there is right heart failure, raised intrathoracic pressure from any cause, or obstruction to the superior vena cava. Increased venous pressure leads to dilatation of veins in the neck. The internal jugular vein can be markedly dilated.

Ventral is the underside, used when speaking of the tongue; thus the ventral surface of the tongue is the underside of the tongue.

Ventricular septal defect (VSD) is the most common type of CHD. There is incomplete sepration of the ventricles. The defect is most commonly present at the junction of membranous and muscular portion of the interventricular septum. VSD can occur alone or can be accompanied by other defects like aortic regurgitation. It results in blood to pass from high pressure left ventricle into low pressure right ventricle. Large defects are associated with early left ventricular failure. Many VSD defects close spontaneously in early childhood.

Vermilion means red.

Verrucal resembles like a wart.

Verrucous carcinoma is a slow growing, exophytic and superficially invasive. It has a low metastatic potential. It occurs over buccal mucosa and gingiva. It is exophytic and papillary in nature. Lesions have folds with deep clefts. Regional lymph nodes are tender and enlarged. Pain and difficulty in mastication are chief complaints. Anaplastic transformation occurs. It mostly develops in tobacco chewing patients. *Clinical features:* commonest site involved are gingiva, alveolar mucosa and buccal mucosa. Surface of the lesion shows multiple deep clefts. Lesion may be single or multiple involving different parts of buccal mucosa. Pain may develop making chewing difficult. It becomes rapidly fixed to underlying bone. Regional lymph nodes are often enlarged. Malignant epithelial cells are usually well differentiated.

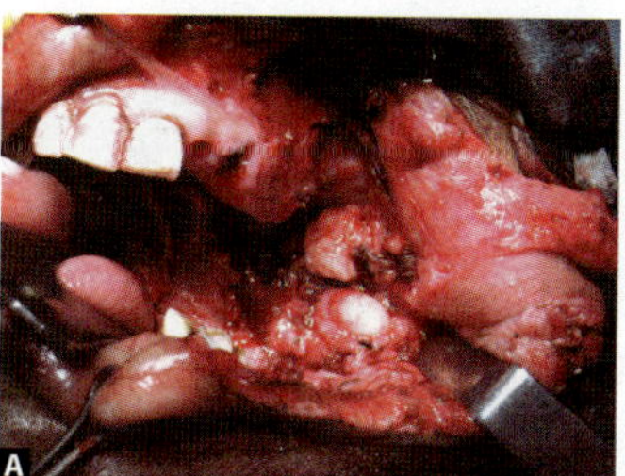

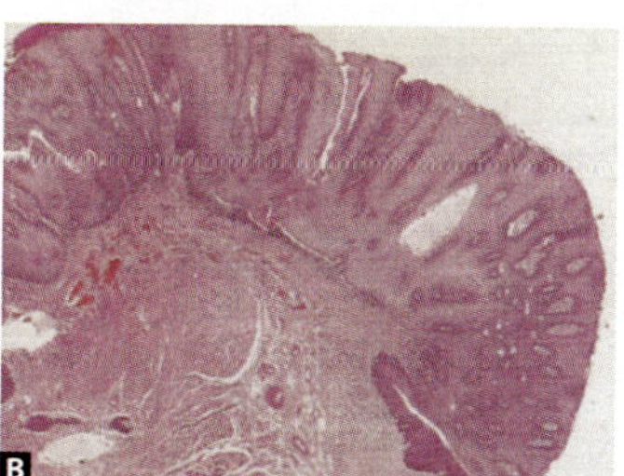

Figs A and B: *Verrucous carcinoma (A) Clinical; (B) Histological*

Vertebral compression fracture may result due to osteoporosis by bending, lifting, coughing or sneezing. There develops acute, severe pain at fracture site. Pain may radiate anteriorly to flank. Pain is typically worse in upright position. Signs include spinal tenderness over fractured spine along with paravertebral muscle spasm. Kyphosis and loss of height will develop. Weakness, sensory deficits incontinence or diminished deep reflexes develop.

Vertebral osteophytes occur due to repeated damage to the posterior joints especially lead to degenerative changes. It is a true osteoarthritic change and lipping of vertebra may take place.

Vertical bone loss is also known as angular bone loss. It does not occur in plane parallel to cementoenamel junction. These bony defects of alveolar process occur in an oblique direction, leaving a hollowed out trough in the bone alongside the root.

Vestibular nuclei are somatic afferent nuclei that lie in the grey matter underlying the lateral part of the floor of the fourth ventricle. They lie partly in the medulla and partly in the pons and receive fibers from end organs in the vestibular part of the internal ear.

Vestibule refers a part between the alveolar processes and the cheeks.

Vestibulocochlear nerve is eighth cranial nerve. It consists of two distinct parts—vestibular and cochlear. Both of them are purely sensory. The vestibular nerve carries impulses necessary for the maintenance of equilibrium from the vestibular part of the internal ear. The cochlear nerve carries impulses of hearing from the cochlear part of the internal ear.

Vibrio cholerae is a microorganism that causes cholera. Their natural habitat is water. Watery diarrhea can be fatal. It is a Gram-negative slender bacilli, comma-shaped with pointed ends. It is highly motile with single flagellum. It is seen under dark field microscopy.

Vimentin is the type of filament that is expressed in mesenchymal cells such as fibroblasts, and in endothelial cells. These fibers often end at the nuclear membrane and

V

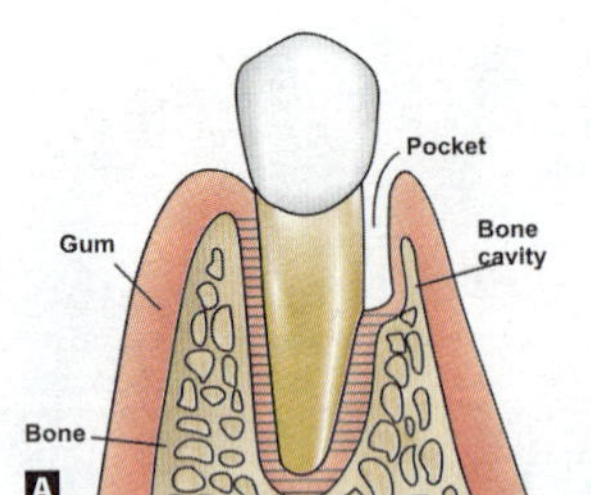

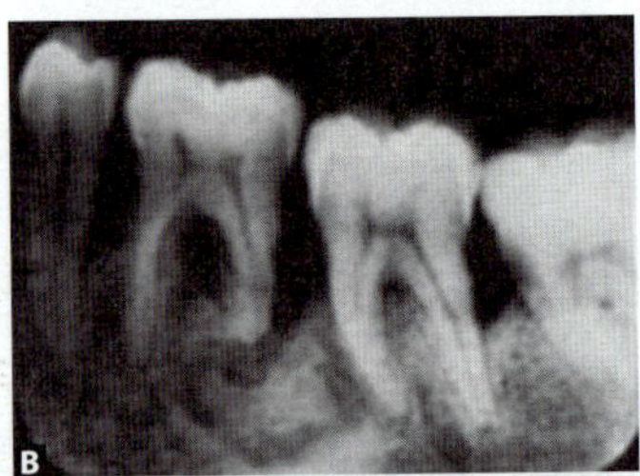

Figs A and B: *Verticle bone loss (A) Schematic; (B) Radiological*

desmosomes. They are closely associated with microtubules, and they form cages around lipid droplets in adipose tissue.

Vincent's angina is a fusospirochetal infection affecting oropharynx and throat, causing a painful ulceration and edema of these areas, also the breaking down of hyperemic patches may extend the lesion to other areas such as larynx and middle ear. There is an acute inflammation of mouth and throat with enlarged lymph glands, pain and fever. Streptococcal sore-throat also produces exudative membrane in throat. Throat becomes sore and extremely painful. Pharynx may show edema and reddening.

Vipeholm dental study was a 5-year investigation of 436 adult inmates in a mental institution at the Vipetional Hospital near Lund, Sweden. The dental caries rate in the inmates was relatively low. The experimental design divided the inmates into seven groups; sugar was introduced either at mealime. The main conclusions of the study were as follows: An increase in carbohydrate definitely increases the caries activity. The risk of caries is greater if the sugar is consumed in a form that will be retained on the surfaces of teeth.The risk of sugar increasing caries activity is greatest if the sugar is consumed between meals and in a form that tends to be retained on the surfaces of the teeth.The increase in caries activity varies widely between individuals. Upon withdrawal of the sugar-rich foods, the increased caries activity rapidly disappears. Caries lesions may continue to appear despite the avoidance of refined sugar and maximum restrictions of natural sugars and dietary carbohydrate.A high concentration of sugar in solution and its prolonged retention of tooth surfaces leads to increased caries activity. The clearance time of the sugar correlates closely with caries activity.

Viperine snake bite: Local symptoms are persistent pain but salivation is rare. There is no paralysis of respiratory organs as in cobra bite. It produces extensive inflammation with cellulitis, discoloration and incessant oozing of hemolysed blood from the punctured point. Signs of collapse may be seen. Pupils are dilated and not reaching to light. There will be multiple hemorrhages, epistaxis, hematuria, hemoptysis and petechial hemorrhages. There may be complete unconsciousness. Death takes place due to cardiac failure within 1-2 days.

Viral fever is caused by influenza virus. Transmission is through inhalation of infected nasopharyngeal secretions.

Viral hepatitis is an acute parenchymal necrotizing lesion where liver cell necrosis of hepatitis includes agents A, B, C, D, E, etc. During active disease one develops fever, nausea, vomiting fatigue, anorexia, headache and chills. There will be disturbance of taste. One can develop pruritic rash, arthritis and altered mental status. Urine will be dark and stools will be clay colored. Liver will be enlarged and tender.

Viral infection is an infection due to virus mumps is caused by a paramyxovirus. It may complicate gonads, CNS, pancreas and myocardium. Clinical features include sudden fever, malaise and anorexia. To start one sided parotid gland is involved then second is involved. Parotid gland enlarges for 2-3 days and return to normal within seven days. Submandibular gland may also be involved. Most of the causes are self-limiting within a week. In some children meningitis or encephalitis may develop. Antibiotics and cortisone avoid complications.

Viral oral ulcer may be primary herpetic gingivostomatitis. Virus is transmitted by saliva and direct contact. Primary infection is subclinical. Multiple oral ulcers will result in painful gums, tongue and sore-throat. Lips may be crushed with blood. Swallowing, eating, talking will be painful. Fever, nausea and vomiting may develop. Initially develop as vesicles which rupture later on. Ulcers are multiple and size is 2 to 3 mm.

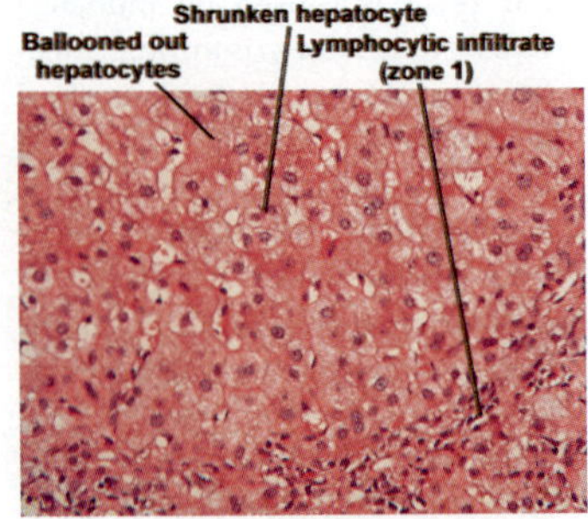

Fig.: *Viral hepatitis*

Virgin B-lymphocytes refer to resting.

Virgin teeth are those teeth that are free from decay or restorations.

Virulence is the strength or disease producing capacity of a pathogen. The virulence of HIV is much less than that of hepatitis B virus. Needle prick involving blood from HBV carrier is 5 to 30% while from HIV positive is only 1%.

Virulent is capable of causing infection or disease.

Virus infections cause disease in mankind. Viruses are obligatory parasites. They cannot reproduce outside living cells. Diseases caused by virus include common cold, measles, chicken pox, mumps, AIDS, poliomyelitis and hepatitis.

Visceral pain is transmitted mainly in the fibers which may accompany sympathetic nerves, most visceral pain impulses travel with sympathetic nerves.

Visceral structures are the tissues that make up the internal organs like the heart, lungs or stomach. These include the lining epithelial of hollow viscera, and smooth muscle including smooth muscle in the walls of blood vessels.

Viscosity is the ability of the material to flow. Thick or viscous liquids flow poorly while thin fluids flow easily. Impression materials have viscosities between 100,000 and 100,000 CP.

Visible luminescent spectroscopy: The visible emission spectra and the fluorescent lifetimes for decayed and non-decayed regions of teeth differ. Quasi-monochromatic light from a tungsten source dispersed with a grating monochromator is focused on the teeth. Although, how exactly it works is unknown, this is a non-radiological, non-invasive clinical method to detect dental caries.

Visual agnosia is a failure to identify objects by sight alone even though visual acuity and cerebral functions are normal. Patient may be able to recognize shape and form but not the image or object as a whole. He can match two identical things but cannot recognize the object as a whole.

Vital staining is technique involves administration of certain dyes to the experimental animal, which gets incorporated to bone. It is possible to study the manner in which one is laid down, site of growth, and the directions.

Vital statistics can be referred as a systematic approach to collect and compile in numerical form the information related to vital events. It is useful for maintaining records, to maintain control during execution of program or to create administrative standard of health.

Vital theory considered dental caries as originating within the tooth itself, analogous to the bone gangrene. At the end of eighteenth century this theory remained dominant until the middle of the nineteenth century. A clinically well-known type of caries is characterized by extensive penetrations into the dentin, and even into the pulp, but with a barely detectable catch or a fissure.

Vitamin A is a fat soluble Vitamin, although Vitamin A was not discovered until 1913, cod liver has been in use for centuries. It was chemically synthesized in 1930. Retinal is found only in foods of animal origin. Herbivorous obtain the vitamins from its precursor, i.e. carotenoid pigment. Conversion of beta-carotene into retinal in small intestine is only 30 percent. Absorption of both retinal and carotene is facilitated by bile salts. Vitamin E prevents the destruction of Vitamin A in the body. It plays a crucial role in normal vision

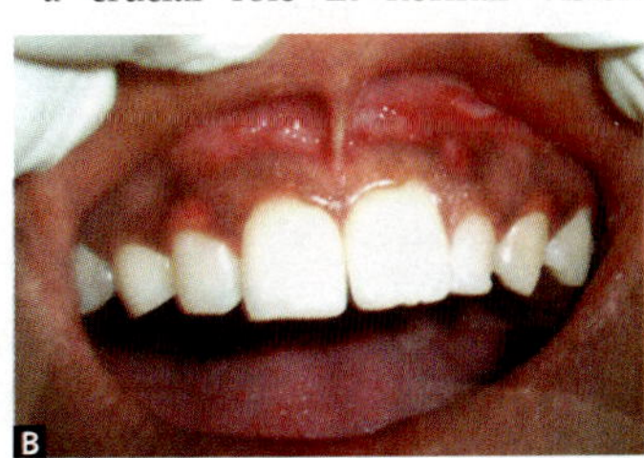

Figs A and B: *Viral herpetic gingivostomatitis*

and plays role in immunological defence mechanism. Liver, egg yolk, butter, milk and fish are good sources of Vitamin A. yellow colured carrots 'pumpkin, papaya and mango are rich source of Vitamin A. Its deficiency may cause night blindness, dry skin and scaly skins. Lack of Vitamin A first causes night blindness or inability to see in dim light. Mother can easily detect in children. Conjuctival xerosis is the first clinical sign of Vitamin A deficiency. Conjunctiva becomes dry and nonwettable. Instead of looking smooth and swing it looks muddy and wrinkled. Bitot's spots are triangular, yellowish foamy spots on bulbar conjunctiva on either side of cornea.

Vitamin B_1 *see* Thiamine.

Vitamin C is an ascorbic acid and it is a white crystalline colorless compound readily soluble in water. It is a strong reducing agent. It is comparatively stable in acid medium but is destroyed by heat and catalysts such as copper. Each cigarette smoked uses up to 25 mg of Vitamin C equivalent of one orange. Being water soluble it cannot be stored in body. Vitamin C is a cementing material which holds the body cell in place. It helps in absorption of calcium and iron. Deficiency of it delays wound healing. Animal food is a poor source of it and amla is a richest source. Daily requirement is 50 mg and has to be consumed daily. It has been claimed that each cigarette smoked uses up to 25 microgram of Vitamin C which is equivalent of one orange. Animal food is a poor source of Vitamin C. Amla is one of the richest sources of Vitamin C. Lemon and oranges are good source of it. Guava and drumsticks have high ascorbic acid content. Leafy vegetables such as cabbage contain lesser quantities. Sprouting converts part of carbohydrate and pulses into Vitamin C.

Vitamin D a fat soluble vitamin is intimately connected with the metabolism of calcium and phosphorus. It promotes the absorption of calcium and phosphorus. It promotes the absorption of calcium from intestine and helps in mineralization of bones. It was synthesized in 1935. Exposing the skin to the sun enables the ultraviolet rays to react on the skin's surface oil to produce Vitamin D.

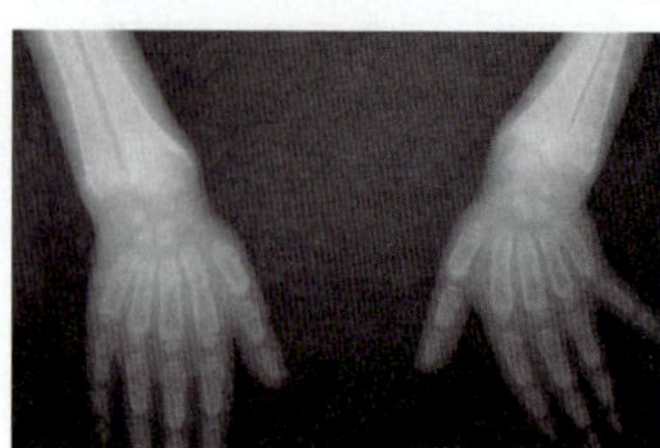

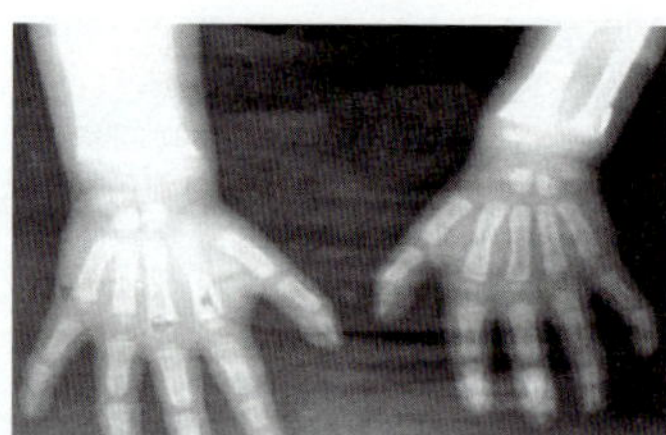

Figs A and B: *Vitamin D Rickets showing cupping and fraying of metaphyses*

The result is not achieved unless you "strip off" since an intervening layer of clothing or of glass impedes the production of Vitamin D. Vitamin D is found in small quantities and in a few animal foods. Foods of plant origin do not contain Vitamin D. It exists in two forms; ergocalciferol (Vitamin D_2) and cholecalciferol (Vitamin D_3). Ergocalciferol is derived from plants (the ergot fungus found especially on rye) and cholecalciferol is synthesized in the skin from 7-dehydrocholesterol under the influence of ultraviolet rays present in sunlight or is synthetically produced. Vitamin D is stored largely in fat depots. Cholecalciferol is converted to active forms by hydroxylation in the liver and subsequently in kidneys. In the liver, it is converted to 25-hydroxycholecalciferol (25 [OH] D_3) and in kidney, to most potent metabolite 1, 25-dihydroxy-cholecalciferol (1, 25 [OH] 2 D_3) or calcitriol. People with mental retardation, cerebral palsy, epilepsy and other neurological conditions closely related to mental retardation which originates prior to age 18 and constitutes a substantial handicap in the year 1975 amendments.

Vitamin E was isolated from wheat germ oil in 1936. It is also known as antisterility vitamin. Chemically, it is identified as tocoferol. This vitamin decreases oxygen require-ment of the body. Foods rich in poly-unsaturated fatty acids are often rich in Vitamin E. Vegetable oils, wheat germ oil and egg yolk are rich in Vitamin E. It minimizes wrinkles. It allows great storage of Vitamin A. It is destroyed by food refining.

Vitamin K was isolated in 1939 by Damin and his Colleagues. Coagulation or clotting of blood is a Vitamin K's role function and in cases of deficiency hemorrhage occurs. Limited stores in liver are maintained. Green vegetables contain it well so deficiency does not occur. Soya bean, unrefined cereals, tomatoes, honey and wheat germ also supply it. It is resistant to heat.

Vitamins are organic compounds required by the body for variety of essential metabolic functions made of carbon, hydrogen and O_2. These are grouped as water-soluble and fat-soluble vitamins. Fat soluble vitamins are Vitamins A, D, E and K. Water-soluble vitamins are thiazine (B_1), riboflavin (B_2), niacin (B_3), pyrido-xine (B_6), cobalamin (B_{12}), folate, pantothenic acid, biotin and L-ascorbic acid (Vitamin C). Vitamins are not synthesized at all or are inadequately synthesized in the body; hence they are required in the diet. Niacin refers to nicotinic acid, nicotinamide and their derivatives. It serves as a precursor of nicotinamide adenine dinucleotide (NAD) and nicotinamide adenine dinucleotide phosphate (NADP) which are involved in many oxidation-reduction reactions.

Vitiligo is a condition where there is partial or complete loss of pigment producing melanocytes within epidermis. Lesions are already seen in darkly pigmented individuals. Histologically, there is loss of melanocytes.

Volatile anesthetic agents refer to the agents that are liquid at room temperature but evaporate easily. Basic properties of these agents are—(i) liquid at room temperature, (ii) potent in low concentration and (iii) more soluble in blood, cell water and fat than anesthetic agents. Because of solubility of these, equilibration is retarded and induction is slow.

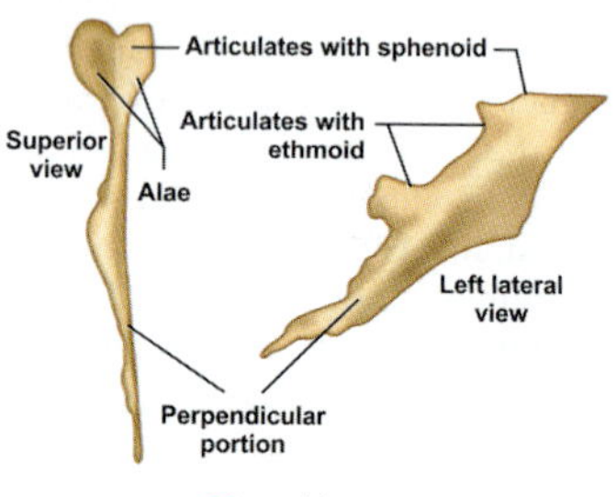

Fig.: *Vomer*

Volvulus is the rotation of a segment of intestine on an axis formed by its mesentery. Cecal volvulus causes colicky pain in right abdomen, obstruction and vomiting with abdominal distension. Plain X-ray will show hugely dilated ovoid cecum. To start single fluid level may be seen.

Vomer is a flat plate of bone that forms part of the nasal septum.

Von Willebrand's disease is a rare hemorrhage disorder inherited as a Mendelian dominant. There is an excessive capillary fragility. Post-operative dental hemorrhage is a potential hazard.

Von–Sallman syndrome is a hereditary benign intraepithelial dyskeratosis. It is rare autosomal dominant trait. Patient shows oral mucosal thickening with superficial gelatinous looking plaques on bulbar conjunctiva. Cytological scrapings show 'cells within cells'.

Vulcanite is a hard rubber prepared by vulcanizing India rubber with sulfur. Previously, it was used for making removable dentures.

Waddling gait is a myopathic gait peculiar to progressive muscular dystrophy. It occurs due to weakness of muscle of pelvic bone. It is also known as rolling gait as the pelvic is unstabilized due to weakness of gluteus medius. Congenital dislocation of hip also results in these. Opposite pelvis drops and trunk is tilted to that side.

Walking: When the sole of the foot is pressed against the couch, the body tries to walk. It persists as a voluntary standing.

Walking of the probe is a probing technique where the probe should be inserted parallel to the vertical axis of the tooth and is 'walked' circumferentially around each surface of the tooth to detect areas of deepest penetration.

Wallace's "Rule of 9" is the most common technique for assessing the TBSA (total body surface area). This divides the body surface into eleven equal areas each of which is 9% of the total or in multiples of 9, e.g.: each upper limb is 9% of the TBSA, each thigh is 9% of TBSA, each lower leg is 9% of TBSA, head and neck is 9%, front of chest is 9%, back of chest is 9%, front of abdomen is 9% and back of trunk is 9%. The perineal area is remaining 1% of TBSA. However this technique cannot be applied for children because of the proportionately larger surface area of head and neck and smaller area of limbs. Hence modification is done for calculating BSA burned in children.

Wallerian degeneration as the degenerative changes of peripheral nerve fiber that occurs due to the biochemical and morphological alterations following trauma which occur in a nerve due to loss of continuity of axon.

WAND local anesthesia system is computer-automated injection system which allows precise delivery

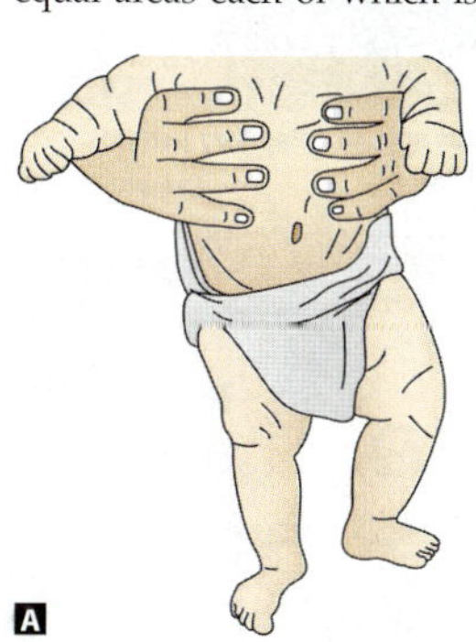

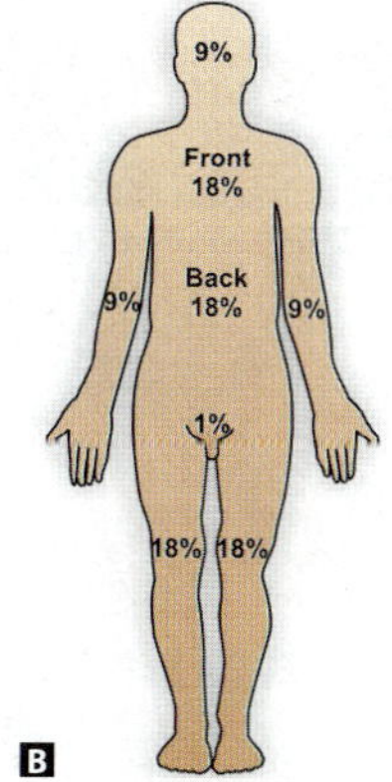

Figs A and B: *(A) Walking reflex; (B) Rule of nine*

of anesthesia at a constant flow rate despite varying tissue resistance.

Warthin tumor is a common benign tumor of salivary gland. These arise from the lymph nodes with ectopic salivary tissue. Microscopically it shows an admixture of glandular and papillary epithelial structure.

Warty dyskeratoma is a benign epidermal proliferation that involves face, scalp and neck, more oral lesions are rare but do occur. These are small, whitish areas of mucosa with a central depression. Lesion is to be treated by surgical excision. There is no malignant transformation.

Wasting is defined as any gradual loss of tooth substance which is characterized by the formation of smooth, polished surface. The various forms of wasting are erosion, abrasion and attrition.

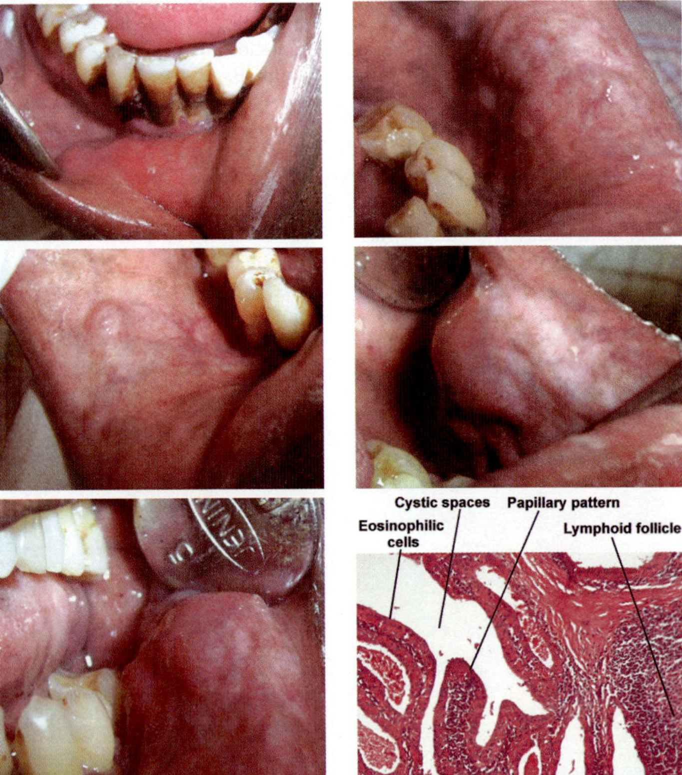

Fig.: *Warthin tumor of minor salivary gland*

Watch winding is back and forth oscillation of the endodontic instrument (file or reamer) right and left as it is advanced into the canal. The angle of rotation is usually 30 to 60 degrees. This technique is efficient with K-type instruments. This motion is quite useful during biomechanical preparation of the canal. Watch winding motion is less aggressive than quarter turn and pull motion because in this motion, the instrument tip is not forced into the apical area with each motion, thereby reducing the frequency of instrumental errors.

Water is a transparent fluid that forms the major constituents for the body fluids. 55 to 70% of total body weight is water. In old age water content decreases. Fat people contain less water. Urine contains 87% of water. Water is required for many chemical changes. Daily requirement is of 2 to 2.5 liters. Hypothalamus controls water balance. Any loss more than 10% of water is serious.

Water fluoridation is a process of adding fluid to commonly water in order to reduce and prevent the incidence of dental caries at community level. It was the result from the Grand Rapids experiment in 1943 that first showed conclusive evidence of the success of water fluoridation. 1 ppm added to the community water supply and used over 15 years reduced caries experience. By 50%, the amount of fluoride varies with the temperature of the area and can be calculated using the formula: Conc. of F (PPM) = 0.34/E, where E = 0.038 + 0.0062, temperature of the area in F. In colder climates where water consumption is reducing, the concentration of F may be from 1 ppm whereas in hotter climates only up to 0.7 ppm is needed. In moderate temperature the optimum pH conc. is 1 PPM.

Water hammer pulse also known as collapsing or jerky pulse and is seen as is having rapid upstroke and descent of pulse wave. It occurs in the case of aortic regurgitation, increased stroke volume results in abrupt upstroke.

Water-soluble vitamins are those vitamins which are filtered through the kidneys and excreted in urine when consumed in excess. These are generally nontoxic and to be supplied daily. Body reserve of these vitamins is minimal, hence toxicity does not develop. Water-soluble vitamins include Vitamin C and B complex including thiamine, niacin, riboflavin, pyridoxine, biotin, cynacobalamine and folate.

Water sorption refers to a material that absorbs water.

Water ratio is the mixing proportion of plaster expressed as a decimal fraction. If 100 gm. of plaster is to be mixed with 50 gram of water the W/P ratio is 0.50.

Wavelength refers to distance between any two corresponding points in the wave. A measurement of physical size, which is important with respect to how the laser light is delivered to the surgical site and to how it reacts with tissue.

Wavelength is measured in meters; microns (10^{-6}m) and nanometers (10^{-9}m).

Wedge fracture are fracture of vertebra results from a flexion force. Posterior elements are intact. Reduction is not required.

Wegener's granulomatosis was first described by Wegener 1936. It is of unknown etiology involving vascular, renal and respiratory system. It may occur at any age. It may develop rhinitis, sinusitis and otitis or ocular symptoms. Hemorrhage or vascular skin lesions are common. It is characterized by necrotizing granulomatous vaculitis of the respiratory tract and kidneys. *Oral Manifestations:* Oral mucosal ulceration, abnormal tooth mobility, spontaneous exfoliation of teeth, delayed healing, gingival enlargement may be localized to a single papilla or generalized. It appears as a florid, exospheric growth with a granular surface. Gingival is reddish purple in color and bleeds on provocation. Appearance is that of "over-riped strawberry".

Weldability is an ability of a substance that has the capability of being joined by the passage of a strong electric current.

W

Well-circumscribed lesion is described when the borders of lesion are specifically not defined. Margins and extent of lesions are well seen.

Wernicke's aphasia refers to language disorder where the speech is fluent and effortless but comprehension is impaired. Speech is without any meaning. Reading is impaired and writing is full of spelling mistakes. In global aphasia all parameters of language are impaired due to lesion involving territory of middle cerebral artery. There is an extensive lesion of posterior superior temporal region.

Wernicke's encephalopathy is a cerebral form of thiamine deficiency. It presents acutely in thiamine deficiency. Patient is confused and bilateral symmetrical ophthalmoplegia, nystagmus and ataxia may be present. There may develop permanent memory defect.

Wet gangrene develops when both arterial and venous supply are blocked suddenly. Wet gangrene is rare except in diabetes. Gangrene of internal organs is wet type strangulated hernia, torsions and intestinal adhesions may cause gangrene of bowel. Lesions of lung cause irregular greenish black cavities with foul smell.

Wetting is the spreading of a liquid drop on the surface of a solid.

Wheal is a red raised area around the injured skin.

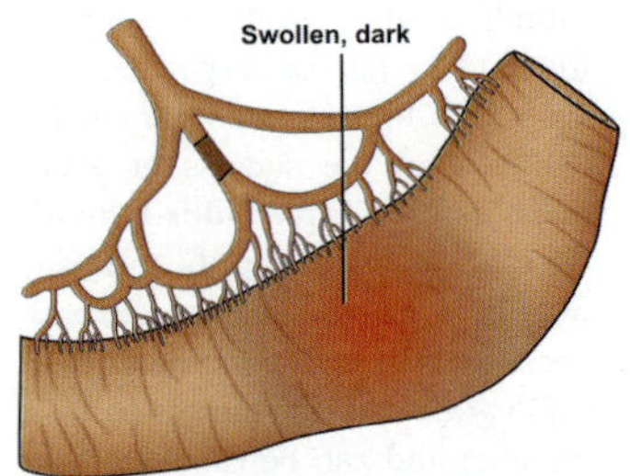

Fig.: *Wet gangrene (bowel)*

Wheezing is a high-pitched continuous musical sound heard due to narrowing of airways. This may be noticed by the patient or relatives or others as in case of asthma. A low-pitched inspiratory sound heard in the obstruction of larynx or trachea is known as "stridor."

White gold alloy is an alloy containing gold and white metal, e.g. silver or palladium that imparts a white appearance to entire mass.

White matter is made up of modulated nerve fibers and supporting glial cells. There are 3 types of fibers. Transverse fibers interconnect two cerebral hemispheres making up corpus collosum. Projection fibers connect the cerebral cortex with lower portions of brain and spinal cord. The short association fibers connect adjacent gyri.

White object is an object that reflects all incident color lights.

White sponge nevus is also known as Cannon's disease. It is an autosomal dominant condition that affects only oral mucosa. Buccal mucosa is the site of lesions. Lesions are asymptomatic. Friction from mastication may strip off the keratotic layer. Cytological study will show empty epithelial cells. Centrally placed are pyknotic nuclei. Oral lesion may be wide-spread involving checks, palate, gingiva and tongue. Mucus appears thick and folded with a spongy texture with white hue. Ragged white areas may be removed by gentle rubbing without bleeding. Numerous pedigrees of families may show it. There is no treatment for the condition. There is no evidence of lesions being transformed into malignancy.

Whitlow is a purulent infection involving end of finger.

Whooping cough a respiratory illness also known as pertussis bacteria known as bordetella pertussis caused by Gram negative toccobacillus and principally affects younger person and children. Focal atelectasis, emphysema and peribronchial infiltration

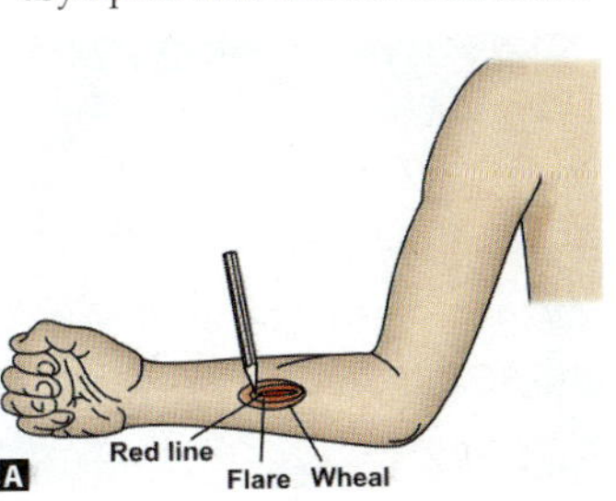

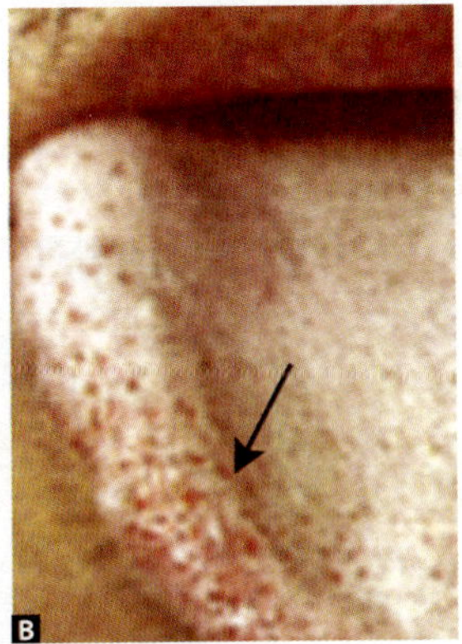

Figs A and B: *(A) Wheal; (B) White spongy nevus*

by lymphocytes are common. Incubation is 7-16 days. It has 3 stages. In catarrhal stage, clinical picture resembles respiratory catarrh. In paroxysmal stage the, diurnal cough becomes paroxysm of 15-20 short coughs followed by deep inspiration with closed glottis producing whoop. Engorged conjunctiva and petechial hemorrhage in forehead and epistaxis are common. Erythromycin is a drug of choice.

Wickham's striae refer to white raised areas on the buccal gingival and palatal soft tissues. Fungal infection, oral leukoplakia and lineal albicans are also white but have different associations and should be differentiated.

Widening of sella turcica takes place due to acromegaly or brain tumor. AP dimension ranges about 11 mm. and vertical measure about 8 mm.

Wine is produced by conversion of sugar present in fruits of different varieties into alcohol and CO_2. Grapes contain 10 to 20% sugar. Fermentation is carried out in vats with the help of selected enzymes. Agreeable aroma and flavor are due to various aromatic principles present in fruits. The special bouquets develop only after wine has been aged for periods varying from four to five years to several decades. Alcoholic content varies from 10 to 20%.

Wisdom tooth means third molar and appears later in life between 17-25 years of age. In many persons these may remain imbedded in jaw bone and are said to be impacted. These have to be removed otherwise; remain the source of infection.

Words in combinations make sentences, allowing for complex communication.

Working length is defined as "the distance from a coronal reference point to a point at which canal preparation and obturation should terminate".

Working range of wire is the maximum deflection of a wire within the elastic range.

Working time is the duration from the start of mixing to the time when a test rod leaves a permanent identification in the material upon withdrawal.

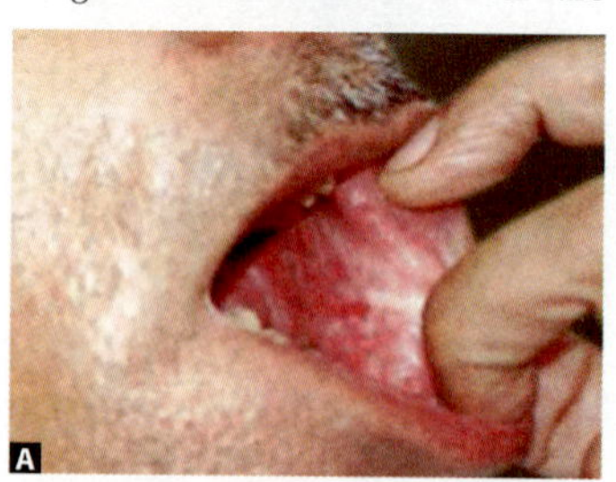

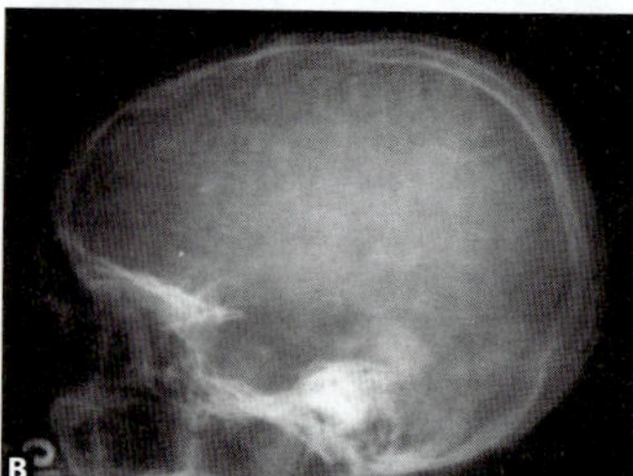

Figs A and B: *(A) Wickham's striae; (B) Widening of sella turcica*

W

Worm's theory is one of the ancient theories of dental caries. According to the ancient Sumerian text, toothache was caused by a worm that drank the blood of the teeth and fed on the roots of the jaws. This legend of the worm was discovered on one of many clay tablets excavated. Niffer, Ur, and other cities within the Euphrates valley of the lower Mesopotamian area and estimated to date from about 5000 BC. The idea that caries is caused by a worm was almost universal at one time, as evidenced by the writing of Homer and popular lore of China, India, Finland, and Scotland.

X

Xenograft refer heterograft.

Xerophthalmia means where the sebaceous and hair follicles of skin and tear glands of eye become blocked with horny plugs of keratin so that their secretion diminishes. Lack of tears and heaping up of epithelium on the sclera and conjunctiva. In conjuctival xerosis conjunctiva looks muddy and wrinkled instead of transparent and clear. It becomes dry.

Xeroradiography is a technique that uses modified xerographic copying techniques to record images produced by diagnostic X-rays. They have an additional feature called "edge enhancement" effect. Due to these small structures and areas of subtle density differences are made more visible. They contain uniformly charged selenium plates. Advantages—(i) Half of X-ray radiation is required. (ii) It produces real image. (iii) Reflected light is used. (iv) No need for chemical processing in dark room. (v) This technique is extensively used in the diagnosis of diseases of breast. (vi) It is economical.

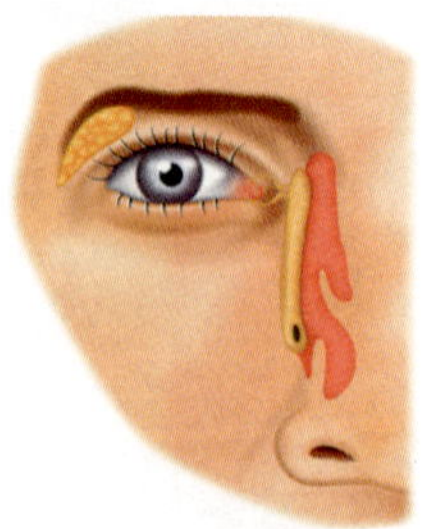

Fig.: *Xerophthalmia*

Xerostomia is defined as the perception of oral dryness. There is a dryness of mouth and all degrees of dryness occur. It is often due to a reduction in salivary flow rates of the major and minor salivary glands. Humans suffering from decreased or lack of salivary secretions often experience an increased rate of dental caries and rapid tooth destruction. Mucosa will appear dry and atrophic. It may be pale and translucent. Tongue may show fissuring and cracking. It may result in rampant dental caries.

X-ray absorptiometry is a diagnostic test where bone thickness is usually measured with bone density scan. Dual energy X-ray absorptiometry is a common test to measure bone thickness in spine, hips and wrists. This test gives two scores. T-score and X-score. T-score compares your bone thickness to the thickness of a healthy 30 years old. While X-score compares your bone thickness to the bone thickness of other person of your age. T-score lower than -2.5 means you have osteoporosis and T-score between -1 and -2.5 shows osteopenia.

Xylitol is the best nutritive sucrose substitute with respect to caries prevention. It is non-acidogenic, hence non-cariogenic. It is also non-cariogenic by inhibiting the growth of certain bacteria (*S. mutans*) stimulating salivary flow and increasing salivary calcium concentration.

Y

Yellow brow film is a processing error, where the film appears brown–yellow due to exhausted developer or fixer.

Yellow lesions give yellow color and are caused by carotene, accumulation of pus, exudation of serum and aggregation of lymphoid tissue. Yellow color is seen in ulcers or pustules. Serum is normally a yellow or straw-colored fluid. Normal lipid containing structures such as Fordyce's granules usually appear yellow.

Yellow stains generally occur from the food pigments and are also associated with the presence of bacterial plaque; it has a dull, light yellow appearance due to bacterial plaque which is common to all ages and more prominent in patients where personal oral hygiene is neglected.

Yield stress is the stress at which dislocation motion and permanent deformation and plastic flow begin.

Young's frame is a U-shaped metal or plastic form used to hold a dental dam in place.

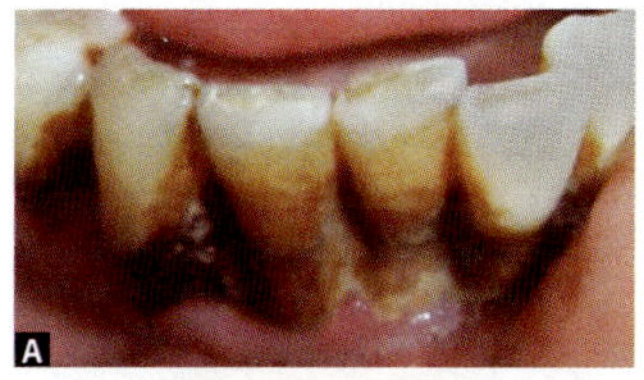

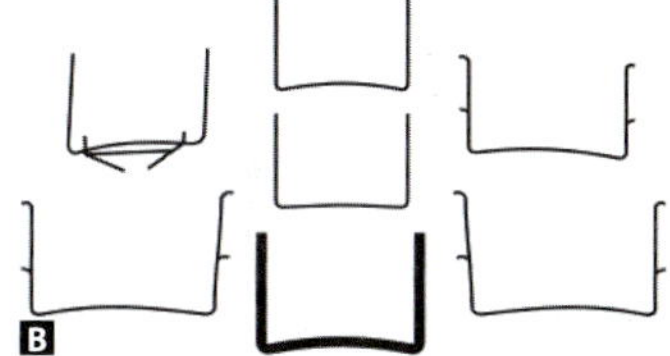

Figs A and B: *(A) Yellow stains; (B) Young rubber dam frame*

Z

Z score is a deviation score divided by the standard deviation. It indicates how many standard deviations the raw score is above or below the mean.

Zimmerman Leband syndrome is a rare autosomal dominant congential disorder in which patient develops gingival fibromatosis with defects of ear, nose, bones and terminal phalanges. Joints become hypermobile. Spleen is enlarged.

Zinc is a mineral present in human body. Average human body contains 1.4 to 2.3 gram of zinc. Highest concentrations are found in liver, bone, prostate and eye. It is a constituent of insulin. Zinc plasma level is 96 micro grams per 100 ml in adults. Daily requirement is 5 to 10 mg. Deficiency of it results in anorexia, pernicious anemia, thalassemia. It maintains normal taste.

Zinc oxide eugenol is a dental material that is generally used suitable as a base under metallic restorations due to its sealing quality. Eugenol has bacteriostatic property. Within 8 weeks period an increasing amount of reparative dentin is noted. Although it causes only a slight pulp response and yet promotes reparative dentin formation in deep cavities. It is a material of choice for use over injured pulps or as a base in deep cavity preparation.

Z-track technique is a method of giving injection that prevents medication from leaking outside the muscle.

Zygomatic arch is a bar of bone lying horizontally on the lateral aspect of the skull. It has 2 parts, i.e. Posterior part which is formed by the zygomatic process of the temporal bone and anterior part by the temporal process of the zygomatic bone.

Zygote: The fertilized ovum.

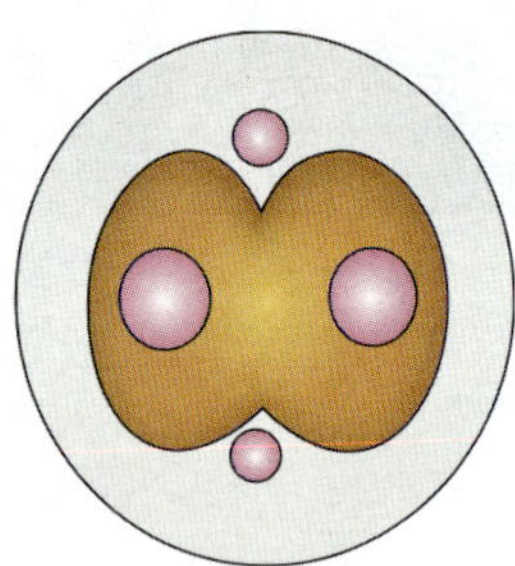

Fig.: *Zygote*

Section 2

Appendices

Annexures

Annexure – I	History of Dentistry
Annexure – II	Syndromes
Annexure – III	Causes of Dental Diseases
Annexure – IV	Synonyms/Alternatives
Annexure – V	Tooth Numbering System
Annexure – VI	Tables
Annexure – VII	Nutritional Values
Annexure – VIII	A. Blood Investigations and Interpretations
	B. Blood Chemistry
	C. Urine Investigations and their Interpretation
	D. Stool Investigations and their Interpretation
Annexure – IX	Miscellaneous

Annexure-I

HISTORY OF DENTISTRY

Dentistry—Past and Present

Dental diseases have remained almost similar throughout history. Decay, toothaches, periodontal disease and premature tooth loss were documented in history. The exact time that dentistry has made its presence felt is not known but there are sufficient evidences of its existence among the various civilizations. Since Dental History is such a broad field, a few of the highlights of dentistry will be mentioned in order of importance and chronology.

Pre-historically

- Life consisted of simple creatures of the sea, which consisted of protoplasmic cells.
- They survived by engulfing themselves around a desired morsel, they were able to absorb food. Later a slit developed the forerunner of the oral cavity and great gut.
- Then there was development of tentacles and feelers developed around this slit, which helped them to carry the food to the slit, oral cavity and great gut.
- Then nature took the outer layer of skin and carried it inward to the oral cavity. This skin contained tentacles which were the forerunners of our teeth. These tentacles, also called shagreen, were calcified.
- Some of these sea creatures developed lungs and became amphibians.
- Some began to spend time on land. At first they crawled on their bellies, later they developed limbs and feet and arose from the ground. Faced with a new environment including a mixed diet, the creatures evolved into stronger animals made up of hard bone and tough muscle fiber. Originally three single tentacles fused and became tri-conodonts.
- These tri-conodonts later changed into teeth very similar to the catarrine apes. The descendants of these apes have the similar dental formula as humans.
- Fire and its benefits were discovered. Cooking made seafood more palatable. Fish and shellfish became the staple diet as well as nuts, fruits, and the flesh of animals; then the cultivated grains such as rice, wheat and barley were added to the diet.
- If we go back to the beginning of history at 4000 BC, toothaches can be traced to the earliest records. In the Egyptian manuscripts known as Eber's Papyri, which dates back to 3700 BC, where dental diseases such as toothaches and sore gums are mentioned.

- 3000 years ago, the Chinese manuscripts of that period, at least nine dental diseases were listed and also along with them were listed the prescriptions for their treatment. Ancient skulls showed the presence of decay. In the Giza Pyramids, skulls were found with evidence of tooth decay.
- People of early ages had odd beliefs concerning teeth. The Egyptians believed that the mouse was under the direct protection of the sun therefore if one had a toothache, the split body of a warm mouse was applied to the affected side. In India, the cuspid of Buddha was enshrined in a famous temple (at Kandy) and prayed to in fertility rites. Prayers were offered to saints for the relief of pain. St Apollonia of Alexandria, 249 AD, was one such saint. She is known as the Patron Saint of Dentistry.

Egyptians

- The first known dentist was an Egyptian named Hesi-Re (3000 BC). He was the chief dentist to the Pharaohs. He was also a physician, indicating an association between medicine and dentistry but in the 5th century BC Herodatus, a historian, described the medical art in Egypt: "The art of medicine is distributed thus: Each physician is a physician of one disease and no more; and the whole country is full of physicians, for some profess themselves to be physicians of the eyes, others of the head, teeth, stomach, and others of more obscure ailments". Dentistry today is somewhat specialized and is divided into eight specialities that are as follows:
    - 1901 Orthodontics
    - 1918 Oral surgery
    - 1918 Periodontics
    - 1918 Prosthodontics
    - 1927 Pedodontics
    - 1937 Public health
    - 1946 Oral pathology
    - 1963 Endodontics.
- The first evidence of a surgical operation was found in Egypt. A mandible with two perforations just below the root of the first molar indicated the establishment of drainage of an abscessed tooth.
- Egyptians practiced the splinting of teeth which dates back to 2750 BC where it shows two molars fastened with heavy gold wire.

Chinese

- The Chinese were known to have treated dental ills with knife, cautery, and acupuncture, a technique whereby they punctured different areas of the body with a needle. There is no evidence of mechanical dentistry at that time.
- Marco Polo in 2700 BC stated that the Chinese did cover teeth with thin gold leaf only for esthetic purposes.

- The earliest practice of the prosthetic arts was among the ancient Phoenicians circa 500 BC Hammarabi, ruler of all lower Mesopotamia (1760 BC), established a state controlled economy in which fees charged by physicians were set.

Greeks

Greeks contributed mostly on the medical side. The ancient Greek physician:

- **Aesculapius (1250 BC)** gained great fame for medical knowledge and skill. Apollo was listed as his father. He originated the art of bandaging and use of purgatives. He also advocated cleaning of teeth and extractions.
- **Hippocrat (500 BC)** was supposed to be a descendant of Aesculapius. Hippocrates became famous both as practitioner and writer on medical subjects. He did not believe in magic and stressed nature's role in healing. Hippocrates raised the art of medicine to a high level. Also in one of his texts (Peri-Arthron) he devoted 32 paragraphs to the dentition. He appreciated the importance of teeth. He accurately described the technique for reducing a fracture of the jaw and also for replacing a dislocated mandible. He was familiar with extraction forceps for this is mentioned in one of his writings.
- **Aristotle (384 BC)** who follows Hippocrates, accurately described extraction forceps and in his book "De Partibus Animation" and also devoted a complete chapter to the teeth. He also stated that figs and soft sweets produce decay. He called it a putrefactive process instead of fermentative.

Etruscans

Etruscans (100–400 BC) made their greatest contribution in restorative dentistry. In Italian museums there are numerous, specimens of crowns and bridges. In 1870, the dental engine was invented. A very unusual specimen is a bridge that was constructed about 2500 years ago. This consists of several gold bands fastened to natural teeth and supporting three artificial teeth. Etruscan art, seen at its best in Florence, reflects some oriental influence but essentially it is their own. Conquered in 309 BC, they were absorbed by the Roman Empire.

Romans

Famous Roman physicians are named below:

- **Celsus (25 BC–50 AD)** Hippocrates did not believe in magic but Celsus believed that general physical deterioration caused dental diseases. For toothaches, he prescribed:
  - Hot water fermentations
  - Narcotics
  - Mustard seed
  - Counter irritants
  - Use of the cautery

- Alum for soft tissue disease
- Extraction of badly broken down teeth. He recommended filling the cavity with lead prior to extraction as a means of lessening the chance of fracturing the crown.
- Introduced the technique for reducing fractures.
- Introduced first technique for tooth straightening or positioning.

- **Archigenus (100 AD)**
  - Pulpitis was recognized by him.
  - Invented the dental drill to enter into pulp chamber.
- **Galen (200 AD)** was considered to be the greatest physician since Hippocrates was the first to recognize that a toothache could be due to:
  - Pulpitis (inflammation of the pulp)
  - Pericementitis (inflammation of radicular portion of the tooth)
  - He classified teeth into centrals, cuspids and molars.
- **Hebrews** gave first evidence of dentistry among the Jews:
  - Relief of toothache and artificial restorations may be found in a collection of books known as the Talmud (352 AD–407 AD).
  - The worm was blamed for decay. Also stated that gum disease started in the mouth but ended in the gut.
  - As for extractions — all cultures expressed anxiety about removing a cuspid for fear of eye injury. This superstition continues today.

The Middle Ages

- 410 AD, the clever and rational approaches of Hippocrates and Celsus had disappeared; magic and superstitious dominated. Then came the **Albucasis**, (1013 AD). He was considered the great exponent of dental surgery in the middle ages. In his book the first illustration of dental instruments was found which was as follows:
  - Surgical elevators
  - Surgical forceps
  - scalers
  - Cautery
  - Dental saws and files for caries removal

Besides being a famous surgeon and competent writer, he was also a greater teacher and believed in the referred pain theory. He accurately described technique for extractions, with special emphasis on careful manipulation of soft tissue. He also described treatment for partially luxated teeth.

The Barber-Surgeons

At the onset of the middle Ages, monks became physicians and dentists. Barbers had acted as assistants to the monks. When the Pope in 1163 ruled that any operation involving the shedding of blood was incompatible with the priestly office, the barber took over the practice of surgery. The barber surgeons were not the only ones doing extractions; another group made up of vagabonds were known as tooth drawers. They plied their trade in public squares. For a while then, dentistry was carried on by Barber-surgeons both in France and England. However, in France (1700) anyone desiring to practice oral surgery and restorative dentistry had to take a regular prescribed examination.

Founding of Universities and Introduction of Dental Texts

Chirurgia Magna was written by the famous French surgeon **Guy de Cahuliac** in 1386. In this text, he devoted some space to pathology and therapeutics of the teeth. Cahuliac was first to coin the term **dentator** and **dentists**. The English term dentist came from his original terms. Following Cahuliac came **Giovanni de Arcoli** in 1400. His opinions and instruments were somewhat modern. His pelican for extraction of teeth was used for years and his root forceps could be used today. He advised good oral cleaning habits and to avoid hot and cold substances as well as sweet stuff. He was first to mention filling teeth with gold.

Famous Scientists

Vesalius (1500 AD) of Belgium, became an anatomist at the University of Padua, Italy. In medical profession he, laid the foundation for true scientific research which is the basis of our present-day medical practice. He accurately described the teeth and pulp chambers.

Fallopius was another anatomist, a pupil of Vesalius. He is credited with the descriptions of the dental follicle, trigeminal nerve, auditory nerve, glossopharyngeal nerve the hard and the soft palate. He stated that teeth were not true bone.

Eustachius (1500 AD) gave the complete anatomical description of teeth and their development. He was credited with the first complete dental book, ninety five pages of anatomy, embryology, physiology, blood and nerve supply of the teeth. In this text, he completely describes the anatomy of the teeth, their development, the alveolus and the periodontal membrane.

Leonardo da Vinci (end of 15th Century) described the anatomy of the jaws, teeth and maxillary sinus. These drawings are the first to accurately describe the maxillary sinus. However, credit has been given to **Dr Nathaniel Highmore** of England (1650 AD).

Ambrose Pare (16th Century) was a Barber-Surgeon at 16 years of age and became a member of the College of Surgeons at the age of 37. He was the first to describe Palatal Obturators and transplant techniques. His instruments, though crude, could be used today.

Malpighi (17th Century) a great anatomist and the founder of histology, had made great use of the microscope for tissue studies.

Leeuwenhoek (17th Century) invented the microscope. He described the dentinal tubuli and was the first to see organisms of the mouth.

Purman of Breslau (middle 17th Century) is known for wax impressions.

Philip Pfaff (18th Century) introduced plaster for pouring up models.

Pierre Fauchard (18th Century - 1728) Father of Scientific Dentistry wrote a great text "Surgeon Dentist". He not only wrote a complete work on Odontology in two volumes but also recognized the intimate relationship between oral conditions and general health. He advocated the use of lead to fill cavities. He removed all decay and if the pulp was exposed, and used the cautery. He prescribed oil of cloves and cinnamon for pulpitis. He also described partial dentures and full dentures in his text and constructed dentures with springs and used human teeth. Gold dowels were used in root canals filled with lead. He was also known as Father of Orthodontics.

Robert Bunon (1743) printed the first dental therapeutics text, dentistry's first pharmacopeia.

Thomas Berdmore (1768) wrote "Disorders and Deformities of Teeth and Gums".

John Hunter (1771) wrote "Natural History of the Human Teeth".

Joseph Fox wrote Pupil of Hunter; wrote text, same title "Natural History of the Human Teeth".

John Greenwood (1789) dentures for George Washington were made by him.

Charles Goodyear (1840) discovered vulcanite rubber. It was used for denture bases. This discovery led to false teeth for the millions. Dentures were called vulcanite dentures.

EJ Dunning (1844) made plaster of Paris impressions, first shown in America.

M Bourdet (mid-18th Century) described use of gold for base plates.

Role of Women in Dentistry

The first woman dentist in England was a widow of Dr Povey (1719). When he died she took over his practice. The first woman dentist in the United States was Emeline Rupert Jones of Connecticut. She too, took over her husband's practice after he died. After his death, she took over and practiced for at least 50 years. She was accepted in both the Connecticut State Dental Society in 1893 and National Dental Association in 1914. The honor of being the first woman graduate dentist goes to Dr Lucy Hobbs (1865). She graduated from the Ohio Dental College.

Famous Scientists

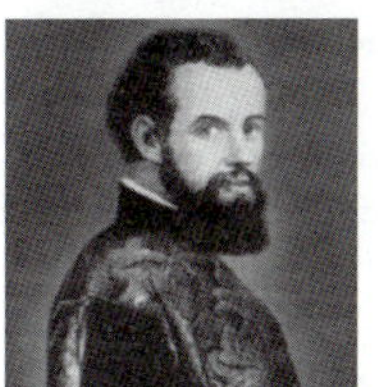
Vesalius

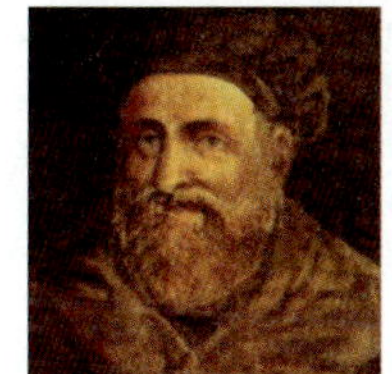
Fallopius

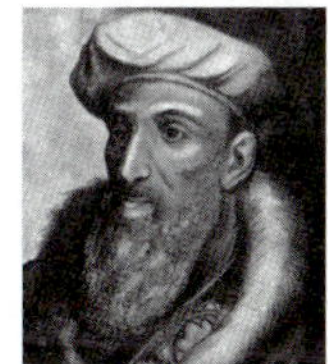
Eustachius

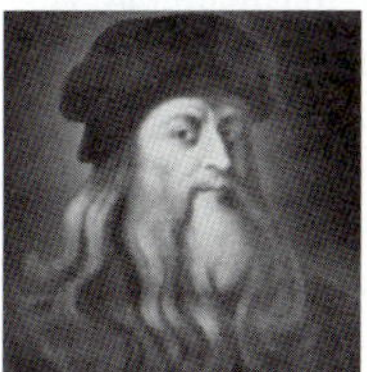
Leonardo da Vinci

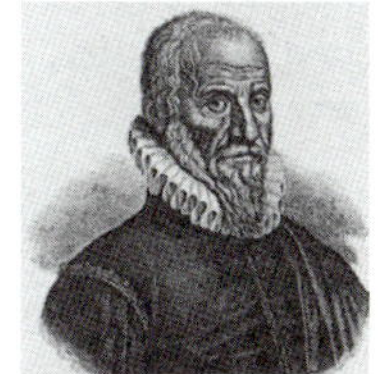
Ambrose Pare

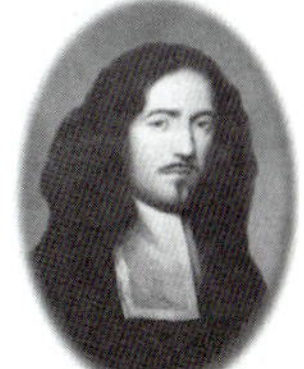
Malpighi

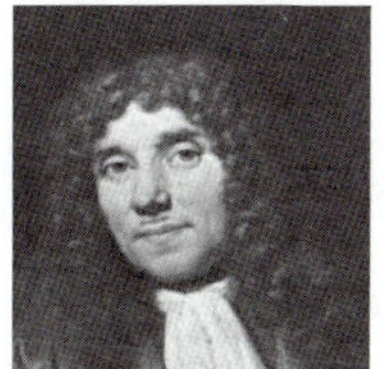
Leeuwenhoek

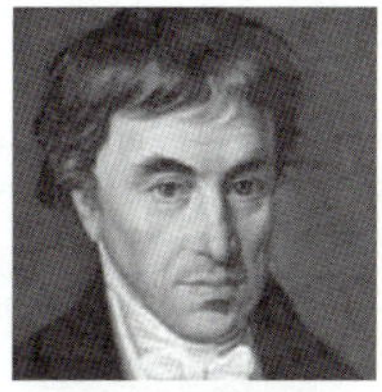
Philip Pfaff

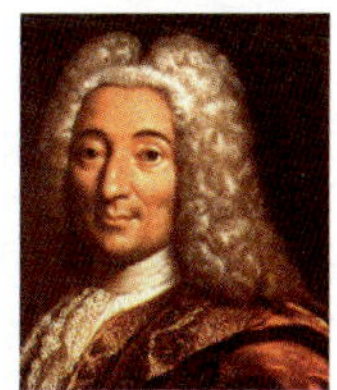
Pierre Fauchard

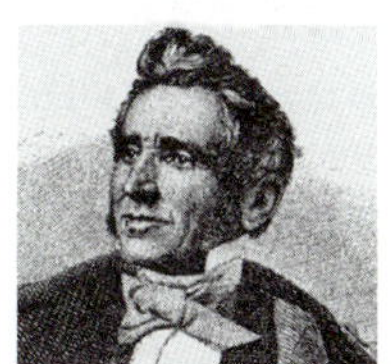
John Hunter

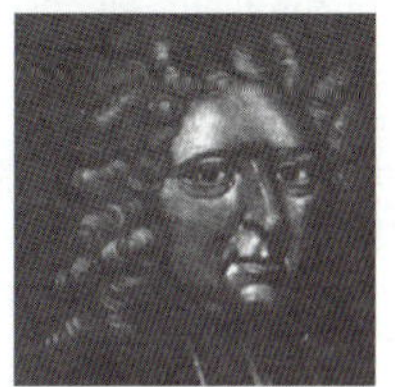
Robert Bunon

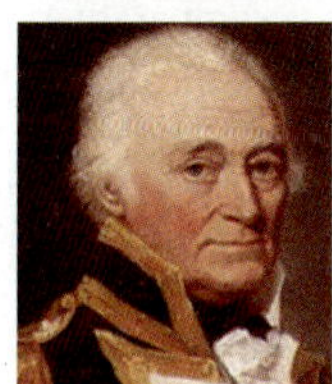
Thomas Berdmore

HISTORICAL EVENTS OF DENTISTRY IN CHRONOLOGICAL ORDER

- 2750 BC–Mandible of the ancient period shows evidence of having had a surgical operation to relieve an alveolar abscess.
- 2500 BC–Egyptian, earliest evidence of simple retentive dental prosthesis as found in Tomb 984 at Gizeh, the linking together of the lower left second and third molar with gold wire woven around the gingival margins of the teeth.
- 1900 BC–Code of **Hammurabi** established the civil and penal responsibility of the physician, dental penalties as to the extraction of teeth.
- 1700 BC–**The Edwin Smith** Surgical Papyrus transcribed from an earlier manuscript contains methods for reducing fractures of the mandible.
- 700-510 BC–Etruscan period of dentistry, i.e. Middle Italy, few examples of their fixed or removable bridgework has been preserved in various museums.
- 669-626 BC–**King Ashurbanipal** had a Collection of Babylonian cuneiform tables and a library. Tooth worm theory. 5th Century Examples of Phoenician simple retentive dental prosthetics found at Sidon.
- 490-425 BC–**Herodotus**, the Greek historian and traveller, describes Egypt as being the home of medical specialists. Confirmation of this was done by **Hermann Junker** in 1914.
- 480 BC–Roman period begins. Dentistry was probably practiced before medicine.
- 460-370–BC **Hippocrates**, the founder of Medicine was first to recognize the teeth *in utero*, humoral pathology, use of gold wire for fractures and instruction on how to handle instruments.
- 450 BC–**Roman Laws** of the Twelve Tables and the permission to bury the dead with gold dental work with which the teeth may be bound together. The use of Centuries BC gold shell crowns.
- 384-322 BC–**Aristotle**, pupil of Plato was the first to make a study of comparative anatomy of the teeth. He also mentioned the extraction of teeth with forceps.
- 30 AD–Celsus wrote his De Medicina, is the earliest to mention the filling of teeth with lint or lead, however, to extract the tooth more readily and not for its preservation. He suggested the binding of teeth in fractures of the jaw and orthodontic treatment.
- 48-117 AD–Archigenes of Apameia, a Roman physician recommended the use of the drill in filling teeth "right down to the center of the tooth, to give vent to the accumulated pus."

- 130-201 AD **Galen**, the Prince of Physicians, in 162 began to practice in Rome and in 168 was appointed as the imperial physician. His treatise (Venice 1490) was a standard textbook for centuries. He was also the earliest to mention the nerves of teeth. He recommended the use of file in removing the carious defect, he also mentioned about pulpitis and pericementitis.
- 249 AD **St Apollonia**, the Patron Saint of Dentistry, had her teeth extracted in Alexandria.
- 936-1013 AD **Albucasis** a physician born near Cordova, was one of the most learned physicians and surgeons of his time. His Dechirurgia, one of the great surgical treatises, contains illustrations of both surgical and dental instruments with detailed description of the use of them. He described a method of transplanting teeth and the use of gold wire to ligate loose ones. Besides improving the type of extracting forceps, he devised many elevators and scalers. He was also one of the earliest to devise a method to correct deformities in the mouth and dental arches.
- 1308-1745 AD France, Guild of Barber-Surgeons founded and remained active until 1745.
- **Guy de Chauliac** completed his celebrated work on surgery (published in 1478) and therein we obtained a clear and concise idea of the condition of dentistry during the fourteenth century. He coined the term dentators.
- 1452-1519 AD **Leonardo da Vinci**, who inspired the work of **Vesalius**, was an anatomist and original dissector of the human body. His manuscript presents the earliest accurate drawings of the skull, teeth, associated structures and maxillary sinus.1460 AD Earliest English medical manuscript Guy de Cahuliac's Surgery.
- 1468 AD **Barbers** in England obtained charter from King Edward IV.
- 1498 AD Invention of the modern toothbrush by the Chinese on June 24.
- 1514 AD Publication of **Giovanni's da Vigo's** work on surgery that passed through innumerable editions wherein we find the earliest printed record of the filling of teeth with gold foil after first excavation and shaping the cavity.
- 1538 AD **Andreas Vesalius**, the famous anatomist, was the first to use wood cuts to illustrate his writings; therein is to be found much relating to the tooth.
- 1542 AD **Ambroise Pare**, famous military surgeon, revived the old method of compression of nerve trunks to produce local anesthesia. He also mentioned transplantation, filling of teeth and ligation of teeth with gold wire. He described palatal obturators as well.
- 1543 AD **Andreas Vesalius** gave important observations on the development of teeth.
- 1561 AD **Gabriel Fallopius** wrote about the dental follicle and development of teeth.

- 1651 AD **Nathaniel Highmore** described maxillary sinus in the superior maxillary bone (1673) microorganisms (animalcules) in teeth and described their tubular construction.
- 1683 AD **Antonie van Leeuwenhoek** discovered the use of microscope
- 1728 AD First edition of **Pierre Fauchard** (founder of Modern Dentistry) textbook on "The Surgeon's Dentist."
- 1728 AD **Pierre Fauchard** great work "Le Chirurgien Dentiste"
- 1733-1735 AD **James Reading** and **James Mills** first tooth-drawers in New York and perhaps in America.
- 1756 AD **Philip Pfaff** made plaster models and described taking the bite. He also practiced capping the pulp.
- 1759 AD The designation Dentist first began to be used.
- 1763 AD **John Baker,** MD, Surgeon Dentist was the earliest qualified dentist to practice in Boston and in America.
- 1766 AD **Robert Woofendale**, pupil of Berdmore, arrives in America and locates in New York. Thomas Berdmore of London published the first English dental textbook in which he claimed the use of sugar to be deleterious. He became the Dentist to his Majesty.
- 1769 AD Title of Doctor began to be used.
- 1771 AD **John Hunter**, comparative anatomist and surgeon, published his classic description of the anatomy of the human teeth, he demanded the removal of the pulp before filling the teeth in the case of transplantation.
- 1774 AD Introduction of porcelain into dentistry by French apothecary **Duchatenu**.
- 1778 AD Body of General Joseph Warren identified by dental work done in the mouth by **Paul Revere**.
- 1779 AD **Isaac Greenwood, Sr.,** began to practice Dentistry in Boston.
- 1784 AD **Isaac Greenwood, Jr.,** began his dental practice in New York.
- 1788 AD Improvement and development of porcelain dentures by **deChemant**.
- 1791 AD Establishment of the first dental clinic in the Dispensary of the City of New York.
- 1793 AD **Benjamin Bell's** interest in dental pathology and therapy led him to important observations on the pulp and pericementum.
- 1794 AD Earliest use of mineral paste teeth in America by **Le Breton**. **John Greenwood** began to swage gold bases for dentures. He made George Washington's dentures.
- 1801 AD First dental book to be published in America by **Richard Cortland Skinner**.
- 1806 AD Individual porcelain teeth with baked-in metal pins, invented by **Fonzi**.

- 1819 AD Mixing of coin silver fillings and mercury into a silver paste, by **Tavenu** in France.
- 1832 AD **Snell** - first dental chair.
- 1836 AD Arsenic introduced by **Spooner** for the killing of pulps.
- 1839 AD First dental periodical, the American Journal of Dental Science.
- 1840 AD The American Society of Dental Surgeons, first national dental organization. The Baltimore College of Dental Surgery, the first school in the world for the training of dentists was founded by Harris and Harden.
- 1842 AD **Crawford W Long** discover anesthetic agent, but did not publicize it.
- 1844 AD Beginning of large scale manufacture of porcelain teeth by **SS White**. Discovery of nitrous oxide anesthesia by **H Wells** and the use of plaster of Paris for impressions.
- 1851 AD Patent for hard rubber (Vulcanite) granted to **Nelson Goodyear**.
- 1855 AD Cohesive gold foil for filling teeth, introduced by **Robert Arthur**.
- 1859 AD Organization of American Dental Association on a representative basis.
- 1863 AD Organization of National Association of Dental Examiners.
- 1864 AD Rubber dam suggested by **Sanford C Barnum**.
- 1866 AD Organization of college faculties.
- 1866 Tiny multiple cysts of palate in fetus and neonates were first described by **Heinrich Bohn** and by **Alois Epstein** in 1880.
- 1868 AD Combination of nitrous oxide and oxygen for prolonged anesthesia, by **Edmund Andrews**.
- 1872 AD First foot-engine, invented by **Morrison**.
- 1877 AD Hydraulic chair invented by **Wilkinson**.
- 1884 AD **Keller** suggested cocaine hydrochlorate for topical anesthesia. **WS Halstead** used conductive anesthesia for the mandible.
- 1885 **Malassez** named the term adamantinoma.
- 1887 AD Gutta percha root canal points.
- 1888 Mikulicz disease was described by **Mr Mikulicz**
- 1890 A.D **WD Miller** described microorganism of the human mouth.
- 1891 AD Extension for prevention and scientific cavity preparation suggested by **GV Black**.
- 1892 AD The establishment of a three-year course in dental colleges.
- 1893 **Garre** described thickening of periosteum of long bones due to infection.
- 1893 AD System of dental nomenclature by **GV Black**
- 1895 A.D **Roentgen** discovered the X-ray. **GV Black** developed the balanced amalgam alloys.
- 1896 AD **C Edward Kells** demonstrated use of Roentgen rays in dentistry.

- 1897 AD **BF Philbrook**, presented paper on "Cast Gold Fillings," the **Taggart** inlay method. American Dental Association and Southern Dental Association consolidated under the name of National Dental Association.
- 1899 AD One year of high school's a requirement for admission to dental school.
- 1901 AD **Weston A Price** recommended the use of X-ray in root canal work.
- 1903 AD Four years course in dental colleges established.
- 1906 AD **Einhorn** recommended novocaine and adrenaline combination for local anesthesia.
- 1907 AD **William H Taggart** demonstrated the cast gold inlay.
- 1909 AD Dental Educational Counsel of America organized.
- 1912 AD National Dental Association organized on a district basis.
- 1913 The term Taur odontin was originated by **Sir Arthur Keith**. Body of tooth is enlarged at the cost of roots.
- 1914 AD J **Leon Williams** developed typical tooth forms.
- 1915 AD **McKay** and **Black** published results of investigation of fluoride in drinking water.
- 1916 Mottled enamel was described by **GV Black** and **F Mackay**.
- 1920 Dentin dysplasia was described by **Ballschmiede**.
- 1922 AD National Dental Association changed name to American Dental Association.
- Association publication changed from National to Journal of the American Dental Association.
- 1933 The retrocuspid papilla was first described by **Hirshfeld** as a small, elevated nodule.
- 1936 Neonatal line in deciduous teeth was described by **Schour**.
- 1938 Dentinogenesis imperfecta was diagnosed by **Finn, Hodge** and his **co-workers** confirmed in 1939.
- 1939 **Dodd** and her colleagues isolated herpes simplex virus from gingivostomatitis.
- 1939 **Parker** and **Jackson** described reticulum cell sarcoma.
- 1939-40 **Gall, Mallory, Jackson** and **Parker** developed classification for malignant lymphoma.
- 1940 The term eosinophilic granuloma of bone was introduced by **Lichtenstein** and **Jaffe** in 1940.
- 1942 Benign chondroblastoma of bone was named by **Jaffe** and **Lichtenstein**.
- 1942 **Stout** and **Murray** suggested the term hemangiopericytoma.
- 1945 Mucoepidermoid carcinoma was described by **Stuart Foote**.
- 1945 **Dublin** and **Johnson** described benign osteoblastoma.

- 1946 **Jaffe** and **Lichtenstein** described chondromyxoid fibroma.
- 1947 Adenoid squamous cell carcinoma was described by **Lever**.
- 1948 Verrucous carcinoma was defined by **Ackerman**.
- 1949 **Mccarthy** described pyostomatitis vegetans.
- 1952 **Christopherson** described alveolar soft part sarcoma.
- 1953 AD **Dr Nelson's** turbo-jet drill, 60,000 RPM.
- 1956 Clear cell carcinoma was described by **Coridan.**
- 1956 **Pindborg** was first to describe calcified epithelial odontogenic tumor.
- 1956 AD Air-rotor drill, 250,000 RPM by **Dr Robert Borden**.
- 1957 Chronic granulomatours disease was identified.
- 1958 **Robinson** and his **co-workers** first described hand, foot and mouth disease.
- 1958-59 **Burkitt** reported African Jaw lymphoma.
- 1960 **Cooke** described recurrent herpetiform ulcer.
- 1962 **Steigman** found out a strain of coxsackie virus causing acute lymphonodular pharyngitis.
- 1962 **Gorlin** and **co-workers** described calcified odontogenic cyst.
- 1963 Odontogenic keratocyst was described by **Philipsen.**
- 1967 Monomorphic adenoma was described by **Kleinsasser.**
- 1971 Verruciform xanthoma was first described by **Shafer.**
- 1975 **Pullon** reported squamous odontogenic tumor.
- 1988 **Sir William Osler,** in 1888, first described hereditary form of angioneurotic edema.

INDIVIDUAL HISTORICAL BACKGROUND IN DENTISTRY

Gold Foil

- **Giovanni d Arcoli**, 15th Century described filling of cavity with gold leaf.
- **Pierre Fauchard**, 1728, used gold for restorations, and denture bases.
- In 1812, a manufacturer in **Hartford**, Connecticut specialized in beaten gold leaf for dental purposes.
- In 1855, **Dr Arthur** described a technique for using cohesive gold foil. the passing of gold foil through a flame would remove impurities and cause it to adhere to each other. One important condition for perfect cohesiveness was that the cavity had to be free of saliva. This wasn't overcome until **Dr Barnum** invented the rubber dam in 1864. The dam plus the dental engine helped gold foil achieve a high degree of perfection. In the early 1900s a leading authority on gold foil was **Dr Charles Woodbury** who taught for many years at Creighton.

Amalgam

First used as a silver paste by M Taveau of Paris in 1826, amalgam at first, had its drawbacks. Some mixtures caused expansion resulting in fractured teeth. GV Black experimented with silver amalgam and developed a suitable formula which met all requirements. He found in his research that if alloy fillings are heated to a certain temperature, they would remain stable for a long period.

Gutta Percha

A rubber-like material which came into use in 1848. It is used as a temporary filling and also extensively used in Endodontics.

Zinc Oxyphosphate Cement

- Came into use in 1880.
- Used in cementing crowns, inlays, and as a protective base over nearly exposed pulps.

Porcelain

- Used since the 1800s for denture teeth.
- All porcelain crowns used since 1900, generally unacceptable.
- Porcelain fused to metal crowns developed in late 1950s.

Gold Inlay

- A new and accurate method of casting gold inlays was announced by **Dr William H Taggart** in 1907.
- This technique was called the disappearing wax technique. He patented this technique but lost his patents when it was discovered that **Dr Philbrook** of Denison, Iowa, had written an article concerning gold inlay castings 25 years earlier. A copy of this article was found in the dental library of the University of Iowa.

Composite

- In 1938 **Castan** invented epoxy resins formed the basis for composite resins.
- Acrylic **Resin** was used for anterior filling in the 1940s, but was unacceptable because of leakage.
- In 1948 an incremental layering technique involving an auto-cured acrylic resin was introduced. Later light-curing catalysis based an alpha-diketones amines were invented in Britain.
- Unfilled resins which were the predecessors of composite resins were introduced in late 1940s and early 1950s. They evolved as a restorative material because they are insoluble, esthetic, insensitive to dehydration,

inexpensive and relatively easy to manipulate but they were found to be only partially successful in meeting the requirements of a durable esthetic restorative material for anterior teeth. High polymerization shrinkage, co-efficient of thermal expansion and lack of abrasion resistance led to clinical deficiencies and permanent failure.

- In 1950, acrylic filling materials containing alumina silicate glass filler were formulated. Here silicate glass was precoated with polymer. Although this process improved the material's physical properties but it was still hard to manipulate.
- In an effort to improve the physical characteristics of unfilled acrylic resin, Development of Modern Dental Composite Restorative material started in the late 1950s early 1960s by **Dr Raefel Bowen** to resolve the deficiencies caused by high polymerization shrinkage and high co-efficient of thermal expansion. Inert filler particles were added to reduce the volume of the resinous component but performance of composites were not too successful because the filler particles were not chemically bonded to the resin matrix. This resulted in fluid leakage, unacceptable surface appearance and poor wear resistance.
- A major advance occurred when **Bowen** developed a new type of composite material. His main innovations are Bisphenol A glycidyl methacrylate, (BISGMA), a dimethacrylate resin or Bowen's resin and use of a silane to coat filler particles that could bond chemically to resin.
- The improved matrix properties and matrix bonding yielded a restorative material that was clearly superior to the unfilled resins. Since the early 1970's the composites have virtually replaced the unfilled acrylics for tooth restorations.
- The first commercial composites were introduced in early 1960s which include TD71 (Dental Filling Ltd) and Addent (3M).

Bleaching

- Bleaching was unsuccessfully used in the middle ages.
- Modern bleaching technique began in 1918. **Abbot** used the combination of superoxol and heat.
- 1958 **Prarson** introduced intrapulpal bleach.
- 1967 **Nutting** and **Poe** introduced walking bleach.
- 1989 **Haywood** and **Hayman** gave night guard vital bleaching,10% carbamide peroxide.
- 1996 Laser tooth whitening officially started with the approval of ion laser technology, Argon and CO_2 lasers to be used with a potential system of chemicals.

Lasers

- The idea and concept of laser capability was first acknowledged in 1917. **Albert Einstein** first conceptualized the use of stimulated emission, which serves as the foundation of a laser. In the early to mid-1950s, Bell Labs' **Arthur L Schawlow**, and **Charles H Townes** invented the MASER (microwave amplification by stimulated emission of radiation), by means of ammonia gas and microwave radiation.
- The MASER was invented prior to the optical laser, yet the technology is very comparable.
- On May 16, 1960, **Theodore Maiman's** ruby laser became the first working laser in history.
- In the 1960s, **Dr Ali Javan** invented the first gas laser with Helium-Neon.
- Four years later, the carbon dioxide laser was successfully shaped by **Kumar Patel** in 1964.
- A new realization of commercial and research opportunities through laser technology became widespread, and substrates and ions such as rare earths (Nd, Pr, Tm, Ho, Er, Yb, Gd, and Ur) were all eventually successfully "lased".
- Over the years, **goldman** and other researchers documented the ability of various types of lasers to cut, coagulate, ablate and vaporize biologic tissues.
- In 1968, **L'Esperance** was the first to report clinical use of an argon laser in ophthalmology.
- In 1972, **Strong** and **Jako** reported the first clinical use of a CO_2 laser in otolaryngology.
- **Kiefhaber** et al documented the first clinical use of Nd: YAG laser in 1977 in gastrointestinal surgery.
- Historically, the first lasers to be marketed for intraoral use generally were CO_2 lasers with otorhinolaryngologic clearance authorized by FDA. In May 1990, the FDA cleared it for intraoral soft tissue surgery. A pulsed Nd: YAG laser developed by **Myers** and **Myers**, recognized as the first laser designed specifically for general dentistry.
- Other lasers and researches followed, and today lasers are used routinely across a broad spectrum of medical disciplines, including dentistry.

Caries Indices

- In 1931, **Bodecker CP** and **Bodecker HWC** described Caries Index. This Caries Index was found to be sensitive but too complex for use in epidemiological surveys.
- **Bodecker** modified this Caries Index later, where, in addition, counting the surfaces decayed, an extra count was allotted for those surfaces that could experience multiple caries attacks. But this was also not used in major epidemiological studies.

- The approach to measuring caries by counting the numbers of teeth in the mouth visibly affected by caries was used in a systematic manner, by **Dean** and associated in their historical studies of the dental caries/fluoride relation.
- **Mellanby M** in 1934 described the carious lesions depending upon the degree of severity and numerical, expressed it as follows:
  1 = Slight caries
  2 = Moderate caries
  3 = Advanced caries.
- However, the first systematic description of what is now known as the DMF index is usually attributed to **Henry Klein** and **Carole Paler** while carrying out their studies of dental caries in **Hagerstown**.

Retrograde Restorative Materials

- Mid-18th century- **Pfaff and Berdmore** performed root-end resection and performed root-end restorations with wax, lead or gold.
- 1880 **Brophy** provided a report on root-end resection, root canal fill and management of the apical filling.
- 1884 **Farrar** first reported of placing a root-end amalgam filling prior to resection.
- 1912 **Faulhaber** and **Neumann** used amalgam to fill root canals from resected root ends.
- 1913 –**Schuster** first reports of using gold foil.
- 1915-1920 Dental Literature carried articles with emphasis on sealing the gutta percha at the root apex with hot burnisher after resection.
- 1916-1919 - **Lucas** in a series of articles indicated that he first polished the resected root end, and then prepared a self-retentive cavity with a small bur in the root end for placement of amalgam.
- 1917- **Ivy** and **Howe** recommended the sealing of the apical resected tubules with silver nitrate.
- In 1935- **Fernando Gracia** indicated an equal choice between amalgam and zinc oxide eugenol, first indication of use of zinc oxide eugenol.
- In 1939- **Castenfeldt** published an article on root-end filling, a total seal with amalgam was recommended by removing all dentinal tubules at the resected root surface. A bevel was cut in the dentin from the canal orifice to the cemental junction.
- 1946- **Sommers** presented a technique for a root end fill with a silver cone. The cone was inserted into the canal at the resected root end, tapped to place with a chisel, and cut off and smoothened or burnished.
- Amalgam was the material of choice among dentist all over in the next seven decades.

- However, reports in the 1960s, 1970s and 1980s continued to recommend the use of gold foils because of the ease of manipulation, marginal adaptation, surface smoothness and tissue biocompatibility.

Topical Fluorides

- Fluorine is an extremely reactive gas and is never found in its pure state, but always combined with other elements (fluorides). Before 1900, most water was consumed directly from the source, and had very little treatment. In some western cities, it was noted that people (especially children) who had grown up in these communities had teeth mottled with white or brown spots. Anecdotally, in the late 1800s, it was noted that many of these people with mottled teeth had few cavities. Much later is was found that this mottling was caused by an excess of natural fluoride in the water.
- In 1901, **Dr Fredrick McKay** of Colorado (USA) accidentally discovered that many of his patients had an apparently permanent stain on their teeth that was often referred to as **'Colorado Stain'** by the local inhabitants.
- In the year 1908, as a first systemic endeavor, he presented a case at the annual meeting of state Dental Association in Boulder and found that the condition was not only confined to Colorado but extended to other towns as well.
- In 1912 **McKay** came across an article written by **Dr JM Eagar** (1902), a U.S. Marble hospital surgeon stationed in Italy, who reported that a high proportion of Italian residents in Naples, had ugly brown stains on their teeth known as 'denti di chiaie'.
- In 1916, **McKay** and **Black** examined 6,873 individuals in USA and reported that an unknown causative factor of mottled enamel was possibly present in domestic water during the period of teeth calcification.
- In 1930, **Kemp** and **McKay** observed that no mottling occurred in people who grew up in Bauxite prior to 1909, the year in which Bauxite had changed its supply from shallow wells to deep-drilled wells.
- In 1931, **Churchill HV**, chief chemist of the aluminum company in New Kensington, Pennsylvania, after thorough spectrographic analysis of the rare element noted that fluoride was present in Bauxite water at a level of 13.7 ppm.
- In the same year, 1931, shoe leather survey by **Trendley H Dean**, the most convincing evidence and direct proof was further established in depths.
- **Trendley H Dean** was assigned the job to continue McKay's work and to find out the extent of geographical distribution of mottled enamel in the US by the US Public Health Service.
- Observations on 5,824 white Children in 22 cities of 10 states revealed that, where water concentration was 3 ppm or more, mottling was wide spread.

Thus Dean established that concentration of fluoride in drinking water was directly correlated with the severity of fluoride in enamel.

- In 1934, **Trendley H Dean** introduced the mottling index, which is popularly known as Dean's index for fluorosis.
- Simultaneously in 1940s, it was demonstrated that extracted teeth when exposed to dilute solutions of fluoride ion for a few seconds were found to have completely bound fluoride on the enamel surface, which subsequently was less soluble than the original enamel surface. These two facts brought forth the idea of topical application of fluoride solution for dental caries prevention.
- The classical study by **Dean** (1941) proved that individuals continuously living in a fluoride rich area had less caries as compared to the individuals who had lived in the same fluoride rich areas during calcification of teeth but had shifted to non-fluoride areas thereafter, which led to a stage of speculation that this effect after the completion of calcification of teeth may be because of repeated continuous contact of teeth with water-containing fluoride.
- The year 1941 began the era of topical fluorides when the first clinical study of NAF was carried out by **Bibby**, using a 0.1% NAF solution.
- In 1942, the important milestone discovery was made by **Dean et al.** that at 1 ppm fluoride in drinking water, 60% reduction in caries experience was observed and only "sporadic instances of the mildest form of dental fluorosis of no practical or esthetic significance, was observed".
- In 1945, world's first artificial fluoridation plant at Grant Rapids, USA was set up.
- In 1946, **Klein** examined children of Japanese ancestry who had been transferred from a community containing 0.1 ppm fluoride or less to Arizona, where water contained 3 ppm of fluoride. It was observed that teeth in process of eruption received maximum benefits from fluorides. Teeth exposed to fluoride shortly after eruption were protected but to a lesser degree.
- From all the above-mentioned studies and findings, fluoride was identified as the essential element for reducing dental caries and this led to introduction of various methods of topical application of fluoride.
- Subsequently over the years various other topical fluoride agents have been evolved in sequential order are SnF2 (1947), APF (1963), sodium mono-fluorophosphate (NaMFP) (1963), amine fluoride (1969) and varnish containing fluoride (1964).

Systemic/Water Fluoridation

- 1901- **Dr Frederick McKay:** Permanent stains present on the teeth of the local inhabitant of Colorado Spring, USA, known as 'Colorado Stains' noticed. Stains characterized by minute white flecks, yellow or brown spots scattered all over the surface of the tooth were termed as mottled enamel (most obviously and unmistakably defective enamel.

- In **1902, Dr JM Eager** described similar stains seen on the teeth of certain Italian emigrants embarking at Naples as 'denti di chiaie", denti scritti" – teeth with writing, "denti neri" – black teeth.
- In **1925, Dr F McKay:** Change of water supply from spring water of the Great Salt Lake of Oakley, Idaho city, showed no brown stains in children, who were born after changes of the water supply.
- In **1933, Dr H Trendley:** Shoe Leather Survey conducted in 97 localities with the help of questionnaire with the aim to find out minimal threshold of fluoride, the level at which it began to blemish the teeth.
- **Dean (1941)-21 cities study:** Children of 12–14 yrs, who were lifelong residents in 8 suburban areas of Chicago, where the water supplies were stable, but at various levels were examined. Moreover, data obtained from 13 other cities were included and showed a substantial difference in caries experience when the fluoride concentration in the water rose from 0.1–0.2 ppm F to 1-2 ppm F.
- **1944-1959—Dean, Francies Arnold, Philip Jay and John Knutson (First artificial water fluoridation – 25th Jan, 1945)**
  (Grand Rapids-Muskegon Study) (water fluoridation)—Grand Rapids as experimental town and sodium fluoride was added to water at 1 ppm and Muskegon as control. First crucial step proved caries reduction from 12.48 to 6.2. DMF indicating that previously observed inverse relationship of fluoride in water and dental caries was a cause and effect relationship.
- **1945–1955-David et al:** Newburgh-Kingston (Control) Study - 10-year study. Newburgh children showed caries declined from 23.5 to 13.9% after water fluoridation.
- **1967(1946–1960)–Drs JR Blayney, TN Hill, SO Zilmmerman:** Evanston-oak Park (Control) Study - ***14-year study.*** Fluoridation in Evanston showed a 49% reduction of caries.
- **1951 - Hutton et al, 1965 - Brown and Poplove:** Canadian study (Brantford) (artificial fluoridation), Sarina (control) and Stratford]. Stratford with naturally present 1.3 ppm fluoride in water was auxiliary control. After 17 year of fluoridation, Brantford showed a 50% reduction in caries than the control Sarina group.
- **1958- World Health Organization** recommended for the first time 1 ppm fluoride in drinking water for a practicable and effective public health measure. This was reaffirmed in the report of the WHO Director General in 1975: fluoridation of communal water supplies where feasible should be cornerstone of any national program of dental caries prevention.

- **1961–Backer Dirks et al:** Dutch study (Tiel-Culemborg control). Tiel was fluoridated at the level of 1.1 ppm. Culemborg with 0.10 ppm served as a control. 13 years study showed 88% reduction in smooth surface caries and 31% in pit and fissure caries.
- **1965–Ludwig:** New Zealand study. Study carried out in Hastings from 1954 to 1964-5 showed a DMF decline from 16.5 to 8.5 with reduction of approximal caries by 73% and occlusal caries by 39%.
- **Wideman et al. (1963):** Reported no radiographic evidence of skeletal abnormality in persons consuming water supply containing up to 4 ppm of fluoride throughout their lives.
- **Hodge (1963):** Observed no evidence of kidney or thyroid damage in persons who, throughout their lives, ingested water-containing 11ppm of fluoride.
- **Erricson (1978):** Compared the cancer mortality statistics in USA cities, with and without fluoridated water supplies and found no differences in the morbidity rates. Neither the United States Centre for Disease Control (Rogot et al., 1978) nor the National Heart Lung and Blood Institute (Upton, AC, 1977) could find any evidence-linking fluoride with cancer.

Pulp Therapy

- Pulp therapy for primary and young permanent teeth has, for years, been subject to change and controversy. The history of pulp therapy has been described to encompass four periods:
  1. The empiricl era that is prior to 1870.
  2. The antiseptic era from 1870 to 1921.
  3. The aseptic era ranging from 1921 to 1937.
  4. The present **experimental era** or the **biologic era** from 1937 onwards.
- The reparative and the recuperative powers of dental pulp have long been recognized in dentistry. The young dental pulp, particularly the pulp in primary teeth, has a potential for repair because of high degree of cellularity and vascularity in this tissue prior to advanced physiological resorption of roots.
- In the mid-eighteenth century, **Pierre Fauchard** advised that all caries in deeply carious sensitive teeth should not be removed because of danger of pulp exposure. As early as 1756, **Ptaff** reported placing a small piece of gold over a vital exposure in an attempt to promote healing. Principles of indirect pulp therapy was recognized by 1850 and published by **Foster**. Many medicaments have been tried since **Taft** (1860) and **Hunter** (1883). Hunter recommended covering an exposure with a mixture of Sorghum molasses and droppings of English sparrow.

- The first mention of a pulp treatment specifically for primary teeth was in 1872 in a column titled "Hints and Query", the question, "What shall we do, with deciduous teeth in which pulps are exposed?" was answered by D Cosmos in this manner - "They should be treated in somewhat the same manner as the permanent teeth. A single application of the arsenical preparation in common use will so far destroy the vitality of the pulp in the crown so that it can be removed day after and then filled. Either Hill's stopping or osteoplastic may be used as filling, but no attempts should be made to fill the root".
- **Richardson** recorded the initial report on pulpotomy in 1860. The present-day use of formocresol medicament has evolved from the use of formalin compounds in the past.
- **Hess,** in 1929, reported pulp amputation as a method of treating exposed pulp and used this method most frequently on traumatic exposures and found it clinically successful to a certain extent.
- The formocresol technique used today is a modification of the original method reported by Sweet in 1930. The formocresol technique did not receive wide popularity as it mummified the pulp and was known as nonvital technique during the previous years. It was also overshadowed by the so-called vital pulpotomy using calcium hydroxide, which was introduced by **Teuscher** and **Zander** in 1938.
- With the Biological Era came a new concern for the histological evaluation of the injured and healthy pulp. The use of zinc oxide eugenol was emphasized during this era and has been considered one of the best pulpotomy dressings. **Glass** and **Zander** in 1949 reported that the so-called palliative zinc oxide eugenol preparation produced an acute inflammatory response with associated degeneration of odontoblasts.
- The search for more suitable medicament led investigations to test preparations containing antibiotics or corticosteroids.
- **Cook** and **Rowbotham** (1956) used zinc oxide eugenol only for pulpotomies in primary teeth, while **Seelig,** in 1956, used dentin chips and other materials in pulpotomy procedure.
- After all these periods of using various compounds and medicaments in pulpotomy procedure a real study was taken up with Formocresol, which is one of the widely used medicament by **Massler** and **Mansukhani** in 1959.
- Doyle et al., 1962, introduced two-visit formocresol pulpotomy in human study. For a period of 10 years formocresol was completely dominating the other medicaments but as there is an unending quest for newer materials, investigators like **Hannah** in 1972 used glutaraldehyde. It is a dialdehyde known to be an excellent disinfectant, active against spores and bacteria and is generally used as 2% solution as quoted by s-Gravenmade in 1975.

Shallow pulpotomy or partial pulpotomy was developed by **Granath L.E.** and **Hagman** (1971) and by **Cvek M** (1978).

- Although **Laws A J** reported electrocoagulation on the pulps of teeth in 1957, it was a decade later that Mack became the first US dentist to perform electrosurgical pulpotomy.
- In 1980, **Nevins et al.** in a study demonstrated that cross-linked collagen phosphate gel could be used for regeneration and calcification of the pulp tissue within teeth that were partially pulpotomized. Electrosurgical pulpotomy was supported histologically by **Ruemping** in 1983.
- **Shoji S et al.**, (1985) in a preliminary report on laser pulpotomy, studied the histopathological changes in dental pulp irradiated by CO_2 laser. Freeze-dried bone **(Fadavi et al., 1988)** and demineralized dentin (Nakashima 1989) were tried.
- Bone morphogenetic protein was suggested by **Nakashima** in 1991. **Fei et al.** (1991) suggested ferric sulphate as a substitute for formocresol. **Seow WK et al.,** (1993) evaluated anti-inflammatory agent – tetrandrine as a pulpotomy medicament and gave favorable results. Osteogenic protein was tried in animals by **Rutherford et al.,** (1993).

Glass Ionomer Cements

- During the early and mid-1960s, science and technology of clinical dental materials were those materials that could be used directly by the dental surgeon. Silicate cement, the principal anterior restorative material of those days was recognized as flaw for use in the general dental practice. It had remained essentially the same for 50 years, even the nature of its setting and structure was imperfectly understood.
- This unsatisfactory state of affairs, however, produced a positive response, and the period of the late 1960s and early 1970s was a most creative one in the development of new materials. There was a general recognition that–
  - Adequate physical properties are not enough by themselves.
  - A restorative material should be more than just an inert stopping.
  - Biocompatibility and adhesion are important.
  - New materials and techniques should be developed with these characteristics.
- Scientific development of glass ionomer cement has been in two steps: First, effort was devoted to improve properties to make it a fully practical material for anterior restorations. Second, properties were modified in order to extend its range of application.
- Wilson collaboration with Kent and Lewis found that employing novel glass formulations, hydrolytically stable cements, could be produced **(Wilson and Kent 1972)**.

Pit and Fissure Sealants

- The dental profession has known for some time that susceptibility to caries on tooth surfaces containing pit and fissure is related to the formation and depth of these pit and fissures. The fissure provides a protected reach for plaque accumulations. The rapidity with which dental caries occurs in pits and fissures is most likely related to the fact that the depth of the fissure is close to the DEJ and the underlying dentin, which is highly susceptible to caries.
- In 1803, **Hunter** noted that "caries is often observed on the hollow parts of the molars". In 1895, **Wilson** documented the use of current for blocking fissures in permanent molars.
- During the 1920s, two different clinical techniques were introduced in an attempt to reduce the extent and severity of pit and fissure caries in occlusal and smooth surfaces.
- In 1924, **Thaddeus Hyatt** advocated prophylactic restorations. This procedure consisted of preparing conservative class I cavity that included all pits and fissures at risk for caries development and then placing an amalgam restorations. The rationale for prophylactic restorations of an otherwise caries free surface was that the procedure prevented further insult to the pulp from caries, decreased loss of tooth structure and required less time for restorations when the tooth eventually succumbed to the caries.
- A more conservative approach to prevention of pit and fissure caries was presented by **Bodecker** in 1929. Initially, he advocated cleaning the fissure with an explorer and flowing a thin mix of oxyphosphate current into the fissure – essentially an attempt to "Seal" the fissure. Later, he introduced an alternative method for caries prevention, the **prophylactic odontotomy**, which involved mechanical eradication of fissures into cleansable ones. These 2 techniques, prophylactic restoration and prophylactic odontotomy, were employed until the use of sealants became prevalent.
- The development of pit and fissure sealants was based on the discovery that etching enamel with phosphoric acid increased the retention of resin restorative materials and improved marginal integrity considerably. The initial studies evaluating the effects of acid-etching on enamel were performed by **Buonocore** in 1955.
- The first sealant material that involved the acid etch technique was introduced in the mid-1960s and was a cyanoacrylate substance; cyanoacrylates were not suitable as sealant materials owing to bacterial degradation of the material in the oral cavity over time.
- By the late 1960s, a number of different resin materials had been tested, and a viscous resin was found to be resistant to degradation and produced a tenacious bond with etched enamel. This resin was formed by reacting

Bisphenol A with glycidyl methacrylate, and this class of dimethacrylate resins has become known as BIS-GMA (Bowen 1982).

- Two methods of polymerization have been employed with BIS GMA sealants: Autopolymerization and photoactivated polymerization.
- During the 1970s and early 1980s UV light with a wavelength of 365 nm was used to initiate setting but was abandoned later. In its place, photoactivation of sealant materials with a visible light source was introduced.
- Laser curing of visible light-activated sealant and resin materials has been advocated. In addition to BIS-GMA sealants, conventional glass ionomer materials have also been used as pit and fissure sealants.
- Glass ionomer bond to both enamel and dentin by physio chemical mechanisms following polyacrylic acid conditioning. The primary advantage of glass ionomers over conventional BIS-GMA sealants is the ability of Glass ionomers to release fluoride.
- Hybrid materials composed of a variable mixture of glass ionomer and composite resin have been advocated as possible pit and fissure sealants because of the improved physical characteristics over glass ionomers, relative case of placement, adhesive compatibility with various dental substrates and fluoride releasing capability.

Dental Chairs

- The first dental chair by **James Snell** in 1832.
- The first hydraulic chair by **Wilkerson** in 1877.

Dental Drills

- Hand operated gear-driven by **John Lewis** in 1838.
- The air abrasive drill by **Dr Black** in 1945.
- The first foot or threadle engine by **Dr Morrison** in 1872.
- The first electric dental engine by **Dr Green** in 1874.
- The water-turbine handpiece by **Dr Nelson** in 1954.
- The air-turbine handpiece by **Dr Borden** in 1957.
- Chemical methods, abrasives and lasers have been advocated for tooth removal, but, as yet, have not been sufficiently developed for widespread use.

George Washington's Dentures

- As there were no satisfactory filling materials or procedures at that time, decay usually proceeded until the patient had a toothache. At the time of Washington's (1790), he had only a lower premolar left, which was lost some time after. His diaries record showed many instances of prolonged toothaches, and his dental problems did not end with the loss of his teeth.

Washington employed the best dentists of his day (John Greenwood was his favorite), many dentures made for him were unsatisfactory. Due to poor materials and procedures, the dentures made at that time fit the gingiva poorly. Although plaster was used to take impressions of the arches, the denture bases were carved or hammered to only approximate fit.

- The upper fit so poorly and had no retention; springs were attached to the upper and lower plates and pushed them against the tissue. It may be due to that there was little understanding of occlusion, so the uppers did not fit the lowers well. This type of denture could not have been comfortable. Although these dentures were mainly cosmetic, he still attempted to wear them for official occasions and dinners, although this did limit his speaking engagements.
- Even with these dentures, his mouth was badly sunken and the ivory used for the teeth stained quickly, common people of that time probably did not attempt to have dentures fitted, and even with their fame and affluence, Washingtons did not have a very satisfactory prosthodontic result.
- Until the late 1800s, catalogues listed "masticators", which crushed food so that it could be consumed by those without teeth. Naturally retained upper dentures seem to have been discovered accidentally, as one of the cases was documented by **Dr Gardette of Philadelphia** in 1800. Gold was the preferred material for these bases, obviously at some cost. These were known as "suction dentures" and preceded vulcanite dentures.

Vulcanite Dentures

- Before restorative dental care came into picture or became popular, the only treatment for dental pain was extraction which resulted in partial or complete edentulism. Unfortunately in those times, there were neither materials nor techniques for the fabrication of satisfactory dentures and the lack of durable material added to the problem. It was **Nelson Goodyear** in 1851 who discovered how to make hard rubber products. This hard rubber was named vulcanite. This product found wide popularity in fabrication of denture bases, where it soon replaced all previously used materials, being far superior in cost and function. The fit of these bases allowed self-retaining dentures, making earlier spring type dentures obsolete. These vulcanite dentures were the first functional, durable and affordable dentures, marking a great advance in dental treatment. After a lot of legal procedures, the Goodyear Company obtained a patent for vulcanite dentures in 1864. They proceeded to license dentists who used their material, and charged a royalty for all dentures made. Dentists who would not comply were sued. Although many dentists bought licenses, the dental profession, as a whole, opposed the patent and licensure of vulcanite denture.

- The struggle came to an end when Goodyear hired Josiah Bacon to prosecute noncompliant dentists, which he did across the country with almost malicious vigor. Once he filed suit against was a well-respected dentist named **Samuel Chalfant**. Chalfant was so distressed that he shot and killed Bacon in California in 1879. Chalfant served 10 years for second degree murder and resumed his practice upon his release. The Goodyear patents expired in 1881, and the company did not again seek to license dentists or dental products.
- Vulcanite dentures were very popular until the 1940s, when acrylic (pink plastic) denture bases replaced them.

Amalgam

- In spite of having great success stories, mercury-silver amalgam material has always been a part of controversy since its earliest days. Many metallic powders (most commonly silver alloys), can be mixed with mercury to form amalgams, which are soft and then harden to metallic solids. Early attempts to use amalgam as a dental restoration were often failures, however. Silver was obtained from many sources, often shaved from coins. First, the ingredients and proportions were usually inconsistent, leading to early breakdown of the filling or tooth fracture from excessive expansion, and then the proportions and mixing procedure with mercury were also variable. The other problem was that the tooth preparation was usually haphazard, both from poor instrumentation and inadequate dental training. Because of these failures, in the middle to late 1800s, the amalgam was subjected to many conflicts in the dental profession and was known as "amalgam wars".
- **GV Black's** greatest success was in the development of usable amalgams around 1900. After many studies and researches, he determined the correct proportions of silver, zinc, copper and tin and the proper processing of the powder. He also determined the right percentage of mercury and the proper mixing procedure.
- Along with the material he developed a systematic and scientific approach to cavity preparation, which was equally responsible for success. GV Black's amalgam and tooth preparation system, for the first time, it was possible to successfully repair cavities quickly and inexpensively.
- While other restorative materials were also in successful use during that period, they were not as widely used because of the time required and the cost. Throughout most of the 20th century, dental amalgam was the predominant material for the general repair of carious teeth. Although amalgam continues to develop and improve through the present time, it is not without problems. Perhaps the greatest disadvantage is the silvery or dark appearance, which is somewhat acceptable in posterior teeth but very unesthetic in the anterior teeth.

- The other concern is the mercury toxicity in amalgam. While some forms of mercury are very toxic and harmful, there has been no scientific evidence that the mercury in dental amalgams causes health problems in the general population. Nonetheless, many individuals and groups ascribe a wide variety of ills to the presence or release of mercury from amalgam restorations with the press often giving credence to these theories, so the controversy continues.

First Use of Inhalation Anesthesia

- Since prehistoric times, man has sought ways to lessen pain. With varying degrees of success, he has utilized: mandrake, opium and other poppy extracts, fermented and distilled beverages, nerve compresses, cold, extreme fatigue from prohibiting sleep, bleeding to the point of fainting shock and hypnosis.
- One of these parties (ether frolics) in 1842, a young physician. **Crawford W Long** of Georgia conceived the idea of administering to patient sufficient ether to inhale so that an operation could be performed without pain to the patient. After selecting his patient, Dr Long removed a tumor from the neck while the patient was under the influence of ether. In that year, 1842, Dr Long claimed three administrations of ether. Since that year, up to 1849, he had performed one or more surgical operations annually on patients under the influence of ether.
- **Dr Horace Wells** of Hartford, Connecticut. A young conscientious dentist. Being a very sensitive individual, the suffering he caused during the extraction of teeth troubled him greatly. These feelings prompted him to give considerable thought to the subject of pain relief during extractions. In 1838, he wrote, "An Essay on Teeth, Comprising a Brief Description of their Formation, Diseases, and Proper Treatment".
- Horace Wells was constantly enhanching his knowledge and attended a lecture on chemical phenomena by **Gardner Q Colton** in 1844. After manufacturing some nitrous oxide, known as "laughing gas", Mr Colton invited spectators to come forward and inhale the fumes. Horace noticed that no sign was exhibited when the volunteers, under the influence of nitrous oxide, stumbled and scraped their shins on the heavy benches. Immediately, Wells conceived the idea of inhalation anesthesia. Though history notes that **Sir Humphrey Davy**, in 1799, published an account of his research and experiments with nitrous oxide, Horace Wells was not aware of it.
- Later Wells spoke with Colton and asked him to bring a bag of the gas to his office the next day. Wells had an aching tooth and felt that by inhaling sufficient nitrous oxide, the tooth could be extracted painlessly. Colton at first had objected as the gas might prove fatal.

- In 1844, Wells, sitting in his own dental chair, inhaled the gas until he lost consciousness. **Dr Riggs**, a friend and former pupil of Dr Wells, stepped forward and extracted the arching third molar (wisdom tooth). On regaining consciousness, Wells exclaimed, "A new era in tooth pulling". After experimenting for weeks, he went to Boston, the medical center of the New England States. There, **William TG Morton** arranged the lecture and demonstrated nitrous oxide before the medical students of John C Warren. However, this demonstration was a failure.
- Wells continued to use nitrous oxide and taught other dentists to use it. **William Thomas Green Morton** received the idea of inhalation anesthesia from Well's demonstration. He extracted a tooth for a patient under its influence. Morton saturated a handkerchief with it, giving it to the patient, he remarked that it was something better than mesmerization. The patient inhaled it and soon was unconscious. The tooth was removed painlessly. This took place in 1846.
- Morton then demonstrated ether as a practical anesthetic to the Harvard medical class. The surgeon incharge was **Dr John C Warren**. He is the man credited with giving both Morton and Wells their big opportunity to demonstrate publicly their anesthetic agents. Morton patented the ether under the name of Letheon and secretly promised to pay a percentage to Jackson.
- Morton, wealthiest of the three, gave up dentistry and became the first specialist in anesthesia. Wells, deranged by his self-experimentation with chloroform, committed suicide in 1848. In 1864, the American Dental Association gave full credit to Horace Wells for the discovery of practical anesthesia and its introduction to the United States of America.

Local Anesthesia

- Local anesthetics were first used in 1884. It was then that Koller, a young intern and house surgeon, first announced the use of cocaine to anesthetize the eye. That same year, William S. Halstead, surgeon at John Hopkins Hospital, demonstrated that the injection of a nerve trunk in any part of its course is followed by local anesthesia in its entire peripheral distribution. The nerve he first blocked was the mandibular branch of the trigeminal.
- Novocaine (procaine hydrochloride) was introduced by Professor Braun in 1905. Novocaine is a comparatively weak anesthetic agent possessing a low degree of toxicity. It is still potent enough to provide a safe, sure analgesia under practically all circumstances. When infiltrated around free nerve endings and fibers, onset of analgesia is almost immediate. At most, the onset is from 3 to 5 minutes. A two percent solution of novocaine is recommended for use in dental practice. This percentage will give approximately 12-15

minutes of analgesia. The addition of epinephrine 1:100,000 per milliliter prolonged analgesia to 30-45 minutes. A 1:50,000 per milliliter produces 60-90 minutes of analgesia. Dental surgery performed under these conditions on a cardiac patient will present no special hazards. Novocaine is now seldom used. It has been replaced by stronger anesthetics such as: Primacaine, 1.5% solution, which is four times more potent than novocaine and slightly more toxic.

- Lidocaine (Xylocaine) Hydrochloride 2% solution was discovered in 1943 by two Swedish chemists, Nils Lofgren and Bengt Lundqvist. After many experiments, Xylocaine was introduced to the medical and dental professions. Its acceptance by the dental profession of the United States in 1950 was rapid and dramatic. Soon afterwards, it was made available to hospitals. Xylocaine did not just happen, its recognition as one of the greatest contributions to the field of local anesthesia constitutes a success story but unlimited credit must be given to first, its discoverers, and the countless number of scientists and clinicians whose untiring efforts established the effectiveness and safety of xylocaine. Lidocaine (Xylocaine) diffuses readily through the tissues, and nerve sheath giving a rapid onset of analgesia. It is detoxified in the liver and possesses slight vaso-constricting properties. Xylocaine has an early cortical depressant effect and it, thereby, potentiates the hypnotic effect of barbiturates. Therefore, in cases of pre-medication with barbiturates, the dosage should be decreased if xylocaine is used. Xylocaine has been used effectively and safely in dentistry and in various specialties of medicine such as: Urology, Ophthalmology, Otorhinolaryngology, Proctology, and Dermatology.
- Xylocaine is rapidly replacing novocaine. It has been widely accepted by obstetricians who have become aware of its effectiveness and safety. The spread of xylocaine has been phenomenal. It has even replaced novocaine in the field of intravenous anesthesia, the advantages being many, such as: a very low incidence of postoperative nausea, vomiting and chest complications. The idea of using anesthetic solutions or drugs in cartridges was developed by Harvey Cook. The idea was conceived from the cartridges used in rifles. Dr Cook fashioned his own syringes and cartridges. From this humble beginning, new agents and different types of syringes have sprung.

Annexure-II

SYNDROMES

1. **Acute coronary syndromes** comprise the spectrum of unstable cardiac ischemia from unstable angina to acute myocardial infarction. Many patients may show ST segment elevation, ST segment depression on T-wave flattening or inversion. Chest pain is the commonest complaint.
2. **AIDS** (Acquired Immunodeficiency Syndrome) is a condition where acute infection occurs 3 to 6 weeks after initial contact with HIV (Human Immuno deficiency Virus). Initially non specific syndrome occurs during which joints pain, gastrointestinal symptoms and a macular rash predominate, and then these self-limiting symptoms persist for 2-3 weeks. Eights to twelve weeks after infection, antibody to HIV can be detected in serum. After acute infection, person enters the symptomatic phase of the disease. The average time from infection to development of disease is 8 to 10 years. During this period, T_4 lymphocytes come down from 800mm^3 to 50mm^3. Oral manifestations in HIV-infected patients are oral candidiasis that occurs in 30% to 90% cases. Persistent ulcers of mouth in AIDS should be biopsied for deep fungal infections. Hairy leukoplakia has been noted in HIV positive homosexuals. Recurrent herpes simplex virus progresses to large chronic oral lesions. Ulcers are surrounded by raised white border. Lesions may co-exist with genital and anal lesions. Painful oral ulcers caused by cytomegalovirus may be seen. Kaposi's sarcoma is the most common oral neoplasm in AIDS. Early lesions look like hemangiomas, flat or raised discolorations. Generalized gingivitis and periodontitis are also seen.
3. **Albright's syndrome** is like fibrous dysplasia of bone. There is replacement of spongy bone by a peculiar fibrous tissue. Radiographs will show radiopacity and radiolucency, some will appear like compact bone and other like cystic

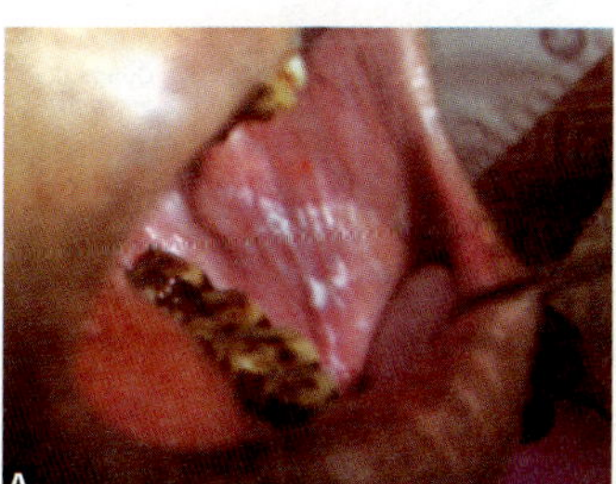

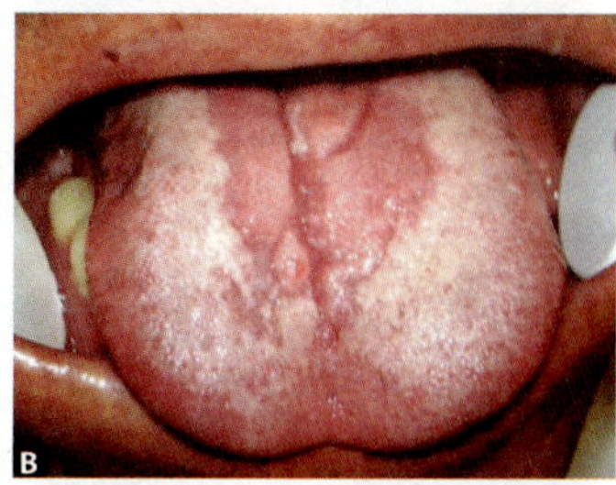

Figs A and B: *(A) Oral candidiasis; (B) Hairy leukoplakia*

bone. The cause of endocrine manifestation in Albright's syndrome is not known. Transformation to malignancy occurs. Radiotherapy is not advised (*see* **Figure on page 619**).

4. **Aldrich syndrome** is rare hereditary disease transmitted as an X-linked recessive trait. It is characterized by thrombocytopenic purpura, eczema and increased susceptibility of disease. Spontaneous bleeding of gingiva is common. Palatal petechiae may be present.
5. **Amelo-onychohypohidrotic syndrome** can be manifested by defective nails with subungal hyperkeratosis is seen with hypofunction of sweat gland and severe hypoplastic-hypocalcified crowns.
6. **Amnesic syndrome** is said to have occurred where it becomes difficult to retaining new information. There may be polyneuritis.
7. **Auriculotemporal syndrome** develops due to damage of auriculotemporal nerve and subsequent reinnervation of sweat glands. There is flushing and sweating of involved side of face during eating. Sweating may increase with tart food. Also known as Frey's syndrome.
8. **BK Mole syndrome** was described by Clark and co-workers. This autosomal dominant condition is characterized by large pigmented nevi. There is higher risk of development of melanoma.
9. **Behcet's disease** is an idiopathic disorder characterized by triad of symptoms, i.e. recurrent oral ulcers, genital ulcers and eye lesions. Development of vasculitis of medium sized blood vessels is seen. Eye lesions consist of

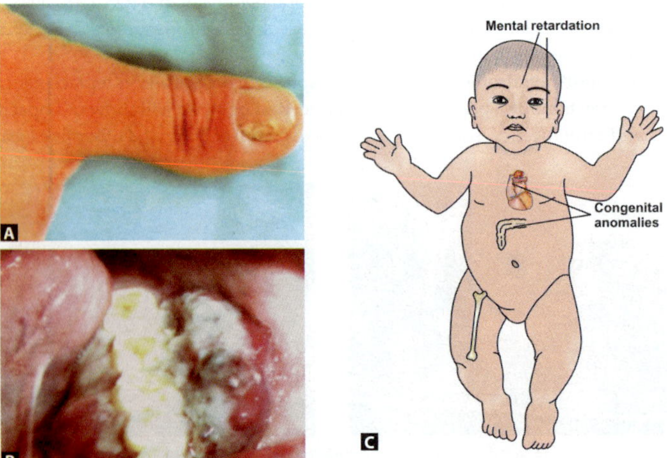

Figs A to C: *(A) Herpetic whitlow; (B and C) Kaposi sarcoma*

uveitis, retinal infiltrates, edema and vascular occlusion. Skin lesions are large papular lesions. Pustules may be formed in 24 hours. Ulcers may also be present on scrotum, penis or vulva. Cyclosporine with cortisone is useful.

10. **Bloch Sulzberger syndrome** is a disease that generally appears shortly after birth and is characterized by erythematous and vesicobullous lesion on trunk. There will be marked eosinophilia. Dental changes include delayed tooth eruption, peg or cone-shaped crowns and congenitally missing teeth.
11. **Branchial arch syndrome** is clinically manifested by heterogeneous group of malformation including antimongoloid palpebral fissures, deficiency of eyelashes, hypoplasia of facial bones, malformations of malar bones, facial clefts and skeletal deformities. Facies are characteristics.
12. **Burning mouth syndrome** is characterized by painful, burning sensation localized in the tongue or affecting other areas of the oral mucosa. The pain of burning tongue is rated similar to that of toothache. Tongue temperature is decreased. Some evidence suggests the existence of oral somatosensory and special sensory deficits.
13. **Chediak-Higashi syndrome** is a congenital autosomal recessive defect. It is a fatal disease in early life. Defect is of granule containing cells as granulocytes and melanocytes. Clinical features include oculocutaneous albinism, photophobia, nystagmus and recurrent infections. Hypopigmentation will be seen in skin and hair. Some may develop neuropathy. Child dies before the age of 10 due to recurrent infection. Lymph nodes, spleen, liver and

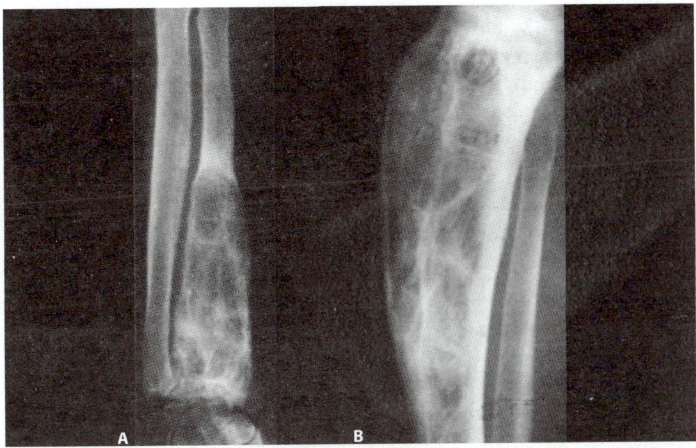

Figs A and B: *Albright's syndrome*

bone marrow are infiltrated with lymphohistiocyte cell. Oral lesions include ulcerations of oral mucosa, severe gingivitis, glossitis and periodontal breakdown are common. Early loss of teeth is noted. There is no specific treatment.

14. **Cleidocranial dysplasia** is a hereditary disorder. There is an abnormal growth of bones of face, skull and clavicles. There is failure of tooth eruption. There is autosomal dominant trait. There is spontaneous mutations. *Clinical Features:* There is hypermobility of shoulder joint, frontal bossing is seen, underdevelopment of mid-face, nose is wide, flat without bridge, multiple unerupted and impacted teeth, supernumerary teeth are seen and clavicle is hypoplastic.
15. **Complex regional pain syndrome** after an injury, patients sometimes, develop a variety of persistent unpleasant sensation in the previously injured area. Pain is severe and burning loss of hair may develop, complex regional pain syndrome typically occurs after nerve trauma, fractures and periods of immobilization pain may lead to reflex sympathetic dystrophy.
16. **Cowden's syndrome** There is hamartomas involvement of many organs with a potential of neoplastic transformation. It is inherited as autosomal dominant character. Multiple cysts over lips and gingiva are seen. Papilloma like lesions as well as pebbly lesion and fibromas at various sites in oral cavity are seen. Tongue is also fissured. Hemangiomas and neuromas are also seen.
17. **Cracked tooth syndrome** can be manifested by development or presence of a crack in a restored or an unrestored tooth due to excessive occlusal forces. There is a sharp pain on biting. Pain is similar to that of trigeminal neuralgia. Radiographs are unable to show cracked tooth.
18. **CREST syndrome** is one of the forms of systemic sclerosis. Its findings include Raynaud's phenomenon, esophageal dysfunction, sclerodactyly and telangiectasia. Calcinosis cutis may also be there. Etiology is not known. Early mild edema of tongue, soft palate and larynx are seen. Tongue often becomes stiff and board like. Dysphagia and choking sensations are seen. Bone resorption of angle of mandibular ramus is noted.

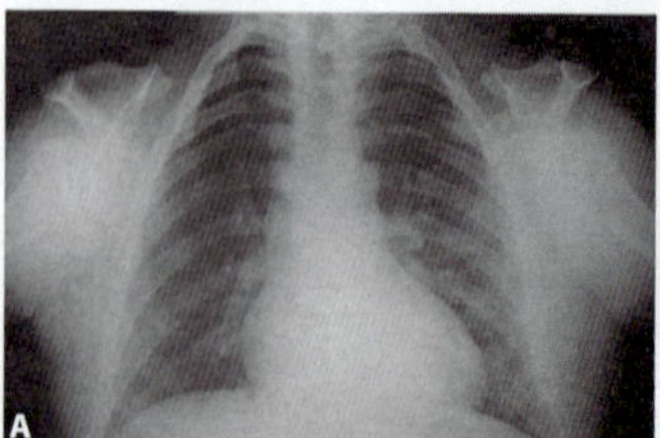

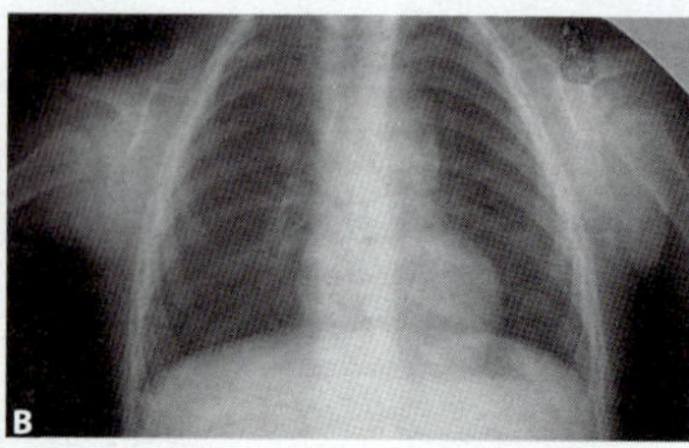

Figs A and B: *Cleidocranial dysplasia*

19. **Crouzon syndrome** is known as craniofacial dysostosis. Signs are due to early synostosis of the sutures. There is protuberant frontal region. There will be hypoplasia of maxillae with mandibular prognathism and a high arched palate.
20. **Cushing's syndrome** is seen due to adrenal hyperactivity. Patient may be hypertensive and hypoglycemic and may have moon face appearance. Gingiva, palate and buccal mucosa may appear blotchy due to melanin granules.
21. **de Quervain's syndrome** in 1985 Swiss doctor named Fritz de Quervain described pain syndrome involving tendons. Injury to nerve or repetitive wrist motions can cause swelling of tunnel through which tendon passes. Diabetes, thyroid disease, rheumatoid arthritis may also cause inflammation in this tunnel. Swelling irritates the tendon and causes pain. This syndrome causes pain at the base of thumb.
22. **Down syndrome/Mongolism**/Trisomy 21 is a congenital disease caused by chromosomal abnormalities, it is characterized by mental deficiency and growth retardation. The birth prevalence of Down syndrome is generally stated to be 1 in 650 live births, but is known to vary in different populations from 1/600 to 1/2,000 live births. Oral manifestations present are periodontal disease with periodontal pockets, diastema, crowding and high frenal attachment.
23. **Dyskeratosis congenital (Zinsser – Engman Cole Syndrome)** is a rare X-linked disorder characterized leading to atrophic, leukoplakic oral mucosa. Tongue and cheek are adversely affected. Oral lesions starting before the age

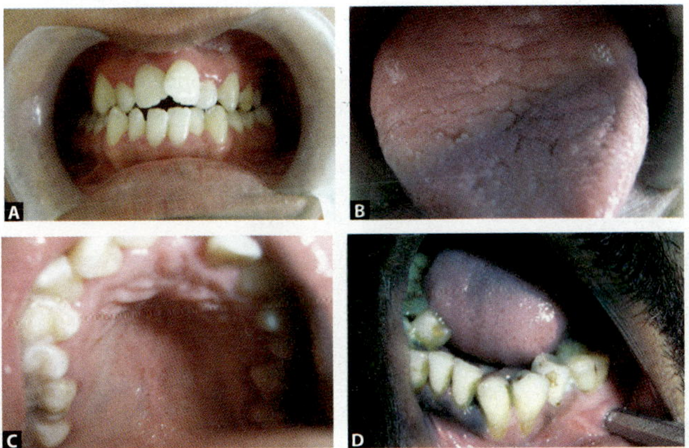

Figs A to D: *Down syndrome/Mongolism*

of 10 present as vesicles and white necrotic patches with Candida, ulcerations and erythroplakic changes.

24. **Ectodermal dysplasia** is an X-linked recessive disorder affecting essentially males. Defect is seen in all ectodermally derived structures. Patients exhibit decreased sweating, sparse hair, many congenitally missing teeth. Hypodontia involves most stable teeth like maxillary central incisor and first molars.
25. **Gardner's syndrome** consists of multiple polyposis of large intestine, osteomas of bone, especially jaw and skull. There is occasional occurrence of desmoids tumors. Multiple epidermoid or sebaceous cysts of skin are noted.
26. **Godtfredsen's syndrome** consists of ophthalmoplegia and trigeminal neuralgia with paralysis of tongue. Tumor is located in cavernous and lateral sinus.
27. **Goltz-Gorlin syndrome** is a hereditary condition transmitted as an autosomal dominant trait. Cutaneous anomalies include plantar keratosis and dermal calcinosis. Dental and osseous abnormalities include odontogenic keratocysts, mandibular prognathism and rib anomalies. Ophthalmic abnormalities include wide nasal bridge, dystopia canthorum while sexual abnormalities include hypogonadism. Patient will develop gingival and other mucosal papillomatous lesions. Lips and teeth develop defects. Associated features include poikiloderma, syndactyly and adactyly.
28. **Gorham's syndrome** is a condition where spontaneous progressive resorption of bone is seen. Etiology is not known but there is an active hyperemia of bone. Osteolysis is most common in older children. Mandible and other bones may be involved. Patient may present with pain and facial asymmetry. There is a replacement of bone by connective tissue containing thin walled blood vessels.
29. **Gardner's syndrome** There is carcinomatous transformation of adenomatous intestinal polyps. There may be osteomas of jaw and accompanying cysts are indictors of Gardner's syndrome and bowel should be examined.
30. **Grinspan's syndrome** is a triad of lichen planus, diabetes mellitus and hypertension. It may predispose to squamous cell carcinoma.

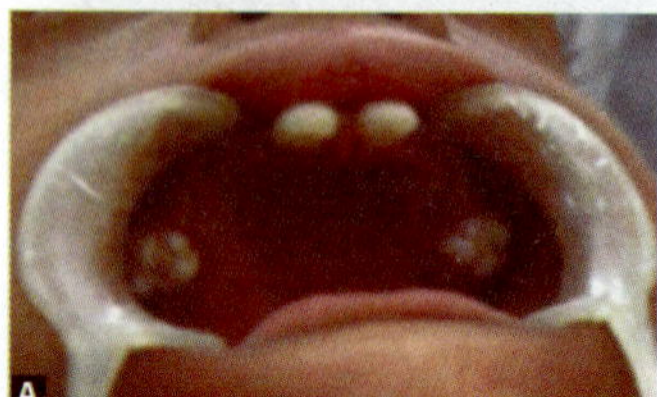

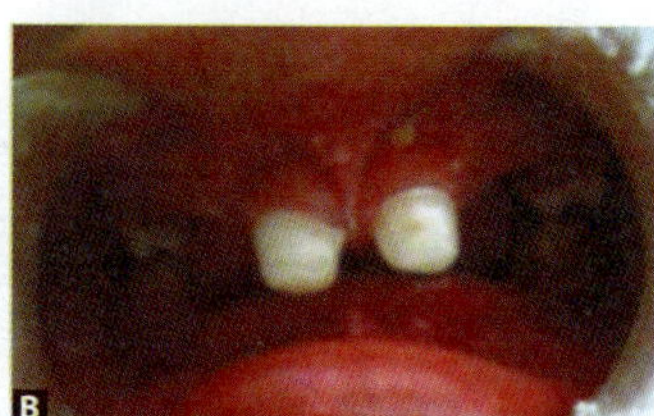

Figs A and B: *Ecodermal dysplasia*

31. **Guillain Barré syndrome** is caused by progressive demyelinating neuropathy. It is an autoimmune following a nonspecific disease. Impaired swallowing or paresthesia of mouth and face is the early sign. There may be ascending anesthesia and paralysis of legs and trunk. In severe case respiration is compromised.
32. **Jadassohn-Lewandowsky syndrome** causes congenital gross thickening of finger and toe nails. Along with it leukokeratosis is noted. Nail lesion is noted just after birth with a horny brownish material at nail bed. Oral leukokeratosis affects dorsum of tongue which becomes thickened and grayish white. Histologically these are similar to white sponge nevus. Frequent oral aphthous ulceration may develop.
33. **James Ramsay Hunt's syndrome** is clinically manifested by facial paralysis as well as pain in external auditory meatus. In addition, vascular eruption may occur in oral cavity. There may be hoarseness of voice.
34. **Jaw-Winking syndrome** may be hereditary. It may be seen after peripheral facial syndrome. On opening mouth, eye is closed. During chewing, tears may flow.
35. **Klinefelter's syndrome** includes taurodontism, i.e. peculiar dental anomaly at the expense of roots. Such males have one more extra X-chromosome.
36. **Lysosomal storage syndrome** is manifested by formation of childhood gingival enlargement, widened alveolar ridges and widely spaced teeth. Certain viscera are also enlarged.
37. **Maffucci's syndrome** is characterized by development of multiple hemangiomas of skin and oral mucosa. Multiple chondromas of jaw bone are seen. They represent calcification of organized blood clots in dilated vascular spaces.

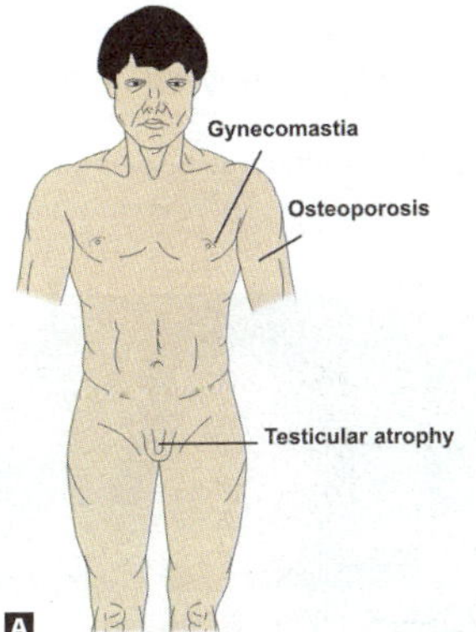

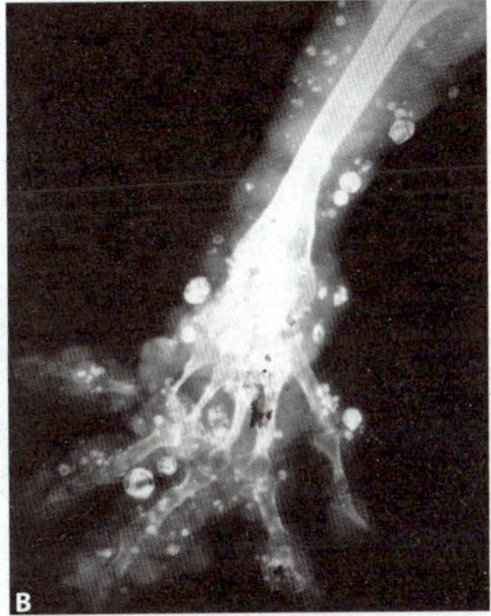

Figs A and B: *(A) Klinefelter's syndrome; (B) Maffucci's syndrome*

38. **Marfan-Achard syndrome** is basically a disease of connective tissue and defective organization of collagen. There will be excessive length of tubular bones, shape of skull and face is long and narrow. There is hyperextensibility of joints and habitual dislocations. High arched palate vault is very common. Bifid uvula is very common. Temporomandibular dysarthrosis is noted.
39. **Meckel's syndrome** is characterized by midline clefting of tongue. Tongue is also thrown into multiple nodular or papillomatous projections.
40. **Median cleft face syndrome** includes hypertelorism, median cleft of premaxilla and palate. There will be bifidum occultum. It has no clinical manifestation.
41. **MEN syndrome** is a group of syndromes characterized by tumors of various endocrine organs.
42. **Miescher's syndrome** is characterized by development of diffuse swelling of lip. Swelling may take place on vermilion border. Formation of scaling, fissuring, vesicle or pustule may take place.
43. **Mobius syndrome** is manifested by facial diplegia with bilateral paralysis of ocular muscles. Child is not able to close the eye during sleep. Lips are everted and mouth may remain open. There is difficulty in mastication and drooling of saliva may be seen. Mental defects and epilepsy may develop.
44. **Mucocutaneous lymph node syndrome** is a disease of unknown etiology. It is a self-limiting febrile illness. Some think it is a collagen vascular disease. There may be dryness, redness and fissuring of lips. There may be acute, nonpurulent swelling of cervical lymph glands.
45. **Myofacial pain dysfunction syndrome (MPDS)** is characterized by pain and limited movements of TMJ. It may be caused by spasm of muscles of mastication and fatigue. Habitual grinding of teeth may also result in the condition. Clinical manifestations are generally seen as most of the females being the sufferer between the age group of 30-40 years, pain in temporomandibular joint, muscle tenderness, limitation of movements, sometimes, clicking sound will be produced.
46. **Neck-Tongue syndrome** is characterized by unilateral upper nuchal or occipital pain with or without numbness in these areas. There is simultaneous numbness of tongue on the same side.

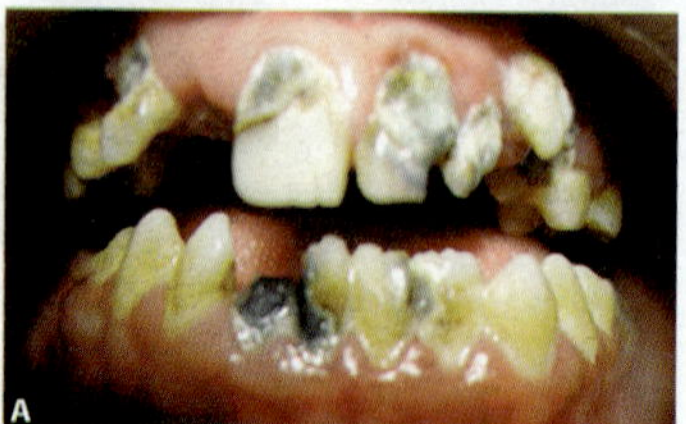

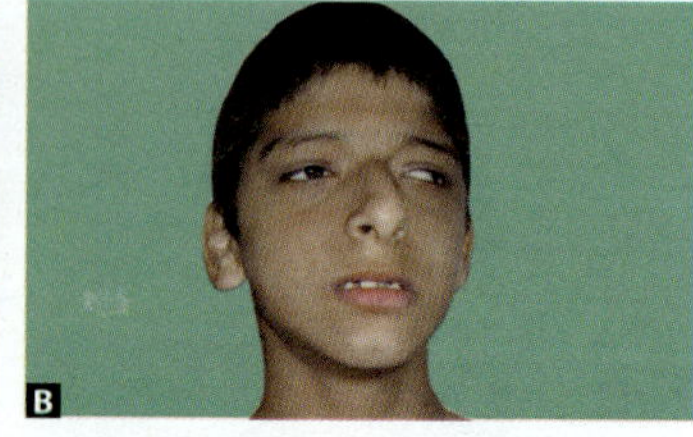

Figs A and B: *Marfan—Achard syndrome*

47. **Nevoid basal cell carcinoma syndrome** Individuals parent with jaw cysts, facies, calcification, bifid ribs and skin lesions. Multiple pink to brown papules appear on face. In 50% cases pitting of soles and palms is seen.
48. **Nursing bottle syndrome** occurs in babies who are on bottlefeed that contains more of sugar. It results in multiple number of caries in many teeth mostly the lower one.
49. **Oculo-dento-osseous dysplasia** is characterized by micro-ophthalmus, iridal anomalies, bony anomalies of the digits and syndactyly, with enamel hypoplasia. The teeth show large multifocal hypoplastic defects and pitting yielding a moth-eaten pattern radiographically.
50. **Oral-facial digital syndrome** is characterized by cleft tongue as one of the part of this syndrome in association with thick fibrous bands in lower anterior mucobuccal fold. It is of little significance.
51. **Papillon-lefevre syndrome** is characterized by hyperkeratotic skin lesion, severe periodontal destruction, destruction of alveolar bone involving both deciduous and permanent dentitions. Inflammatory gingival enlargement, gingival ulceration, formation of deep pockets are frequently present and calcification of the dura, the cutaneous. The dural changes generally occur before the age of 4 years. The syndrome is inherited and appears to follow an autosomal recessive pattern. Parents are not affected and may occur in siblings; males and females are equally affected.
52. **Paratrigeminal syndrome** is a disease with severe headache or pain in area of distribution of trigeminal nerve. Cause of disease is not known. Some of the signs may be of Horner's syndrome.
53. **Peutz-Jegher's syndrome** is characterized by an oral pigmentation. Multiple focal, melanotic brown macules are concentrated on lips. Macules may go upto 3-5 cms in size. Anterior tongue may be involved. Histologically these show basilar melanogenesis without melanocytic proliferation.
54. **Pierre-Robin syndrome** consists of cleft palate, micrognathia and glossoptosis. There is hypoplasia of mandible. Patient may have congenital heart defects and ocular lesions.

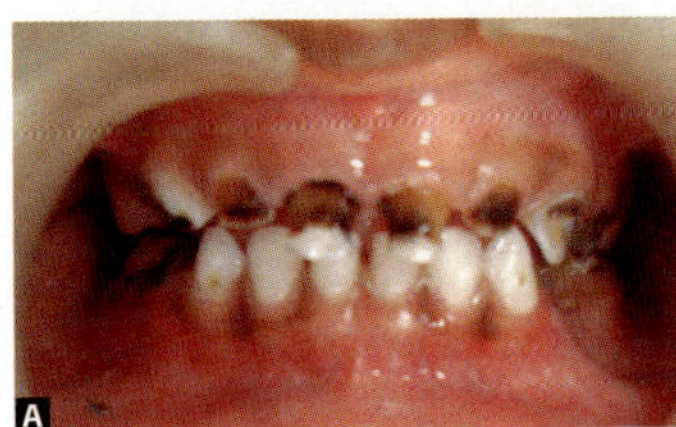

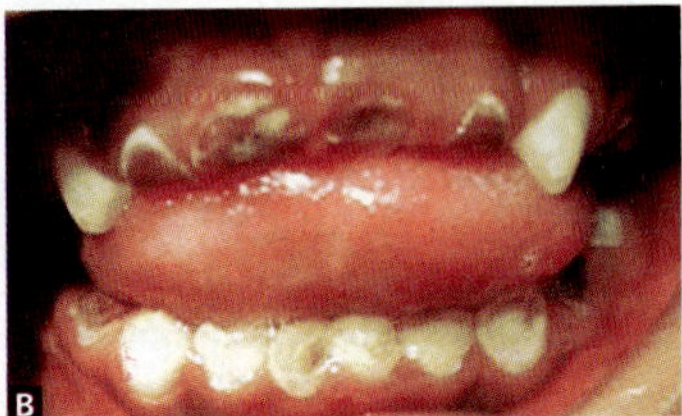

Figs A and B: *Nursing bottle syndrome*

55. **Plummer-Vinson syndrome** develops chiefly in women of fourth and fifth decade of life. Clinically it may be manifested by the presence of anemia, cracks or fissures at corners of mouth, smooth red painful tongue with atrophy of filiform and later fungiform papillae. Mucous membrane and esophagus are atrophic and show loss of keratinization. Koilonychias develop. Blood will show hypochromic microcytic anemia.
56. **Pterygopalatine fossa syndrome** is caused by metastatic tumor to pterygopalatine fossa. It consists of maxillary dental pain, infraorbital and palatal anesthesia. There may also be associated blindness and paralysis of pterygoid muscle.
57. **Romon syndrome** can be clinically described where patient develops gingival and alveolar enlargement, microophthalmia. Cornea becomes cloudy. Hypopigmentation results with athetosis. Mental retardation is rare.
58. **Rubinstein-Taypi syndrome** is manifested by talon cusp being the main feature along with development retardation, broad thumbs and great toes. Facial features are characteristics. Head circumference and bone age are below fifth percentile.
59. **Rutherford syndrome** is characterized by congenitally enlarged gingiva, delayed tooth eruption and superior corneal opacities. Patient may have mental retardation, aggressive behavior and dentigerous cysts.
60. **Scheuthauer-Marie sainton syndrome** is also known as cleidocranial dysplasia, patient may have high narrow arched palate. Maxilla is under-developed. Mandible may be larger. There may be prolonged retention of deciduous tooth.
61. **Sinus of Morgagni syndrome** consists of mandibular nerve pain, palatal immobilization and trismus. There may be unilateral deafness. It may be due to carcinoma.
62. **Sipple's syndrome** is characterized by parathyroid hyperplasia or adenoma but no tumors of pancreas. There is no peptic ulcer but may have pheochromocytomas of adrenal medulla.
63. **Sjögren's syndrome** is a multisystem autoimmune disorder of exocrine glands which may be associated with neuropathy and lymphoproliferative disorder with acinar destruction of glands. It is a condition originally described as triad consisting of keratoconjunctivitis sicca, xerostomia and rheumatoid arthritis, i.e. Lacrimal and salivary glands are affected. In primary Sjögren's syndrome only salivary and lacrimal glands are involved. In this, mouth and eyes become dry. In secondary Sjögren's syndrome along with above symptoms rheumatoid arthritis may also develop. Some may develop arthalgia. Person feels tired. Histological hallmark is focal lymphocytic infiltration of exocrine glands. Epstein-Barr or a type A retrovirus is the causative organism. Xerostomia is a major complaint in most patients as it results in difficulty in

swallowing and talking. Taste sensations may also be distorted. Mucosa becomes red and parchment like look. Dorsum of tongue becomes red and atrophic. There may be fissuring. Parotid gland enlargement is seen along with enlargement of submandibular gland. There may be symptoms of rheumatoid arthritis. Kidney involvement is noted **(*see* Figure under).**

64. **Solitary median maxillary central incisor syndrome** presents with a single central incisor in the midline. This condition may be associated with other midline disturbances such as cleft lip and palate, imperforate anus, umbilical hernia, choanal stenosis.
65. **Stevens-Johnson syndrome** is also known as erythema multiforme when the vesicles and bulla involve skin, mouth, eyes and genitals. Generally young adults are involved. Discrete macula, papule or vesicles are distributed symmetrically over hands and arms, face and neck. Oral mucous membrane lesions are very painful and mastication may not be possible. Mucosal vesicles rupture leaving surface covered with thick, white, yellow exudates. Erosions of pharynx are common. It may also occur secondary to a drug reaction. It can slough skin and mucosa. Electrolyte imbalance may develop.
66. **Sturge–Weber syndrome** is described as where patients develops orofacial and meningeal angiomatosis with secondary mental deficiency. There may be seizures, hemiplegia and mild to severe enlargement of gingiva. Hyperplastic

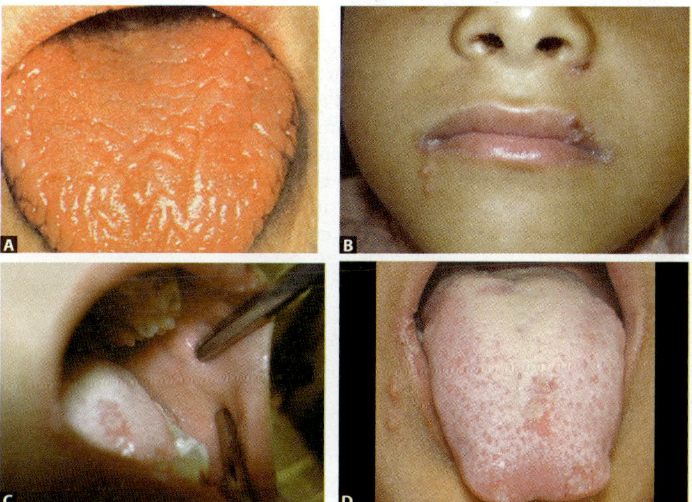

Figs A to D: *(A) Sjögren's syndrome; (B) Steven johnson syndrome (extra oral lesions; (C and D) Steven johnson syndrome (intra oral lesions)*

vascular gingival blanch on pressure. Bony hemangiomas and delayed tooth eruption may be noted.

70. **Sweat Retention syndrome** can be described as an extravasation of sweat in the tissue with subsequent inflammation, there is also keratin plug formation in sweat glands.
71. **Tietze syndrome** is a painful costochondral function syndrome. There is no palpable abnormality and pain is identified in medial quadrant of breast. It is generally unilateral and may develop at any age. Antiinflammatory drugs may give comfort.
72. **Trichodento-osseous syndrome** also shows enamel defects in conjunction with morphologic dental anomalies. These patients have tightly curled kinky hair with osteosclerosis of bone cortices. The enamel is hypoplastic and hypocalcified, lacking mesiodistal contact with pitting.
73. **Trisomy** – 13 develops due to multiple abnormalities of various organs. Child dies within a year. There may be bilateral cleft lip and palate, small or no eye at all. Superficial hemangioma of forehead, delayed growth, mental retardation, polydactyly of hands and fest are noted.
74. **Uremic syndrome** is a disease where signs and symptoms of kidney failure is seen, one of them is decreased creatinine clearance. As disease progresses, glomerular filtration rate falls and blood urea nitrogen rises. Person may develop impaired ability to concentrate urine, nocturia and mild anemia. Advanced uremia is associated with pericarditis, pericardial effusion and neuropathies.
75. **Von–Sallman syndrome** is a hereditary benign intra-epithelial Dyskeratosis. It is rare autosomal dominant trait. Patient shows oral mucosal thickening with superficial gelatinous looking plaques on bulbar conjunctiva. Cytological scrapings show 'cells within cells'.
76. **Zimmerman–Lebarnd syndrome** is characterized when patient develops gingival fibromatosis with defects of ear, nose, bones and terminal phalanges. Joints become hyperexible. Spleen is enlarged.

Annexure-III

CAUSES OF DENTAL DISEASES

Causes of Pulpitis

- Fracture of crown/cusp
- Dental caries
- Thermal/chemical irritation.

Causes of Resorption of Permanent Teeth

- Impacted teeth putting pressure on adjacent teeth
- Periapical periodontitis
- Replanted teeth
- Neoplasm
- Idiopathic resorption.

Causes of Exacerbating Gingivitis

- Dental irregularities
- Restorations resulting in stagnation area
- Pregnancy
- Medication
- Uncontrolled diabetes.

Causes of Persistence of Plaque

- Overhanging restorations
- Calculus
- Mouth breathing
- Pocketing
- Irregular teeth.

Causes of Premature Periodontal Tissue Destruction

- Severe uncontrolled diabetes
- Leukopenia

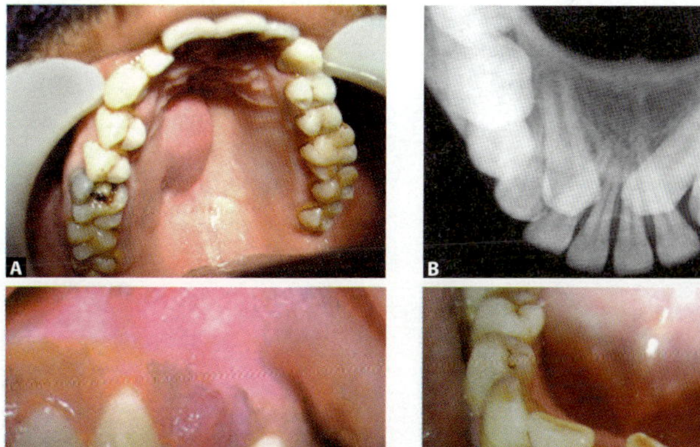

Figs A to D: *Causes of (A) Pulpitis; (B) Resorption of permanent teeth; (C) Persistence of plaque; (D) Premature periodontal tissue destruction*

- HIV infections
- Hypophosphatasia.

Causes of Gingival Enlargement

- Genetic
- Drugs associated phenytoin
- Calcium channel blockers
- Pregnancy
- Inflammatory
  - Leukemia
  - Sarcoidosis
  - Scurvy.

Causes of Cyst-Like Areas of Jaw

- Ameloblastoma
- Hyperparathyroidism
- Pseudocysts
- Giant cell granuloma.

Causes of Swellings of Jaw

- Odontogenic tumors
- Odontogenic cysts
- Giant cell lesion
- Metastatic neoplasm
- Fibro-osseous lesions.

Drugs Causing Lichenoid Reactions

- Beta blockers
- Allopurinol
- Methyldopa
- Antimalarials
- Captopril
- Penicillamine.

Causes of Macroglossia

- Cretinism
- Amyloidosis
- Lingual thyroid
- Down's syndrome.

Causes of Xerostomia

- Functional causes
  - Dehydration
  - Hemorrhage
  - Anxiety/depression
  - Psychogenic
- Organic causes
  - Mumps
  - HIV infection
  - Sarcoidosis
  - Amyloidosis
- Drugs
  - Excessive diuretic
  - Atropine
  - Decongestants
  - Bronchodilators.

Causes of Ptyalism

- False ptyalism
  - Bell's palsy

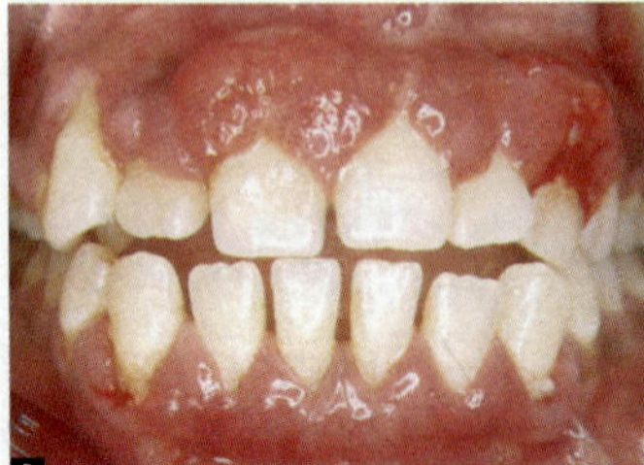

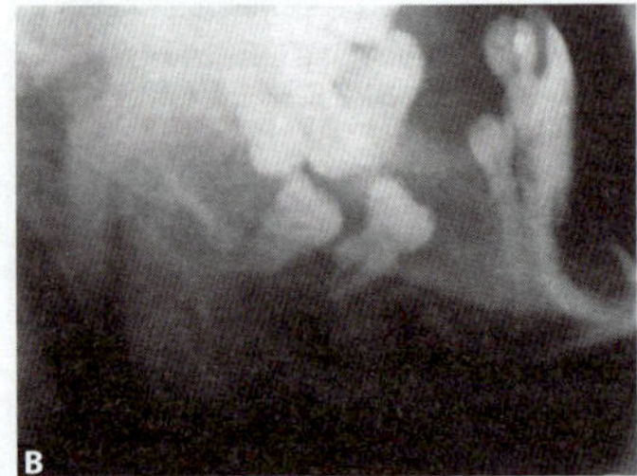

Figs A and B: *Causes of* (A) *Gingival enlargement; (B) Cyst like areas of jaw*

- Psychogenic
- Stroke
- Parkinsonism

- Local
  - Oral wounds
  - New dentures
  - Oral infections.

Causes of Sialadenosis

- Diabetes mellitus
- Drugs
- Idiopathic
- Alcoholism.

Causes of Dental Pain

- Dull throbbing pain
  - Pericoronitis
  - Late pulpitis
  - Dry socket
  - Herpes zoster
  - Atypical odontalgia
  - Atypical facial pain
- Burning pain
  - Post-herpetic neuralgia
  - Burning mouth syndrome
- Sharp stapping pain
  - Exposed dentine
  - Early pulpitis
  - Trigeminal neuralgia
  - Fractured tooth.

Developmental Defects in Jaws

- Craniofacial anomalies
- Hereditary prognathism
- Cleidocranial dysplasia
- Osteogenesis imperfecta
- Gardner's syndrome.

Classification of Cysts of Jaw

- Inflammatory odontogenic cyst
  - Radicular
  - Paradental.
- Odontogenic developmental cysts
  - Dentigerous
  - Eruption cyst
  - Lateral periodontal
  - Gingival cyst.
- Nonodontogenic developmental cysts
  - Nasolabial cyst
  - Nasopalantine duct cysts.

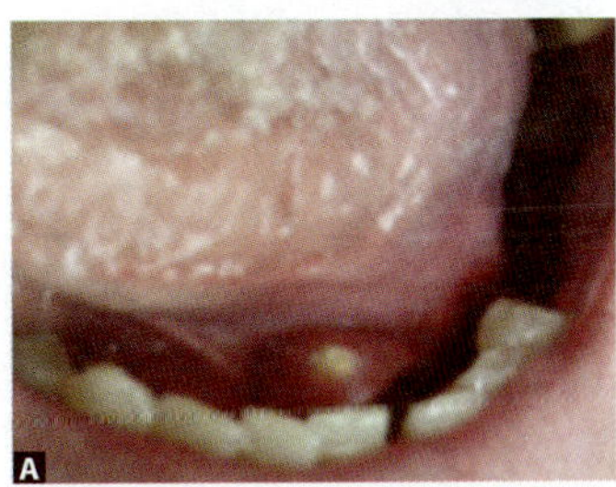

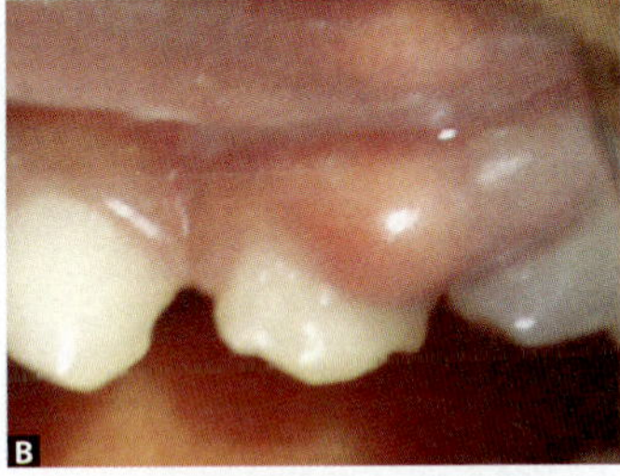

Figs A and B: *Causes of* (A) *Sialodenosis; (B) Classification of cysts of jaw*

Annexure-IV

SYNONYMS/ALTERNATIVES

Perleche	Angular cheilitis
Mucous retention cyst	Mucocele
Dry socket	Alveolitis sicca dolorosa, Alveolar osteitis
Hand Schuller Christian disease	Multifocal eosinophilic granuloma
Histiocytosis	Nonlipid reticuloendotheliosis
Osteomalacia	Adult rickets
Renal rickets	Renal osteodystrophy
Marfan syndrome	Arachnodactyly
Down's syndrome	Trisomy 21 syndrome, Mongolism
Osteopetrosis	Marble bone disease, osteosclerosis
Achondroplasia	Chondrodystrophia fetalis
Osteitis deformans	Paget's disease
Van Buchem disease	Generalized cortical hyperostosis
Massive osteolysis	Vanishing bone
Cherubism	Familial fibrous dysplasia
Osteoarthritis	Degenerative joint disease
Ankylosis	Hypomobility
Pernicious anemia	Addison's anemia
Sprue	Celiac disease
Thalassemia	Cooley's anemia
Polycythemia vera	Erythroblastic anemia
Agranulocytosis	Granulocytopenia
Infectious mononucleosis	Glandular fever
Thrombocythemia	Thrombocytosis
Hemophilia	Disease of King's
Acute necrotizing ulcerative gingivitis (ANUG)	Vincent's infection, Ulcerative gingivitis, Trench mouth

Juvenile Periodontitis	Periodontosis
Migraine headache	Menstrual headache, Sunday headache, Monday morning headache, Sick headache
Acute septic osteitis	Osteomyelitis
Dentinal sclerosis	Transparent dentin
Secondary dentin	Irregular dentin
Hypercementosis	Cementum hyperplasia
Internal resorption	Odontoclastoma, pink tooth of mummery
Scarlet fever	Scarlatina
Sarcoidosis	Boeck's Sarcoid
Uveoparotid fever	Heerfordt's syndrome
Leprosy	Hansen's disease
Botryomycosis	Bacterial actinophytosis
Granuloma inguinale	Granuloma venereum
Rhinoscleroma	Scleroma
Midline lethal granuloma	Malignant granuloma
NOMA	Cancrum oris, Gangrenous stomatitis
Progenic granuloma	Granuloma pyogenicum
Herpes simplex	Herpes labialis
Recurrent aphthous stomatitis	Canker sores
Herpangina	Aphthous pharyngitis
Rubella	German measles
Herpes zoster	Shingles
Mumps	Epidemic parotitis
Poliomyelitis	Infantile paralysis
Coccidioidomycosis	Valley fever
Candidiasis	Moniliasis, Thrush
Periapical granuloma	Atypical periodontia
Apical periodontal cyst	Radicular cyst

Periapical abscess	Alveolar abscess
Condensing osteitis	Chronic focal sclerosing osteomyelitis
Traumatic ulcer	Decubitus ulcer, Sore ulcer
Palatal papillomatosis	Inflammatory papillary hyperplasia
Dental lamina cyst	Gingival cyst, Epstein's pearls, Bohn's nodules
Bifid rib syndrome	Basal cell nevus syndrome, Goltz syndrome
Calcifying odontogenic cyst	Cystic keratinizing cyst
Enameloma	Enamel drop
Ameloblastoma	Adamatinoma multilocular cyst
Primary intraosseous carcinoma	Primary intra-alveolar epidermoid carcinoma
Calcifying epithelial odontogenic tumor (CEOT)	Adenoameloblastoma, ameloblastic adenomatoid tumor
Squamous odontogenic tumor	Benign epithelial odontogenic tumor
Peripheral odontogenic fibroma	Peripheral ossifying fibroma, calcifying fibrous eupilis
Odontogenic myxoma	Myxoma, Myxofibroma, fibromyxoma
Periapical cemental dysplasia	Cementoma, periapical osteofibrosis, Cementifying fibroma, periapical cemental dysplasia, focal cemento-osseusdysplasia
Benign cementoblastoma	True cementoma
Gigantiform cementoma	Familial multiple cementoma
Ameloblastic fibroma	Soft mixed odontogenic tumor, soft mixed odontoma
Ameloblastic fibroma	Ameloblastic sarcoma
Ameloblastic odontoma	Odontoameloblastoma calcified odontoma
Teratoma	Teratoblastoma
Primary lymphoma of bone	Primary reticulum cell sarcoma
African jaw lymphoma	Burkitt's lymphoma

Multiple myeloma	Plasma cell myeloma
Plasma cell myeloma	Plasmacytoma
Angiomyoma	Vascular leiomyoma
Granular cell myoblastoma	Granular cell tumor myoblastic myoma
Traumatic neuroma	Amputation neuroma
Alveolar soft part sarcoma	Malignant granular cell myoblastoma
Multiple endocrine neoplasm	Men syndrome
Neurofibroma	Neurofibromatosis, fibroma molluscum
Neurolemma	Schwannoma, perineural fibroblastoma
Malignant schwannoma	Neurofibrosarcoma
Olfactory neuroblastoma	Esthesioneuroblastoma
Pleomorphic adenoma	Mixed tumor
Papillary cystadenoma lymphomatosum	Warthin's tumor, Adenolymphoma
Oxyphilic adenoma	Oncocytoma, acidophilic adenoma
Mikulicz's disease	Benign lymphoepithelial lesion
Sjogren's syndrome	Sicca syndrome
Malignant pleomorphic adenoma	Malignant mixed tumor pleomorphic adenoma
Adenoid cystic carcinoma	Cylindroma, basaloid mixed tumor, adenocystic basal cell carcinoma
Acinic cell carcinoma	Serous cell adenoma, adenocarcinoma
Dentigerous cyst	Follicular cyst
Apical periodontal cyst	Radicular cyst, periapical cyst, dental root-end cyst
Facial neuritis	Bell's palsy
Ankylosed deciduous teeth	Submerged teeth
Median anterior maxillary cyst	Nasopalatine duct cyst, incisive canal cyst
Nasoalveolar cyst	Nasolabial cyst
Palatal cysts	Epstein's pearls
Benign cervical lymphoepithelial cyst	Branchial cleft cyst, benign cystic lymph node

Keratoacanthoma	Self-healing carcinoma, molluscum sebaceum
Intraepithelial carcinoma	Carcinoma in situ
Basal cell carcinoma	Rodent ulcer
Epidermoid carcinoma	Squamous cell carcinoma
Spindle cell carcinoma	Carcinosarcoma, lane tumor
Adenoacanthoma	Adenoid squamous cell carcinoma
Peripheral ossifying fibroma	Peripheral odontogenic fibroma
Central ossifying fibroma	Central fibro-osteoma
Osteoclastoma giant cell epulis	Peripheral giant cell granuloma
Verruciform xanthoma	Histiocytosis 'Y'
Hemangioma	Vascular nevus
Sturge-Weber syndrome	Encephalotrigeminal angiomatosis
Rendu-Osler-Weber disease	Hereditary hemorrhagic telangiectasia
Nasopharyngeal	Juvenile nasopharyngeal fibroma, angiofibroma
Benign chondroblastoma	Codman's tumor
Benign osteoblastoma	Giant osteoid osteoma
Kaposi's sarcoma	Angioreticuloendothelioma
Ewing's sarcoma	Round cell sarcoma, endothelial myeloma
Osteosarcoma	Osteogenic sarcoma
Labial/oral melanotic macule	Ephelis, focal melanosis, solitary labial lentigo
Focal epithelial hyperplasia	Heck's disease
Fibromatosis gingiva	Elephantiasis gingivae, hereditary gingival fibromatosis
Fissured tongue	Scrotal tongue
Medium rhomboid glossitis	Central papillary atrophy of tongue
Benign migratory glossitis	Geographic tongue, erythema migrans, wandering rash of tongue
Lymphoid hamartoma	Angiofollicular, lymph node malformation

Angiolymphoid hyperplasia	Kimura's disease, eosinophilic folliculitis
Lymphoepithelial cyst	Branchial cyst, branchiogenic cyst
Aplasia	Agenesis
Dens in dente	Dens invaginatus, dilated composite odontome, occlusal enamel pearl
Amelogenesis imperfecta	Hereditary brown opalescent teeth, hereditary enamel dysplasia
Dentinogenesis imperfecta	Hereditary opalsescent dentin, Odontogenic imperfecta
Regional odontodysplasia	Ghost teeth
Plasma cells	Effector cells
Rickett's E line	E-line
Bell's palsy	Facial neuritis
Accessory cusp	Supernumerary cusp
Gumma	Tertiary syphilitic oral ulcer
Vitamin B_1	Thiamine
Endogenous malodor	True oral malodor
Vasodepressor syncope	Vasovagal syncope
Angular defects	Vertical defects
Cannon's disease	White spongy nevus
Sterility	Infertility
Nursing bottle caries	Infancy caries
Soother caries	Infancy caries
Kissing disease	Infectious mononucleosis
Infracristal pocket	Infrabony pocket
Infra-alveolar pocket	Infrabony pocket
Centric occlusion	Intercuspal position
Papillary gingival	Interdental gingiva
Supracontact	Interference
Apoplexy	Intracerebral hemorrhage
Chronic microcytic	Iron deficiency anemia, hypochromic anemia

Juvenile periodontitis	Localized juvenile periodontis, Early onset periodontitis, localized aggressive periodontitis
Warty dyskeratoma	Keratosis follicularis
Kirkland knives	Periodontal knives, gingivectomy knives
Le Fort I	Low-level fracture
Le Fort II	Pyramidal fracture, subzygomatic fracture
Le Fort III	High transverse fracture, suprazygomatic fracture
Migratory glossitis	Geographic tongue
Sulcular fluid	Gingival fluid
Polyalkenoate cements	Glass ionomer cements (GICs)
Miescher's syndrome	Granulomatous cheilitis
Bicuspidization	Hemiseptum
Witkop von Sallman syndrome	Hereditary benign intraepithelialdys-keratosis
Thyrotoxicosis	Hyperthyroidism
Mucoperiosteal flap	Full thickness flap
German measles	Rubella
Septic theory	Parasitic theory
Partial thickness flap	Mucosal flap, split thickness flap
Servo system	Petrovic's hypothesis
Branchial arches	Pharyngeal arches
Compomers	Polyacid – modified composite resins
Orthostatic hypotension	Postural hypotension
Dentinoid	Predentin
Deciduous dentition	Primary dentition
Unethical act	Professional misconducts
Thrush	Pseudomembranous candidiasis
Takayasu's disease	Pulseless disease

Pyelonephritis	Pyelitis
Progressive systemic sclerosis	Scleroderma
Cartilaginous theory	Scott's hypothesis
Fissured tongue	Scrotal tongue
Diode lasers	Semiconductor lasers
Steiner's line	S-line
Incomplete fracture	Split tooth
Contact stomatitis	Stomatitis venenata
Suprabony pocket	Supracristal pocket, supra-alveolar pocket
Neutrophilis	Polymorphonuclear, Leukocytes, microphage
Monocytes	Macrophages
Unattached gingival	Marginal gingiva
Transitional dentition	Mixed dentition

Annexure–V

TOOTH NUMBERING SYSTEM

I. American Numbering System

A Permanent Teeth

Upper Teeth

1. Maxillary right third molar
2. Maxillary right second molar
3. Maxillary right first molar
4. Maxillary right second premolar
5. Maxillary right first premolar
6. Maxillary right canine
7. Maxillary right lateral incisor
8. Maxillary right central incisor
9. Maxillary left central incisor
10. Maxillary left lateral incisor
11. Maxillary left canine
12. Maxillary left first premolar
13. Maxillary left second premolar
14. Maxillary left first molar
15. Maxillary left second molar
16. Maxillary left third molar.

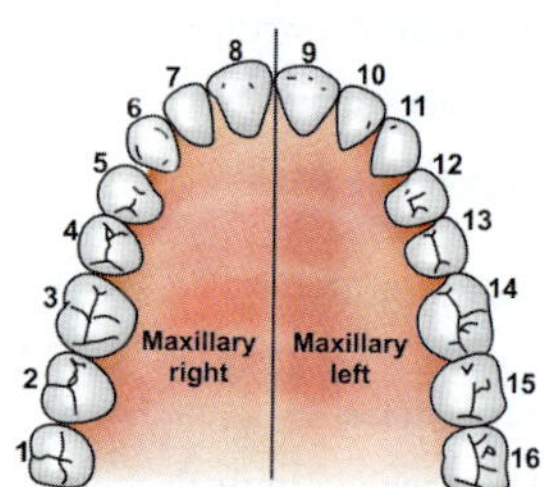

Lower Teeth

17. Mandibular left third molar
18. Mandibular left second molar
19. Mandibular left first molar
20. Mandibular left second premolar
21. Mandibular left first premolar
22. Mandibular left canine
23. Mandibular left lateral incisor
24. Mandibular left central incisor
25. Mandibular right central incisor
26. Mandibular right lateral incisor
27. Mandibular right canine

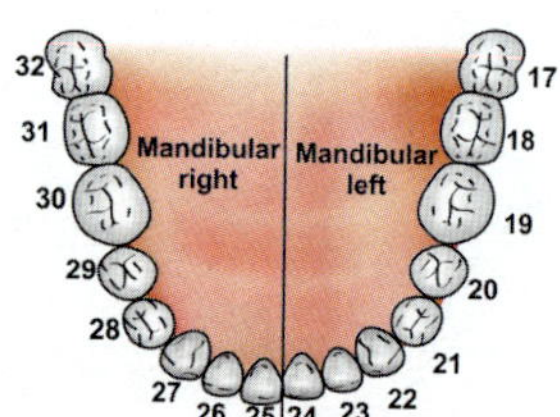

28. Mandibular right first premolar
29. Mandibular right first premolar
30. Mandibular right first molar
31. Mandibular right second molar
32. Mandibular right third molar.

B Primary Teeth

Upper Teeth

A. Maxillary right second molar
B. Maxillary right first molar
C. Maxillary right canine
D. Maxillary right lateral incisor
E. Maxillary right central incisor
F. Maxillary left central incisor
G. Maxillary left lateral incisor
H. Maxillary left canine
I. Maxillary left first molar
J. Maxillary left second molar.

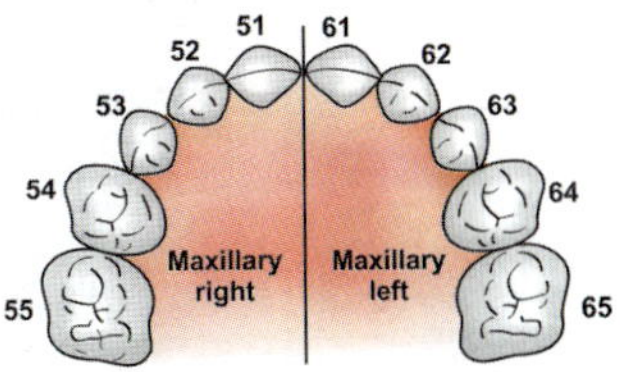

Lower Teeth

K. Mandibular left second molar
L. Mandibular left first molar
M. Mandibular left canine
N. Mandibular left lateral incisor
O. Mandibular left central incisor
P. Mandibular right central incisor
Q. Mandibular right lateral incisor
R. Mandibular right canine
S. Mandibular right first molar
T. Mandibular right second molar.

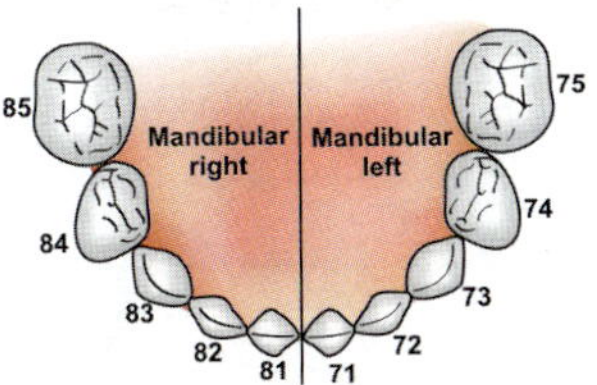

Federation Dentaire Internationale System

A. Permanent Teeth

Quadrant number	*Quadrant identification*
1	Maxillary right
2	Maxillary left
3	Mandibular left
4	Mandibular right

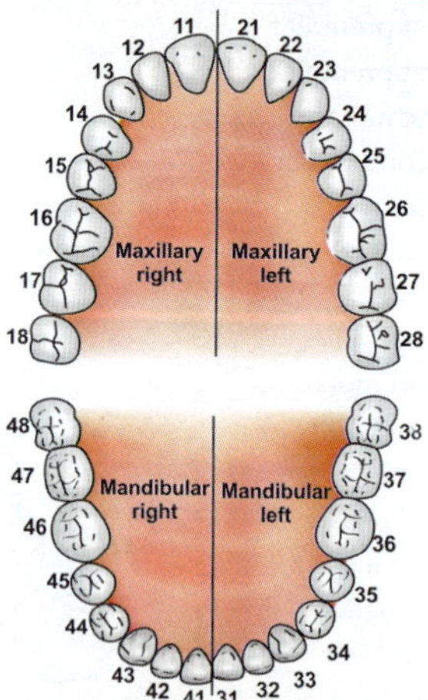

Fig.: *Federation dentaire internationale numbering system for permanent dentition*

Federation Dentaire Internationale System

B. Primary Teeth	
Quadrant number	*Quadrant identification*
5	Maxillary right
6	Maxillary left
7	Mandibular left
8	Mandibular right

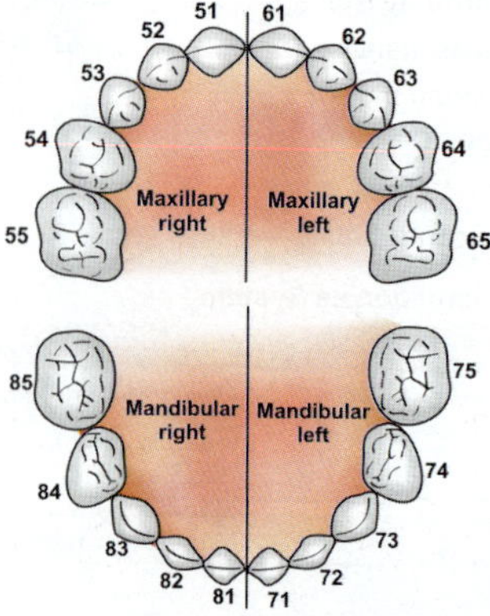

Fig.: *Federation dentaire internationale numbering system for primary dentition*

III. Zsigmondy-Palmer system

It identifies specific teeth by using a grid system.

Upper right	Upper left
Lower right	Lower left

(A) Zsigmondy-palmer System for Deciduous Dentition

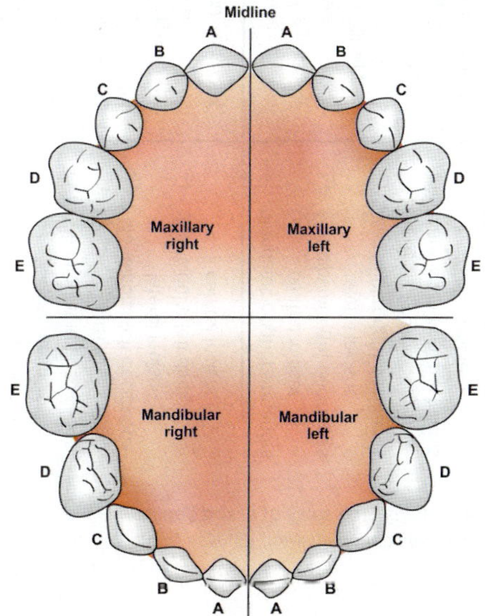

(B) Zsigmondy-palmer System for Mixed Dentition

A

6	E	D	C	B	A	A	B	C	D	E	6
6	E	D	C	B	1	1	B	C	D	E	6

B

Maxillary right	Maxillary left
6 Maxillary right permanent first molar	A Maxillar left deciduous central incisor
E Maxillary right deciduous second molar	B Maxillar left deciduous lateral incisor
D Maxillar right deciduous first molar	C Maxillar left deciduous cuspid
C Maxillary right deciduous cuspid	D Maxillar left deciduous first molar
B Maxillary right deciduous lateral incisor	E Maxillar left deciduous second molar
A Maxillary right deciduous central incisor	6 Maxillar left deciduous first molar

Mandibular right	Mandibular left
6 Mandibular right deciduous first molar	1 Mandibular left deciduous central incisor
E Mandibular right deciduous second molar	B Mandibular left deciduous lateral incisor
D Mandibular right deciduous first molar	C Mandibular left deciduous cuspid
C Mandibular right deciduous cuspid	D Mandibular left deciduous first molar
B Mandibular right deciduous lateral incisor	E Mandibular left deciduous second molar
1 Mandibular right permanent central incisor	6 Mandibular left permanent first molar

B

FigsA and B: *(A) Schematic display of mixed dentition using Zsigmondy Palmer tooth identification system; (B) Key to display shown in A.*

(C) Zsigmondy-palmer System for Permanent Dentition

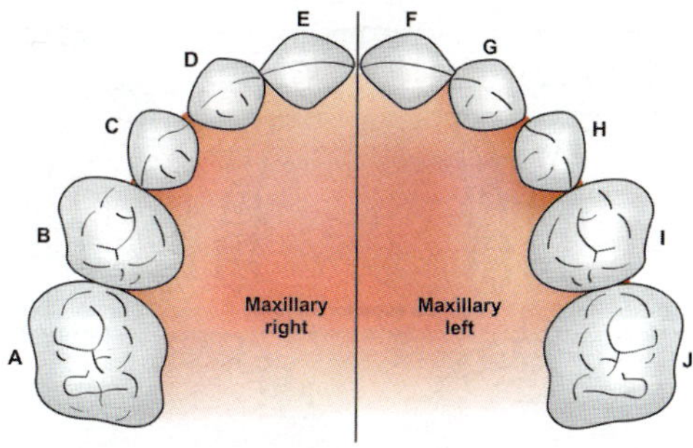

Fig.: *Number eight represents third molars, Number one represents central incisors*

Sites for the Administration of Anesthesia

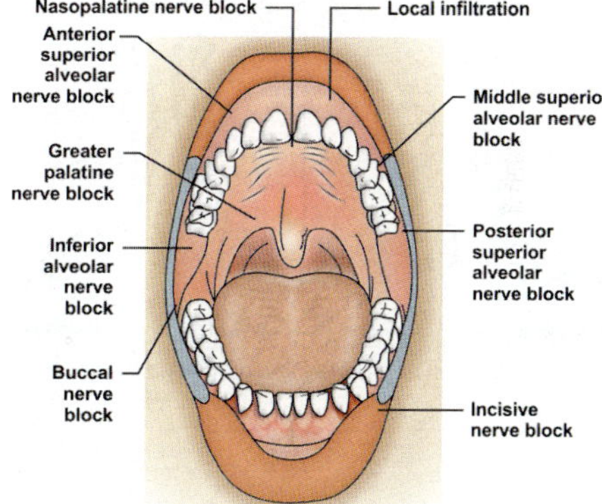

Areas Affected Post-Administration of Local Anesthesia

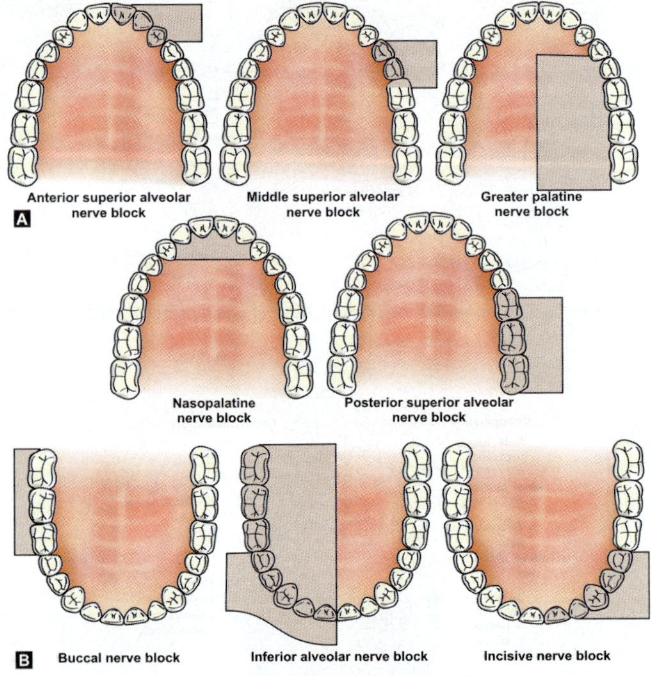

Figs A and B: *(A) Mandibular; (B) Maxillary*

Annexure–VI

TABLES

Lypmph Nodes of the Head and Neck	
Lymph nodes of the head	**Drainage**
Retroauricular nodes	Skin of ear and posterior parietal region of scalp
Preauricular nodes	Auricle of ear and temporal region of scalp
Parotid nodes	Root of nose, eyelids, anterior temporal region, external auditory meatus, tympanic cavity, nasopharynx, and posterior portions of nasal cavity
Facial nodes	
Infraorbital nodes	Eyelid and conjunctiva
Buccal nodes	Skin and mucous membrane of nose and cheek
Mandibular nodes	Skin and mucous membrane of nose and cheek
Submandibular nodes	Chin, lips, nose, nasal cavity, cheeks, gums, inferior surface of palate and anterior portion of tongue.
Submental nodes	Chin, lower lip, cheeks, tip of tongue, and floor of mouth
Superficial cervical nodes	Inferior part of ear and parotid region
Deep cervical nodes	
Superior deep cervical node	Posterior head and neck, auricle, tongue, larynx nodes, esophagus, thyroid gland, nasopharynx, nasal cavity, palate and tonsils
Inferior deep cervical node	Posterior scalp and neck, superficial pectoral region, and part of arm

Muscles of the Face

Muscles	Origin	Action and comments
Orbicularis oris	Muscle fibers surrounding mouth	Closes lips, presses lips against teeth, protrudes lips and shapes lips in speech
Zygomaticus minor	Zygomatic bone	Elevates upper lip
Major	Zygomatic bone	Draws angle of mouth upward and outward.
Levator labii superioris	Maxilla and zygomatic bone	Raises upper lip and turns it outward.
Depressor labii inferioris	Mandible	Draws lower lip downward and a little laterally.
Depressor anguli oris	Mandible	Draws angle of mouth downward and laterally.
Buccinators	Mandible and maxilla in region near molars	Compresses cheeks against teeth, provides a stable lateral wall to oral cavity for pressure in speech, sucking and mastication.
Levator anguli oris	Canine fossa of maxilla	Raises angle of mouth.
Mentalis	Incisor fossa of mandible	Draws lower lip downward and a little laterally.
Risorius	Facial of masseter muscle	Retracts angle of mouth.
Masseter	Maxilla, zygomatic arch	Elevates mandible, closing jaw.
Temporalis	Temporal fossa	Elevates mandible, closing jaw; draws mandible backward after protrusion, assists in lateral movements.
Lateral pterygoid	Greater wing of the sphenoid bone and lateral pterygoid plate	Helps in opening mouth, protrusion of jaw, and grinding movements.
Medial pterygoid	Pterygoid plate, palatine bone, and maxilla	Elevation and protrusion of mandible and side-to-side movements of jaw.

Muscles of the Neck

Muscle	Origin	Insertion	Action and comments
Superficial lateral cervical muscles			
Platysma	Fascia covering pectoralis major and deltoid muscles skin and subcutaneous tissue of lower part of face	Body of mandible	Wrinkles skin in neck, assists in lowering mandible, draws down lower lip and angle of mouth.
Trapezius			
Sternocleidomastoid	Manubrium of sternum and clavicle cervical nerves	Mastoid process of temporal bone	Singly: tilts head toward shoulder of same side, rotates head to face opposite side; together; draws head forward, flexes cervical part of vertebral column; if head is fixed, they help to raise the thorax in forced inspiration.
Suprahyoid muscles			
Digastric	Mastoid portion of temporal bone, symphysis of mandible	Hyoid bone, occasionally mandible	Depresses mandible, can elevate hyoid bone.

Contd...

Contd...

Muscle	Origin	Insertion	Action and comments
Stylohyoid	Styloid process of temporal bone	Hyoid bone	Elevates the hyoid bone and draws it back, elongating the floor of the mouth. Can stabilize hyoid bone for tongue muscle action.
Mylohyoid	Mylohyoid line on mandible	Hyoid bone median raphe	Elevates floor of mouth in the first phase of swallowing elevates hyoid bone or depresses mandible.
Geniohyoid	Inferior mental spine on mandible	Body of hyoid bone	Elevates hyoid bone and draws it forward; depresses mandible when hyoid bone is fixed.
Infrahyoid muscles			
Sternohyoid	Manubrium of the sternum	Bone of hyoid bone	Depresses hyoid bone after it has been raised as in swallowing.
Sternothyroid	Manubrium of sternum and cartilage of first rib	Lamina of thyroid cartilage	Draws larynx downward after it has been elevated as in swallowing.

Major Arteries of the Head and Neck		
Artery	**Major branches**	**Region supplied**
External carotid artery	Superior thyroid artery	Thyroid gland and adjacent muscles
	Lingual artery	Tongue and floor of the mouth, oropharynx, sublingual gland, and neighboring muscles
	Facial artery	Muscles and tissues of the face below the level of the eyes, the submandibular gland, tonsil, and soft palate
	Occipital artery	Muscles, skin, and other tissue in the region behind the ear and the back part of the scalp
	Posterior auricular artery	Parotid gland, muscles, skin and other tissues of the ear and posterior scalp regions
	Superficial temporal artery	Parotid gland, temporomandibular joint, outer ear, forehead, temporal region of the scalp, adjacent muscles
	Maxillary artery	Upper and lower jaws, teeth, muscles of mastication, palate, nose, and dura mater
Internal carotid artery	Hypophyseal artery Ophthalmic artery	Pituitary gland eye, lacrimal gland, ocular muscles, nasal cavity, forehead
Right and left subclavicular arteries	Vertebral artery	Spinal cord, vertebrae and surrounding tissues, deep neck structures
	Thyrocervical trunk	Thyroid gland, neck muscles, trachea, esophagus
	Costocervical trunk	Muscles at the back of the neck, vertebral canal, first intercostals space

Major Branches from Various Segments of the Aorta		
Artery	**Major branches**	**Region supplied**
Inferior mesenteric artery	Left colic artery	Transverse and descending colon
	Sigmoid arteries	Descending and sigmoid colon
	Superior rectal artery	Rectum
Lumbar arteries		Muscles and skin of the back, vertebral canal, and its contents intercostals
Median sacral artery		Sacral vertebrae, rectum
Common iliac arteries		Pelvic region and legs
	External iliac	Leg
	Internal iliac	Viscera and walls of the pelvis, perineum, and gluteal region

Cranial Nerves (Major Components)			
No.	**Name**	**Peripheral distribution**	**Functions**
I	Olfactory	Mucous membrane of olfactory region of nose	Smell
II	Optic	Retina of eye	Vision
III	Oculomotor	Muscles (superior, inferior, and medial rectus; inferior oblique; and levator palpebrae Pupillary constrictor and ciliary muscles of eye	Eye movements, raises upper eyelid Regulation of pupil size, accommodation of lens
IV	Trochlear	Superior oblique muscle	Eye movements
V	Trigeminal	Face, greater part of scalp, teeth, mouth, nasal cavity Muscles (medial and lateral pterygoid, masseter, temporalis)	Sensory from face, nose, and mouth Chewing movements
VI	Abducent	Lateral rectus muscle	Eye movements
VII	Facial	Anterior part of tongue and soft palate Muscles of face, scalp, and outer ear Submandibular and sublingual salivary glands, lacrimal glands, glands of nasal and palatine mucosa	Taste Facial expression Secretions

contd...

No.	Name	Peripheral distribution	Functions
VIII	Acoustic	Hair cells of organ of corti, semi-circular canals, maculae, and saccule	Hearing, balance, change of rate of motion of head
IX	Glosso-pharyngeal	Back of tongue, pharynx, carotid sinus, and body Stylopharyngeus muscle Parotid salivary gland	Taste and other sensations of tongue, changes in levels of blood pressure and gases Swallowing movements Secretions
X	Vagus	Taste buds on epiglottis; larynx, trachea, pharynx, heart, lungs, esophagus, small intestine, part of colon Smooth muscle of bronchi, esophagus, stomach, and intestines; heart; striated muscles of pharyngeal constrictors and intrinsic muscles of larynx	Pain, stretching, changes in levels of blood pressure and gases, taste Movement and secretion by the organs supplied
XI	Accessory	Muscles of larynx, trapezius, sternocleidomastoid	Shoulder movements, turning head, voice production
XII	Hypoglossal	Muscles of tongue	Tongue movements

National Immunization Schedule	
At birth	**BCG and OPV**
At 6 weeks	DPT-1, OPV-1 and Hepatitis B_1
At 10 weeks	DPT-2, OPV-2 and Hepatitis B_2
At 14 weeks	DPT-3, OPV-3 and Hepatitis B_3
At 9th month	Measles
16 and 24 months	DPT and OPV
At 10 and 16 years	Tetanus toxoid second dose after 1 month
For pregnant women	$T_1 - TT_2$ after one month in first trimester

Milestone in Vaccination			
Year	**Vaccine**	**Year**	**Vaccine**
1798	Small pox vaccine	1949	Mumps vaccine
1885	Rabies vaccine	1954	Salk's polio vaccine
1892	Cholera vaccine	1957	Sabin's live oral polio vaccine
1913	Toxin/Diphtheria	1960	Measles vaccine
1921	BCG	1962	Rubella vaccine
1923	Diphtheria toxoid	1968	Type C meningococcal vaccine
1923	Pertussis vaccine	1976	Hepatitis – B vaccine
1937	Influenza vaccine		

Periods of Isolation	
Disease	**Duration of isolation**
Measles	Catarrhal stage to 3rd day of stage
Chicken pox	Usually till 6 days
German measles	Women should not be exposed in first trimester
Cholera/Diphtheria	3 days after antibiotic
Shigellosis	Until stool becomes negative repeatedly
Hepatitis A	3 weeks
Influenza	3 weeks after onset
Polio	2 weeks adult and six weeks children

Methods for Sterilizations		
Method	**Used for**	**Advantages/Disadvantages**
Hot air	2 hours, 160°C used for all instruments of root kits	It kills all microorganisms; It is too long a procedure very limited use.
Flaming autoclave	Immediate 3 minutes 134°C Most metal instruments, swab, towels, rubber, plastics handpieces	Kills all organisms/Equipment may be costlier.

Impression Material		
Material	**Use**	**Advantages/Disadvantages**
Alginate	Edentulous	Accuracy but dimension may change
Elastomers	For undercuts soft flabby ridges	Stronger than alginate but more extensive and takes longer to set
Impression compound Impression paste	Edentulous impressions Lining base plates	Economical but dose not record the minute details Accuracy but sticks to lips/skin

Temporary Fillings

Fillings	Uses	Advantages	Disadvantages
Zinc oxide and eugenol cement	1. Temporary filling 2. Lining deep cavities 3. Sedative dressing for dry socket 4. Gingivectomy 5. Obturating material for primary teeth	1. Economical 2. Easily available 3. Can be used in deep cavities 4. Rate of resorption is closer to the primary tooth	1. Soft 2. Slow-setting 3. Irritant to soft tissue
Gutta-percha	1 Permanent filling for root canals 2. Vitality tests 3. Temporary obturator for cleft palates and cyst cavities 4. Lining for gunning splints	1. Inert 2. No mixing as a foreign body	1. Too soft 2. Periapically can act
Zinc phosphate cement	1. Thick mix: cavity lining: temporary filling 2. Thin mix: adhesive cement for inlays and crowns	1. Hard 2. Rapid set 3. Adhesive	1. Irritant in deep cavities
Polycarboxylate	1. Thick mix: cavity lining: temporary filling 2. Thin mix: adhesive cement for inlays, crowns and orthodontic bands	1. Less irritant 2. More adhesive	1. May be difficult to manipulate
Calcium hydroxide	1. Cavity lining 2. Endodontic treatment 3. Antibacterial 4. Pulp capping agent 5. Root induction procedures 6. Intracanal medicament	1. Non-irritant 2. Can be used in deepest cavities 3. Compatible with all materials 4. Restorable 5. Can be used in periapical areas	1. Sublining only, in deep cavities under metal fillings 2. Contraindicated in primary dentition as it causes internal resorption

Comparison of Permanent Filling

Filling	Uses	Advantages/Disadvantages
Glass ionomer cement	Permanent restoration for primary anterior teeth	• It is cariostatic and non-irritant. It develops chemical bond to tooth. • But it is too dark and opaque and is too soft for back teeth.
Amalgam	Permanent filling for posterior teeth	• It sets rapidly. Technique is simple but it requires lining.
Composite	• Permanent filling for front teeth • Fissure sealants brackets	• Good strength suitable for large and complicated restorations. • It is good for undercut, and • Bonding with teeth • But for back teeth, it is not good.
Gold	Crown for back teeth	• It is much stronger but takes more time

Elastic Modulus of Some Dental Materials

Materials	Pounds/inch^2
Human enamel	1,20,00,000
Dental amalgam	40,00,000
Gold alloy	1,40,00,000
Zinc phosphate cement	20,00,000
Glass ionomer cement	8,00,000
Human dentin	2,70,00,000

Tensile Strength of Some Dental Materials

Materials	Tensile strength (Pounds/inch^2)
Human enamel	5000
Dental amalgam	7000
Gold alloy	60,000-120,000
Porcelain	5000
Nikel-chromium alloy	61000

Properties of Alloying Elements

	Platinum	Gold	Silver	Copper
	Pi	Au	Ag	Cu
Color	White	Yellow	White	Reddish
Tarnish resistance	Excellent	Excellent	Poor	Fair
Chemical activity	Inert	Inert	Active	Very active
Density	21.5	19.3	10.5	9

Different Alloys Used for Orthodontic Wires

	Co-Cr	Stainless steel	B-T1
Elastic limit	1100	1300	900
Stiffness	185 high	180 high	72 medium
Maximum flexibility	low	low	medium
Formability	medium	high	medium

Hardness Values

Materials	Hardness
Cementum	40
Composite	30
Dentin	70
Amalgam	90
Gold alloy	100
Enamel	340
Porcelin	595
Tungsten	1900
Diamond	7000

Cranial Nerves

Cranial Nerves	Function	Physical Findings
I (Olfactory)	Smell	No smell
II (Optic)	Vision	Decreased visual acuity
III (Oculomotor)	Eye movement Pupillary constriction	Failure to move eye in fild of motion of muscle Pupillary abnormalities
IV (Trochlear)	Eye movement	May be difficult to detect anything if 3rd nerve intact
V (Trigeminal)	Facial, nasal and oral sensation Jaw movement	Absent corneal reflex, weakness of masticatory muscles
VI (Abducens)	Eye movement	Failure of eye to abduct
VII (Facial)	Facial movement	Asymmetry of facial contraction
VIII (Auditory and vestibular	Hearing Balance	Decreased hearing Nystagmus, Ataxia
IX (Glossopharyngeal)	Palatal movement	Asymmetric palate
X (Vagus)	Palatal movement Vocal cords	Asymmetric palate Brassy voice
XI (Spinal accessory)	Turns neck	Paralysis of sterno-cleidomastoid muscle
XII (Hypoglossal)	Moves tongue	Wasting and fasciculation or deviation of tongue

The Muscles acting on the Temporomandibular Joint

Muscles	Main actions
Temporalis	Elevates mandible, closing jaws; its posterior firbers retrude mandible after protrusion.
Masseter	Elevates and protrudes mandible, thus closing jaws; deep fibers retrude it.
Lateral pterygoid	*Acting together*, protrudes mandible and depresses chain *Acting alone* and alternately, it produces side-to-side movements of mandible.
Medial pterygoid	Helps to elevate mandible, closing jaws *Acting together*, helps to protrude mandible *Acting alone*, it protrudes side of jaw.

Annexure–VII

NUTRITIONAL VALUES

Nutrition Ready Reckoner

These are average values for standard recipes found in most books and used in Indian kitchens

	Calories (Kcal)	Proteins (g)	Fats (g)	Carbo-hydrates (g)	Fiber (g)	Calcium (mg)	Iron (mg)	Caro-tene (mcg)	Retinol (mcg)	Vit B_1 (mg)	Vit B_2 (mg)	Niacin (mg)	Vit C (mg)	Serving Portion
BEVERAGES														
Hot Tea	34	0.6	1.0	5.7	0.0	31.0	0.0	0.0	7.00	0.01	0.01	0.0	0	1 Tea Cup
Instant Coffee	149	1.0	13.3	6.3	0.0	31.0	0.0	0.0	7.00	0.01	0.01	0.0	0	1 Tea Cup
Cold Coffee (with Cream)	279	3.9	17.0	27.7	0.0	144.0	0.3	487.0	183.00	0.06	0.23	0.1	2	1 Tall Glass
Banana Milk Shake	228	6.2	7.5	33.8	0.0	223.0	0.5	40.0	101.00	0.11	0.37	0.4	7	1 Tall Glass
Mango Milk Shake	237	6.2	7.7	35.6	0.8	227.0	1.3	2067.0	608.00	0.15	0.41	9.0	16	1 Tall Glass
Lemonade	107	0.3	0.3	25.7	0.5	21.0	0.1	0.0	0.00	0.01	0.00	0.0	12	1 Glass
BREAKFAST CEREALS														
Cracked Wheat Porridge	292	10.0	10.4	39.7	2.5	296.0	1.5	152.0	39.00	1.29	0.49	1.3	5	1 Bowl
Semolina Porridge	293	9.8	10.2	40.4	0.0	291.0	0.8	139.0	36.00	1.24	0.47	0.6	5	1 Bowl
Vermicelli Porridge	294	9.4	10.2	41.1	2.5	292.0	0.9	139.0	36.00	1.24	0.47	0.6	5	1 Bowl
Oat Meal Porridge	217	6.6	6.6	32.8	2.0	154.0	1.0	70.0	18.00	0.80	0.26	0.3	2	1 Bowl
Cornflakes with Milk	291	9.8	10.8	38.7	1.2	290.0	0.9	157.0	41.00	1.28	0.48	0.6	5	1 Bowl

Contd...

Contd...

	Calories (Kcal)	Proteins (g)	Fats (g)	Carbo-hydrates (g)	Fiber (g)	Calcium (mg)	Iron (mg)	Caro-tene (mcg)	Retinol (mcg)	Vit B_1 (mg)	Vit B_2 (mg)	Niacin (mg)	Vit C (mg)	Serving Portion
Semolina Upma	147	2.3	7.7	17.1	9.9	11.0	0.5	1.0	0.00	0.04	0.01	0.4	2	1 Bowl
Vermicelli Upma	296	4.0	15.2	35.7	5.4	24.0	1.2	2.0	1.00	0.10	0.03	0.9	5	1 Bowl
Vegetable Upma	192	4.4	9.7	21.7	1.5	22.0	0.9	107.0	27.00	0.20	0.02	1.6	4	1 Bowl
Poha	158	2.8	7.3	20.2	1.5	10.0	4.2	6.0	1.00	0.10	0.02	2.0	3	1 Bowl
Vegetable with Poha	202	4.9	9.3	24.7	2.1	21.0	4.6	111.0	28.00	0.18	0.03	3.1	5	1 Bowl
EGGS														
Boiled Egg	87	6.7	6.7	0.0	0.0	25.0	0.7	300.0	180.00	0.05	0.20	0.1	0	1 Egg
Poached Egg	87	6.7	6.7	0.0	0.0	25.0	0.7	300.0	180.00	0.05	0.20	0.1	0	1 Egg
Fried Egg	160	6.7	14.8	0.0	0.0	25.0	0.7	620.0	260.00	0.05	0.20	0.1	0	1 Egg
Scrambled Egg	172	6.7	15.8	0.8	0.0	57.0	0.7	620.0	267.00	0.06	0.22	0.1	0	1 Egg
Baked Egg	124	6.7	10.8	0.0	0.0	25.0	0.7	460.0	220.0	0.05	0.20	0.1	0	1 Egg
Fluffy Omelette	160	6.7	14.8	0.0	0.0	25.0	0.7	620.0	260.00	0.05	0.20	0.1	0	1 Egg
Cheese and Mushroom Omelette	308	12.9	27.1	3.0	0.0	182.0	1.3	780.0	373.00	0.09	0.42	1.5	1	1 Egg
SOUPS														
Minestrone Soup	90	1.4	5.2	9.4	1.2	43.0	0.7	491.0	123.00	0.07	0.03	0.5	17	1 Bowl
Chicken Soup Corn Soup	322	25.5	13.5	24.6	6.0	23.0	2.6	10.7.0	93.00	0.21	0.34	8.6	6	1 Bowl
French Onion Soup	208	4.8	11.6	21.1	2.4	102.0	0.8	321.0	110.00	0.08	0.05	0.6	8	1 Bowl

Contd...

Contd...

	Calories (Kcal)	Proteins (g)	Fats (g)	Carbo-hydrates	Fiber (g)	Calcium (mg)	Iron (mg)	Caro-tene (mcg)	Retinol (mcg)	Vit B_1 (mg)	Vit B_2 (mg)	Niacin (mg)	Vit C (mg)	Serving Portion
Tomato Soup	82	2.1	4.5	8.3	2.3	101.0	1.3	862.0	216.00	0.25	0.21	0.8	55	1 Bowl
Green Pea Soup	185	9.0	6.4	23.1	2.2	70.0	1.9	375.0	109.00	0.28	0.08	1.1	11	1 Bowl
Spinach Soup	561	3.9	8.9	116.2	5.9	81.0	1.5	5902.0	1475.00	0.06	0.27	0.08	29	1 Bowl
Mixed Vegetable Soup	145	3.3	9.2	12.5	1.4	124.0	0.9	779.0	225.0	0.11	0.16	0.6	23	1 Bowl
Cream with Tomato Soup	245	5.4	16.6	18.5	2.3	180.0	1.5	984.0	287.00	0.32	0.25	1.0	45	1 Bowl
Cream with Spinach Soup	307	8.5	23.2	16.0	5.1	200.0	2.2	6214.0	1644.0	0.20	0.52	0.9	32	1 Bowl
Cream with Carrot Soup	250	4.6	16.2	21.5	2.0	172.0	1.4	1935.0	531.00	0.17	0.17	0.9	6	1 Bowl
Cream of Pea Soup	342	12.4	18.2	32.2	2.6	132.0	2.4	590.0	188.00	0.44	0.17	1.4	15	1 Bowl
Cream with Potato Soup	282	5.4	13.1	35.7	3.1	118.0	1.1	415.0	144.00	0.24	0.17	1.6	21	1 Bowl
Cream with Mixed Vegetable Soup	263	7.5	13.4	28.0	3.2	179.0	2.0	1160.0	331.00	0.33	0.24	1.5	45	1 Bowl
Cream with Mushroom Soup	308	6.6	22.4	19.9	0.7	136.0	1.5	554.0	189.00	0.13	0.41	2.9	6	1 Bowl
Hot and Sour Soup	181	11.2	9.3	13.2	1.6	65.0	2.8	86.0	22.00	0.22	0.25	23	6	1 Bowl

Contd...

Contd...

	Calories (Kcal)	Proteins (g)	Fats (g)	Carbo-hydrates	Fibre (g)	Calcium (mg)	Iron (mg)	Caro-tene (mcg)	Retinol (mcg)	Vit B_1 (mg)	Vit B_2 (mg)	Niacin (mg)	Vit C (mg)	Serving Portion
CEREALS														
Chapati	273	9.7	1.4	55.5	5.6	38.0	3.9	23.0	5.00	0.39	0.14	3.40	0	3 or 4 Med.
Plain Parantha	363	9.7	11.4	55.5	5.6	38.0	3.9	23.0	6.00	0.39	0.14	3.40	0	3 Medium
Potato-Stuffed Parantha	632	11.2	31.5	75.8	7.9	56.0	4.4	42.0	10.00	0.49	0.15	4.50	16	3 Medium
Pea Parantha	693	20.7	31.5	75.8	7.9	78.0	6.3	148.0	37.00	0.78	0.15	4.70	16	3 Medium
Cauliflower Parantha	577	12.0	31.7	60.9	7.1	74.0	5.0	47.0	12.00	0.44	0.22	4.30	47	3 Medium
Radish Parantha	574	10.8	31.5	61.8	8.2	90.0	4.5	27.0	7.00	0.48	0.16	4.10	20	3 Medium
Daal Parantha	665	16.2	33.1	75.6	9.0	65.0	5.6	62.0	15.00	0.55	0.19	4.20	3	3 Medium
Sprouted Dal Parantha	727	22.1	32.0	87.6	10.2	85.0	6.0	48.0	12.00	0.64	0.24	4.70	2	3 Medium
Paneer Parantha	713	20.9	43.9	58.5	5.9	173.0	4.0	243.0	61.00	0.45	0.15	3.50	4	3 Medium
Onion-Green Chilli Parantha	594	10.9	31.5	66.6	7.1	85.0	4.5	23.0	6.00	0.57	0.15	3.80	11	3 Medium
Keema Parantha	712	24.8	42.1	58.4	5.9	169.0	6.2	25.0	13.00	0.55	0.25	9.00	3	3 Medium
Methi Parantha	652	14.2	32.4	75.8	8.1	293.0	7.2	1230.0	303.00	0.52	0.32	4.50	0	3 Medium
Pooris (10 g oil absorbed)	375	9.2	12.1	57.4	4.0	28.0	3.0	42.0	11.00	0.24	0.10	2.70	0	3 Medium
Daal Stuffed Pooris	427	12.8	12.3	66.3	51.5	5.0	3.6	47.0	12.00	0.31	0.13	3.00	0	4 or 5
Palak Pooris	388	10.2	12.4	58.8	64.9	6.0	3.6	2832.0	708.00	0.26	0.23	2.9	14	4 or 5

Contd...

Contd...

	Calories (Kcal)	Proteins (g)	Fats (g)	Carbo-hydrates (g)	Fiber (g)	Calcium (mg)	Iron (mg)	Caro-tene (mcg)	Retinol (mcg)	Vit B_1 (mg)	Vit B_2 (mg)	Niacin (mg)	Vit C (mg)	Serving Portion
Besan Pooris	380	11.2	13.0	54.6	5.5	35.0	3.6	62.0	16.00	0.32	0.12	2.7	0	4 or 5
Pooris	431	13.6	12.1	66.9	5.0	40.0	3.9	91.0	23.00	0.39	0.10	3.2	5	4 or 5
Pea Kachori (10 g oil absorbed)	215	6.9	7.4	30.2	1.8	17.0	1.6	49.0	13.00	0.16	0.03	1.1	5	2
Khasta Kachori (10 g oil absorbed)	441	11.4	18.9	56.3	3.2	45.0	2.4	163.0	41.00	0.16	0.8	1.8	0	2
Naan	200	6.7	2.1	38.5	1.5	60.0	1.4	31.0	9.00	0.19	0.10	1.2	1	1
Bhatura	176	5.6	3.8	29.9	1.2	28.0	1.2	51.0	27.00	0.06	0.07	0.1	0	2 or 3
Boiled Rice	277	6.0	0.8	61.4	3.6	8.00	2.6	2.0	0.40	0.17	0.13	3.1	0	1 Full plate
Curd Rice	484	15.1	12.5	77.8	5.3	253.0	3.8	66.0	26.00	0.33	0.41	3.7	2	1 Full plate
Zeera Pulao	400	8.2	10.5	68.1	4.4	25.00	2.9	78.0	45.00	0.22	0.18	3.5	6	1 Full plate
Mixed Vegetable Pulao	523	17.6	9.0	92.9	7.2	71.0	5.2	126.0	32.00	0.60	0.15	4.6	21	1 Full plate
Pea Pulao	510	12.1	9.1	94.8	8.1	108.0	4.6	1033.0	258.00	0.44	0.17	4.8	28	1 Full plate
Channa Daal & Vegetable Pulao	529	15.1	10.1	94.3	8.5	102.0	5.3	1014.0	254.00	0.47	0.19	4.6	14	1 Full plate
Black Channa Pulao	464	10.9	10.2	82.1	7.5	82.00	4.0	49.0	11.00	0.28	0.17	4.1	6	1 Full plate
Mushroom Pulao	411	9.7	9.7	71.2	4.3	38.00	4.4	2.0	0.40	0.31	0.55	8.1	9	1 Full plate
Paneer Pulao	520	13.3	20.4	70.9	4.3	272.0	4.9	2.0	0.40	0.21	0.13	3.3	6	1 Full plate
Mutton Pulao	622	22.6	28.5	68.7	4.3	216.0	5.1	13.0	12.00	0.37	0.29	8.8	6	1 Full plate
Chicken Pulao	661	27.9	30.5	68.7	4.3	110.0	4.6	88.0	90.00	0.33	0.34	11.4	6	1 Full plate

Contd...

Contd...

	Calories (Kcal)	Proteins (g)	Fats (g)	Carbo-hydrates (g)	Fiber (g)	Calcium (mg)	Iron (mg)	Caro-tene (mcg)	Retinol (mcg)	Vit B_1 (mg)	Vit B_2 (mg)	Niacin (mg)	Vit C (mg)	Serving Portion
Idli	157	6.7	0.5	31.5	2.5	33.00	1.6	8.00	2.00	0.14	0.08	1.4	0	3 or 4
Plain Dosa	261	7.1	4.6	47.8	3.2	28.00	1.6	166.0	41.00	0.17	0.08	2.2	0	2
Masala Dosa	208	3.0	4.2	39.5	4.5	39.00	1.1	36.0	9.00	0.19	0.02	2.0	31	1
Mixed Vegetable Dosa	184	4.8	4.4	31.2	4.2	79.00	1.8	624.0	156.00	0.20	0.10	1.8	43	1
Paneer Filling	130	3.8	8.8	8.9	1.3	144.0	0.6	176.0	44.00	0.10	0.00	0.4	19	1
Uttapam	316	7.8	8.7	51.6	3.9	55.00	2.1	465.0	116.00	0.20	0.10	2.5	23	2
Beans and Macaroni	352	12.1	16.8	38.0	3.7	243.0	2.2	673.0	242.00	0.20	0.20	1.5	40	1 Plate
Spaghetti Bolognese	346	14.6	14.9	38..3	33.0	174.0	3.2	867.0	236.00	0.28	0.21	4.8	30	1 Shallow dish
Chicken Chowmein	542	31.4	24.2	49.6	3.9	104.0	5.6	9.8	333.00	0.39	0.36	8.1	59	1 Shallow dish
PULSES														
Dal Moong	104	7.3	0.4	17.9	2.6	23.0	1.2	15.0	4.00	0.14	0.06	0.7	0	1 Curry bowl
Cumin Seed Baghar	47	0.0	5.0	0.5	0.0	0.0	0.0	100.0	25.00	0.00	0.00	0.0	0	
Onion Tomato Baghar	59	0.4	5.1	2.8	0.5	17.0	0.2	153.0	38.00	0.03	0.01	0.1	6	
Mustard Seed Baghar	45	0.0	5.0	0.0	0.0	0.0	0.0	100.0	25.00	0.00	0.00	0.0	0	
Urad Sp.	94	7.9	5.5	3.3	3.1	78.0	1.5	82.0	21.00	0.19	0.08	0.9	11	1 Curry bowl

Contd...

Contd...

	Calories (Kcal)	Proteins (g)	Fats (g)	Carbo-hydrates (g)	Fiber (g)	Calcium (mg)	Iron (mg)	Caro-tene (mcg)	Retinol (mcg)	Vit B_1 (mg)	Vit B_2 (mg)	Niacin (mg)	Vit C (mg)	Serving Portion
Dehusked Dry Arhar Daal with Spinach	159	7.7	5.9	18.7	4.4	58.0	1.4	2830.0	707.00	0.50	0.19	1.1	14	1 Curry bowl
Channa Daal with Ghia	117	6.3	1.7	19.1	3.4	27.0	1.8	39.0	10.00	0.16	0.06	0.8	0	1 Curry bowl
Sambar	119	5.6	2.5	18.4	3.2	45.0	1.7	88.0	22.00	0.13	0.08	0.9	19	1 Curry bowl
Green Gram Whole	100	7.2	0.4	17.0	1.2	37.0	1.3	28.0	7.00	0.14	0.08	0.6	0	1 Bowl
Dry Khatta Channa	232	6.0	11.7	25.6	4.8	83.0	1.9	369.0	91.00	0.16	0.07	1.3	14	1 Bowl
Rajma Curry	268	10.5	11.0	31.8	3.7	162.0	2.6	193.0	49.00	0.29	0.12	1.2	20	1 Bowl
Lobia Curry	259	10.9	10.9	29.3	2.8	89.0	4.1	182.0	46.00	0.31	0.12	0.9	19	1 Bowl
Besan Gatte Curry	497	21.3	30.6	34.0	5.5	255.0	2.9	367.0	96.00	0.34	0.22	1.4	14	1 Bowl
Besan Kadhi with Pakoris	408	9.9	30.2	24.1	3.7	140.0	2.2	73.0	23.00	0.21	0.19	1.0	1	1 Bowl
Meats														
Keema Matar	411	26.9	23.7	22.6	2.8	215.0	4.9	298.0	84.00	0.53	0.19	8.0	29	1 Bowl
Roganjosh	404	25.0	30.6	7.2	0.8	276.0	4.0	114.0	45.00	0.31	0.27	8.0	12	1 Bowl
Mutton Korma	439	24.0	34.7	7.7	0.8	259.0	3.7	149.0	54	0.30	0.22	8.50	6.0	1 Bowl
Palak Meat	374	19.1	28.4	10.6	5.2	290.0	3.8	5600.0	1410	0.24	0.46	620	34.0	1 Bowl
Shahi Keema Kofta Curry	508	23.8	41.3	10.2	1.5	238.0	4.3	217.0	65	0.34	0.21	8.70	23.0	1 Bowl

Contd...

Contd...

	Calories (Kcal)	Proteins (g)	Fats (g)	Carbo-hydrates (g)	Fiber (g)	Calcium (mg)	Iron (mg)	Caro-tene (mcg)	Retinol (mcg)	Vit B1 (mg)	Vit B2 (mg)	Niacin (mg)	Vit C (mg)	Serving Portion
Boti Kabab	365	23.6	27.8	5.0	0.5	232.0	3.6	8.0	19	0.24	0.22	8.30	9.0	1 Bowl
Shammi Kabab	435	25.0	25.8	25.8	3.6	180.0	3.4	890.0	58.00	0.29	0.21	7.4	3.7	1 Bowl
Shepherd's Pie	486	23.8	34.5	20.0	2.2	206.0	3.5	339.0	98.00	0.31	0.18	9.2	15	1 Bowl
Roast Chicken	297	25.3	21.8	0.0	0.0	18.0	2.0	334..0	166.0	0.13	0.20	10.0	0	1 Bowl
Chilli Chicken	464	27.3	35.5	8.8	1.9	46.0	3.1	222.0	135.0	0.35	0.31	10.9	50	1 Bowl
Chicken Sweet and Sour	420	27.0	33.3	3.1	0.8	39.0	2.7	270.0	181.0	0.28	0.35	10.6	30	1 Bowl
Chicken Korma	493	28.1	36.4	13.2	2.1	188.0	3.2	94.0	127.0	0.23	0.32	10.2	11	1 Bowl
Bengal Fish Curry	296	18.4	17.5	16.3	1.6	731.0	1.7	22.4	7.00	0.14	0.11	1.1	35	1 Bowl
Tandoori Fish	174	25.7	6.8	2.4	0.0	7.0	3.1	10.0	11.00	0.01	0.02	0.0	0	1 Bowl
Fried Fish with Chips	443	26.3	26.2	25.4	2.3	307.0	3.3	165.0	94.00	0.09	0.11	0.9	9	1 Bowl
Fish in Coconut Milk	371	27.0	17.1	27.2	3.2	150.0	3.2	4.0	1.00	0.06	0.03	0.5	7	1 Bowl
Prawn Curry	342	30.1	19.9	10.5	2.7	509.0	9.3	3.0	0.80	0.05	0.18	7.5	4	1 Bowl
Crispy Baked Fish	390	32.3	15.1	31.2	4.1	461.0	4.1	496.0	153.00	0.13	0.13	1.3	16	1 Bowl
Vegetables and Paneer														
Nutri Nugget Sweet and Sour	252	12.8	18.3	9.1	8.0	22.0	1.0	180.0	79.00	0.16	0.16	1.0	30	1 Bowl
Nutri Nugget Korma	347	14.2	23.4	20.0	2.1	217.0	1.4	28.0	12.00	0.11	0.13	0.6	11	1 Bowl

Contd...

Contd...

	Calories (Kcal)	Proteins (g)	Fats (g)	Carbo-hydrates (g)	Fiber (g)	Calcium (mg)	Iron (mg)	Caro-tene (mcg)	Retinol (mcg)	Vit B1 (mg)	Vit B2 (mg)	Niacin (mg)	Vit C (mg)	Serving Portion
Mashroom Matar	239	10.3	10.8	25.2	2.8	68.5	3.3	298.0	75.00	0.41	0.30	4.1	31	1 Bowl
Nutri Nugget Matar	283	18.4	10.5	28.6	2.8	68.5	2.4	298.0	75.00	0.35	0.05	1.0	29	1 Bowl
Palak Mushroom	161	5.2	10.6	11.3	7.7	149.0	2.9	708.0	2177.00	0.17	0.59	3.0	60	1 Bowl
Vegetable Nargisi Kofta Curry	394	17.1	33.1	6.8	6.7	188.0	2.0	146.0	103.0	0.30	0.06	2.6	43	1 Bowl
Paneer Makhani	659	9.5	61.3	17.4	3.0	305.0	2.9	2046.0	580.0	0.36	0.19	1.3	64	1 Bowl
Pea Potato Curry	267	8.9	10.3	34.6	4.1	62.8	2.2	165.0	41.00	0.37	0.03	1.7	30	1 Bowl
Pea Paneer Curry	351	17.3	20.8	23.6	2.8	162.0	2.0	153.0	94.00	0.36	0.04	1.1	23	1 Bowl
Pea Curry	311	15.3	10.3	39.2	4.5	78.0	3.5	236.0	60.00	0.60	0.04	2.0	30	1 Bowl
Pea/Cholia Vadi Curry	309	11.7	15.3	31.0	3.7	68.0	2.8	195.0	49.00	0.50	0.03	1.5	26	1 Bowl
Potato Curry	221	2.5	10.2	29.9	3.6	47.7	1.0	94.0	23.60	0.17	0.03	1.5	29	1 Bowl
Egg Curry	314	15.5	17.6	23.3	2.8	85.0	2.8	483.0	237.00	0.38	0.25	1.2	21	1 Bowl
Dahi Aloo	260	4.2	12.2	33.4	3.9	119.0	1.0	169.0	58.00	0.22	0.12	1.8	35	1 Bowl
Dum Aloo	291	2.1	21.1	23.2	2.5	41.5	0.5	29.0	8.00	0.11	0.03	1.2	17	1 Bowl
Ghia Kofta Curry	273	3.6	20.9	17.5	2.9	70.0	1.9	122.0	31.00	0.17	0.05	0.9	15	1 Bowl
Potato Kofta Curry	290	2.9	15.3	35.1	4.1	51.0	1.3	101.0	25.00	0.19	0.03	1.80	33	1 Bowl

Contd...

Contd...

	Calories (Kcal)	Proteins (g)	Fats (g)	Carbo-hydrates (g)	Fiber (g)	Calcium (mg)	Iron (mg)	Caro-tene (mcg)	Retinol (mcg)	Vit B_1 (mg)	Vit B_2 (mg)	Niacin (mg)	Vit C (mg)	Serving Portion
Cabbage Kofta Curry	297	5.9	21.0	21.0	4.0	85.0	2.1	210.0	52.00	0.20	0.14	1.1	136	1 Bowl
Paneer Kofta Curry	383	11.2	30.7	15.5	1.5	149.0	0.9	74.0	74.00	0.13	0.04	0.6	15	1 Bowl
Aloo Methi	221	5.8	11.0	24.7	4.1	404.0	2.5	2361.0	590.00	0.12	0.32	1.8	66	1 Bowl
Gajar Methi	180	5.2	11.0	15.0	3.5	460.0	2.8	3854.0	963.00	0.08	0.33	1.3	55	1 Bowl
Sarson Ka Saag	157	8.5	6.7	15.7	3.2	200.0	25.0	6734.0	1682.00	0.22	0.14	0.5	66	1 Bowl
Palak Paneer	240	11.2	17.5	9.4	7.7	228.0	2.1	8545.0	2180.00	0.16	0.43	1.1	59	1 Bowl
Palak Aloo	230	5.1	11.3	27.0	9.7	153.0	2.5	8564.0	2141.00	0.20	0.40	2.0	72	1 Bowl
Mooli Bhujia	144	4.6	10.6	7.6	2.3	294.0	0.8	5300.0	2.00	0.23	0.49	1.2	91	1 Bowl
Bathua Bhujia	152	6.0	10.7	7.8	0.3	236.0	6.8	2614.0	1.00	0.04	0.22	1.0	55	1 Bowl
Peas and Cabbage Subzi	122	5.5	5.2	13.2	2.2	50.0	1.7	164.0	41.00	0.19	0.10	0.8	129	1 Bowl
Dry Arbi (Fried)	254	3.6	15.2	25.6	1.6	62.0	0.9	79.0	14.00	0.14	0.04	0.6	8	1 Bowl
Masala Arbi	187	3.0	10.1	21.1	1.0	40.0	0.4	24.0	0.00	0.09	0.03	0.4	0	1 Bowl
Bingan Bhartha	192	2.8	15.5	10.4	4.5	55.0	0.9	216.0	54.00	0.12	0.19	1.6	29	1 Small Bowl
Stuffed Tomatoes	233	6.0	15.6	17.1	2.8	138.0	1.5	829.0	228.00	0.27	0.08	1.1	41	2 Tomatoes
Bhindi Subzi	189	2.6	15.0	11.0	6.3	93.0	0.7	62.0	16.00	0.11	0.12	0.8	19	1 Bowl
Stuffed Bhindi	132	2.3	10.2	7.7	5.9	79.0	0.5	62.0	16.00	0.08	0.12	0.7	16	1 Bowl
Stuffed Karela (Wet)	225	1.9	20.2	8.9	2.6	39.0	1.0	101.0	25.00	0.10	0.08	0.6	76	1 Bowl
Stuffed Karela (Dry)	156	1.3	15.2	3.4	1.8	16.0	0.5	100.0	25.00	0.06	0.07	0.4	70	3 Pcs
Kathal (Dry)	300	2.2	20.3	27.0	7.1	89.5	1.3	201.0	51.00	0.15	0.02	1.1	12	1 Bowl

Contd...

Contd...

	Calories (Kcal)	Proteins (g)	Fats (g)	Carbohydrates (g)	Fiber (g)	Calcium (mg)	Iron (mg)	Carotene (mcg)	Retinol (mcg)	Vit B_1 (mg)	Vit B_2 (mg)	Niacin (mg)	Vit C (mg)	Serving Portion
Cauliflower, Peas and Potato Subzi	196	5.1	10.3	20.7	2.9	49.0	1.6	143.0	36.00	0.21	0.07	1.4	42	1 Bowl
Stuffed Ghia	456	21.3	31.8	21.1	2.5	323.0	2.9	632.0	304.00	0.22	0.34	4.1	3	1/2 Marrow
Rost Potatoes	191	2.4	5.0	34.0	3.8	15.0	0.8	228.0	57.00	0.15	0.01	1.8	26	1-2 Potatoes
Stuffed Baked Potato	334	7.1	18.8	34.0	3.8	33.0	1.3	698.0	248.00	0.19	0.16	1.8	26	1-2 Potatoes
Creamed Spinach	429	21.4	29.8	18.8	9.3	458.0	3.5	11812.0	3195.00	0.25	1.00	1.4	58	1 Small bowl
Creamed Spinach and Mushrooms	363	13.4	25.8	19.2	7.1	366.0	2.9	8692.0	2284.00	0.23	0.90	3.5	45	1 bowl
SALADS														
Russian Salad	959	19.7	85.6	27.5	3.3	100.0	3.8	879.0	333.00	0.38	0.33	5.4	39	1 Small bowl
Beetroot and Egg Salad	366	8.9	30.8	13.4	3.6	62.0	2.1	300.0	180.00	0.12	0.29	0.6	15	1 Small bowl
Tossed Green Salad	153	1.5	12.2	9.2	2.0	50.0	0.9	225.0	57.00	0.18	0.04	0.5	43	1 Small bowl
Cucumber and Yogurt Salad	29	1.3	1.3	2.9	1.0	53.0	0.5	10.0	4.00	0.04	0.05	0.2	6	1 Small bowl
French Dressing	722	0.0	80.0	0.4	0.0	1.0	0.0	0.0	0.00	0.00	0.00	0.01	1	3/4 Cup
Mayonnaise	1220	7.1	131.8	1.3	0.0	56.0	1.4	380.0	229.00	0.08	0.26	0.0	4	1 Cup
Mayonnaise without Eggs	886	7.7	90.1	11.0	0.0	288.0	0.5	139.0	36.00	1.20	0.46	0.3	6	1 Cup

Contd...

Contd...

	Calories	Proteins	Fats	Carbo-	Fiber									
	Calcium (Kcal)	Iron (g)	Caro- (g)	Retinol hydrates (g)	Vit B_1 (g)	Vit B_2 (mg)	Niacin (mg)	Vit C tene (mcg)	Serving (mcg)	(mg)	(mg)	(mg)	(mg)	Portion
RAITAS														
Tomato Onion Raita	79	3.7	4.1	6.7	0.6	173.0	0.5	120.0	36.00	0.10	0.18	0.3	11	1 Bowl
Cucumber Raita	68	3.3	4.1	4.5	0.8	155.0	0.6	32.0	14.00	0.07	0.16	0.2	5	1 Bowl
Carrot Raita	85	3.6	4.1	8.3	0.9	189.0	0.7	977.0	250.00	0.07	0.17	0.4	3	1 Bowl
Ghia Raita	67	3.2	4.1	4.3	0.3	159.0	0.4	32.0	14.00	0.06	0.17	0.2	1	1 Bowl
Potato Raita	110	3.9	4.1	14.3	1.3	154.0	0.5	44.0	17.00	0.10	0.17	0.7	10	1 Bowl
Spinach Raita	143	7.7	8.7	8.5	4.9	231.0	1.6	5616.0	1410.00	0.17	0.43	2.6	29	1 Bowl
Bathua Raita	147	9.3	8.4	8.5	0.4	308.0	4.7	1776.0	15.00	0.15	0.31	2.7	36	1 Bowl
Sprouted Green Gram Raita	105	5.8	4.1	11.2	1.2	166.0	0.7	37.0	15.00	0.11	0.18	0.4	3	1 Bowl
Boondi Raita	224	7.3	15.0	15.0	2.1	160.0	1.3	58.0	21.00	0.15	0.20	0.6	1	1 Bowl
Pineapple Raita	84	3.3	4.1	8.4	0.0	159.0	1.4	41.0	16.00	0.15	0.22	0.2	21	1 Bowl
Banana Raita	118	3.7	4.1	16.6	0.4	158.0	0.4	71.0	24.00	0.08	0.20	0.4	5	1 Bowl
Mango Raita	97	3.4	4.2	11.5	0.5	156.0	0.9	1404.0	357.00	0.09	0.20	0.6	9	1 Bowl
Grape Raita	91	3.4	4.2	10..0	1.4	159.0	0.5	33.0	14.00	0.06	0.17	0.2	2	1 Bowl
DESSERTS														
Rice Kheer	257	7.2	8.3	38.3	0.4	241.0	0.7	12.0	104.00	0.12	0.40	0.6	4	1 Bowl
Sevian Kheer	271	7.9	9.2	39.2	1.2	273.0	0.6	12.0	111.00	0.12	0.40	0.4	4	1 Bowl
Carrot Kheer	218	6.9	8.3	29.0	0.9	280.0	0.9	957.0	340.00	0.12	0.38	0.5	6	1 Bowl
Apple Kheer	244	6.5	8.5	35.4	0.6	245.0	0.8	12.0	104.00	0.10	0.38	0.2	5	1 Bowl
Phirni	258	7.1	8.3	38.8	0.4	241.0	0.5	12.0	104.00	0.11	0.39	0.4	4	1 Bowl
Carrot Halva	472	8.3	24.5	54.5	2.7	443.0	1.6	3137.0	844.00	0.14	0.30	1.0	7	1 Small Bowl

Contd...

Contd...

	Calories (Kcal)	Proteins (g)	Fats (g)	Carbohydrates (g)	Fiber (g)	Calcium (mg)	Iron (mg)	Carotene (mcg)	Retinol (mcg)	Vit B_1 (mg)	Vit B_2 (mg)	Niacin (mg)	Vit C (mg)	Serving Portion
Suji Halwa	380	3.6	23.2	39.1	0.8	16.0	0.7	400.0	100.00	0.04	0.04	0.6	0	1 Small Bowl
Moong Dal Halwa	545	13.8	28.2	59.0	2.7	310.0	1.2	415.0	149.00	0.22	0.27	0.9	2	1 Small Bowl
Vanilla Ice Cup Cream	288	2.3	22.9	18.2	0.0	90.0	0.2	415.0	139.00	0.03	0.14	0.1	0	1 Ice Cream
Strawberry Ice Cup Cream	288	2.3	22.9	18.2	0.0	90.0	0.2	415.0	139.00	0.03	0.14	0.1	0	1 Ice Cream
Chocolate Ice Cup Cream	288	2.3	22.9	18.2	0.0	90.0	0.2	415.0	139.00	0.03	0.14	0.1	0	1 Ice Cream
Cocochip Ice Cup Cream	288	2.3	22.0	18.2	0.0	90.0	0.2	415.0	139.00	0.03	0.14	0.1	0	1 Ice Cream
Coconut Ice Glass Cream	460	5.5	30.5	40.8	0.0	106.0	1.0	411.0	414.00	0.10	0.18	0.4	2	1 Sundae
Fruit Ice Cream Glass	323	2.6	23.0	26.5	0.3	95.0	0.4	832.0	246.00	0.05	0.16	0.3	5	1 Sundae
Cold Lemon Dish Souffle	534	6.9	41.9	32.3	0.4	41.0	0.8	1000.0	355.00	0.05	0.20	0.1	8.8	1 Sooffle
Cold Orange Dish Souffle	594	7.8	42.0	46.2	1.5	64.0	1.2	2656.0	769.00	0.05	0.20	0.1	45	1 Souffle

Contd...

Contd...

	Calories (Kcal)	Proteins (g)	Fats (g)	Carbo-hydrates (g)	Fiber (g)	Calcium (mg)	Iron (mg)	Caro-tene (mcg)	Retinol (mcg)	Vit B_1 (mg)	Vit B_2 (mg)	Niacin (mg)	Vit C (mg)	Serving Portion
Cold Pineappple Souffle	525	6.7	42.0	30.00	0.0	25.0	0.7	1000.0	355.00	0.00	0.20	0.1	0	1 Souffle dish
Cold Vanila Souffle	536	7.3	42.7	30.6	0.0	57.0	0.7	1000.0	362.00	0.06	0.20	0.1	0.2	1 Souffle dish
Cold Chocolate Souffle	536	7.3	42.7	30.6	0.0	57.0	0.7	1000.0	362.00	0.06	0.20	0.1	0.2	1 Souffle dish
Bread and Butter Pudding	222	7.4	11.3	22.7	1.0	124.0	0.7	316.0	177.00	0.08	0.27	0.2	2	1 Small plate
SNACKS														
Gulabjamuns	329	6.7	12.9	46.6	0.2	279.0	0.2	145.0	36.00	0.23	0.17	0.3	2	2 Pcs
Chenna Murkhi	275	9.3	10.6	35.6	0.0	110.0	0.0	186.0	47.00	0.06	0.02	0.0	2	10 Pcs
Plain Barfi	276	10.0	13.0	29.8	0.0	478.0	0.0	249.0	63.00	0.12	0.21	0.2	3	2 Pcs
Coconut Barfi	472	11.7	28.6	41.9	4.3	578.0	2.0	249.0	63.00	0.14	0.21	1.0	5	2 Pcs
Besan Burfi	266	5.3	13.9	30.0	2.7	14.0	1.3	282.0	71.00	0.12	0.05	0.6	1	2 Pcs
Khoya Laddoo	375	10.7	22.2	33.0	1.8	441.0	1.4	206.0	52.00	0.14	0.21	0.8	3	2 Pcs
Besan Laddoo	286	5.8	16.4	28.7	2.8	15.0	1.4	332.0	83.00	0.13	0.05	0.7	1	2 Pcs
Suji Laddoo with Nuts	290	3.4	16.7	31.4	0.8	16.0	0.8	306.00	77.00	0.09	0.03	0.5	0	2 Pcs
Suji Laddoo with Khoya	355	5.6	20.1	38.0	1.9	125.0	0.6	312.00	78.00	0.07	0.07	0.5	1	2 Pcs
Til Laddoo	158	3.2	7.2	20.0	0.0	256.0	2.0	10.0	3.00	0.18	0.07	0.8	0	6 Pcs
Gujia	272	4.8	13.2	33.6	1.3	114.0	0.9	121.0	31.00	0.05	0.06	0.7	1	6 Pcs
Peanut Brittle (Chikki)	229	5.2	8.1	33.7	0.9	44.0	1.3	7.00	2.00	0.20	0.06	4.1	0	5 Pcs

Contd...

Contd...

	Calories (Kcal)	Proteins (g)	Fats (g)	Carbo-hydrates (g)	Fiber (g)	Calcium (mg)	Iron (mg)	Caro-tene (mcg)	Retinol (mcg)	Vit B_1 (mg)	Vit B_2 (mg)	Niacin (mg)	Vit C (mg)	Serving Portion
Til and Channa Chikki	217	5.2	3.3	41.7	2.1	110.0	2.3	29.00	7.00	0.16	0.09	0.8	0	5 Pcs
Murmura Chikki	139	0.7	0.0	34.0	0.4	28.0	1.3	0.0	0.00	0.03	0.03	0.4	0	5 Pcs
Vegetable Pakoras	333	7.8	21.9	26.2	5.2	49.0	2.3	1166.0	291.00	0.19	0.13	1.3	23	5 Pcs
Masala Onion Pakoras	343	7.5	21.8	29.1	4.7	64.0	2.2	39.0	10.00	0.20	0.06	1.1	11	5 Pcs
Paneer Pakoras	425	15.5	32.1	18.6	3.2	121.0	1.6	222.0	56.00	0.18	0.06	0.7	2	5 Pcs
Bread Pakoras	489	11.8	22.2	60.5	8.6	28.0	2.5	51.00	13.00	0.24	0.06	1.7	9	5 Pcs
Egg Pakoras	380	13.0	28.4	18.0	3.2	42.0	2.3	339.00	190.00	0.19	0.25	0.8	0	2 Pcs
Chicken Pakoras	451	22.6	31.8	18.7	3.2	29.0	3.0	1.1	78.00	0.23	0.18	7.2	1	2 Pcs
Fish Cutlets	373	19.7	22.8	22.2	3.2	538.0	2.6	41.00	10.00	0.19	0.11	1.3	18	2 Pcs
Bondas	457	10.7	25.8	45.5	6.4	45.0	2.5	66.00	7.00	0.35	0.08	4.0	20	2 Pcs
Vegetable Cutlets	216	4.6	10.3	26.2	3.0	36.0	1.2	600.00	150.00	0.13	0.02	1.0	9	2 Pcs
Paneer Cutlets	330	14.5	24.7	12.3	1.2	148.0	0.3	257.00	65.00	0.07	0.02	0.2	2	2 Pcs
Sago Cutlets	293	1.7	10.2	48.7	2.5	13.0	0.9	24.00	6.00	0.10	0.01	1.2	17	2 Pcs
Chirwa Cutlets	325	6.8	10.7	50.4	2.6	41.0	9.1	593.00	148.00	0.19	0.03	2.2	4	2 Pcs
Fish Cutlets	470	19.1	31.6	27.2	2.3	658.0	1.6	13.00	3.00	0.12	0.08	1.5	31	2 Pcs
Keema Cutlets	307	1.8	23.6	21.9	1.1	155.0	3.0	1.00	9.00	0.21	0.14	7.2	0	2 Pcs
Vegetable Samosas	246	4.4	12.0	30.2	1.0	19.0	1.1	131.00	33.00	0.13	0.02	1.3	12	2 Pcs
Paneer Pea Samosas	255	6.2	16.5	20.5	0.8	110.0	0.9	119.00	30.00	0.08	0.02	0.9	3	2 Pcs
Keema Samosas	262	10.0	17.0	17.3	2.8	80.0	1.7	164.00	45.00	0.13	0.08	3.3	6	2 Pcs

Contd...

Contd...

	Calories (Kcal)	Proteins (g)	Fats (g)	Carbo-hydrates (g)	Fiber (g)	Calcium (mg)	Iron (mg)	Caro-tene (mcg)	Retinol (mcg)	Vit B_1 (mg)	Vit B_2 (mg)	Niacin (mg)	Vit C (mg)	Serving Portion
Mathri	223	2.8	15.3	18.5	2.1	6.0	0.7	6.00	21.00	0.03	0.02	0.6	0	2 Pcs
Masala Vada	179	6.6	8.6	18.7	2.8	24.0	1.3	39.00	10.00	0.15	0.06	0.8	1	2 Pcs
Plain Urad Daal Vada	171	7.2	7.9	17.8	2.1	46.0	1.1	11.00	3.00	0.13	0.06	0.06	0	2 Pcs
Masala Urad Daal Vada	198	7.5	10.0	19.6	2.8	51.0	1.3	11.00	3.00	0.14	0.07	0.07	1	2 Pcs
Mint and Coriander Chutney	17	0.6	0.1	3.4	0.3	28.0	1.7	43.00	108.00	0.01	0.02	0.1	8	1 T
Tomato Ginger Chutney	6	0.3	0.1	1.0	0.3	12.0	0.2	88.00	22.00	0.03	0.02	0.1	7	2 T
Sandwiches														
Tomato and Cheese	268	7.2	11.8	33.3	4.6	88.0	0.9	460.0	145.00	0.09	0.06	0.6	11	2 Pcs
Tomato and Cucumber	231	5.2	8.6	33.1	4.9	28.0	1.0	460.0	115.00	0.10	0.02	0.6	12	2 Pcs
Tomato Grilled	313	9.6	15.0	34.8	5.0	160.0	1.2	530.0	192.00	0.12	0.12	0.6	16	4 Pcs
French Toast	443	14.6	27.6	34.0	4.6	144.0	1.7	1088.0	407.00	0.15	0.20	0.6	11	2 Pcs
Cheese Open	340	11.7	18.6	31.5	7.4	196.0	1.1	328.0	168.00	0.14	0.11	1.5	0	2 Pcs
Danish Luncheon	350	16.2	17.5	31.9	4.6	42.0	2.1	620.0	260.00	0.24	0.22	1.2	3	2 Pcs
Chicken and Corn Open	340	15.6	15.0	35.6	5.5	18.0	1.8	362.0	124.0	0.12	0.11	4.6	3	2 Pcs

Contd...

Contd...

	Calories (Kcal)	Proteins (g)	Fats (g)	Carbohydrates (g)	Fiber (g)	Calcium (mg)	Iron (mg)	Carotene (mcg)	Retinol (mcg)	Vit B_1 (mg)	Vit B_2 (mg)	Niacin (mg)	Vit C (mg)	Serving Portion
CAKES														
Sponge Cake	177	6.2	4.6	27.8	0.5	20.2	0.9	202.0	120.00	0.05	0.14	0.4	0	1 Pc
Sponge Chocolate Cake	156	5.5	4.5	23.3	0.3	18.8	0.7	201.0	120.00	0.05	0.14	0.3	0	1 Pc
Pineapple Pastry	279	7.1	13.2	32.9	0.6	23.1	1.0	390.0	176.00	0.06	0.16	0.5	0	1 Pastry
Chocolate Pastry	228	5.5	12.5	23.3	0.3	19.0	0.7	361.0	160.00	0.05	0.14	0.3	0	1 Pastry
Chocolate Cream Cake	223	3.1	13.1	23.2	0.4	9.0	0.5	526.0	158.00	0.03	0.06	0.3	0	1 Pc

Annexure-VIII

A. BLOOD INVESTIGATIONS AND INTERPRETATIONS

Blood Values

Types of Leukocytes

Lymphocytes	20-40%	Non granulocytes
Monocytes	2–6%	
Neutrophils	60-70%	
Eosinophils	1-4%	Granulocytes
Basophils	0.5-1%	

Leukocytes–Normal 5–10 million/cu mm	
Increased level	**Decreased level**
(About 10 million/cu mm) • Severe infection • Hemorrhage • Trauma • Malignancy • Uremia • Leukemia	(Below 4000 cu/mm) • Viral disease • Hypersplenism • Bone marrow depression • Antithyroid drugs • Myeloma • Aplastic anemia

Eosinophilia–Normal 1–4%	
Increased level	**Decreased level**
>5% total count 500 • Allergies • Parasitic • Hodgkin's/lymphoma • Polyarteritis nodosa • Ulcerative colitis/Crohn's disease • Lowest count is in morning • Stress will decrease counts • Steroid therapy can mask eosinophilia	• Increased steroids • Cushing's syndrome • Infection with neutrophilia • Neutropenia

Basophis–Normal 0.5–1% of total count	
Increased level	**Decreased level**
• Allergy • Inflammation	• Hyperthyroidism • Stress

Contd...

Contd...

• Polycythemia	• Myocardial infarction
• Splenectomy	• Prolonged steroid use
• Bleeding peptic ulcer	

Monocytes–Normal 2 to 6%	
Increased level	**Decreased level**
• Recovery stage of illness	• Prednisolone use
• Viral infections	• Rheumatoid arthritis
• Malaria	• HIV infection
• Collagen diseases	

Lymphocytes–Normal 20 to 60% total leukocytes	
Increased level	**Decreased level**
• Mumps, rubella	• Hodgkin's disease
• Infectious hepatitis	• ACTH
• Tuberculosis	• After burns
• Grave's disease	• Chronic uremia
• Acute lymphocytic leukemia	• TB
• Aplastic anemia	

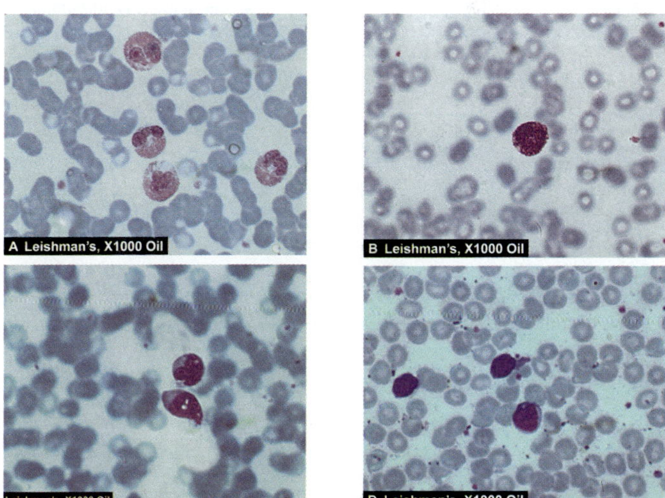

FigsA to D: *(A) Eosinophilia; (B) Basophils; (C) Monocytes; (D) Lymphocytes*

Red Blood Cells–Normal Male–4.8 Million/cu mm Female 4.3 million/cu mm	
Increased level	**Decreased level**
• Polycythemia • Dehydration • Acute poisoning • Hemorrhage - just after • Leukemia • Extreme exercise and excitement produce higher count • RBC count in newborn is higher • In pregnancy, lower count • Gentamicin/methyldopa increases RBCs	• Hodgkin's • Multiple myeloma • Leukemia • Rheumatic fever

Packed Cell Volume (PCV) – Men 40–54%, Women 37–47%	
Increased level	**Decreased level**
• Polycythemia • Erythrocytosis • Severe dehydration • Shock	• Anemia • Hyperthyroidism • Cirrhosis • Acute massive blood loss

Hemoglobulin–Normal Men 13–16 gm, Women 12–15 gm	
Increased level	**Decreased level**
• Severe burns • Congestive heart failure • Chronic obstructive • Polycythemia vera • Burns to start • Excessive fluid intake will decrease value • At high altitude values are increased	• Anemia • Hodgkin's • Leukemia • Sarcoidosis

Reticulocyte–Normal	Men Women	0.5–1.5% of total RBCs 0.5–2.5% of total RBCs
Increased level		**Decreased level**
• Hemolytic anemia • Toxin exposure • Hypersplenism • Parasitic infection		• Iron deficiency anemia • Chronic infection • Radiation treatment • Tumor

MCHC (Mean Corpuscular Hb. Concentration) - 31–38 gm Hg b/dl	
Increased level	**Decreased level**
• Spherocytosis • Thalassemia • Hypochromic anemia	• Iron deficiency

MCH (Mean Corpuscular Hemoglobin) – Normal values 26–34 picogram cell	
Increased level	**Decreased level**
• Macrocytic anemia • Hyperlipidemia	• Microcytic anemia

Ferritin–Normal values	Men Women	15–300 ng/ml 12–150 ng/ml
Increased level		**Decreased level**
• Malignancy • Hepatitis • Inflammatory disease • Iron overload		• Iron deficiency anemia

Erythrocyte Sedimentation Rate (ESR) – Normal values

i. Wintrobe method

Men	0–9 mm/hour
Women	0–15 mm/hour
Children	0–13 mm/hour

ii. Westergren method

Men	0–15 mm/hour
Women	0–20 mm/hour
Children	0–10 mm/hour

Increased level	Decreased level
• Infections • Carcinoma • Toxemia • Nephritis • Rheumatoid arthritis	• Congestive heart failure • Sickle cell anemia • Polycythemia vera • Spherocytes

Bleeding Time–Normal values 3–10 minutes

Bleeding liver prolonged	Time decreased
• Severe liver disease • Leukemia • Vascular • Aplastic anemia • Aspirin	

Prothrombin Time–Normal values 10–14 seconds. It varies from lab to lab

Increased level	Decreased level
• Prothrombin deficiency • Vitamin K deficiency • Liver diseases • Biliary obstruction • Hypervitaminosis – A	• Hemolytic anemia • Allergic conditions • Cancer therapy • HIV infection • Bone marrow lesions

Fibrinogen–Normal value - 200–400 mg/dl

Increased level	Decreased level
• Multiple myeloma • Cancer DIC • Uremia • Pregnancy • Burns	• Dysfibrinogenemia • DIC • Liver disease

B. BLOOD CHEMISTRY

Calcium–Total 8.8–10 mg/dl	
Increased level	**Decreased level**
• Hyperparathyroidism • Cancer • Addison's disease • Hyperthyroidism • Paget's disease • Excess intake of Vitamin D	• Hypoparathyroidism • Osteomalacia • Acute pancreatitis • Osteomalacia • Rickets • Diarrhea

Phosphate–Normal values: Adults 2.7–4.5 mg/dl	
Increased level	**Decreased level**
• Hypoparathyroidism • Hypocalcemia • Excessive intake of alkali • Bone tumors • Addison's disease	• Hyperparathyroidism • Rickets • Diabetic coma • IV glucose ++

Magnesium–Normal Adults 1.3–2.1 mEq/L	
Increased level	**Decreased level**
• Chromic renal disease • Hemodialysis • Chronic pancreatitis • Diuretics • Ulcerative colitis • Hyperthyroidism	• Renal failure • Diabetic acidosis • Addison's disease • Dehydration • Hypothyroidism • Controlled diabetes

Potassium – Normal value 3.5–5 mEq/l	
Increased level	**Decreased level**
• Renal failure • Oliguria • Burns • Surgery • Acidosis • Uncontrolled diabetes • Addison's disease	• Diarrhea • Pyloric stenosis • Starvation • Severe vomiting • Diuretics • Steroids

Sodium – Normal values: Adults 135–148 mmol/l	
Increased level	**Decreased level**
• Dehydration	• Severe burns
• Coma	• Severe diarrhea
• Cushing's disease	• Severe nephritis
• Diabetes insipidus	• Diabetic acidosis
• Primary aldosteronism	• Edema

Glucose (Fasting Blood Sugar) – Normal Fasting 70–110 mg/dl	
Increased level	**Decreased level**
• Diabetes	• Overdose of insulin
• Cushing's disease	• Bacterial sepsis
• Acute stress	• Hepatic necrosis
• Pituitary adenoma	• Hypothyroidism
• Pancreatitis	• Psychogenic disorder
• Hyperthyroidism	
• Chronic liver disease	

2-Hour Postprandial Blood Sugar–Normal value less than 120 mg/dl	
Increased level	**Decreased level**
• Malnutrition	• Ant. pituitary tumor
• Advanced cirrhosis	• Addison's disease
• Cushing's syndrome	• Steatorrhea
• Myocardial infarction	
• Anxiety	
• Pregnancy	
• Some malignancies	

Glycosylated Hemoglobin –

Normal	– 4 to 7.0%
Diabetic	– >7%
Good control	– <9%
Fair control	– 9.0 – 12.0%
Poor control	– >12.0%

Serum Bilirubin – Normal 0.2 to 1 mg/dl

Bilirubin increased

i. Hepatocellular jaundice
   - Viral hepatitis
   - Cirrhosis
   - Reaction of chlorpromazine

ii. Obstructive jaundice
  - Bile duct stone
  - Neoplasm.

iii. Hemolytic jaundice
  - Rh/ABO incompatibility
  - Pernicious anemia

A. **Elevated conjugate and nonconjugate**
  - Cirrhosis
  - Hepatic metastasis
  - Lymphoma
  - Hepatitis

B. **Elevated nonconjugate bilirubin**
  - Hemolytic anemia
  - Hemorrhagic pulmonary infarcts

C. **Elevated conjugated bilirubin**
  - Choledocholithiasis
  - Cancer of head of pancreas.

Blood Urea Nitrogen (BUN)–Adult 7–18 mg/dl	
Increased level	**Decreased level**
• Shock • Dehydration • Diabetes • Infection • Impaired renal function • Chronic gout	• Liver failure • Negative nitrogen balance • Nephritic syndrome • Pregnancy

Blood creatinine – Normal	Adult 0.6–1.2 mg/dl Child 0.3–0.7 mg/dl
Increased level	
• Chronic nephritis • UTI obstruction • Gigantism • Poliomyelitis • Diabetic acidosis • Hyperthyroidism • Muscular dystrophy	

Blood Uric Acid–Normal	Men	3.4–7.2 mg/dl
	Children	2.5–5.5 mg/dl

Increased level	Decreased level
• Gout • Leukemia • Lymphoma • Shock • Alcoholism • Multiple myeloma • Diabetic ketoacidosis	• Neoplastic disease • Wilson's disease • Drugs–allopurinol probenecid

Alkaline Phosphatase–Normal	Adult	20–70 u/l
	Child	20.150 u/l

Increased level	Decreased level
• Obstructive jaundice • Biliary cirrhosis • Liver metastasis • Paget's disease • Metastatic bone disease • Hyperparathyroidism • Leukemia	• Hypophosphatasia • Hypothyroidism • Milk alkali syndrome

Amylase–Normal values 50–150 u/l

Increased level	Decreased level
• Acute hemorrhagic pancreatitis • Pancreatic duct obstruction • Mumps • Alcoholism	• Hepatitis • Liver cirrhosis • Severe burns • Severe thyrotoxicosis

Serum Glutamic–Oxaloacetic Transaminase (SGOT) – Normal

Men	8–20 u/l
Children	25–75 u/l
Women	6–18 u/l

Increased level	Decreased level
• Myocardial infarction • Severe angina • Acute hepatitis • Active cirrhosis • Hepatic necrosis	• Uncontrolled diabetes • Beri Beri

Contd...

Contd...

Increased level
• Acute pancreatitis • Acute renal disease • Severe burns • Brain trauma

Serum Glutamic Pyruvic Transaminase (SGPT) – Normal

Men	7–24 u/l
Women	7–17 u/l
Child	5–28 u/l

Increased level	Decreased level
• Hepatocellular disease • Metastatic liver • Myocardial infarction • Severe burns • Trauma/shock • Pancreatitis	• Active cirrhosis

Proteins: Albumin and Globulin AG Ratio

Total proteins	6.8 gm/dl
Albumin	3.8–5.0 gm/dl
Globulin	2.3–3.5 gm/dl
A/G ration	> 1

Increased level	Decreased level
• Hemoconcentration • Eclampsia • Nephrosis • Third degree burns • Starvation	• Malabsorption

Decrease in total protein

Increased loss of albumin urine
Insufficient protein intake

Increase in globulin

• Rheumatoid arthritis • Chronic infections • Chronic alcoholism • Shock • TB • Rheumatic fever	• Severe liver disease • Diarrhea • Severe burns

Serum Cholesterol–Normal	Adult 140–220 mg/dl Child 70–175 mg/dl
Increased level	**Decreased level**
• Atherosclerosis • Nephrosis • Uncontrolled diabetes • Nephritic syndrome • Obesity	• Liver disease • Anemia • Hyperthyroidism • Antibiotics

High Density Lipoproteins (HDL) – Normal	
Men 35–70 mg/dl Women 35–86 mg/dl Children 30–65 mg/dl	
Increased level	**Decreased level**
• Very high in liver disorder • Long-term aerobic exercise • Moderate alcohol • Cigarette smoking • Contraceptive pills	• Hyperthyroidism • Diabetes • Obesity

Very Low Density Lipoproteins–Normal	
Men <130 mg/dl High risk above 160 mg/dl	
Increased values of LDL	**Increased values of VLDL**
• Saturated fats • Familial • Hypothyroidism • Multiple myeloma • Familial	• Alcoholism • Obesity • Diabetes • Pancreatitis • Birth control pills.

Free Thyroxine T_4 – Normal value	
Men 0.8–2.4 ng/dl	
Increased values of LDL	**Increased values of VLDL**
• Grave's disease • Thyrotoxicosis due to T_4	• Primary hypothyroidism • Thyrotoxicosis due to T_3

Free Tyrosine T_3–Normal value	
Adult 230–660 pg/dl	
Increased values of LDL	**Decreased values of VLDL**
• Hyperthyroidism • T_3 toxicosis	• Nephrosis • Hypothyroidism

Thyroid Stimulating Hormone – Normal value	
Adult 0.5–6 milli/IU/l	
Increased values of LDL	**Decreased values of VLDL**
• Primary hypothyroidism • Secondary and tertiary hypothyroidism	• Hyperthyroidism

(C) URINE INVESTIGATIONS AND THEIR INTERPRETATION

Specific Gravity of Urine – Normal value	
1.003–1.035 1.025–1.030 concentrates urine	
Increased specific gravity	**Low-specific gravity**
• Diabetes mellitus • Nephrosis • Dehydration/diarrhea • Fever	• Diabetes insipidus • Glomerulonephritis • Severe renal damage

- Color of urine:
  - Yellow is the normal color
  - Straw-colored urine is due to low specific gravity
  - Amber-colored urine is due to high specific gravity
- Colorless urine:
  - Large fluid intake
  - Chronic interstitial nephritis
  - Diabetes insipidus
  - Diuretic therapy
- Smoky red color urine:
  - Red blood cells
- Orange-colored urine:
  - Fever
  - Concentrated urine
  - May be bile pigment
- Green-colored urine:
  - Due to biliverdin bile pigment
  - Pseudomonas
- Dark brown urine:
  - Melanotic tumor
- Addison's disease
- Port-wine colored urine:
  - Methemoglobin
  - Oxyhemoglobin.

Odor of Urine

Normal odor is aromatic.

- Infected urine gives unpleasant odor.
- Sweet smell of acetone can be due to diabetic acidosis.
- Long-standing urine gives pungent odor.

pH – Normal value 4.6–8. pH is acidic.

Acidic urine is found in

- Acidosis
- Uncontrolled diabetes
- Dehydration
- Diarrhea
- High protein diet.

Alkaline Urine (pH more than 7)

It is found in–

- Pyloric stenosis
- Salicylates
- Chronic renal failure
- On standing, the pH of urine becomes alkaline.

Turbidity

- Normal urine is clear or slightly hazy.
- Pathological urine is cloudy.
- Turbidity results due to urinary infection.

- Phosphates may produce cloudiness.

Hematuria

It is found in:

- Glomerulonephritis
- Malignant hypertension
- Lower urinary tract infection
- Heavy smoking.

Hemoglobinuria

- Extensive burns
- Fever
- Malaria
- Hemolytic anemia
- Poisoning.

Protein

Normal value 10–140 mg/l in 24 hours. Proteinuria occurs in–

- Nephritis
- Polycystic kidney
- TB of kidney
- Pyelonephritis
- Fever
- Toxemia
- Hyperthyroidism
- Liver disease.

Bence-Jones Protein

- It is found in urine in case of:
- Multiple myeloma
- Amyloidosis
- Tumor metastasis to bone
- Malignant lymphoma.

Ketone Bodies in Urine

Normal urine does not contain ketone bodies. Ketone bodies in urine may be present in:

- Excessive fat metabolization
- Fever
- Starvation
- Fasting
- Diabetes
- High protein diets
- Drugs–Levodopa, metformin, pyridium, phenformin.

Urobilinogen

Normal value 0.1–1 Ehrlich unit/ml

- Urobilinogen increases in
  - Hemolytic anemia
  - Pernicious anemia
  - Malaria
  - Infectious/Toxic hepatitis
  - Hemolytic jaundice
- Urobilinogen decreases in
  - Cholelithiasis
  - Cancer head of pancreas
  - Severe inflammatory disease.

Urine–Sediments

Bacteria	Urinary tract infection
Epithelial	Tubular degeneration
Granular/ waxy	Renal parenchymal disease
Hyaline	Acid urine
Red cell	Acute glomerulonephritis
Fat bodies	Nephrotic syndrome
Leukocytes	Urinary tract infection Pyelonephritis.

Red Cell Cast

This is found in:

- Renal infarction
- Collagen disease
- Acute glomerulonephritis
- Subacute bacterial endocarditis.

Red Cells in Urine

- Trauma to kidney
- Pyelonephritis
- Renal spiky stones
- Cystitis
- Tuberculosis
- Malaria
- Malignant hypertension.

White Cells and White Cell Cast

Normal

- WBC 0–4/high power field
- WBC cast – None

WBCs in urine are found in

- Fever
- Urinary tract disease – cystitis
- Strenuous exercise
- Chronic pyelonephritis
- Tuberculosis

White cell cast is found in

- Pyelonephritis
- Acute glomerulonephritis.

Epithelial Cast

It is found when tubular epithelium is damaged in:

- Amyloidosis
- Glomerulonephritis
- Acute tubular necrosis
- Nephrosis
- Poisoning of heavy metals.

Hyaline Cast

Occasional hyaline casts per low-power field are found. It is found in:

- Malignant hypertension
- Chronic renal disease
- Congestive heart failure
- Emotional stress.

Granular Cast

Normal–Occasional granular cast is found. It is found in:

- Advanced glomerulonephritis
- Pyelonephritis
- Lead poisoning

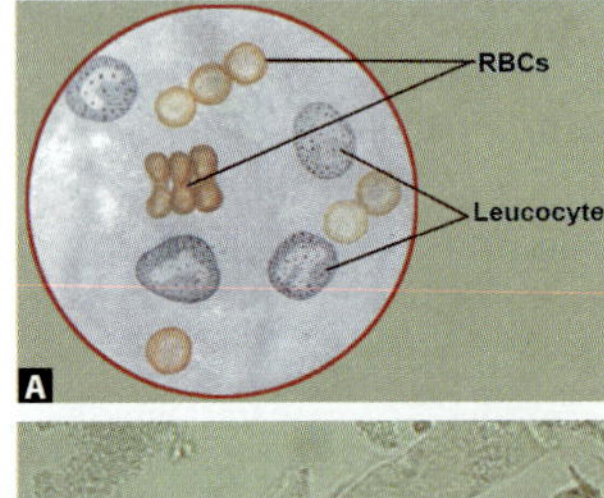

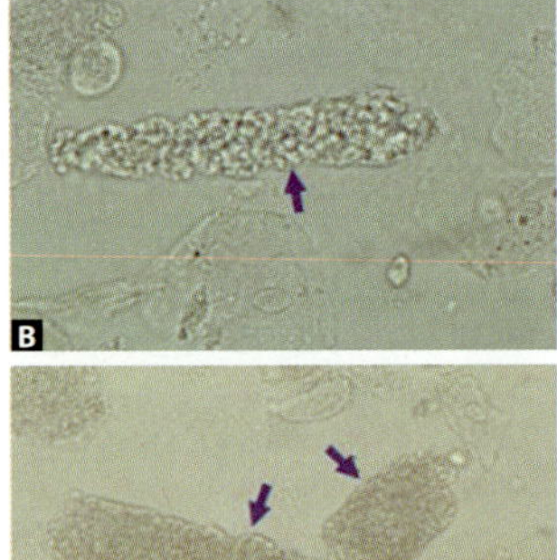

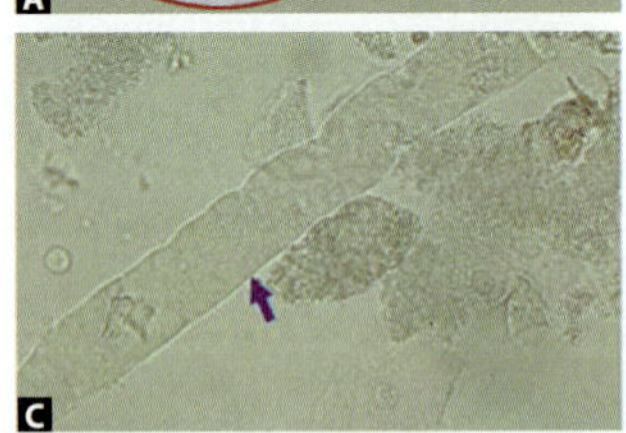

Figs A to D: *(A) Red cells in urine; (B) White cell cast; (C) Hyaline casts; (D) Granular casts*

- Acute tubular necrosis.

Waxy Cast

This is found in:

- Tubular degeneration
- Localized nephron obstruction
- Chronic renal failure.

Crystals

Normal acidic urine may show:

- Uric acid crystals
- Amorphous urates
- Calcium oxalate.

Alkaline urine may show crystals of

- Calcium phosphate
- Amorphous phosphate
- Calcium carbonate.

Abnormal crystals

- Cystine
- Leucine
- Cholesterol
- Sulfonamides.

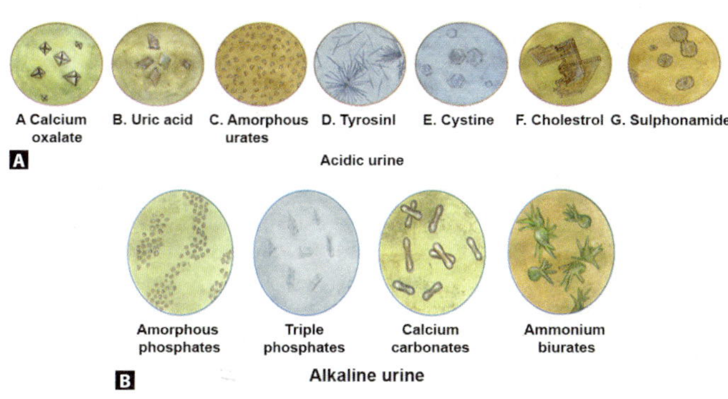

Figs A and B: *(A) Granular cast; (B) Crystals in urine*

(D) STOOL INVESTIGATION AND THERE INTERPRETATION

- Diarrhea mixed with mucus
  - Typhoid
  - Cholera
  - Amoebiasis
  - Large bowel cancer
- Diarrhea mixed with mucus + white blood cells
  - Ulcerative colitis
  - Salmonellosis
  - Intestinal tuberculosis
  - Regional enteritis

Alteration of Shape

- A narrow ribbon like stool is seen in
  - Spastic bowel
  - Rectal narrowing
  - Stricture
  - Partial block
  - Decreased elasticity
- Large earlier stool indicates dilatation of viscous
- Small round hard stool is seen in
  - Habitual constipation

Color of Stool

Normal color – Brown

- Different colors of stool
  - Green - Severe diarrhea
  - Black - Upper G.I. bleeding
  - Clay colored - Blockage of bile duct
  - Red - Bleeding from lower G.I.
- Certain drugs which may change the color of stool
  - Yellow - Santonin
  - White color - Antacid
  - Black - Iron salts
  - Red - Pyrvinium phenol-phthalein
  - Green - Spinach
  - Yellow brown - Senna
  - Green to blue - Dithiazanine

Occult Blood

It may be seen in

- Diverticulitis
- Gastic carcinoma
- Gastritis

Drugs that May Cause False Positive

- Bromides
- Colchicines
- Iodine
- Oxidizing agents

Mucus in Blood

Normal value-Negative

- Translucent gelatinous mucus
  - Spastic constipation
  - Mucus colitis
  - Emotionally disturbed
  - Excessive straining
- Mucus + Pus and blood
  - Ulcerative colitis
  - Ulcerative cancer

- Acute diverticulitis
- Intestinal tuberculosis

- Large amount of pus
  - Chronic ulcerative colitis
  - Chronic bacillary dysentery
  - Localized abscess
- Primary polymorph in stool
  - Shigellosis
  - Salmonellosis
  - Ulcerative colitis
  - Invasive E coli diarrhea
- No leukocytosis in stool
  - Cholera
  - Viral diarrhea
  - Amoebic colitis
  - Parasites.

Annexure-IX

MISCELLANEOUS

Properties of Artificial Teeth		
	Acrylic resin	**Porcelain**
Density (gm cm^{-3})	2.4	1.2
Coefficient of thermal expansion	7	8.0
Modulus of elasticity	80	2.5
Hardness	500	20

Radiopaque Denture Base Material	
Radiopaque additive	**Description**
Barium sulfate	• Weakens base at high concentration • Insufficient opacity
Powdered metals	• Weak base • Appearance is poor
Barium acrylate	• Poor mechanical properties

Thermal Conductivity	
Material	**Thermal conductivity**
Dentin	0.63
Enamel	0.91
Dental amalgam	23.02
Zinc phosphate cement	1.17
Zinc oxide	0.46
Gold	291.70
Porcelain	1.05

Properties of Elastomeric Impression Material				
Property	Condensation silicones	Polysulphides	Addition silicones	Polyethers
Elasticity	Very good	Viscoelastic	Very good	Adequate

Contd...

Contd...

Viscosity	Available in 4 viscosities	3 viscosities	4 viscosities	Single viscosity
Dimensional stability	Pouring should be quick	Quick pouring	Very good	Very good

Teeth-Age Verification

Primary Teeth	Eruption	Complete calcification of tooth
Central incisors (lower)	6–8 months	1½ to 2 years
Central incisors (upper)	7–9 months	1½ to 2 years
Lateral incisors (upper)	7–9 months	1½ to 2 years
Lateral incisors (lower)	10–12 months	2 to 2½ years
First molar	12–14 months	2 to 2½ years
Canines	17–18 months	2½ to 3 years
Second molars	20–30 months	3 to 3½ years

Permanent Teeth

Teeth	Eruption	Complete calcification of tooth
First molars	6–7 years	9–10 years
Central incisors	6–8 years	10 years
Lateral incisors	8–9 years	11 years
First bicuspid	9–11 years	12–18 years
Second bicuspid	10–12 years	13–14 years
Canines	11–12 years	13–15 years
Second molars	12–14 years	14–16 years
Wisdom	17–25 years	17–25 years

Crude Death Rate

It is defined as the number of deaths per 100 estimated mid-year population in one year, in a given place. It is calculated from the formula.

$$= \frac{\text{No. of deaths during the year}}{\text{Mid-year population}} \times 100$$

Case Fatality Rate

It represents the killing power of a disease. It is simply the ratio of death to cases. It can be calculated as–

$$= \frac{\text{Total no. of deaths due to disease}}{\text{Total no. of specific disease}} \times 100$$

Incidence

This rate is defined as the number of new cases occurring in defined population during a specified period of time. It is calculated as–

$$= \frac{\text{No of new cases of specific disease during a specific period}}{\text{Population at risk during that period}} \times 1000$$

Prevalence

Disease prevalence refers specifically to all old and new current cases existing at a given point in time. It is calculated as–

$$= \frac{\text{No. of current cases}}{\text{Estimated population at the time}} \times 1000$$

Strain

Strain has no physical dimensions but can be seen as a measure of fractional change in length caused due to an applied force.

$$\text{Strain} = \frac{\text{Chain in length}}{\text{Original length}}$$

Refractive Index

$$N = \frac{\text{Velocity of light in air}}{\text{Original Velocity}}$$

Mental Age

Binet and Simon (1896) developed concept of mental age. The child who could be five year test was credited with mental age of 5 years. It gives level of intelligence but is not indicative of dullness/brightness. While IQ is equal to

$$IQ = \frac{\text{Mental age}}{\text{Chronological age}} \times 1000$$

Levels of Intelligence

- Idiot 0–24 IQ
- Imbecile 25–49 IQ
- Moron 50–69 IQ

- Border line 70–79 IQ
- Low normal 90–109 IQ
- Superior 110–119 IQ
- Very superior 120–139 IQ
- Near genius 140 and above IQ

Loudness

It is the intensity depending upon the amplitude of vibrations. Loudness is measured in decibel. Noise levels are as follows:

- Whispering 10–20 decibels
- Normal conversation 60 decibels
- Heavy street traffic 70 decibels
- Train passing 110 decibels
- Motor car horn 120 decibels
- Threshold of pain 140 decibels
- Mechanical damage 150+ decibels

Heat Stress Index

It represents the percentage of heat storage capacity of an average man

- 0 – No thermal stress
- 10–30 – Moderate to mild heat strain
- 40–60 – Severe heat strain
- 70–90 – Very severe heat strain
- 100 – Upper limit of heat strain

Vesicular Breath Sounds

Breath sounds will be of normal intensity when lung is inflating normal. Intensity will be reduced when there is airway narrowing. This is low-pitched rustling sounds. There is no distinct pause between end of inspiration and beginning of expiration. In asthma, expiration phase is prolonged.

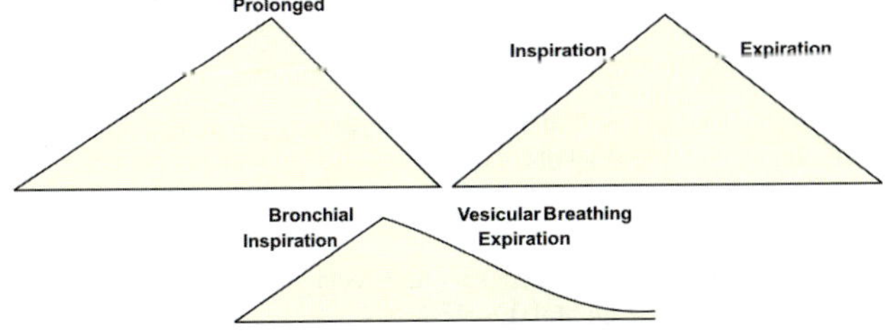

Fig.: *Vasicular breath sounds*

Intensity of Sound

Sound is measured in decibels. At a distance of one meter intensity, is as follows:

❑ Normal conversation	60 dB
❑ Whisper	30 dB
❑ Shouting	90 dB
❑ Discomfort in ear	120 dB
❑ Pain in ear	130 dB

Benedict's Test

To 5 ml of Benedict's reagent add 8 drops of urine, boil for 2 minutes and allow to cool. If a reducing substance is present, a precipitate will appear varying from a light green turbidity to red precipitate. If reduction is due to glucose, test will give–

❑ Light green turbidity	0.1–0.5 gm/dL sugar
❑ Green precipitate	0.5–1.0 gm/dL sugar
❑ Yellow precipitate	1.0–2. gm/dL sugar
❑ Red precipitate	2.0 gm/sugar

Grading of Mottled Enamel

❑ Less than 0.5 ppm	6% population will show mild defect
❑ 0.5 to 1.5 ppm	20% may show mild defects
❑ 2.5 ppm	Effect is moticeable in 50% cases. 10% may show defects.
❑ 4.5 ppm	Effect is of disfiguring. 40% will have moderate and 20% will have severe effect.
❑ 6.0 ppm ++	All persons are affected. 50% will show severe effect.

Grading of Mottled Enamel

❑ Very mild	Paper white areas affecting 25% of an area
❑ Opaque area	Involving up to 50% area
❑ Moderate	Paper white/± brownish area covering whole area
❑ Severe	Enamel is pitted/defective and opaque.

Causes of Malformed Permanent Teeth

❑ Infective	Congenital syphilis
❑ Metabolic	Rickets Hypothyroidism
❑ Drugs	Tetracycline
❑ Fluorosis genetic	Dentigenesis imperfecta Dental dysplasia Odontodysplasia

Quality of Carcinogenic Bacteria

- It is to be acidogenic and can produce pH <5.
- It should be able to decalcify tooth substance.
- It should be able to adhere to smooth surface.
- It should be able to produce adhesive isoluble plaque polysaccharides.

Stages of Formation of Plaque

- Deposition of salivary glycoprotein.
- Bacterial action precipitating salivary proteins.
- Colonization of *S. sanguis* and *S. mutans* in 24 hours.
- Progressive build up of plaque by bacterial polysaccharides.

Important Biopsy Principles

- Choose red area when premalignancy is suspected.
- Avoid necrotic and slough area.
- Don't give local anesthesia in lesion/mass.
- Always include normal tissue margin.
- For large areas many samples may be collected.
- Suture and control any bleeding.

Different Oral Pigmentations

- Brown/black pigmentation
  - Malignant melanoma
  - Pigmented nevi
  - Addision's disease
- Purple or red pigmentation
  - Hemangioma
  - Purpura
  - Lingual varices
  - Giant cell euplis.

Oral Diseases in HIV Cases

- Viral
  - Herpes simplex
  - Leukoplakia
- Bacterial
  - HIV-associated gingivitis
  - Necrotizing gingivitis

- Fungal
  - Thrush
- Tumor
  - Kaposi's sarcoma
- Enlarged glands.

Sweetness/Cariogenicity	
Sweetness	**Cariogenicity**
• Sucrose	Highly cariogenic
• Glucose/fructose	Less cariogenic
• Lactose/galactose	Less cariogenic
• Glucose syrups	Less cariogenic than sugar
• Sorbitol/mannitol	Noncariogenic
• Saccharin	Nonsugar sweetness
• Aspartame	Non cariogenic
• Cyclamate	

Section 3

Schematic Representation of Important Anatomic Landmarks

Plates

- Embryology
- Arteries, Veins and Nerves of Head and Neck
- Cranial Nerves
- Osteology
- Myology
- Miscellaneous

Embryology

Plate 1. *Human embryo at various stages of development. The relative size has been distorted to emphasize coorespondence of parts*

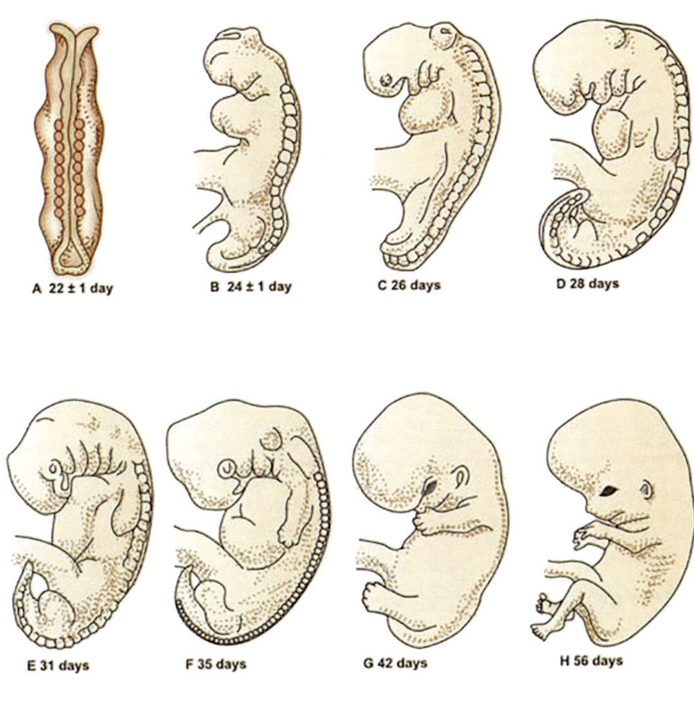

Arteries, Veins and Nerves of Head and Neck

Plate 2. *Arterial* Blood *supply*

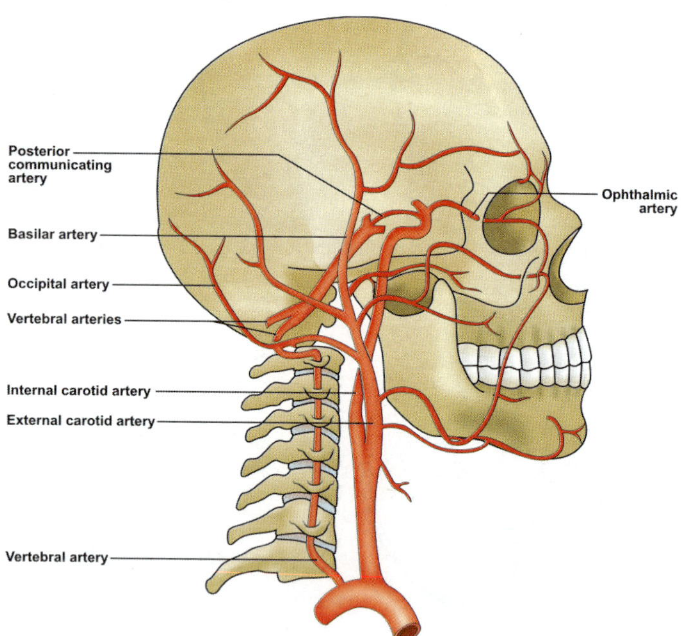

Plate 3. *Venous supply*

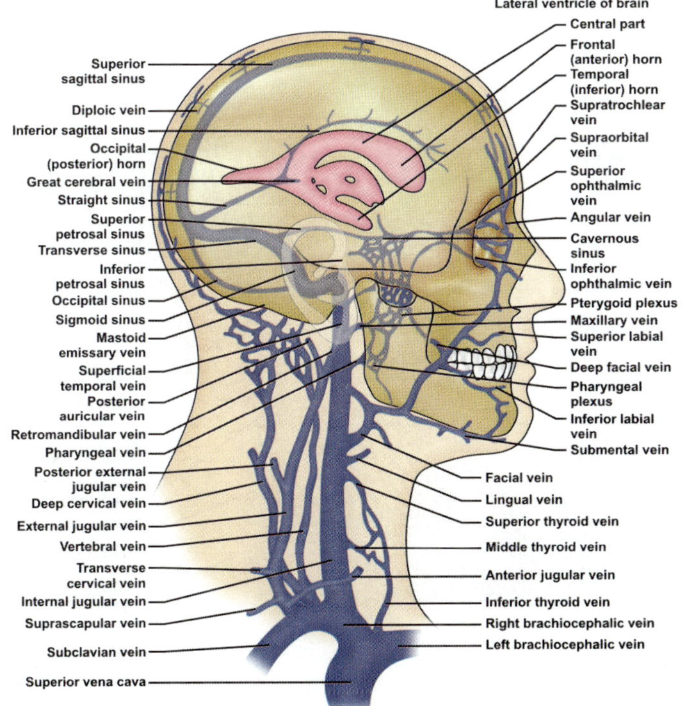

Plate 4. *Nerve supply*

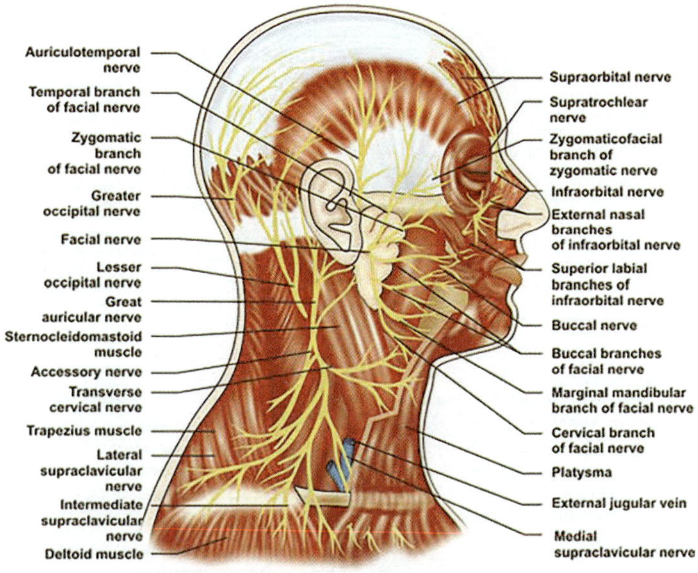

Plate 5. *Arteries of head, neck, base of brain*

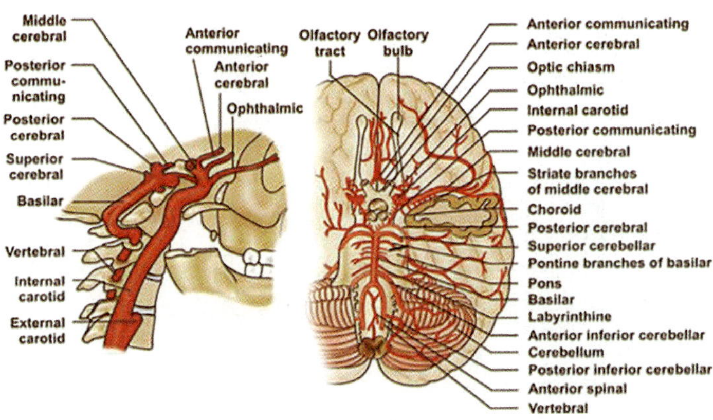

Plate 6. *Circle of Willis*

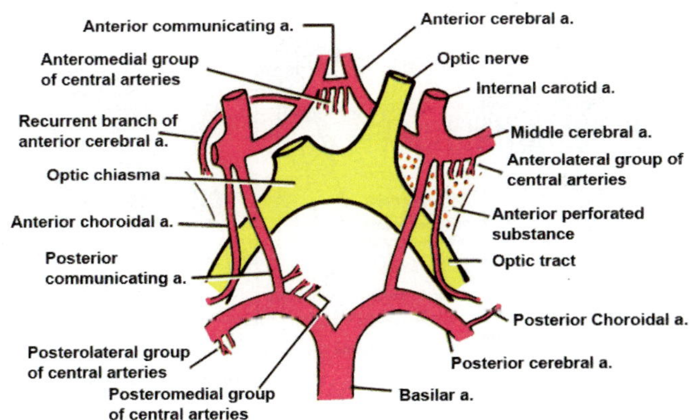

Cranial Nerves

Plate 7. *Olfactory nerve (I)*

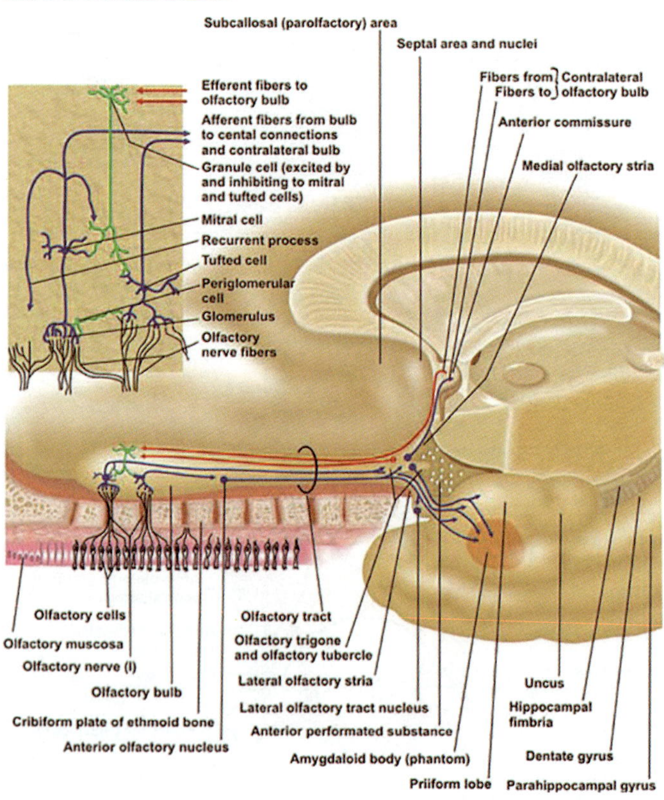

Plate 8. *Optic nerve (II)*

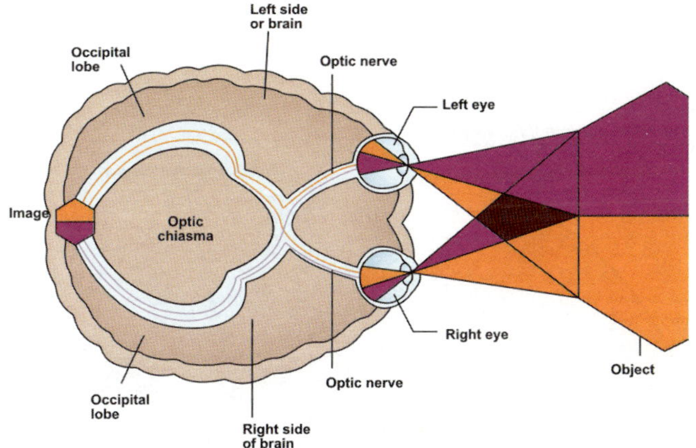

Plate 9. *Occulomotor nerve (III), trochlear nerve (IV), abducent nerve (VI)*

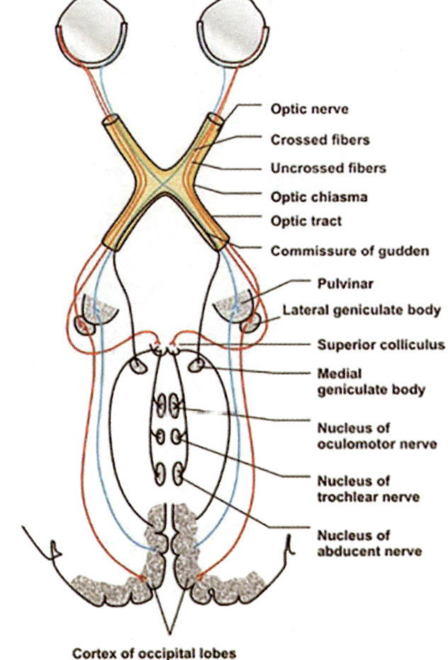

Plate 10. *Trigeminal nerve (V)*

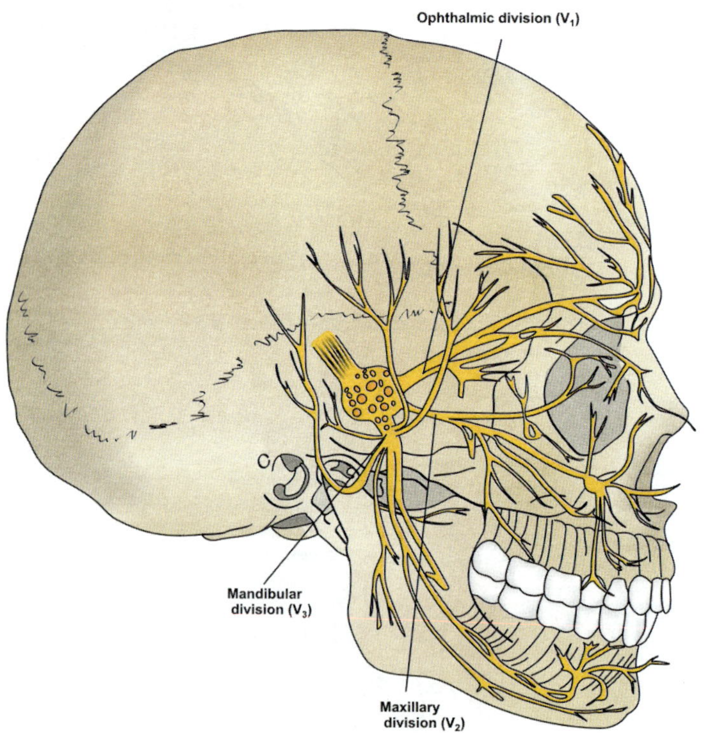

Plate 11. *Trigeminal ophthalmic nerve (V_1)*

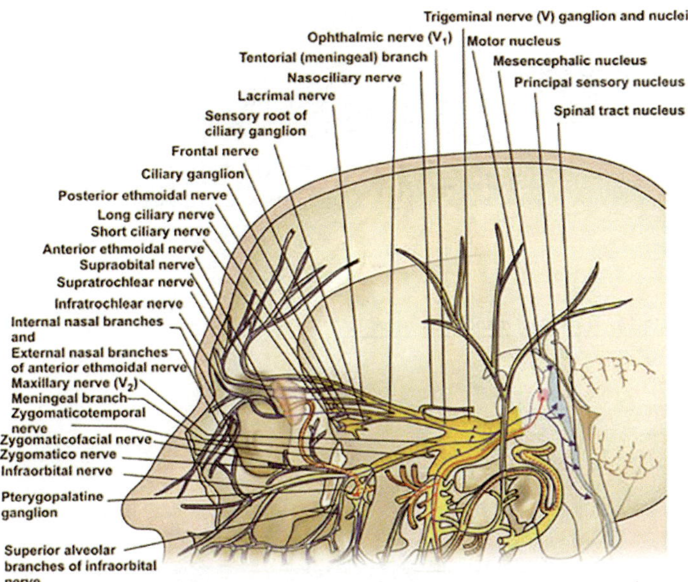

Plate 12. *Trigeminal maxillary nerve (V_2)*

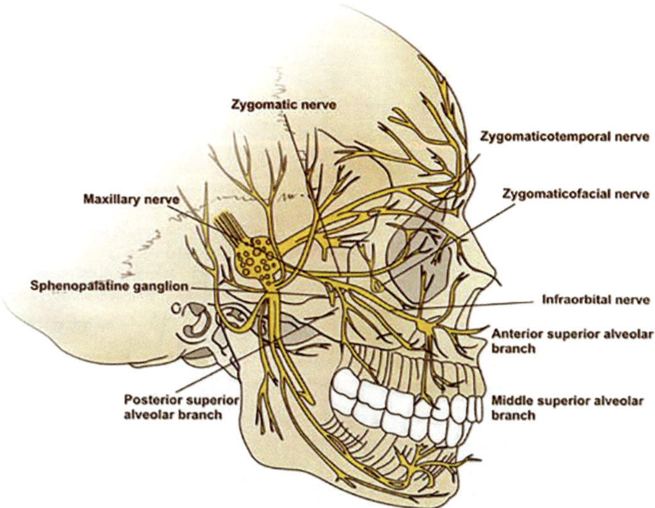

Plate 13. *Trigeminal mandibular nerve (V_3)*

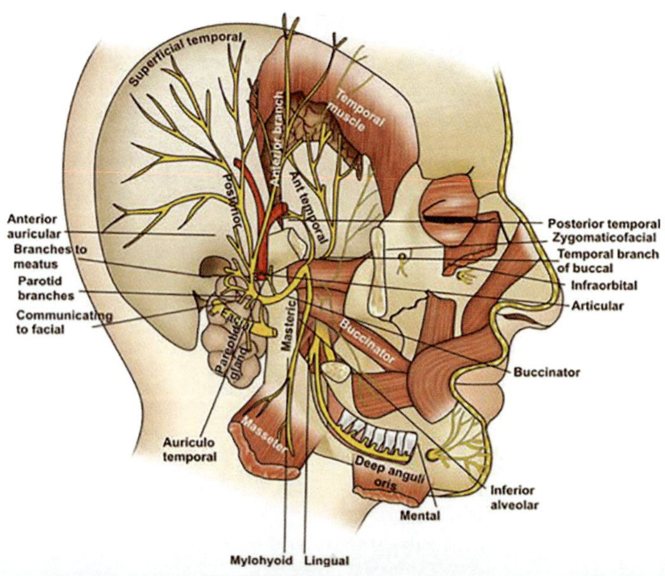

Plate 14. *Facial nerve (VII)*

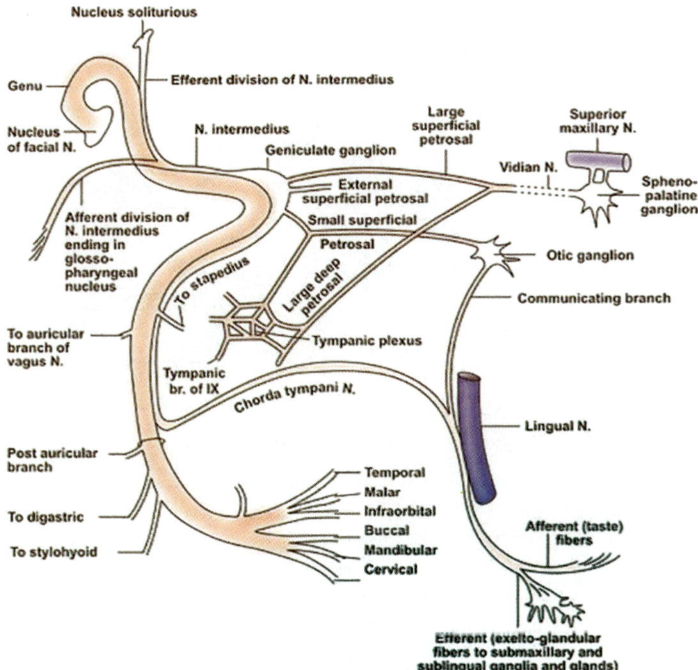

Plate 15. *Vestibulocochlear nerve (VIII)*

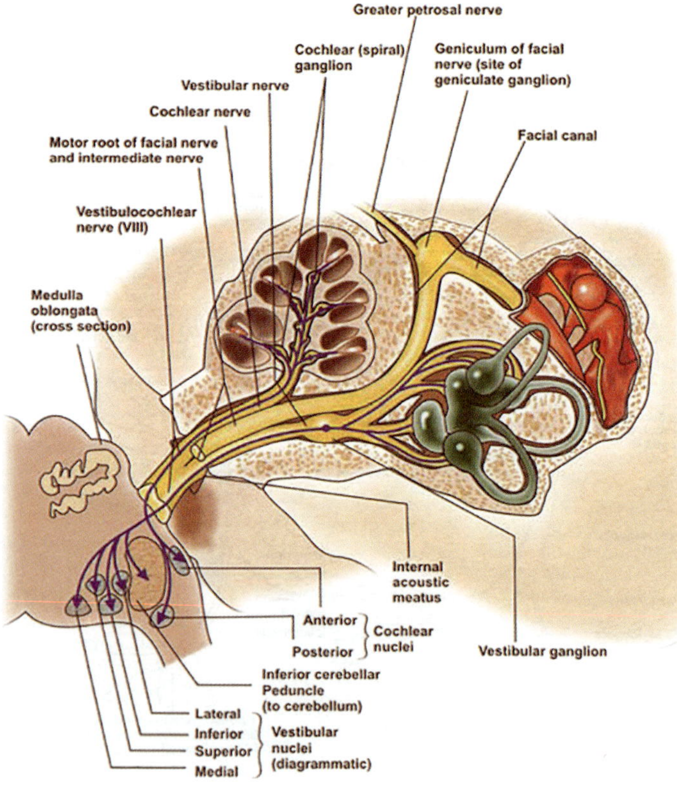

Plate 16. *Glossopharyngeal nerve (IX)*

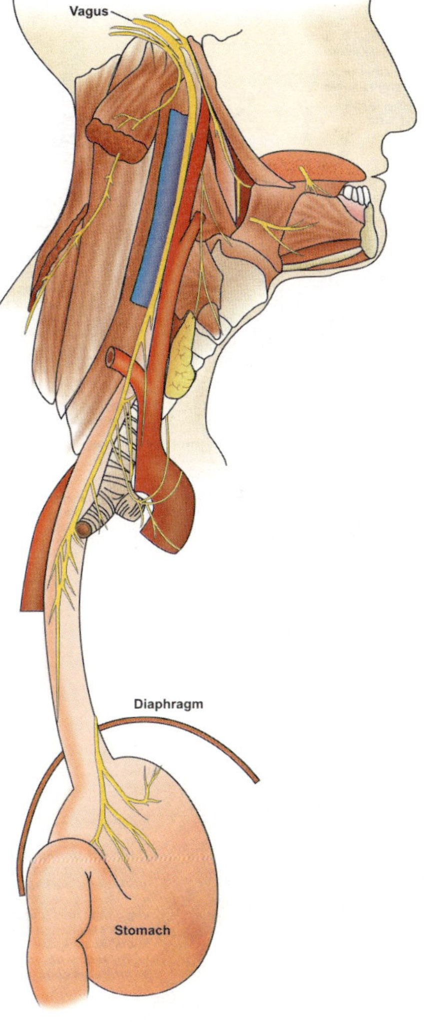

Plate 17. *Vagus nerve (X) schema*

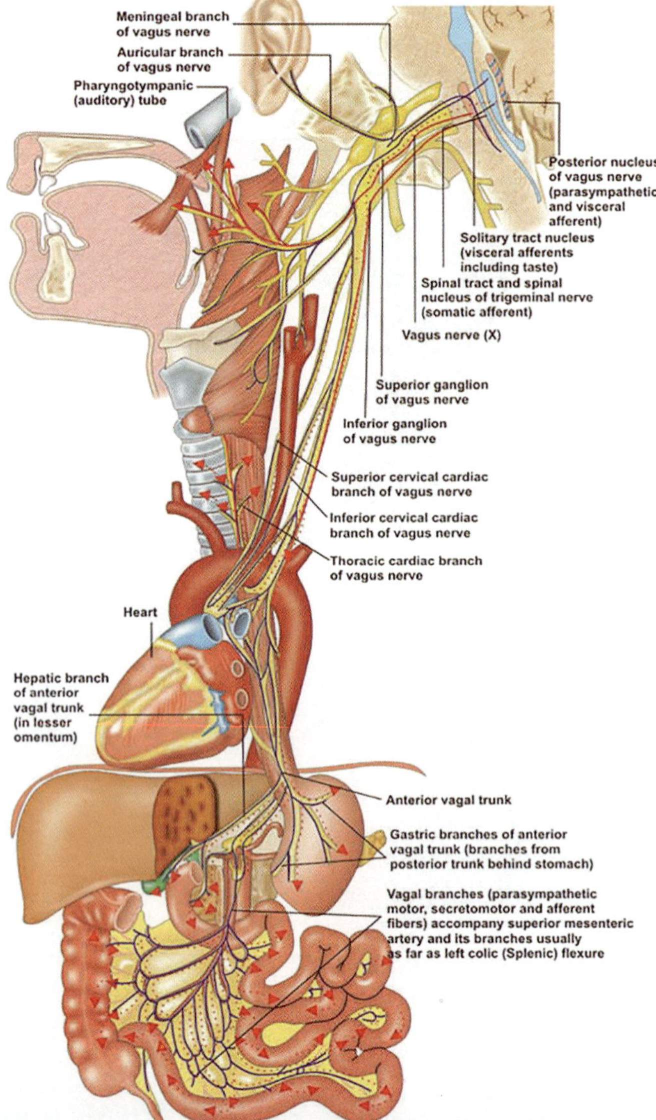

Plate 18. *Accessory nerve (XI)*

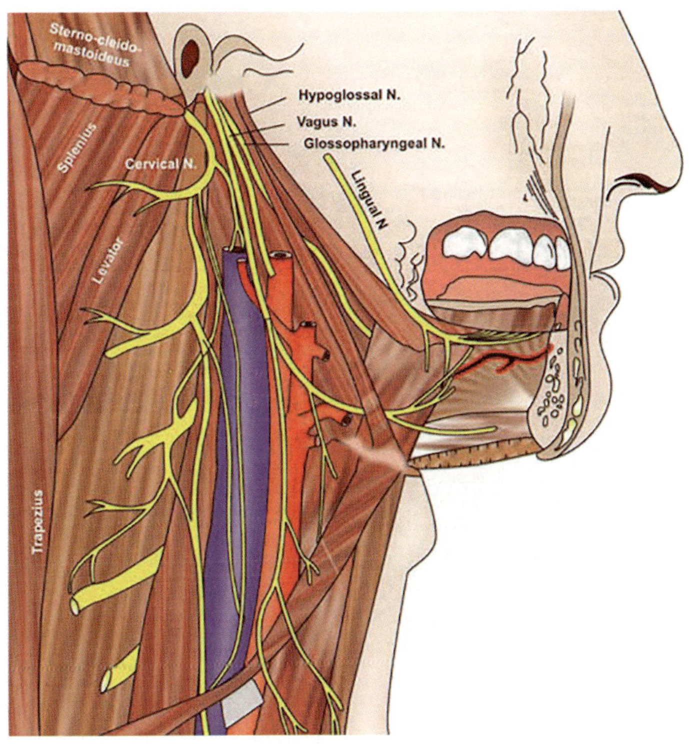

Plate 19 *Hypoglossal nerve (XII)*

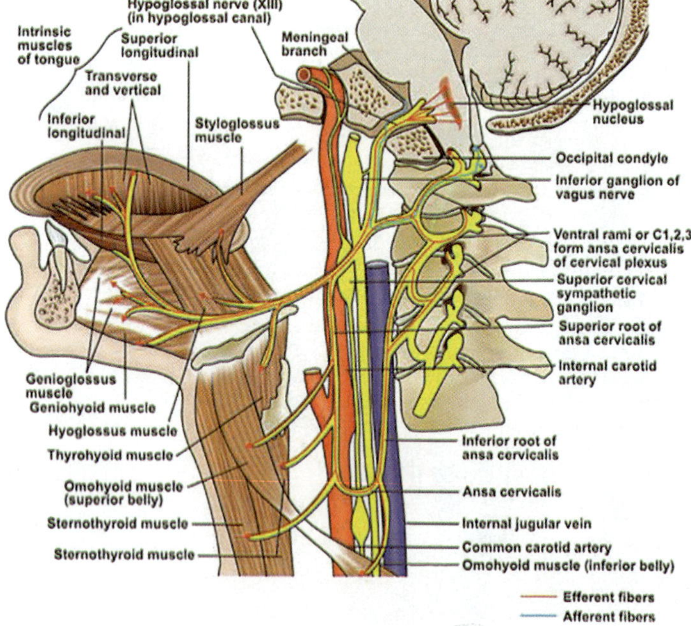

OSTEOLOGY

Plate 20. *The fontanelles*

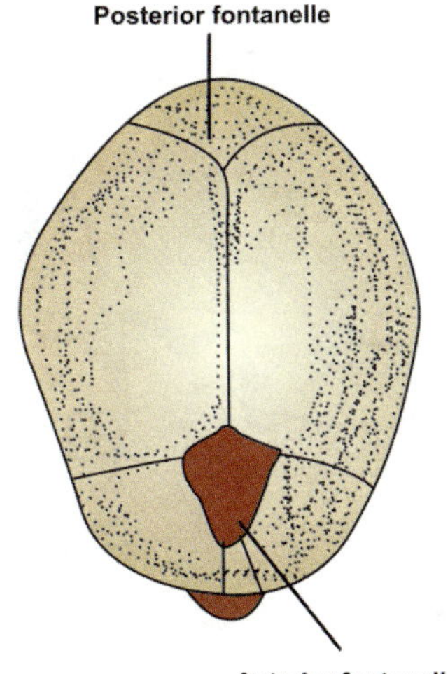

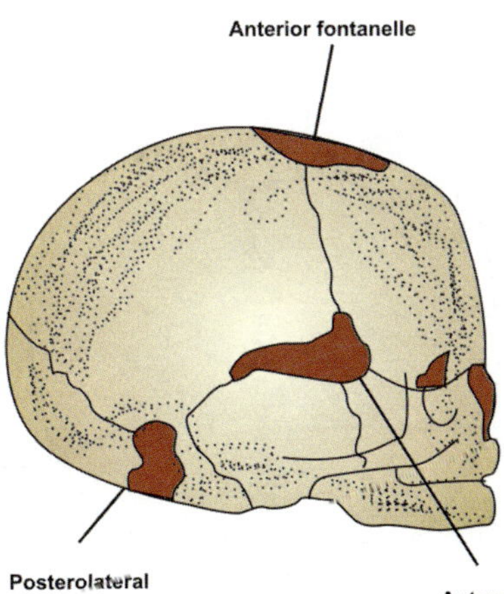

Plate 21. *(A) Skull (Lateral view)*

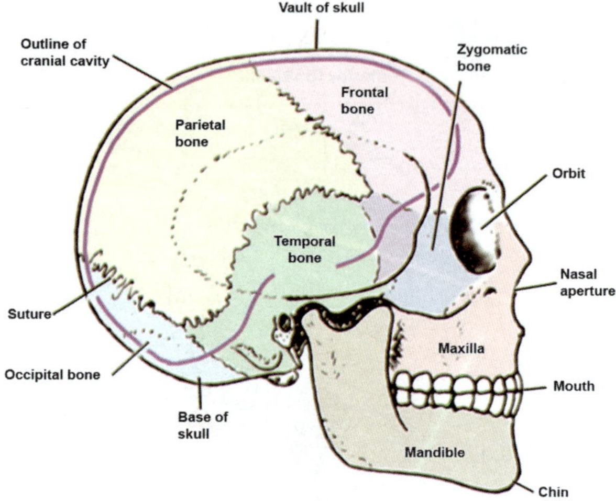

Plate 22. *(B) Skull (Top view)*

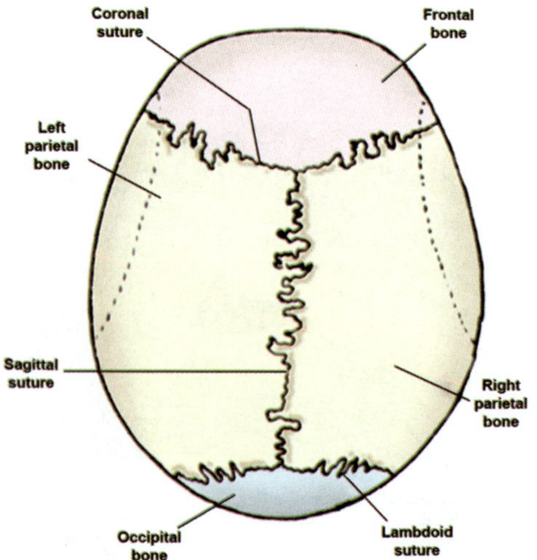

Plate 23. *Maxilla*

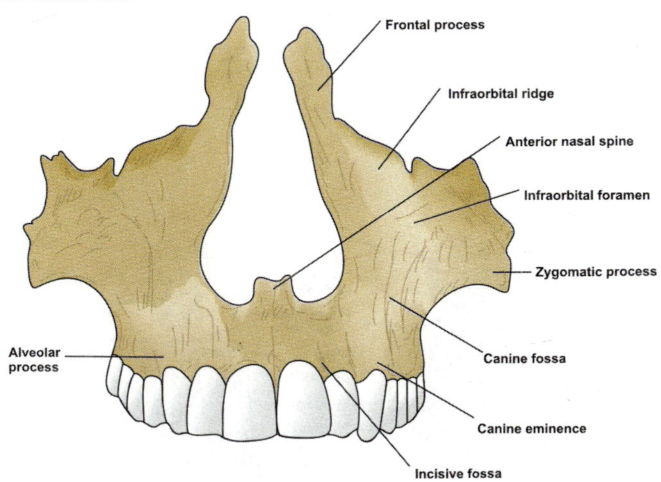

Plate 24. *Mandible (D)*

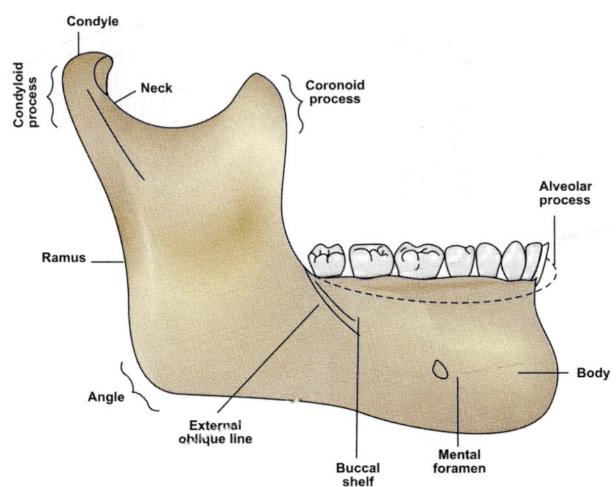

Plate 25. *Anterior and posterior view of the human skeleton*

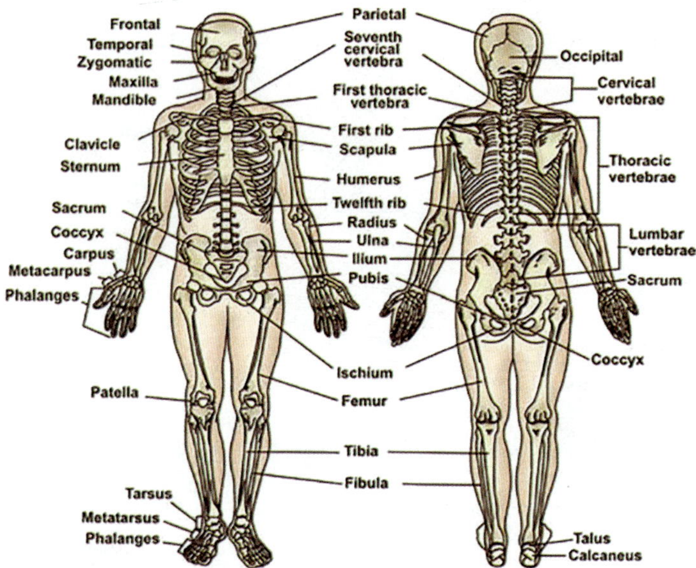

Myology

Plate 26. *Muscles of facial expression*

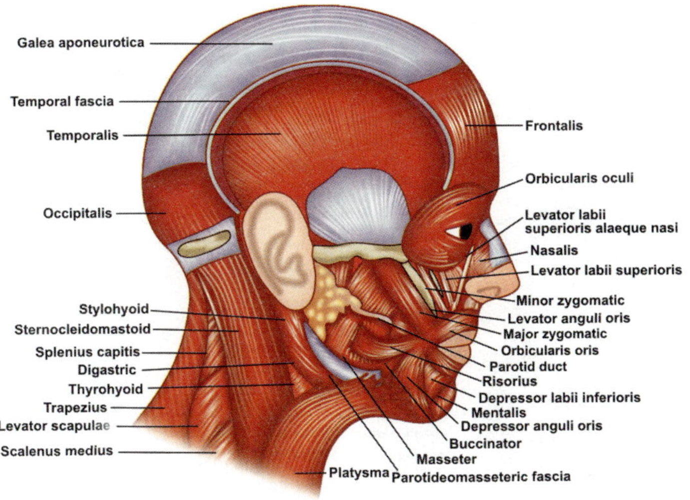

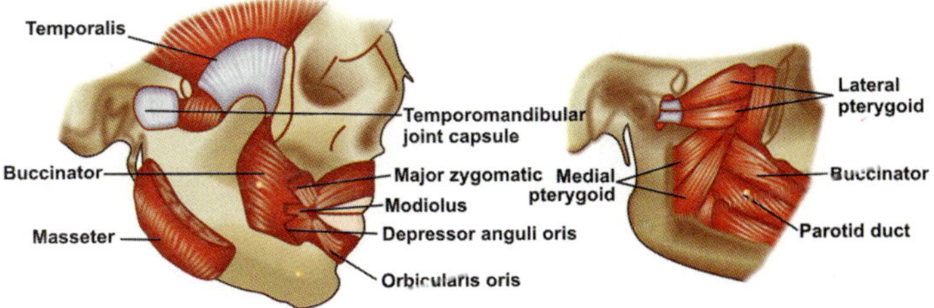

Miscellaneous

Plate 27. *Lymph nodes*

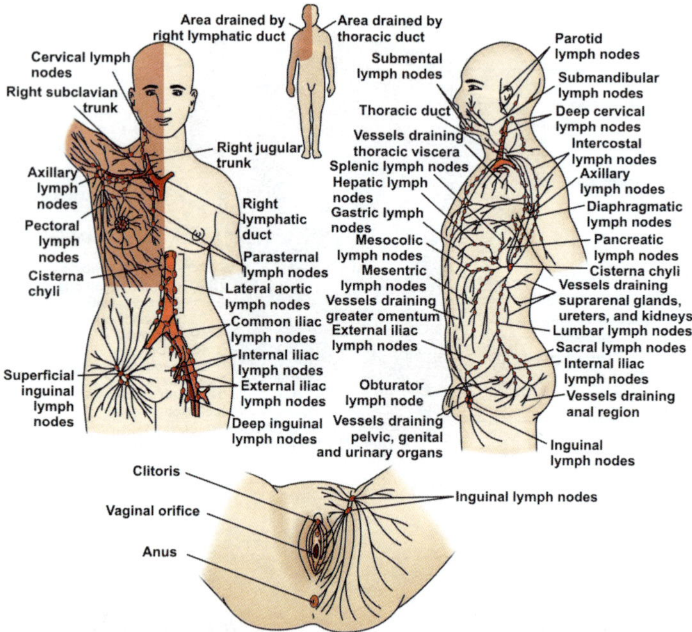

Plate 28. *Salivary glands*

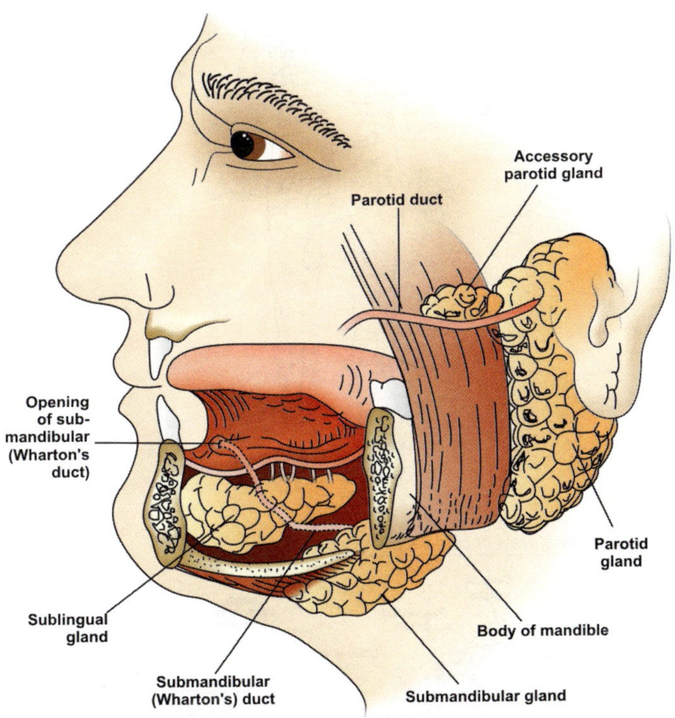

Plate 29. *Anterior and posterior view of dermatomes*

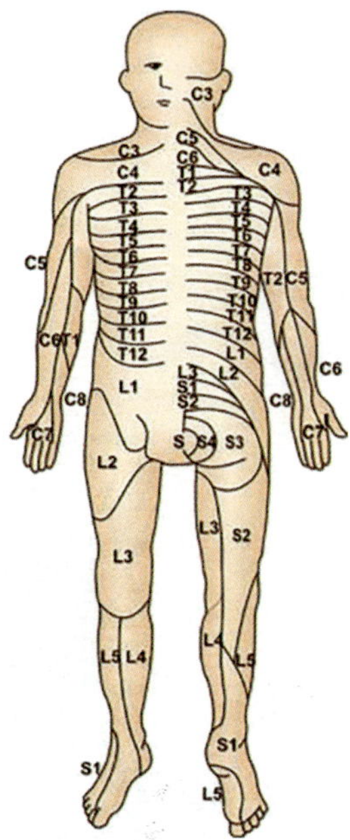

Plate 30. *Lateral view of corticle lobes and ventricles*

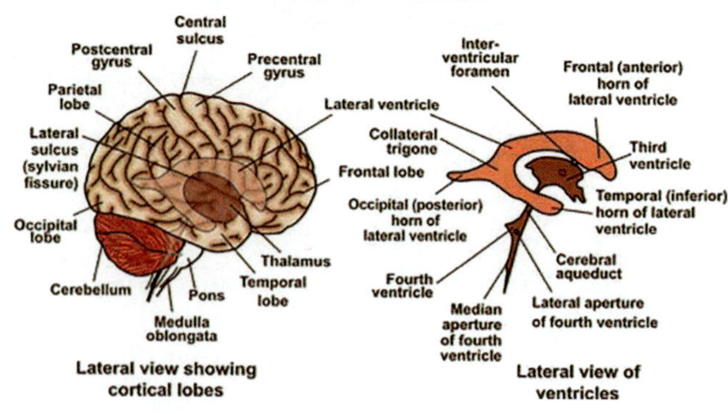

Plate 31. *Motor-sensaory homunculus*

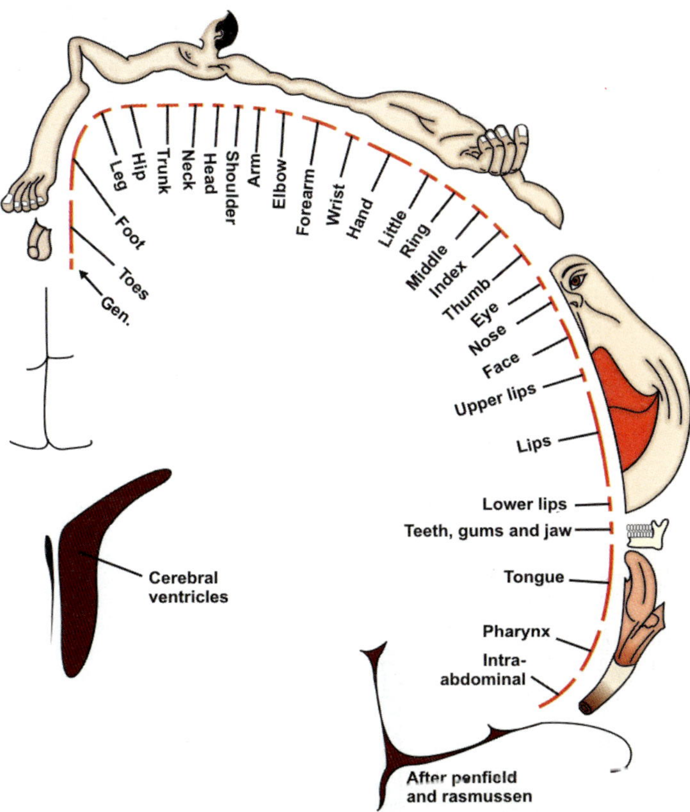

Sensory homunculus demonstrating the relative somatotopical representation in the somesthetic cortex of the brain

Plate 32. *Intrinsic and extrinsic pathways of blood coagulation*

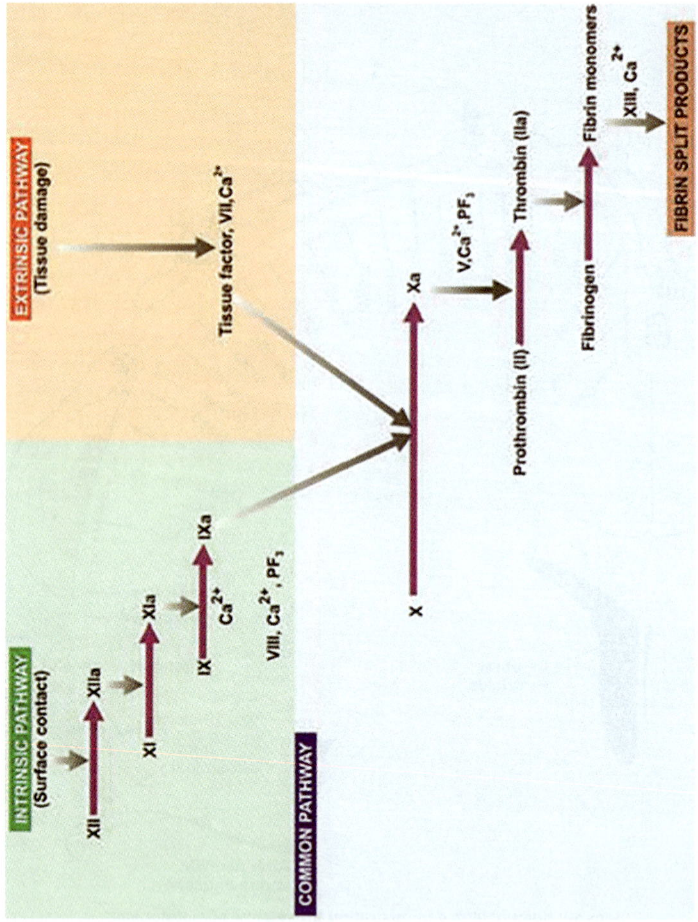

Plate 33. *Branchial plexus*

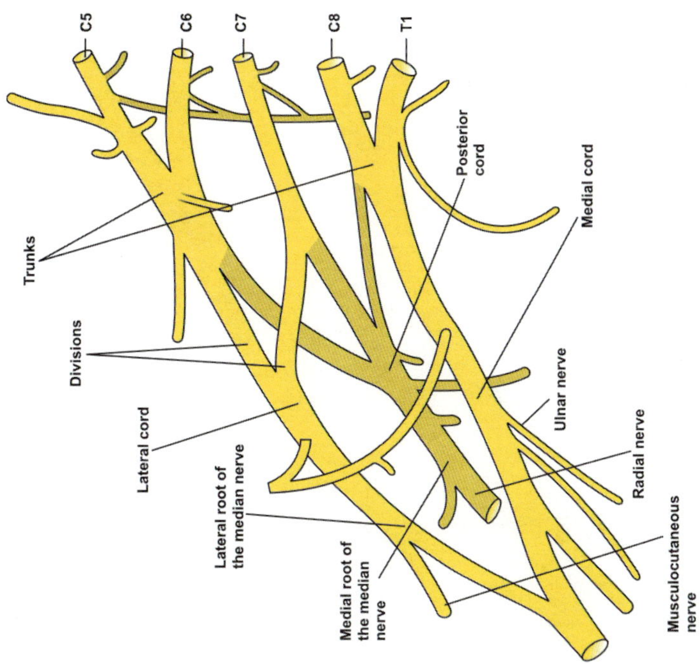